Rare Diseases of the Immune System

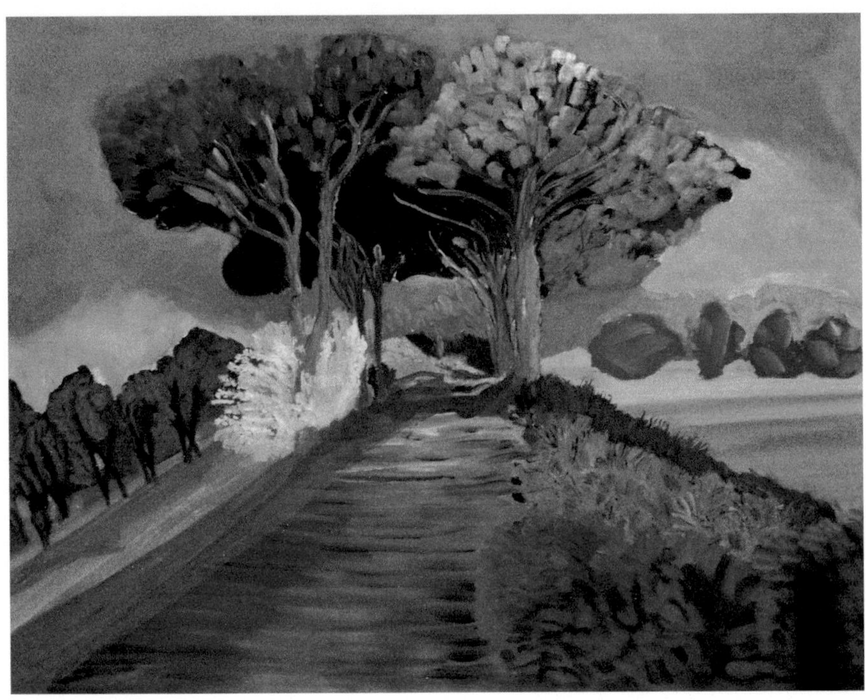

Tramonto in arancione
Laura Maddii Emmi (Private collection)

Dario Roccatello • Lorenzo Emmi
Editors

Connective Tissue Disease

A Comprehensive Guide-Volume 1

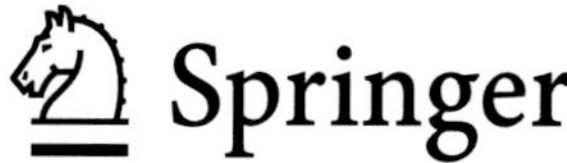

Editors
Dario Roccatello
Nephrology and Dialysis Unit
Department of Rare, Immunologic
Hematologic and Immunohematologic
Diseases, Center of Research of
Immunopathology and Rare Diseases
Coordinating Center of the Network of
Rare Diseases of Piedmont and
Aosta Valley, Giovanni Bosco Hospital, and
University of Turin
Turin
Italy

Lorenzo Emmi
SOD Patologia Medica, Center for
Autoimmune Systemic Diseases
Behçet Center and Lupus Clinic
AOU Careggi
Florence
Italy

ISSN 2282-6505 ISSN 2283-6403 (electronic)
Rare Diseases of the Immune System
ISBN 978-3-319-24533-1 ISBN 978-3-319-24535-5 (eBook)
DOI 10.1007/978-3-319-24535-5

Library of Congress Control Number: 2016932896

Springer Cham Heidelberg New York Dordrecht London

Printed on acid-free paper

Springer International Publishing AG Switzerland is part of Springer Science+Business Media (www.springer.com)

Contents

Part I

Systemic Lupus Erythematosus

1 Introduction

Dario Roccatello

The connective tissue disorders (CTDs) comprise a number of related conditions that include systemic lupus erythematosus, systemic sclerosis, myositis, and Sjögren's syndrome. They are characterized by autoantibody production and other immune-mediated dysfunctions, mainly disturbances of T-cell and B-cell functions.

Basic and clinical research has been advancing rapidly in the field of CTDs, a promising world of new diagnostic tools and pharmacological agents in development that offer patients the real possibility of new therapies and physicians and scientists novel insights into the pathogenesis of these diseases.

Looking back over the past decade, research has mainly focused on the role of B cells and B-cell cytokines in the pathogenesis of CTDs and the use of anti-B-cell/anti-B-cell cytokine agents in their therapy. Looking forward, a number of new themes are emerging, including therapeutic modulation of T/B lymphocyte signaling with so-called target therapies, inhibition of T-cell activation, antibodies to IFN, IL, and anti-CD40L.

This textbook summarizes the critical aspects of the autoimmune conditions facing the clinician in the twenty-first century, including both basic science and clinical science in order to provide a translational medicine model. Two sections deal separately with systemic lupus erythematosus (SLE) and Sjögren's syndrome (SS).

SLE is a complex autoimmune disease, predominantly affecting young women during the prime years of their life. The chronic nature of the disease, its relapsing

D. Roccatello
Nephrology and Dialysis Unit, Department of Rare, Immunologic, Hematologic and Immunohematologic Diseases, Center of Research of Immunopathology and Rare Diseases, Coordinating Center of the Network of Rare Diseases of Piedmont and Aosta Valley, Giovanni Bosco Hospital, and University of Turin, Turin, Italy
e-mail: dario.roccatello@unito.it

D. Roccatello, L. Emmi (eds.), *Connective Tissue Disease: A Comprehensive Guide-Volume 1*, Rare Diseases of the Immune System 5,
DOI 10.1007/978-3-319-24535-5_1

remitting course, and organ damage accrual over time frustrate both the physician and the patient.

To date, lupus has no known cause or cure. Early detection and treatment is the key to a better health outcome and can usually lessen the progression and severity of the disease. Anti-inflammatory drugs, antimalarials, and steroids are often used to treat lupus. Cytotoxic chemotherapies are also used to suppress the immune system in lupus patients.

Sjögren's syndrome is a systemic autoimmune disease whose clinical spectrum extends from sicca syndrome to systemic involvement (extraglandular manifestations). Systemic involvement plays a key role in the prognosis of Sjögren's syndrome, and recent studies have focused on cutaneous, pulmonary, renal, and neurological disease features. The diagnosis of Sjögren's syndrome can be confusing and time consuming. The management can also be a significant challenge for the clinician. However, recent genomic and proteomic developments are unlocking the mystery of the disease process as well as contributing to our ability to define, diagnose, and develop new treatment modalities for patients with this complex disorder.

This volume features very prominent physicians and scientists as contributors who bring their most recent discoveries to the benefit of the readers, who will find introductory contributions regarding general diagnostic and treatment principles, followed by chapters addressing the SLE and SS-specific organ manifestations. This book also offers an update on specific aspects of these diseases, including an emphasis on unifying aspects such as connections between immune system dysfunctions and development of the different types of CTDs, management of high-risk pregnancies, and the role of new target therapies.

This book would be aimed both at the rheumatologist already familiar with CTDs and at the general clinician and practitioner, equipping them to handle the requirements of the unique treatment, as well as rheumatologist trainees and nurses wishing to specialize.

2 Epidemiology of Systemic Lupus Erythematosus

Simone Baldovino and Cristiana Rollino

Systemic lupus erythematosus (SLE) is an often severe autoimmune rheumatic disease of unclear etiology that affects people worldwide. SLE presents with a wide spectrum of clinical patterns and can affect all ages and ethnicities [1]. Regardless of the age of disease onset, the diagnosis relies upon a combination of clinical and laboratory findings which are addressed in more detail in other sections of the book. In this chapter we aim to critically review the epidemiology of SLE.

2.1 Issues in Epidemiological Studies About SLE

Epidemiological studies about SLE are complicated by many issues such as variable disease presentation, the remitting and relapsing nature of the disease, and the presence of different classification criteria. The American College of Rheumatology (ACR) classification is the most widely accepted, and the only validated instrument for "diagnosing" lupus [2–4]; however, these criteria do not represent the full spectrum of disease and other classification criteria have been proposed [5, 6]. These classification criteria were created to identify SLE patients for clinical studies. Patients fulfilling 4 out of the 11 1982 ACR criteria are classified with SLE with

S. Baldovino
Center of Research of Immunopathology and Rare Diseases, Coordinating Center of the Network of Rare Diseases of Piedmont and Aosta Valley, Department of Rare, Immunologic, Hematologic and Immunohematologic Diseases, San Giovanni Hospital, Piazza donatore di Sangue 3, Turin 10154, Italy
e-mail: simone.baldovino@unito.it

C. Rollino (✉)
SCDU Nephrology and Dialysis, San Giovanni Hospital,
Piazza donatore di Sangue 3, Turin 10154, Italy
e-mail: cristiana.rollino@libero.it

D. Roccatello, L. Emmi (eds.), *Connective Tissue Disease: A Comprehensive Guide-Volume 1*, Rare Diseases of the Immune System 5,
DOI 10.1007/978-3-319-24535-5_2

approximately 95 % certainty, although many individuals who meet only two or three criteria are "diagnosed" with SLE.

The use of different and more sensitive criteria for the assessment and the inclusion of milder cases may partly explain the differences in incidence and prevalence observed in different periods. A study conducted in Olmsted County, Minnesota, analyzed SLE incidence rates in two periods. The age- and sex-adjusted incidence rate was higher in the latter period (1.5 and 5.6 per 100,000 person-years, respectively, in 1950–1979 and 1980–1992) [7]. Similar increases were seen in an incidence study in 1980–1984, 1985–1989, and 1990–1994 in Denmark [8].

Moreover, the different study designs can affect estimation of the prevalence, incidence, morbidity, and mortality. Studies based on the use of population registries potentially allow to identify a greater number of cases. However, often the used diagnostic criteria are not sufficiently controlled. On the other hand, studies carried out by reference centers allow a more precise definition of the reported cases but suffer from a selection bias. In fact, often, patients treated at referral centers are more complex and serious and do not represent the full spectrum of the disease.

Another issue is the potential contribution of undiagnosed disease to the total burden within a population. This issue was addressed by a community survey in Birmingham (United Kingdom), combined with antinuclear antibody testing and clinical assessment of "positive" respondents and reported a prevalence of diagnosed SLE in women ages 18–65 years of 54 per 100,000. With the addition of the cases found during the screening, this estimate rose to 200 per 100,000 [9]. These results were confirmed by subsequent studies conducted in Israel and in Michigan [10, 11].

2.2 Incidence and Prevalence of SLE

According to the last available revision of the literature, incidence rates of SLE range from approximately 1 to 10 per 100,000 person-years, and prevalence rates generally range from 20 to 70 per 100,000 [12]. After that review many studies about SLE epidemiology were conducted worldwide [11, 13–30]. Even if SLE occurs throughout the world, many variables such as ethnicity, geography, sex, and age affect the epidemiology of SLE. In the following sections, we will analyze each of these variables.

Kidney involvement plays a pivotal role in the prognosis of patients with SLE, as it deeply affects mortality and morbidity. Thus, in this chapter we will address this aspect with a special emphasis.

2.3 Ethnicity, Geography, and Genetics in SLE

In North America, the lowest incidences of SLE were seen among Caucasian Americans, Canadians, and Spaniards with incidences of 1.4, 1.6, and 2.2 cases per 100,000 people, respectively [12]. A higher incidence is observed among Arab and Chaldean Americans (age-adjusted incidence of 7.6 and 62.6 per 100,000, respectively) [30] and among black people (age-adjusted incidence of 3.2 and 13.4 6 per 100,000 for men and for women, respectively) [19, 31].

Throughout Europe, the highest incidences were found in Sweden (4.7 cases/100,000) [32], in France (3.32 cases/100,000) [22], and in Asian (17.45 cases/100,000) and Afro-Caribbean (31.46 cases/100,000) residents of the United Kingdom [24].

Consistent with data from the United Kingdom, the prevalence of SLE was also high in Puerto Rico, with an overall prevalence of 159 per 100,000 individuals (277 per 100,000 for females and 25 per 100,000 for males) [33].

In Australia some studies focused on the difference in SLE prevalence and clinical and laboratory expression between Aboriginal and non-Aboriginal Australians. Prevalence of SLE was higher in Aboriginal than among non-Aboriginal (52.0–92.8 vs 19.3–39.0 cases per 100,000 population) [25]. Both ethnographic and genetic differences and more complex social factors related to poverty and access to care are likely associated with increased risk of the disease.

A systematic review, published by Osio-Salido and Manapat-Reyes in 2010, identified the epidemiological data for 24 Asian countries. Prevalence falls within 30–50/100,000, with a higher prevalence of 70 in Shanghai and a lower prevalence ranging from 3.2 to 19.3 in India, Japan, and Saudi Arabia. Incidence data were available only for three countries (Japan, Hong Kong, and China) and varied from 0.9 to 3.1 per annum [13].

The influence of genetics is one of the factors implicated in differences in epidemiology and clinical expression of SLE in different populations. The genetic basis of SLE is very complex and recent genome-wide studies have identified more than 50 robust loci associated with SLE susceptibility [34]. One study conducted by Wang and coworkers on 695 Chinese SLE patients estimated that the heritability of SLE should be of 43.6 %. The authors concluded that the genetic model of SLE could be a polygenetic model and major gene mode is the best fitted one [35]. Studies on twin show a concordance rate ranging from 2 to 5 % for dizygotic twins and 24–60 % for monozygotic twins. However, this concordance in twins can be explained by behavior as well as by genetic predisposition [36].

The strongest genetic associations are reported for the human leukocyte antigen (HLA) class II (DR2 and DR3), with relative risks of approximately 2.0, with differing strengths of association in different racial populations, and HLA class III region (MSH5 and SKIV2L) [36, 37]. Other non-HLA genes associated with SLE can be classified by the pathway in which they are involved, such as type I interferon pathway (TLR7, IRF5 and IRF7, IFIH1, STAT4, TYK2, and SLC15A4), nuclear factor kB (TNFAIP3, IRAK1, and possibly MECP2), B- and T-cell signaling (PTPN22, c-Src tyrosine kinase, BANK1, BLK, IL10, and IKZF1), immune complex clearance (FCGR2A,FCGR3A, FCGR3B, ITGAM, a protein involved in forming complement receptor 3, and protein involved in classic pathway of complement, especially C1q), production of oxygen reactive species (NCF2, a protein coding for a NADPH oxidase subunit), cell-cycle regulation (CDKN1B), autophagy (ATG5 and DRAM1), and DNA demethylation (TET3) [34].

2.4 Age, Sex, and SLE

Age at onset defines different subtypes of SLE: neonatal lupus, secondary to passive transfer of antibodies from an affected mother to the child, pediatric lupus (pSLE), adulthood SLE, and late-onset SLE (loSLE) [36].

SLE onset is more common in young adults, between 15 and 40 [36]. Pediatric lupus accounts approximately 10–20 % of cases [38]. The onset of SLE beyond the age of 50 years is reported to occur in 3–18 % of patients [39].

During the child-bearing years, the ratio of women to men with lupus is approximately 9:1. This ratio is less in younger (2:1) and older (3:1) populations, supporting a role for hormonal factors in disease induction and pathogenesis [1, 36]. The higher incidence among women is clearly seen in black people in the United States (crude incidence per 100,000 of 13.6 in women vs 2.6 in men) [19]. A similar pattern is observed in other populations, as seen in a large study from the United Kingdom as well as in smaller studies from the Sweden and Iceland. However, in these populations the highest age-specific incidence rates are generally seen after 40 years of age. Although there are no incident data for Hispanics in the United States or Latin America, some studies suggest they also develop lupus earlier in life [24].

The importance of hormonal and reproductive factor in the highest susceptibility of women to SLE has been proven by few studies that correlate age at menarche with risk to develop SLE (odds 4.6-fold higher for women with menarche at age 10 years versus menarche at age 13 years). Menstrual irregularities were also associated with increased risk of SLE in a Japanese case–control study and in the Carolina Lupus study [36].

Many authors have studied the influence of oral contraceptives on SLE onset but the results are controversial. In addition, the effect of breastfeeding has been analyzed with an apparent protective effect. Finally, early menopausal and postmenopausal hormone therapy seems to be correlated with a higher risk of SLE [36].

2.5 Other Risk Factors for SLE Development

Tobacco smoking has been proposed to be a trigger for the development of SLE. Results of nine studies have been summarized in a meta-analysis by Costenbader and coworkers. The authors revealed a small but significantly increased risk for the development of SLE among current smokers compared with nonsmokers (OR 1.50, 95 % CI 1.09–2.08). They did not observe a similar association for ex-smokers compared with never smokers, concluding that the effect of active smoking on risk appears to be stronger than a past exposure [40]. A subsequent Japanese study showed that the association between smoking and a particular polymorphism of the receptor for TNF, TNFRSF1B, was associated with a greater risk of developing SLE [41]. Moreover, two studies conducted in Japan showed a dose–response relationship between smoking and the risk of SLE [41].

The role of alcohol consumption is more controversial. A meta-analysis conducted by Wang and coworkers showed that moderate alcohol intake has a protective effect on the development of SLE [42]. Heavy alcohol consumption (>4–5 days/week) was shown to be associated with odds of 4.49 (95 % CI, 1.43–14.08) for the occurrence of SLE only in some populations, suggesting that additional genetic or environmental factors can interact with alcohol consumption in SLE development [41].

Some medications, such as procainamide, can induce lupus-like disease, typically without the presence of autoantibodies, in susceptible individuals. To date, the drugs mainly associated with the development of SLE in animal models are estrogen. However, even if some case series described the induction of SLE and disease flares in patients who took combined oral contraceptive pills, a randomized controlled trial found that combined oral contraceptives did not confer a higher risk of disease flares in women with clinically stable SLE. On the other hand, another randomized controlled trial did find a higher risk of mild to moderate lupus flares in postmenopausal women with SLE who used hormone replacement therapy [41].

Other drugs that have been supposed to be associated with SLE induction are anti-TNF used in the treatment of inflammatory arthritis. Even if cases of anti-TNF-induced lupus have been reported, we lack a clear figure of real impact of these agents in SLE induction [43].

The supposed association between LES and vaccines has never been proven [41]. A recent analysis conducted in silico by McGarvey and colleagues suggests that the presence of some genetic variations associated with specific immunological pathways could be associated with a higher risk to develop autoimmune diseases such as SLE as a consequences of vaccination [44]. These preliminary data need confirmation that should necessarily be based on genetic epidemiology studies conducted on large populations.

Many other chemicals, such as crystalline silica, chlorinated compounds, mercury, liquid pesticides, solvents, phthalates (that are also present in lipsticks), and aromatic amines (that are also found in hair dyes), have been associated with SLE onset or flairs [41].

2.6 SLE Mortality, Morbidity, and Clinical Expression

SLE still remains an important cause of morbidity and mortality among young and middle-aged people, but, until the middle of the last century, 5-year survival was <50 % [36].

Owing to improvements in disease management and recognition over the past 20–30 years, patients now live longer, but as a result have increased disease damage.

Such as incidence and prevalence, also the clinical expression, the morbidity, and the mortality of SLE are influenced by ethnicity, geography, sex, and age at the onset.

Few Australian studies investigated the differences in SLE expression between Aboriginal and non-Aboriginal in Australia with heterogeneous results. One study reported that laboratory anomalies and organ involvement were similar in Aboriginal and non-Aboriginal Australians, but another reported differences (not statistically significant) between these populations in clinical manifestations and certain laboratory features, including malar rash, discoid rash, photosensitivity, oral ulcers, pleuritis and anticardiolipin, anti-Smith and anti-ribonucleoprotein antibodies, and lupus anticoagulant. Other analyses investigated SLE features in Asian Australians. Two studies reported that Asian Australians were more affected by SLE than non-Asian Australians in terms of disease severity, renal involvement, photosensitivity, laboratory characteristics, and flares [25].

A recent study from Qian and colleagues explored the correlation between SLE activity and altitudinal variations. The authors performed a retrospective analysis of 1,029 hospitalized patients in China. The study did not found significant correlation between SLE activity (recorded using SLEDAI) and altitudes. However, the authors found a correlation between the age at diseases onset and at hospital admission, the presence of Sm antibodies, and living at high altitudes [45].

Pediatric cases are associated with higher disease severity, more rapid damage accrual (the majority of patients will have developed damage within 5–10 years of disease onset), and atypical presentations than adult-onset SLE. Premature atherosclerosis and osteoporosis have become increasingly prevalent morbidities in pSLE patients. Differential ethnic expression is present in pediatric patients such as in adult with a more severe disease course in patients of African ancestry. The most prevalent manifestations of SLE in pediatric patients are musculoskeletal, ocular, renal, and neuropsychiatric. Furthermore, the presentation of a serious incurable, potentially devastating disease, in a period of important psychosocial development, may result in significant psychosocial stress [38]. The serological pattern of pediatric patients can be characterized by absence of ANA and anti-nDNA antibodies, mostly in SLE secondary to complement deficiencies [46]. Due to the more severe course of disease, patients with pSLE have a higher mortality than patients with adult onset (mortality hazard ratios of 6.29 vs 1.75) [47].

loSLE is usually associated with milder manifestations. The most prevalent manifestations are pulmonary involvement and serositis. Furthermore, late-onset SLE can be associated with Sjogren's syndrome and may present an atypical serological pattern with the presence of rheumatoid factor and of antinuclear antibody and a lower frequency of anti-ribonucleoprotein (anti-RNP) and anti-Sm antibody [39]. Despite the milder presentation, loSLE is associated with poorer survival than early-onset SLE (mortality hazard ratios of 3.44 vs 1.75 in patients with adult onset) [47]. The higher mortality likely reflects the consequences of aging rather than true differences in survival. Importantly, the cause of death in late-onset SLE patients is usually not SLE itself, but rather the more frequent occurrence of infections, cardiovascular disorders, malignancies, or drug-induced complications [39].

Few studies tried to explore the role of socioeconomic factors as risk factors for SLE outcome. Poorer outcomes and higher disease activity have been associated with measures of socioeconomic status (SES) such as insurance, income, and education. It is often difficult to disentangle these from other closely related potential risk factors associated with disease susceptibility such as environmental and toxic exposure. Non-Caucasian race, lower levels of education, and limited access to medical care appear to be associated with SLE-related organ damage and higher morbidity. Broader measures of lower SES, such as the Hollingshead Index, were associated with patients' perceived health outcomes such that lower SES was associated with higher morbidity [36].

Deficiency of vitamin D was demonstrated to be associated with higher lupus disease activity. In a recent study from Petri and colleagues, 1,006 SLE patients were assessed for serum 25(OH)D levels, 76 % of which had levels of 25(OH)D that were <40 ng/ml (insufficient). This percentage was significantly higher among African-Americans (85 %) and among those ages 30–59 (79 %). Moreover, in patients with insufficient 25(OH)D levels, a 20-ng/ml increase in serum was shown to be associated with a 15 % decrease in the odds of clinically important proteinuria (urine protein-to-creatinine ratio >0.5) [48].

2.7 Lupus Nephritis

Renal involvement is a major complication of SLE and a strong determinant of morbidity and mortality. About 60 % of SLE patients develop kidney involvement [49].

A clear definition of what we are referring to as "lupus nephritis" must be introduced. Traditionally, authors refer to lupus nephritis (LN) as the glomerular involvement in the course of SLE. However, the kidney involvement in the context of the disease may be heterogeneous, also including tubulointerstitial nephropathy, which manifests clinically with electrolyte disorders and/or renal acidosis, and different features of vascular disease.

In the following paragraphs, we will refer to the lupus glomerulonephritis as LN. Similarly to other manifestations of SLE, many factors influence LN incidence estimates: location, ethnicity, gender, and method of diagnosis.

The literature reports a frequency of LN among SLE patients ranging from 40 to 70 % [50]. However, this estimation is probably lower than the real one, because of the bias generated by the method of diagnosis. Patients with less severe forms of lupus glomerulonephritis may not undergo renal biopsy ascertainment, hence resulting in incorrect estimate.

Moreover the incidence of LN may have been modified over the recent years by the use of more aggressive treatments.

Most SLE patients develop nephritis early in the course of their disease. The vast majority is younger than 55 years. Children are more likely to develop severe nephritis than elderly patients [51].

2.8 LN Histological Classification

The 2003 edition of the ISN/RPS classification of the modified WHO histological classification of LN [52] has significantly improved management and prognosis of the disease [49].

According to the ISN/RPS classification [52], lupus glomerulonephritis ranges from less severe to highly severe forms. The most active forms, such as class III, IV, and V, are usually ascertained by biopsy. On the contrary, patients with less severe forms (class I, II, and probably some of class III cases) may not be submitted to renal biopsy, so that these forms may elude the epidemiologic estimates.

At this regard, in one study kidney biopsy was offered to all patients with SLE seen at a Japanese hospital over an 11-year period, whether or not clinical signs of renal disease were present [53]. Of the 195 patients who had adequate biopsies, 86 had no clinical renal involvement. Of these 86 patients without clinical renal disease, 13 (15 %) had either class III or IV lupus nephritis and 9 (10 %) had class V disease.

2.9 Immunosuppression and Renal Replacement Advancements

Despite the ancient history of SLE, the renal manifestations were described for the first time in the early 1900s [54] (Fig. 2.1).

Renal failure soon emerged as an important cause of death among SLE patients. Survival rate was less than 50 % at 5 years for LN patients in the late 1950s [55]. Survival of LN patients with end-stage kidney disease (ESKD) was negatively affected by the absence of renal replacement therapies (RRTs) or by their delayed utilization (Fig. 2.1).

Hemodialysis (HD) for LN was first reported only in the mid-1970s and only in the European literature. Initial reports indicated that the outcomes of LN patients with ESKD who underwent RRT seemed to be worse than those of the general

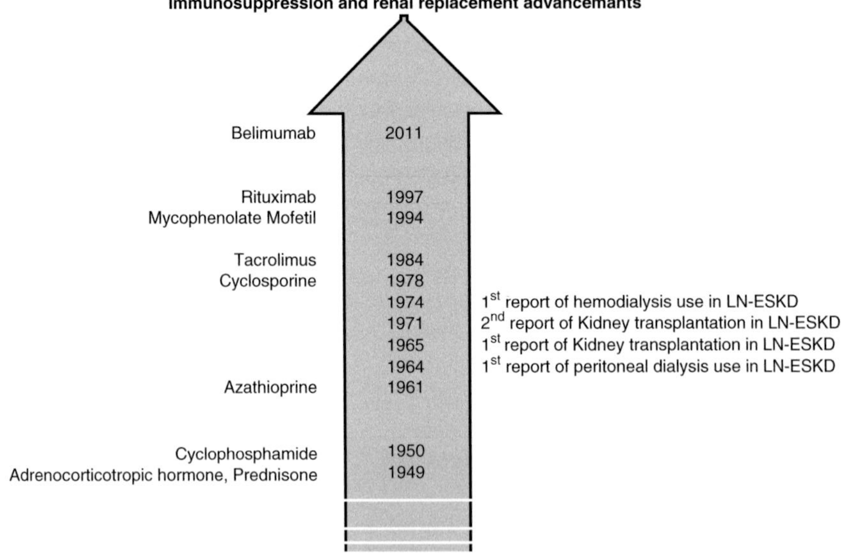

Fig. 2.1 Timeline of immunosuppressions and renal replacement advancements

ESKD population [56]. Morbidity in the SLE group was primarily associated with infection and vascular access problems, but no deaths were directly attributable to SLE activity.

The 5-year survival rate in the early 1980s was reported to be significantly lower in HD-dependent SLE patients than in non-SLE HD patients (58.6 % versus 88.5 %).

With advances in lupus treatment, outcome improved dramatically. Studies from the 1990s reported that more than 93 % of LN patients survived for 5 years and 85 % survived for 10 years [57] and the 5-year survival rate for patients on dialysis increased to 73 % [56, 58]. As the need for a dialytic treatment may be only temporary, dialysis now represents the opportunity for renal recovery.

Hence the almost free availability of dialysis also affects epidemiologic data: the incidence of LN-associated ESKD has increased from 1.16 cases per million in 1982 to 4.9 cases per million in 2004 in the United States [59, 60].

2.10 General Data on Lupus Nephritis

Several data are reported about prevalence and incidence of LN.

The overall annual incidence rate has been rated 0.40 per 100,000 subjects per year (95 % CI 0.24–0.63) [61] and the prevalence ranging from 4.4 per 100,000 inhabitants (95 % CI 3.8–5.0) (in northwest England in 2001-Patel-) to 6.85/100,000 person-years [62].

Prevalence and incidence are increasing over the years. Iseki et al. [63] analyzed 566 SLE patients in Japan over a 20-year period. They found that the annual incidence and prevalence of LN in women had increased from 16.0 per million and 66.0 per million, respectively, in 1972 to 46.7 and 683.3, respectively, in 1991 and that the annual incidence and prevalence in men had increased from 4.2 and 8.3, respectively, in 1972 to 8.3 and 70.0, respectively, in 1991.

It is unclear why the prevalence of end-stage LN increased by nearly tenfold in 20 years. One possible explanation is an improvement in therapeutic option, resulting in a lower patient mortality and a possible longer life span, compatible with a potential development of renal failure.

In a recent retrospective study, male sex, young age (<33 years), and non-European ancestry were found to be determinants of earlier renal disease in patients with SLE [49].

2.11 Gender

The striking prevalence of women affected with SLE is less evident as regards LN.

More severe renal disease, skin lesions, serositis, thrombotic events, and seizures have been reported in males by several authors [64].

Whereas the incidence of SLE among the male population is low when androgen levels are high, the incidence approaches the same of the female population during childhood and old age when androgen levels are low.

In the study of Patel [61], the annual incidence rate was higher in women, at 0.68 per 100,000 per year (95 % CI 0.40–1.10), than in men, at 0.09 per 100,000 per year (95 % CI 0.01–0.32).

The prevalence rates were also higher in women than in men (7.1 per 100,000 [95 % CI 6.1–8.2] versus 1.4 per 100,000 [95 % CI 1.0–2.0], respectively) [61], and this was true for all ethnic groups.

In Saxena study [49], the median age at diagnosis was 35 years (IQR 65.1–65.9) in men.

Male gender was found to be a poor prognostic factor for the clinical course of LN, progression to ESKD, and morbidity [59, 65].

2.12 Ethnicity

It is well known that frequency and severity of LN differ among ethnicities.

Besides a higher SLE incidence, African-American ethnicities may present with more severe presentation and earlier renal disease, as shown in a retrospective study [50].

In the Saxena study [49], a higher proportion of Indo-Asian patients with SLE (27 %) and an even higher proportion of Afro-Caribbean patients with SLE (58 %) were estimated to have LN when compared to the white population, in which the estimated proportion of SLE patients with LN was 10 %. The prevalence estimates were significantly higher in women, in particular, in the Chinese and Afro-Caribbean populations when compared with the white population. Indeed, there was a marked ethnic gradient, with the prevalence estimates increasing from the white population to the Indo-Asian, Afro-Caribbean, and the Chinese populations.

2.13 Socioeconomic Status

A number of studies suggest that LN is both more common and more severe in some ethnic minorities and progression to end-stage renal disease is higher in uninsured and low SES groups [66, 67].

An interesting study based on the Medicaid Analytic eXtract (MAX) administrative data system analyzes LN patients searched on the basis on ≥2 ICD-9 hospital discharge diagnoses of LN from January 1, 2000, to December 31, 2004.

The study was conducted utilizing combined categories: white, black or African-American, Hispanic or Latino, Asian (including Pacific Islander), Native American, and others. Seven SES indicators were taken into account: median household income, proportion with income below 200 % of the federal poverty level, median home value, median monthly rent, mean education level, proportion of people age >25 who were college graduates, and proportion of employed persons with a professional occupation.

From 2000 to 2004, the prevalence of LN was 30.9 per 100,000 (7,388 individuals) or 21.5 % of SLE cases, with higher rates among all non-Caucasian racial/ethnic groups compared to whites.

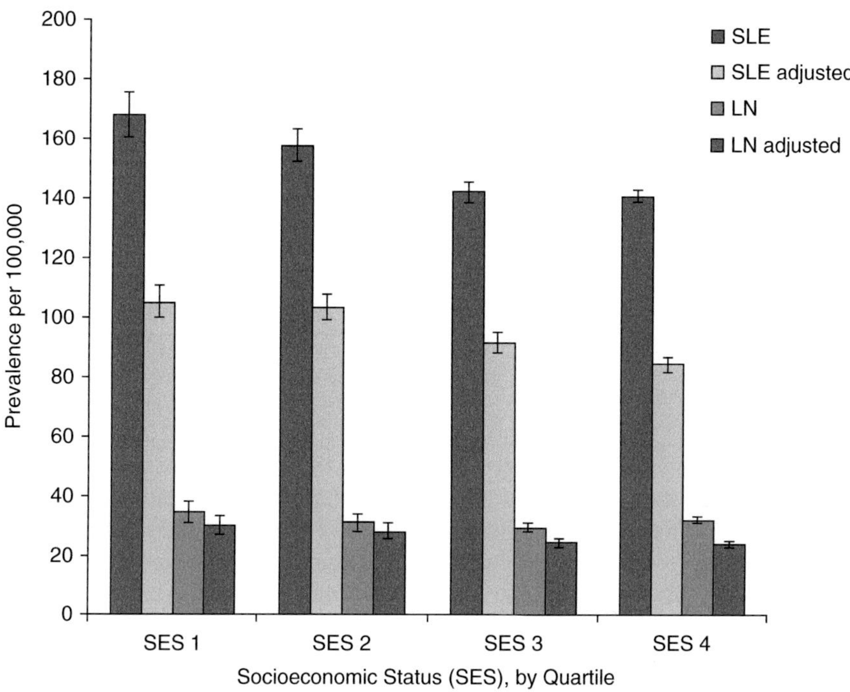

Fig. 2.2 Prevalence of systemic lupus erythematosus (*SLE*) and lupus nephritis (*LN*) per 100,000 US Medicaid enrollees ages 18–65 years, stratified by socioeconomic status (*SES*) quartile (SES 1 [lowest] = –1.62 or below, SES 2 = above –1.62 through –0.74, SES 3 = above –0.74 through 0.26, SES 4 [highest] = above 0.26). Results of crude analyses and analyses adjusted for age group, sex, and race/ethnicity are shown. Bars represent 95 % confidence intervals. (Modified from Feldman et al. [62])

By dividing the population into quartiles of county level SES, statistically significant differences were found between the lowest SES group, which had the highest SLE prevalence (167.9 per 100,000, 95 % CI 160.4–175.7) and the two highest SES quartiles, which had the lowest SLE prevalence. A similar pattern was found after adjusting for age, sex, and race/ethnicity.

On the opposite, the trend of LN prevalence did not differ significantly across SES quartiles. This suggests that genetics may be a more important determinant in the development of LN compared to SLE. It is also possible that once individuals enter into care for their SLE, SES contributes less to disease complications (Fig. 2.2).

2.14 Lupus Nephritis and Progression Toward End Stage Kidney Disease

Overall prognosis of SLE patients has improved in recent decades [59]. However, approximately 10–30 % of patients with proliferative LN progress to ESKD.

The incidence of LN-associated ESKD has increased from 1.16 cases per million in 1982 to 4.9 cases per million in 2004 in the United States (Fig. 2.3) [59, 60].

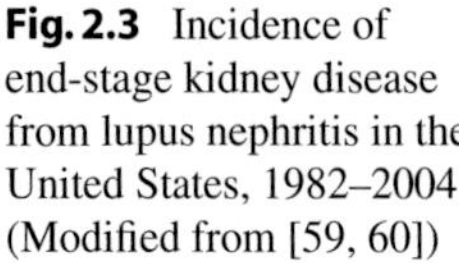

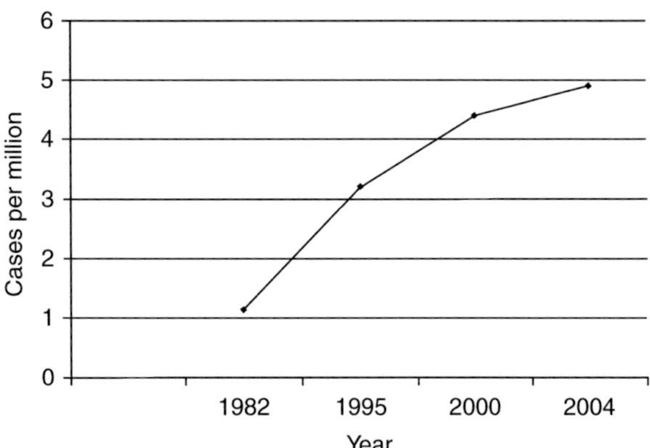

Fig. 2.3 Incidence of end-stage kidney disease from lupus nephritis in the United States, 1982–2004 (Modified from [59, 60])

Analysis of the US Renal Data System from 1996 to 2004 showed that there were 9,199 new cases of ESKD attributable to LN with most patients being of African-American descent and of female sex (49 % and 82 % of cases, respectively) [59, 68]. This increase in the incidence of ESKD due to LN is a cause for concern. Recent epidemiological studies have pointed to several risk factors associated with the progression of LN to ESKD that could affect these estimations.

Young age is one of the primary risk factors for progression to ESKD. It was reported that up to 75 % of children with SLE eventually develop nephritis and 18–50 % show progression to ESKD [69, 70]. The lack of standardized protocols for treating LN in pediatric populations is a challenge in managing treatment.

Delayed renal biopsy [71, 72] and delay in treatment of LN are other important risk factors associated with poor outcomes and progression to ESKD. Specifically, an elapsed time of more than 6 months between urinary evidence of nephropathy and biopsy has been associated with progression to ESKD.

While ESKD in LN appears to have stopped increasing in the last decade, ethnical disparities in outcomes persist: the African-Americans are still more likely to die prematurely [73].

Tubulointerstitial involvement with or without immune deposits along the tubular basement membrane is a common finding in LN, almost always being seen with concurrent glomerular disease [74, 75].

The severity of the tubulointerstitial involvement is an important prognostic sign. In a Chinese study of 313 patients with LN, for example, the presence of tubulointerstitial nephritis was significantly associated with a twofold higher risk of developing end-stage renal disease [76].

In a few cases, tubulointerstitial involvement is the only manifestation of LN. This possibility should be suspected when a patient with SLE presents with a rising plasma creatinine concentration and a urinalysis that is relatively normal or shows only a few red cells and/or white cells. These changes may be accompanied by signs of tubular dysfunction such as metabolic acidosis due to type 1 (distal) renal tubular acidosis, hyperkalemia, or hypokalemia [77, 78].

Involvement of the renal vasculature is not uncommon in LN, and its presence can adversely affect the prognosis of the renal disease [79]. The most frequent manifestations are immune complex deposition, immunoglobulin microvascular "thrombi" [78], a thrombotic microangiopathy [80, 81], vasculitis [82], or atheroembolic disease and atherosclerosis.

Rarely, patients with LN develop renal vein thrombosis [83].

Conclusions

According to the most recent revision of the literature, incidence rates of SLE range from approximately 1 to 10 per 100,000 person-years, and prevalence rates generally range from 20 to 70 per 100,000. Even if SLE occurs throughout the world, many variables such as ethnicity, geography, sex, and age affect the epidemiology of SLE.

Kidney involvement plays a pivotal role in the prognosis of patients with SLE, as still approximately 10–30 % of patients with proliferative LN progress to ESKD.

Prevalence and incidence are increasing over the years. A "big data" approach in perspective studies will enable hitherto unseen connections in SLE epidemiology to emerge.

References

1. Tsokos GC (2011) Systemic lupus erythematosus. N Engl J Med 365(22):2110–2121. doi:10.1056/NEJMra1100359
2. Tan EM, Cohen AS, Fries JF et al (1982) The 1982 revised criteria for the classification of systemic lupus erythematosus. Arthritis Rheum 25(11):1271–1277, http://www.ncbi.nlm.nih.gov/pubmed/7138600. Accessed 13 May 2015
3. Levin RE, Weinstein A, Peterson M et al (1984) A comparison of the sensitivity of the 1971 and 1982 American Rheumatism Association criteria for the classification of systemic lupus erythematosus. Arthritis Rheum 27(5):530–538, http://www.ncbi.nlm.nih.gov/pubmed/6721885. Accessed 13 May 2015
4. Passas CM, Wong RL, Peterson M et al (1985) A comparison of the specificity of the 1971 and 1982 American Rheumatism Association criteria for the classification of systemic lupus erythematosus. Arthritis Rheum 28(6):620–623, http://www.ncbi.nlm.nih.gov/pubmed/4004972. Accessed 13 May 2015
5. Petri M (2005) Review of classification criteria for systemic lupus erythematosus. Rheum Dis Clin N Am 31(2):245–254, vi. doi:10.1016/j.rdc.2005.01.009
6. Petri M, Orbai A-M, Alarcón GS et al (2012) Derivation and validation of the Systemic Lupus International Collaborating Clinics classification criteria for systemic lupus erythematosus. Arthritis Rheum 64(8):2677–2686. doi:10.1002/art.34473
7. Uramoto KM, Michet CJ, Thumboo J et al (1999) Trends in the incidence and mortality of systemic lupus erythematosus, 1950–1992. Arthritis Rheum 42(1):46–50. doi:10.1002/1529-0131(199901)42:1<46::AID-ANR6>3.0.CO;2-2
8. Voss A, Green A, Junker P (1998) Systemic lupus erythematosus in Denmark: clinical and epidemiological characterization of a county-based cohort. Scand J Rheumatol 27(2):98–105, http://www.ncbi.nlm.nih.gov/pubmed/9572634. Accessed 23 May 2015

9. Johnson AE, Gordon C, Hobbs FD et al (1996) Undiagnosed systemic lupus erythematosus in the community. Lancet 347(8998):367–369, http://www.ncbi.nlm.nih.gov/pubmed/8598703. Accessed 23 May 2015
10. Geva E, Lerner-Geva L, Burke M et al (2004) Undiagnosed systemic lupus erythematosus in a cohort of infertile women. Am J Reprod Immunol 51(5):336–340. doi:10.1111/j.1600-0897.2004.00165.x
11. Somers EC, Marder W, Cagnoli P et al (2014) Population-based incidence and prevalence of systemic lupus erythematosus: the Michigan Lupus Epidemiology and Surveillance program. Arthritis Rheumatol (Hoboken NJ) 66(2):369–378. doi:10.1002/art.38238
12. Pons-Estel GJ, Alarcon GS, Scofield L et al (2010) Understanding the epidemiology and progression of systemic lupus erythematosus. Semin Arthritis Rheum 39(4):257–268. doi:10.1016/j.semarthrit.2008.10.007
13. Osio-Salido E, Manapat-Reyes H (2010) Epidemiology of systemic lupus erythematosus in Asia. Lupus 19(12):1365–1373. doi:10.1177/0961203310374305
14. Mok CC (2011) Epidemiology and survival of systemic lupus erythematosus in Hong Kong Chinese. Lupus 20(7):767–771. doi:10.1177/0961203310388447
15. Barnabe C, Joseph L, Belisle P et al (2012) Prevalence of systemic lupus erythematosus and systemic sclerosis in the First Nations population of Alberta, Canada. Arthritis Care Res (Hoboken) 64(1):138–143. doi:10.1002/acr.20656
16. Furst DE, Clarke AE, Fernandes AW et al (2013) Incidence and prevalence of adult systemic lupus erythematosus in a large US managed-care population. Lupus 22(1):99–105. doi:10.1177/0961203312463110
17. Ng R, Bernatsky S, Rahme E (2013) Observation period effects on estimation of systemic lupus erythematosus incidence and prevalence in Quebec. J Rheumatol 40(8):1334–1336. doi:10.3899/jrheum.121215
18. Shim J-S, Sung Y-K, Joo YB et al (2014) Prevalence and incidence of systemic lupus erythematosus in South Korea. Rheumatol Int 34(7):909–917
19. Lim SS, Bayakly AR, Helmick CG et al (2014) The incidence and prevalence of systemic lupus erythematosus, 2002–2004: the Georgia Lupus Registry. Arthritis Rheumatol (Hoboken NJ) 66(2):357–368. doi:10.1002/art.38239
20. Zou Y-F, Feng C-C, Zhu J-M et al (2014) Prevalence of systemic lupus erythematosus and risk factors in rural areas of Anhui Province. Rheumatol Int 34(3):347–356. doi:10.1007/s00296-013-2902-1
21. Simard JF, Sjowall C, Ronnblom L et al (2014) Systemic lupus erythematosus prevalence in Sweden in 2010: what do national registers say? Arthritis Care Res (Hoboken) 66(11):1710–1717. doi:10.1002/acr.22355
22. Arnaud L, Fagot J-P, Mathian A et al (2014) Prevalence and incidence of systemic lupus erythematosus in France: a 2010 nation-wide population-based study. Autoimmun Rev 13(11):1082–1089. doi:10.1016/j.autrev.2014.08.034
23. Ferucci ED, Johnston JM, Gaddy JR et al (2014) Prevalence and incidence of systemic lupus erythematosus in a population-based registry of American Indian and Alaska Native people, 2007–2009. Arthritis Rheumatol (Hoboken NJ) 66(9):2494–2502. doi:10.1002/art.38720
24. Rees F, Doherty M, Grainge M et al (2014) The incidence and prevalence of systemic lupus erythematosus in the UK, 1999–2012. Ann Rheum Dis. doi:10.1136/annrheumdis-2014-206334
25. Nikpour M, Bridge JA, Richter S (2014) A systematic review of prevalence, disease characteristics and management of systemic lupus erythematosus in Australia: identifying areas of unmet need. Intern Med J 44(12a):1170–1179. doi:10.1111/imj.12568
26. Ju JH, Yoon S-H, Kang KY et al (2014) Prevalence of systemic lupus erythematosus in South Korea: an administrative database study. J Epidemiol 24(4):295–303
27. Nasonov E, Soloviev S, Davidson JE et al (2014) The prevalence and incidence of systemic lupus erythematosus (SLE) in selected cities from three Commonwealth of Independent States countries (the Russian Federation, Ukraine and Kazakhstan). Lupus 23(2):213–219. doi:10.1177/0961203313512881

28. Jarukitsopa S, Hoganson DD, Crowson CS et al (2014) Epidemiology of systemic lupus erythematosus and cutaneous lupus in a predominantly white population in the United States. Arthritis Care Res (Hoboken). doi:10.1002/acr.22502
29. Brinks R, Fischer-Betz R, Sander O et al (2014) Age-specific prevalence of diagnosed systemic lupus erythematosus in Germany 2002 and projection to 2030. Lupus 23(13):1407–1411. doi:10.1177/0961203314540352
30. Housey M, DeGuire P, Lyon-Callo S et al (2015) Incidence and prevalence of systemic lupus erythematosus among Arab and Chaldean Americans in southeastern Michigan: the Michigan Lupus Epidemiology and Surveillance Program. Am J Public Health 105(5):e74–e79. doi:10.2105/AJPH.2014.302423
31. Urowitz MB, Gladman DD, Tom BDM et al (2008) Changing patterns in mortality and disease outcomes for patients with systemic lupus erythematosus. J Rheumatol 35(11):2152–2158
32. Ståhl-Hallengren C, Jönsen A, Nived O et al (2000) Incidence studies of systemic lupus erythematosus in Southern Sweden: increasing age, decreasing frequency of renal manifestations and good prognosis. J Rheumatol 27(3):685–691, http://www.ncbi.nlm.nih.gov/pubmed/10743809. Accessed 23 May 2015
33. Molina MJ, Mayor AM, Franco AE et al (2007) Prevalence of systemic lupus erythematosus and associated comorbidities in Puerto Rico. J Clin Rheumatol 13(4):202–204. doi:10.1097/RHU.0b013e318124a8af
34. Deng Y, Tsao BP (2014) Advances in lupus genetics and epigenetics. Curr Opin Rheumatol 26(5):1–11. doi:10.1097/BOR.0000000000000086
35. Wang J, Yang S, Chen JJ et al (2007) Systemic lupus erythematosus: a genetic epidemiology study of 695 patients from China. Arch Dermatol Res 298(10):485–491. doi:10.1007/s00403-006-0719-4
36. Simard JF, Costenbader KH (2007) What can epidemiology tell us about systemic lupus erythematosus? Int J Clin Pract 61(7):1170–1180. doi:10.1111/j.1742-1241.2007.01434.x
37. Deng Y, Tsao BP (2011) Genetic susceptibility to systemic lupus erythematosus in the genomic era. Nat Rev Rheumatol 6(12):683–692. doi:10.1038/nrrheum.2010.176.Genetic
38. Kamphuis S, Silverman ED (2010) Prevalence and burden of pediatric-onset systemic lupus erythematosus. Nat Rev Rheumatol 6(9):538–546. doi:10.1038/nrrheum.2010.121
39. Arnaud L, Mathian A, Boddaert J et al (2012) Late-onset systemic lupus erythematosus: epidemiology, diagnosis and treatment. Drugs Aging 29(3):181–189. doi:10.2165/11598550-000000000-00000
40. Costenbader KH, Kim DJ, Peerzada J et al (2004) Cigarette smoking and the risk of systemic lupus erythematosus: a meta-analysis. Arthritis Rheum 50(3):849–857. doi:10.1002/art.20049
41. Mak A, Tay S (2014) Environmental factors, toxicants and systemic lupus erythematosus. Int J Mol Sci 15(9):16043–16056. doi:10.3390/ijms150916043
42. Wang J, Pan H-F, Ye D-Q et al (2008) Moderate alcohol drinking might be protective for systemic lupus erythematosus: a systematic review and meta-analysis. Clin Rheumatol 27(12):1557–1563. doi:10.1007/s10067-008-1004-z
43. Postal M, Appenzeller S (2011) The role of Tumor Necrosis Factor-alpha (TNF-α) in the pathogenesis of systemic lupus erythematosus. Cytokine 56(3):537–543. doi:10.1016/j.cyto.2011.08.026
44. McGarvey PB, Suzek BE, Baraniuk JN et al (2014) In silico analysis of autoimmune diseases and genetic relationships to vaccination against infectious diseases. BMC Immunol 15(1):1–12. doi:10.1186/s12865-014-0061-0
45. Qian G, Ran X, Zhou CX et al (2014) Systemic lupus erythematosus patients in the low-latitude plateau of China: altitudinal influences. Lupus 23(14):1537–1545. doi:10.1177/0961203314544186
46. Leffler J, Bengtsson AA, Blom AM (2014) The complement system in systemic lupus erythematosus: an update. Ann Rheum Dis 73(9):1601–1606. doi:10.1136/annrheumdis-2014-205287
47. Chen Y-M, Lin C-HC-H, Chen H-H et al (2013) Onset age affects mortality and renal outcome of female systemic lupus erythematosus patients: a nationwide population-based study in Taiwan. Rheumatology 53(1):180–185. doi:10.1093/rheumatology/ket330

48. Petri M, Bello KJ, Fang H et al (2013) Vitamin D in systemic lupus erythematosus: modest association with disease activity and the urine protein-to-creatinine ratio. Arthritis Rheum 65(7):1865–1871. doi:10.1002/art.37953
49. Saxena R, Mahajan T, Mohan C (2011) Lupus nephritis: current update. Arthritis Res Ther 13:240–252
50. Seligman VA, Lum RF, Olson JL, et al (2002) Demographic differences in the development of lupus nephritis: a retrospective analysis. Am J Med 112:726–729
51. Mak A, Mok CC, Chu WP et al (2007) Renal damage in systemic lupus erythematosus: a comparative analysis of different age groups. Lupus 16:28–34
52. Weening JJ, D'Agati VD, Schwartz MM et al (2004) The classification of glomerulonephritis in systemic lupus erythematosus revisited. Am J Kidney Dis 15:241–250
53. Wakasugi D, Gono T, Kawaguchi Y et al (2012) Frequency of class III and IV nephritis in systemic lupus erythematosus without clinical renal involvement: an analysis of predictive measures. J Rheumatol 39:79
54. Osler W (1904) On the visceral manifestations of the erythema group of skin diseases. Am J Med Sci 127:1–23
55. Maroz N, Segal MS (2013) Lupus nephritis and end-stage kidney disease. Am J Med Sci 346:319–323
56. Jarrett M, Santhanam S, Del Greco F (1983) The clinical course of endstage renal disease in systemic lupus erythematosus. Arch Intern Med 143:1353–1356
57. Cervera R, Khamashta M, Hughes G (2009) The Euro-lupus project: epidemiology of systemic lupus erythematosus in Europe. Lupus 18:869–874
58. Mojcik C, Klippel J (1996) End-stage renal disease and systemic lupus erythematosus. Am J Med 101:100–107
59. Ward MM (2009) Changes in the incidence of endstage renal disease due to lupus nephritis in the United States, 1996–2004. J Rheumatol 36:63–67
60. Ward MM (2000) Changes in the incidence of end-stage renal disease due to lupus nephritis, 1982–1995. Arch Intern Med 160:3136–3140
61. Patel M, Clarke AM, Bruce IN et al (2006) The prevalence and incidence of biopsy-proven lupus nephritis in the UK: evidence of an ethnic gradient. Arthritis Rheum 54:2963–2969
62. Feldman CH, Hiraki LT, Liu J et al (2013) Epidemiology and sociodemographics of systemic lupus erythematosus and lupus nephritis among U.S. adults with Medicaid coverage, 2000–2004. Arthritis Rheum 65:753–763
63. Iseki K, Miyasato F, Oura T et al (1994) An epidemiologic analysis of end-stage lupus nephritis. Am J Kidney Dis 23:547–554
64. Andrade RM, Alarcon GS, Fernandez S et al LUMINA Study Group (2007) Accelerated damage accrual among men with systemic lupus erythematosus: XLIV. Results from a multiethnic US cohort. Arthritis Rheum 56:622–630
65. Chen HA, Wang JJ, Chou CT et al (2011) Predictors of long term mortality in patients with and without systemic lupus erythematosus on maintenance dialysis: a comparative study. J Rheumatol 38:2390–2394
66. McCarty DJ, Manzi S, Medsger TA Jr et al (1995) Incidence of systemic lupus erythematosus: race and gender differences. Arthritis Rheum 38:1260–1270
67. Bastian HM, Roseman JM, McGwin G Jr et al (2002) Systemic lupus erythematosus in three ethnic groups. XII. Risk factors for lupus nephritis after diagnosis. Lupus 11:152–160
68. Costenbader K, Desai A, Alarcon G et al (2011) Trends in the incidence, demographics, and outcomes of end-stage renal disease due to lupusnephritis in the US from 1995 to 2006. Arthritis Rheum 63:1681–1688
69. Hiraki L, Lu B, Alexander S et al (2011) End-stage renal disease due to lupus nephritis among children in the US, 1995–2006. Arthritis Rheum 63:1988–1997
70. Bartosh SM, Fine RN, Sullivan EK (2001) Outcome after transplantation of young patients with systemic lupus erythematosus: a report of the North American pediatric renal transplant cooperative study. Transplantation 72:973–978

71. Fiehn C, Hajjar Y, Mueller K et al (2003) Improved clinical outcome of lupus nephritis during the past decade: importance of early diagnosis and treatment. Ann Rheum Dis 62:435–439
72. Esdaile J, Levinton C, Federgreen W et al (1989) The clinical and renal biopsy predictors of long-term outcome in lupus nephritis: a study of 87 patients and review of the literature. Q J Med 72:779–833
73. Sexton DJ, Reule S, Solid C et al (2015) ESKD from lupus nephritis in the United States, 1995–2010. Clin J Am Soc Nephrol 10:251–259
74. Brentjens JR, Sepulveda M, Baliah T et al (1975) Interstitial immune complex nephritis in patients with systemic lupus erythematosus. Kidney Int 7:342
75. Park MH, D'Agati V, Appel GB et al (1986) Tubulointerstitial disease in lupus nephritis: relationship to immune deposits, interstitial inflammation, glomerular changes, renal function, and prognosis. Nephron 44:309
76. Yu F, Wu LH, Tan Y et al (2010) Tubulointerstitial lesions of patients with lupus nephritis classified by the 2003 International Society of Nephrology and Renal Pathology Society system. Kidney Int 77:820
77. Kozeny GA, Barr W, Bansal VK et al (1987) Occurrence of renal tubular dysfunction in lupus nephritis. Arch Intern Med 147:891
78. DeFronzo RA, Cooke CR, Goldberg M et al (1977) Impaired renal tubular potassium secretion in systemic lupus erythematosus. Ann Intern Med 86:268
79. Wu LH, Yu F, Tan Y et al (2013) Inclusion of renal vascular lesions in the 2003 ISN/RPS system for classifying lupus nephritis improves renal outcome predictions. Kidney Int 83:715
80. Kwok SK, Ju JH, Cho CS et al (2009) Thrombotic thrombocytopenic purpura in systemic lupus erythematosus: risk factors and clinical outcome: a single centre study. Lupus 18:16
81. Song D, Wu LH, Wang FM et al (2013) The spectrum of renal thrombotic microangiopathy in lupus nephritis. Arthritis Res Ther 15:R12
82. Abdellatif AA, Waris S, Lakhani A et al (2010) True vasculitis in lupus nephritis. Clin Nephrol 74:106
83. Gelfand J, Truong L, Stern L et al (1985) Thrombotic thrombocytopenic purpura syndrome in systemic lupus erythematosus: treatment with plasma infusion. Am J Kidney Dis 6:154

SLE Pathogenesis: From Apoptosis to Lymphocyte Activation

3

Danilo Squatrito, Giacomo Emmi, Elena Silvestri, Domenico Prisco, and Lorenzo Emmi

3.1 Introduction

Systemic lupus erythematosus (SLE) is considered a typical protean systemic autoimmune disease. It is characterized by multiorgan and multisystem involvement. Virtually, SLE may affect almost any organ during the disease course, and several pathogenic pathways drive SLE inflammation in affected tissues. Recently, the apoptotic process was thoroughly investigated, and in particular the link between apoptotic debris containing autoantigens, innate immunity activation, and maintaining of inflammation has been further elucidated. A better understanding of the pathogenic mechanisms and of the inflammatory cytokine cascade contributed to the recent development of new biological drugs specifically approved for SLE therapy. In this chapter we provide an overview of both the traditional and the more recently discovered immunological pathways that drive inflammation and contribute to organ damage in SLE (Fig. 3.1).

D. Squatrito • E. Silvestri • D. Prisco • L. Emmi (✉)
SOD Patologia Medica, Center for Autoimmune Systemic Diseases,
Behçet Center and Lupus Clinic, AOU Careggi, Largo Brambilla, 3,
Florence 50134, Italy
e-mail: l.emmi@dmi.unifi.it

G. Emmi
Department of Experimental and Clinical Medicine, University of Florence,
Viale Pieraccini 6, Florence 50139, Italy

D. Roccatello, L. Emmi (eds.), *Connective Tissue Disease: A Comprehensive Guide-Volume 1*, Rare Diseases of the Immune System 5,
DOI 10.1007/978-3-319-24535-5_3

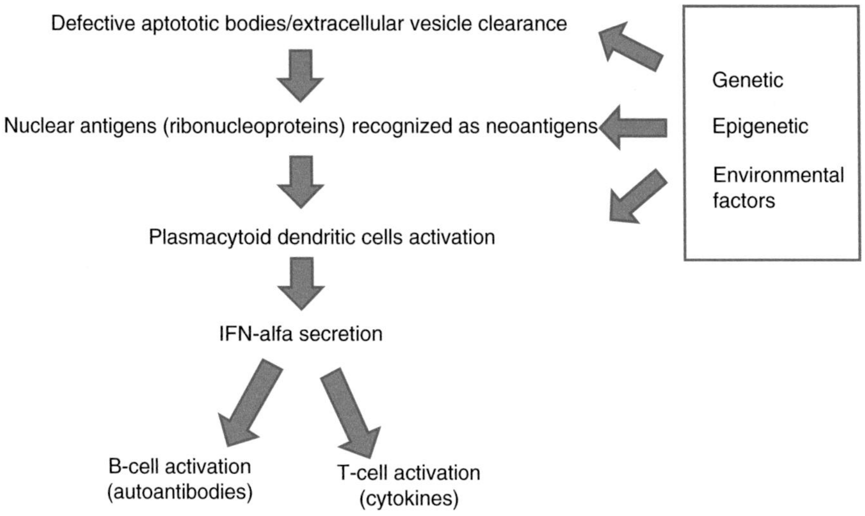

Fig. 3.1 Overview of SLE pathogenesis

3.2 Genetic and Environmental Factors

3.2.1 Genetic Aberrations

Genes that breach immune tolerance and promote autoantibody production may play a crucial role in SLE development. These genes might act with other genetic factors that augment innate immune signaling and IFN-I production, which in turn can generate an influx of effector leukocytes, inflammatory mediators, and autoantibodies into involved organs, such as the kidneys. Genetic factors influence SLE susceptibility and likely affect disease severity as well. In the last years, genetic susceptibility has been extensively investigated in SLE. However, even if the disease is definitely more frequent in certain families compared to others, identical twins show only 50 % concordance. Some major histocompatibility complex classes, in particular in class II genes (HLA-DR, DQ and DP), have been associated with SLE susceptibility [1]. Recently, several other gene polymorphisms have been found more frequently in patients with a more severe disease course [2].

Some genetic aspects however warrant more accurate discussion in SLE since they probably deeply promote both disease onset and subsequent prolonged inflammation.

The identified genes implicated in SLE can be assigned to one of four functional categories: genes that affect lymphocyte activation, particularly B cells; genes that affect innate immune signaling, (NF-κB activation and IFN-I signaling); genes that might function within the kidneys, potentially promoting renal tissue damage; and genes that influence the handling of apoptotic debris, chromatin, and immune complexes bearing these antigens. These categories have been designated on the basis of a priori analysis regarding the cell types in which the identified genes are expressed and their known molecular functions. However, alternative pathways and models cannot be excluded. Although numerous genes have been implicated in SLE, several questions remain. Firstly, the specific causative mutations and subsequent molecular alterations that contribute to the disease phenotype have not been firmly established for many of the identified candidate genes [2].

Among the others, homozygous C1q deficiency and genetic mutations resulting in low levels of C2 and C4 significantly increase the risk of developing SLE. These complement system deficiencies probably contribute to SLE pathogenesis through defective clearance of the apoptotic material, consequently leading to a significant accumulation of potential autoantigens [3].

Genome-wide microsatellite characterization was recently used to screen large-scale single nucleotide polymorphisms (SNPs) and to identify chromosomal loci that are associated with SLE. Among them IRF5, TYK2, STAT4, IRAK1, and PHPRF1 are linked to type I IFN production or IFN-induced cellular response [2].

IFN-I signaling is important in myeloid cells, including monocytes and dendritic cells, and might also have important functions in resident renal cells. Since direct evaluation of circulating IFN-alpha levels is usually very complex and does not always reliably reflect IFN overexpression, recent studies have shown a good correlation between the expression of IFN-inducible genes in peripheral blood mononuclear cells and SLE activity [4]. Microarray techniques showed that peripheral blood mononuclear cells isolated from patients with active SLE indeed display a high degree of IFN-I activity or "signature" [5, 6]. IFN-alpha hyperactivity is detected, though to a lesser extent, in patients with incomplete lupus syndrome or undifferentiated connective tissue disease, and it is even more blunted in first-degree relatives of patients with SLE [7]. Nowadays, IFN signature represents the most significant genetic discovery in SLE since it potentially implies new therapeutic options.

DNA methylation and histone modifications are key mechanisms of human epigenetic control of gene expression. Patients with active lupus were found to have reduced capacity of DNA methylation of several genes, leading to an increase in the transcription of inflammatory proteins such as CD11a, CD70, and CD40L. Perforin overexpression due to gene hypomethylation is also responsible for abnormal CD4+ T-lymphocyte killing activity [8, 9]. Interestingly, some drugs, such as hydralazine or procainamide, which are well known for being associated with drug-induced, new-onset lupus, may affect DNA hypomethylation as well. Other epigenetic mechanisms potentially affecting pathogenesis of SLE include histone acetylation and microRNA (miRNA) expression. Abnormal patterns of miRNAs have been recently detected in the blood of SLE patients [10].

3.2.2 Environmental Factors

Many theories and evidence in the past have indeed linked SLE pathogenesis to environmental factors, in particular hormones, since it is well known that SLE predominantly affects women during their childbearing years.

The first reliable mouse model of renal lupus was described in New Zealand black/white female (NZB/WF) mice [11]. Although there have been subsequent descriptions of lupus even in male murine strains, the NZB/WF mouse model provided the very first strong scientific evidence of the influence of sex hormones on SLE pathogenesis [12]. Moreover, increased production of inflammatory cytokines by T and B lymphocytes (probably via NF-kB activation) has been described after exposure to estrogens. On the other hand, progesterone is able to inhibit Toll-like receptor (TLR) 7 signals, inducing a reduction in inflammatory cytokines [13].

Historically, infections have been considered possible triggers for SLE induction in the early phases and for relapse in the course of the disease [14]. Cross-reactivity between self and non-self microbial epitopes is generally considered an appealing mechanism to explain the break in immune tolerance. For instance, a molecular mimicry has been described between EBV nuclear antigen-1 and self-antigens [15].

Ultraviolet (UV) exposure is a well-known risk factor for lupus development and disease flares [16]. UV-B exposure in particular promotes apoptosis of skin cells in SLE patients, with subsequent plasmacytoid dendritic cell (pDC) recruitment into cutaneous lesions, presentation of apoptosis-associated autoantigens to lymphocytes, and triggering of specific humoral and cellular adaptive responses. Increased levels of IFN-alpha triggered by pDCs have been demonstrated in skin specimens of SLE patients after ultraviolet exposure. Similarly, the production of other inflammatory cytokines, such as IL-1, IL-6, and TNF-alpha, by keratinocytes and lymphocytes has been shown to be influenced by UV [17].

The role of vitamin D on the immune system has also been profoundly investigated, since insufficient circulating levels are often detected in patients with several autoimmune diseases, especially with SLE. Besides influencing bone metabolism and protecting from osteoporosis, 1-25 (OH) vitamin D inhibits cellular T-lymphocyte responses and favors T^{reg} differentiation. Vitamin D deficiency is thought to be a potential susceptibility factor for autoimmune diseases [18].

In summary, as far as the role of genetic and environmental factors in SLE is concerned, a combination of genes rather than a single gene seems to predispose to the disease in the majority of patients, in particular when crucial interactions between such genes and environmental factors occur.

3.3 Apoptosis Disturbances in SLE

Previous research has shown that nuclear antigens are targeted in SLE, which is characterized by a strong serological response to DNA, histones, and ribonuclear proteins. These nuclear antigens are not usually exposed to the immune system as they are sequestered within cellular and nuclear membranes. Consequently, numerous studies have investigated the processes underlying the exposition of nuclear autoantigens and the autoimmune responses associated with SLE. Although several known pathways can lead to cell death, apoptosis remains the dominant mechanism. Apoptosis is a regulated process, which requires energy with ATP consumption, sequential activation of intracellular proteases (caspases), digestion of chromatin and DNA by DNAse enzyme, and lastly cytoskeleton modification through the formation of microparticles from the membrane. Various stimuli, such as DNA damage, UV exposure, or infections, can induce apoptosis in vitro and in vivo [19].

Rapid clearance of apoptotic cells prevents immunogenicity or the ability to initiate an inflammatory response. Experimental evidences suggest that accumulation of apoptotic debris, which can occur as a result of failure of the clearance machinery, is an important contributor to autoimmunity in SLE. Multiple ligands, receptors, opsonins, and other molecules are involved in the clearance of apoptotic cells and their debris. Genetic knockout models and pharmacological studies in mice investigated how genes affecting autoantigen clearance could promote the production of antinuclear autoantibodies and trigger other features of SLE [20]. Murine models with a deficiency of Tyro-3, Axl, and Mertk receptors showed that a decreased capacity in binding to apoptotic cells resulted in autoantibody production, development of arthritis, skin rash, and deposition of immune complexes in glomeruli. Mice deficient in T-cell IgG4 (TIM-4), which binds the phosphatidylserine residues exposed on the surface of apoptotic cells, exhibit anti-dsDNA antibodies and elevated B-cell and T-cell activation. Phosphatidylserine, which is exposed on the external membrane in the early phases of apoptosis, probably plays a pivotal role in phagocyte recognition in SLE. However, the receptors involved in this process are neither completely understood nor have they been fully identified. Noteworthy, the interaction between macrophages and apoptotic cells results in a tolerogenic immunological response that is characterized by the release of TGF-beta and IL-10 into the microenvironment, which ultimately prevents the onset of inflammation and the activation of the immune system.

If phagocytic cells are not effective in removing apoptotic cells, they accumulate and progress into secondary necrosis, which implies an inflammatory reaction. This occurs every time "danger signal" molecules, which are usually enclosed inside the cellular cytoplasm because they could potentially trigger the production of inflammatory cytokines, are released into the extracellular environment after membrane integrity is broken [21]. High-mobility group box protein 1 (HMGB1), which is produced during cell activation and, early, in apoptosis in the attempt to stabilize the nucleosome structure, warrants special consideration. If necrosis occurs, HMGB1 shows strong pro-inflammatory activity when released into the extracellular compartment, acting as an "alarmin" or "danger signal." HMGB1 activates immune responses by interacting with specific receptors of the innate immunity, in particular with TLR2 and TLR4 [22]. Therefore, the efficient clearance of apoptotic remnants remains a key physiological step for preventing the autoimmune manifestations. Apoptosis-derived extracellular vesicles (exosomes, microvesicles, apoptotic bodies) contain large amounts of digested nuclear compounds which represent a potential source of neoantigens if not promptly recognized and removed by phagocytes [23].

3.4 Innate Immune System and SLE

The role of the innate component of the immune system has been reevaluated in SLE based on knowledge of the defective apoptotic clearance in SLE, described above. Immature dendritic cells (DCs) normally express self-antigens on their surface in the absence of co-stimulatory signals, thereby inducing a tolerogenic effect on potentially autoreactive lymphocytes. A pro-inflammatory environment, such as infection, can induce DCs' maturation and the expression of co-stimulatory molecules. In this scenario, self-antigens can be presented to T lymphocytes and an autoimmune response may be potentially triggered [24].

DCs are considered very efficient in recognizing damage-associated molecular patterns (DAMPs) and particularly in recognizing a highly conserved family of pathogen-associated molecular pattern (PAMP) receptors, which can efficiently identify microbiological agents and trigger the earliest inflammatory response.

However, when apoptotic clearance is not effective enough, endogenous components such as DNA, RNA, or ribonucleoproteins may potentially be recognized by specific TLRs. Nucleic acid-sensitive TLRs (TLR3, TLR7, TLR8, and TLR9) are of interest for SLE pathogenesis, since they bind DNA- or RNA-containing antigens. Among these receptors, TLR7 recognizes single-stranded RNA, while TLR9 is considered very efficient in binding unmethylated CpG DNA, both of which are typical of viral genomic material [25].

The strategic location of nuclear-sensitive TLRs inside the cell usually minimizes accidental exposure to endogenous material, so intracellular TLRs are usually activated only by viral- or microbiological-derived DNA or RNA, in particular when they are conjugated with antibodies in the form of immune complexes (ICs).

A second cascade signal coming from an Fc receptor is required to amplify the immunological response. This mechanism is especially relevant in SLE, a condition in which autoantibodies to nuclear antigens are abundantly detected. Many different ICs can activate pDCs, but RNA-containing ICs are probably the best inducers of IFN-alpha secretion owing to the simultaneous recruitment of Fc receptors and intracytosolic TLRs. Both TLR7 and TLR9 efficiently stimulate the production of type I interferon from pDCs using adaptor molecules such as MyD88, an intracellular protein that is critical for IFN-alpha secretion. Increased circulating levels of endogenous DNA, RNA, and nuclear proteins have been observed in predisposed subjects. This apoptotic-derived material or nucleoma is able to activate the IFN-alpha system through TLR7 and TLR9 [26]. It has been also found that HMGB1-DNA compounds and immune complex-containing snRNA can directly activate TLR7 and TLR9 in pDCs in a manner similar to viral RNA or DNA.

The defective apoptotic clearance explains the gap between apoptosis, apoptotic cellular fragments containing nuclear material accumulation, and IFN-alpha production by pDCs [27].

Unlike myeloid dendritic cells (mDCs), pDCs efficiently recognize immune complex containing apoptotic material and are very efficient in producing large amounts of IFN-alpha in response to autoantigen recognition. Although any cell is able to produce type I IFN-alpha in response to certain viral stimuli, pDCs are undoubtedly considered the main producers of this type of cytokine, which indeed encompasses 13 different IFN-alpha isoforms as well as other IFNs. IFN-alpha determines the downstream activation of interferon regulatory factor 5, a transcription factor of pDCs, and the subsequent link to promoter regions and transcription of IFN-alpha target genes [28].

3.4.1 Modulation of IFN-I Signaling

The type I IFN family is characterized by several immunological functions including promotion of B-cell differentiation, immunoglobulin class switch, production of autoantibodies, and increase in activated B- and T-cell survival. IFN-alpha is endowed with pleiotropic effects to target cells. It activates monocytes, NK cells, cytotoxic CD8+, and CD4 Th1 and induces autoantibody production by B-cell potentiating antiviral response. Conversely, T^{regs} are usually suppressed by INF-alpha. IFN-gene signature has also been detected in several tissues obtained from SLE patients, such as glomerular, synovial, and cutaneous tissues suggesting a pathogenetic role of type I IFN family in almost all target organs in SLE [29]. Moreover, lupus-like syndrome is a very well-known complication of recombinant IFN-alpha therapy administered for chronic viral hepatitis or during cancer immunotherapy [30].

Under normal circumstances, IFN-alpha release is usually triggered by viral particles through a time-regulated process which is turned off when the infection resolves. This is not the case with SLE since IFN release is independent on viral stimulus [31].

3.4.2 NETosis

The possible role of neutrophils, the most abundant leukocytes in humans, has been recently suggested in the pathogenesis of SLE. Neutrophils are typically recruited to infection sites during the early phases of inflammatory response and are considered an effective defense against bacterial and fungal infections. They are able to kill pathogens through phagocytosis and release of highly reactive oxygen species or cytotoxic molecules contained in the cytoplasmic granules. Besides, another killing modality has recently been proposed. Neutrophil extracellular traps (NETs) are meshwork structures containing chromatin and peptides with antimicrobial activity, which are externally released from dying cells [32]. This specific form of neutrophil PCD, called NETosis, has been implicated in the pathogenesis of autoimmune diseases [33]. NETosis is a specialized form of cell death that occurs primarily in neutrophils, characterized by NETs' release. NETs comprise a mesh of DNA and histones, as well as the content of cytoplasmic granules and other mediators. Neutrophil-derived structures containing a significant amount of DNA and ribonucleoproteins could potentially stimulate pDCs (via TLR9) to produce significant amounts of IFN-alpha, similarly to apoptotic-derived nuclear material [34]. Interestingly, neutrophil hyperactivation and NET release have been recently linked to an increased risk of developing deep venous thrombosis in systemic vasculitis and other autoimmune diseases [35].

3.5 Adaptive or Acquired Immunity in SLE: Focus on T Cells

Both CD4+ or "helper" and CD8+ or "cytotoxic" T cells have been traditionally considered key players in SLE pathogenesis and inflammation.

CD4+ T^helper cells can be subdivided into Th1 and Th2, depending on the pattern of cytokine production and their immunological functions (mainly allergic reactions for Th2 and defense against infections for Th1). IL-12 is the main cytokine driving the differentiation of naïve CD4+ T cells into Th1 cells, which primarily produce IFN-gamma, IL-2, and TNF-alpha. On the other hand, IL-4, IL-5, and IL-13 cytokines produced by Th2 lymphocytes are involved in several T- and B-cell functions including proliferation, activation, and isotype switching.

Previous studies suggested that SLE was a Th2-driven disease since increased levels of IL-10 and IL-4 are usually detected in the lymphocytes isolated from SLE patients [36]. Subsequently, increased levels of both Th1 and Th2 cytokines have been described in humans and mice, underlying the complex heterogeneity of SLE that probably determines the diversity of lymphocyte subsets in the involvement of various organs.

Th1 lymphocytes are probably the key drivers of the inflammatory process in lupus nephritis (LN) [37]. Moreover, T-cell receptor (TCR) hyperactivation after interaction with the MHC-antigen complex has been reported in patients with SLE [38].

Th17 cells are a new subset of T lymphocytes that have been involved in the pathogenesis of a broad spectrum of autoimmune diseases, in particular rheumatoid arthritis, seronegative spondyloarthritis, and inflammatory bowel diseases [39]. They are generated after stimulation of naïve T cells with TGF-beta, IL-6, and IL-23. All these factors act together in preventing the switch of naïve T cells to a Th1 phenotype [40]. Interestingly, besides maintaining ongoing inflammation in target tissues, Th17 cells determine a concomitant downregulation of T^reg function and development [41]. Th17 cells and cytokines of the IL-17 family have also been shown to play a crucial role in SLE, and Th17 cells have been detected in the glomerular tissue of patients with active LN [42].

Recently, Savino et al. showed both in mice and in humans a possible role in SLE pathogenesis for Rai, a member of the Src homology 2 domain adapter family. Rai (−/−) mice develop a lupus-like phenotype with spontaneous activation of self-reactive lymphocytes. Moreover, it has been demonstrated that Rai (−/−) mice present Th1 and Th17 cell infiltrates in the kidneys, suggesting that Rai knockout mice (−/−) are more susceptible than normal mice to LN. Finally, a defect in Rai expression has been shown in T cells derived from SLE patients [43].

In summary, several studies on regulatory T cells showed their potential role in the breakdown of immune tolerance, since both quantitative and qualitative abnormalities of peripheral regulatory T lymphocytes (CD4+ CD25 + ^high) have been described in SLE [44, 45].

3.6 Adaptive or Acquired Immunity in SLE: Focus on B Cells

Considerable data has been collected regarding the function of B cells and their role in both inflammation and in autoimmune diseases [46].

B-lymphocyte involvement in SLE pathogenesis has traditionally been considered in the light of the production of circulating autoantibodies that are typical of

SLE and connective tissue diseases in a broad sense. Noteworthy, such autoantibodies, which are pathogenetic in most cases, are useful to clinicians in the diagnostic work-up and in follow-up [47]. B lymphocytes have been considered fundamental, because of the production of autoantibodies against soluble and cellular components, such as nuclear antigens. However, the role of B cells in autoimmune diseases has recently widely investigated. B lymphocytes are now considered important players of adaptive immunity in the complex chessboard of SLE pathogenesis. It is acknowledged that besides secreting autoantibodies, B lymphocytes efficiently present autoantigens and activate T cells. Therefore, they deeply influence T-cell function and activation [48].

B lymphocytes are classified into two main lineages: B1 and B2 cells. B1 lymphocytes are generated both in the bone marrow and in fetal liver. They are also thought to play a role in removing apoptotic material and debris by linking innate and adaptive immunity together. On the other hand, B2 cells are generated exclusively in the bone marrow, where autoreactive cells are first removed (central tolerance), and then undergo further selection in the spleen microenvironment (peripheral tolerance). After this initial step, B2 cells may follow two different paths. They can become mature follicular cells, migrating to the secondary lymphoid organs and waiting for T-cell-dependent activation, and then they ultimately evolve into plasma cells or memory B cells. Alternatively, B2 cells can colonize the marginal zone (MZ) of the spleen becoming MZ B2 cells, which, similarly to B1 cells, are able to respond to antigens regardless of T-cell help [49].

Although the role of MZ B cells in lupus is still controversial, they are probably involved in some autoimmune cellular responses, such as autoimmune thrombocytopenia, a condition for which splenectomy is usually beneficial [50]. An increased number of MZ B cells have been detected using the NZB/WF1 mouse model of SLE, suggesting an important role for these B lymphocytes in SLE pathogenesis [51]. Interestingly, IFN-alpha is a potent driver of MZ B-cell activation and an efficient enhancer of the co-stimulatory function, making the MZ B cell an important player in the autoantibody response to nuclear autoantigens in the context of pDC hyperactivation [52].

Lastly, B cells can produce important cytokines, such as IL-6 and TNF-alpha and IL-1, therefore contributing significantly to maintaining and amplifying the inflammatory process in SLE. Interestingly, and similar to T cells, BCR hyperactivation has also been described in the B lymphocytes of SLE patients, with increased phosphorylation of several signaling molecules and abnormal calcium influx after antigen recognition [53, 54].

Recently, a regulatory activity has also been described for a subset B lymphocytes. The term *regulatory B cells* or simply *Breg* has been used when referring to such cells [55]. The recently described $CD24^{high}CD27^{++}B$ population probably includes the large proportion of human B^{reg}. The main function of regulatory B cells is to produce IL-10, and currently the identification of this cytokine by intracellular staining is the preferred method for isolating B^{reg} [56]. The immunosuppressive properties of IL-10 have been described in animal models of collagen-induced arthritis and experimental autoimmune encephalitis. However, the role of IL-10 in

SLE is still controversial since both activating and immunosuppressive properties have been attributed to this cytokine.

Despite such premises, IL-10 is currently regarded mainly as an immunosuppressive cytokine, especially in SLE, and B^{reg} is probably one of the main sources [57].

Interestingly, after depletion of B cells using the anti-CD20 monoclonal antibody rituximab, the subsequent repopulation phase is probably constituted mainly of regulatory B cells, and this is especially true in patients who achieve good clinical response after rituximab [58]. However, further data are necessary to better clarify the role of B^{reg} cells and IL-10 in SLE pathogenesis.

In conclusion, as far as the role of lymphocytes in SLE pathogenesis is concerned, the *T-lymphocyte centric hypothesis* has recently been counterbalanced with a newer *B-lymphocyte centric theory*, which has been mainly supported by emerging data from the effects of B-cell target therapies [59].

References

1. Crow MK (2008) Collaboration, genetic associations and lupus erythematosus. N Engl J Med 358:956–961
2. Flesher DL, Sun X, Behrens TW, Graham RR, Criswell LA (2010) Recent advances in the genetics of systemic lupus erythematosus. Expert Rev Clin Immunol 6(3):461–479
3. Bowness P, Davies KA, Norsworthy PJ, Athanassiou P, Taylor-Wiedeman J, Borysiewicz LK, Meyer PA, Walport MJ (1994) Hereditary C1q deficiency and systemic lupus erythematosus. QJM 87(8):455–464
4. Kirou KA, Lee C, George S, Louca K, Peterson MG, Crow MK (2005) Activation of the interferon-alpha pathway identifies a subgroup of systemic lupus erythematosus patients with distinct serologic features and active disease. Arthritis Rheum 52(5):1491–1503
5. Baechler EC, Batliwalla FM, Karypis G, Gaffney PM, Ortmann WA, Espe KJ et al (2003) Interferon-inducible gene expression signature in peripheral blood cells of patients with severe lupus. Proc Natl Acad Sci U S A 100(5):2610–2615
6. Kirou KA, Lee C, George S, Louca K, Papagiannis IG, Peterson MG et al (2004) Coordinate overexpression of interferon-alpha induced genes in systemic lupus erythematosus. Arthritis Rheum 50(12):3958–3967
7. Li QZ et al (2010) Interferon signature gene expression is correlated with autoantibody profiles in patients with incomplete lupus syndromes. Clin Exp Immunol 159:281–291
8. Zhao S, Long H, Qiaanjin L (2010) Epigenetic perspectives in systemic lupus erythematosus: pathogenesis, biomarkers and therapeutic potentials. Clin Rev Allergy Immunol 39:3–9
9. Wen ZK, Xu W, Xu L, Cao QH, Wang Y, Chu YW, Xiong SD (2007) DNA hypomethylation is crucial for apoptotic DNA to induce systemic lupus erythematosus-like autoimmune disease in SLE-non-susceptible mice. Rheumatology (Oxford) 46:1796–1803
10. Stagakis E, Bertsias G, Verginis P, Nakou M, Hatziapostolou M, Kritikos H, Iliopoulos D, Boumpas DT (2011) Identification of novel microRNA signatures linked to human lupus disease activity and pathogenesis: mir-21 regulates aberrant T-cells response trough the regulation of PDCD4 expression. Ann Rheum Dis 70:1496–1506
11. Hudson CA, Cao L, Kasten-Jolly J, Kirkwood JN, Lawrence DA (2003) Susceptibility of lupus-prone NZM mouse strains to lead exacerbation of systemic lupus erythematosus symptoms. J Toxicol Environ Health A 66(10):895–918
12. Hughes GC, Clark EA (2007) Regulation of dendritic cells by female sex steroids: relevance to immunity and autoimmunity. Autoimmunity 40(6):470–481

13. Tayel SS, Helmy AA, Ahmed R, Esmat G, Hamdi N, Abdelaziz AI (2013) Progesterone suppresses interferon signaling by repressing TLR-7 and MxA expression in peripheral blood mononuclear cells of patients infected with hepatitis C virus. Arch Virol 158(8):1755–1764
14. Doria A, Canova M, Tonon M, Zen M, Rampudda E, Bassi N, Atzeni F, Zampieri S, Ghirardello A (2008) Infections as trigger and complications of systemic lupus erythematosus. Autoimmun Rev 8:24–28
15. Poole BD, Scofield RH, Harley JB, James JA (2006) Epstein–Barr virus and molecular mimicry in systemic lupus erythematosus. Autoimmunity 39:63–70
16. Werth VP (2007) Cutaneous lupus: insight into pathogenesis and disease classification. Bull NYU Hosp Jt Dis 65:200–204
17. Kuhn A, Wenzel J, Weyd H (2014) Photosensitivity, apoptosis, and cytokines in the pathogenesis of lupus erythematosus: a critical review. Clin Rev Allergy Immunol 47(2):148–162
18. Mathieu C (2011) Vitamin D and the immune system: getting it right. IBMS BoneKEy Rep 8:178–186
19. Beyer C, Pisetsky DS (2010) The role of microparticles in the pathogenesis of rheumatic diseases. Nat Rev Rheumatol 6:21–29
20. Muñoz LE et al (2010) The role of defective clearance of apoptotic cells in systemic autoimmunity. Nat Rev Rheumatol 6:280–289
21. Mevorach D, Trahtemberg U, Krispin A, Attalah M, Zazoun J, Tabib A, Grau A, Verbovetski-Reiner I (2010) What do we mean when we write "senescence", "apoptosis", "necrosis", or "clearance of dying cells"? Ann N Y Acad Sci 1209:1–9
22. Pisetsky DS, Erlandsson-Harris H, Andersson U (2008) High mobility group box protein 1 (HMGB1): an alarmin mediating the pathogenesis of rheumatic disease. Arthritis Res Ther 10:209
23. Rahman A, Isenberg DA (2008) Systemic lupus erythematosus. N Engl J Med 358(9):929–939
24. Fransen JH, van der Vlag J, Ruben J, Adema GJ, Berden JH, Hilbrands LB (2010) The role of dendritic cells in the pathogenesis of systemic lupus erythematosus. Arthritis Res Ther 12:207
25. Marshak-Rothstein A (2006) Toll-like receptors in systemic autoimmune disease. Nat Rev Immunol 6:823–835
26. Pisetsky DS, Ullal AJ (2010) The blood nucleome in the pathogenesis of SLE. Autoimmun Rev 10:35–37
27. Theofilopoulos AN et al (2010) Sensors of the innate immune system: their link to rheumatic diseases. Nat Rev Rheumatol 6:146–156
28. Ronnblom L, Alm GV, Eloranta ML (2011) The type I interferon system in the development of lupus. Semin Immunol 23:113–121
29. Nzeusseu Toukap A et al (2007) Identification of distinct gene expression profiles in the synovium of patients with systemic lupus erythematosus. Arthritis Rheum 56(5):1579–1588
30. Wilson LE et al (2002) Autoimmune disease complicating antiviral therapy for hepatitis C virus infection. Semin Arthritis Rheum 32(3):163–173
31. Ronnblom L, Elkon KB (2010) Cytokines as therapeutic targets in SLE. Nat Rev Rheumatol 6:339–347
32. Branzk N, Papayannopoulos V (2013) Molecular mechanisms regulating NETosis in infection and disease. Semin Immunopathol 35(4):513–530
33. Knight JS, Kaplan MJ (2012) Lupus neutrophils: 'NET' gain in understanding lupus pathogenesis. Curr Opin Rheumatol 24:441–450
34. Garcia-Romo GS et al (2011) Netting neutrophils are major inducers of type I IFN production in pediatric systemic lupus erythematosus. Sci Transl Med 3:73ra20
35. Tobias A et al (2012) Neutrophil Extracellular Trap (NET) impact on deep vein thrombosis. Arterioscler Thromb Vasc Biol 32:1777–1783
36. Funauchi M, Ikoma S, Enomoto H, Horiuchi A (1998) Decreased Th1-like and increased Th2-like cells in systemic lupus erythematosus. Scand J Rheumatol 27(3):219–224

37. Masutani K, Akahoshi M, Tsuruya K et al (2001) Predominance of Th1 immune response in diffuse proliferative lupus nephritis. Arthritis Rheum 44(9):2097–2106
38. Scheinecker C, Bonelli M, Smolen JS (2010) Pathogenetic aspects of systemic lupus erythematosus with an emphasis on regulatory T cells. J Autoimmun 35:269–275
39. Truchetet ME, Mossalayi MD, Boniface K (2013) IL-17 in the rheumatologist's line of sight. Biomed Res Int 2013:295132
40. Ghoreschi K et al (2011) T helper 17 cell heterogeneity and pathogenicity in autoimmune disease. Trends Immunol 32(9):395–401
41. Chen X, Oppenheim JJ (2014) Th17 cells and Tregs: unlikely allies. J Leukoc Biol 95(5):723–731
42. Nalbandian A, Crispı'n JC, Tsokos GC (2009) Interleukin-17 and systemic lupus erythematosus: current concepts. Clin Exp Immunol 157(2):209–215
43. Savino MT, Ulivieri C, Emmi G, Prisco D, De Falco G, Ortensi B, Beccastrini E, Emmi L, Pelicci G, D'Elios MM, Baldari CT (2013) The Shc family protein adaptor, Rai, acts as a negative regulator of Th17 and Th1 cell development. J Leukoc Biol 93(4):549–559
44. Valencia X, Yarboro C, Illei G, Lipsky PE (2007) Deficient CD4+ CD25 high T regulatory cell function in patients with active systemic lupus erythematosus. J Immunol 178:2579–2588
45. Bonelli M et al (2008) Quantitative and qualitative deficiencies of regulatory T cells in patients with systemic lupus erythematosus (SLE). Int Immunol 20:861–868
46. Crispín JC et al (2010) T cells as therapeutic targets in SLE. Nat Rev Rheumatol 6:317–325
47. Meroni PL, Biggioggero M, Pierangeli SS, Sheldon J, Zegers I, Borghi MO (2014) Standardization of autoantibody testing: a paradigm for serology in rheumatic diseases. Nat Rev Rheumatol 10(1):35–43
48. Grammer AC, Lipsky PE (2003) B cell abnormalities in systemic lupus erythematosus. Arthritis Res Ther 5:S22–S27
49. Dorner T, Radbruch A, Burmester GR (2009) B-cell directed therapies for autoimmune disease. Nat Rev Rheumatol 5(8):433–441
50. Lopes-Carvalho T, Kearney JF (2005) Marginal zone B cell physiology and disease. Curr Dir Autoimmun 8:91–123
51. Wither JE, Roy V, Brennan LA (2000) Activated B cells express increased levels of costimulatory molecules in young autoimmune NZB and (NZB 9 NZW)F(1) mice. Clin Immunol 94(1):51–63
52. Wang JH, Wu Q, Yang P, Li H, Li J, Mountz JD, Hsu HC (2011) Type I interferon-dependent CD86 (high) marginal zone precursor B cells are potent T cell costimulators in mice. Arthritis Rheum 63(4):1054–1064
53. Jenks SA, Sanz I (2009) Altered B cell receptor signaling in human systemic lupus erythematosus. Autoimmun Rev 8(3):209–213
54. Liossis SN, Kovacs B, Dennis G, Kammer GM, Tsokos GC (1996) B cells from patients with systemic lupus erythematosus display abnormal antigen receptor-mediated early signal transduction events. J Clin Invest 98(11):2549–2557
55. Goode I, Xu H, Ildstad ST (2014) Regulatory B cells: the new "it" cell. Transplant Proc 46(1):3–8
56. Iwata Y, Matsushita T, Horikawa M et al (2011) Characterization of a rare IL-10-competent B-cell subset in humans that parallels mouse regulatory B10 cells. Blood 117:530–541
57. Matsushita T, Horikawa M, Iwata Y, Tedder TF (2010) Regulatory B cells (B10 cells) and regulatory T cells have independent roles in controlling experimental autoimmune encephalomyelitis initiation and late-phase immunopathogenesis. J Immunol 185:2240–2252
58. Sanz I, Lee FE (2010) B cells as therapeutic targets in SLE. Nat Rev Rheumatol 6:326–337
59. Dörner T et al (2009) B-cell-directed therapies for autoimmune disease. Nat Rev Rheumatol 5:433–441

Systemic Lupus Erythematosus: Clinical Aspects

4

Savino Sciascia and Maria Josè Cuadrado

4.1 Introduction

Systemic lupus erythematosus (SLE) is a multisystem autoimmune disorder that results from a combination of genetic, environmental, and hormonal factors. The disease is characterized by a heterogeneous clinical presentation, a different course in different individuals, and a variability in the disease progression/fluctuations within the same patient.

Patients with SLE are mostly young women, adolescents, and some ethnic groups are more prone to a severe course of disease. The unpredictable and fluctuating flares of disease, the need for long-term treatment, and the side effects and damage caused by the disease itself severely reduce quality of life (QoL).

The clinical picture of SLE is extremely variable and may be related to disease activity, organ damage, drug toxicity, and quality of life. Assessment of patients with SLE in clinical practice relies upon the experience of the treating doctor and thus is subject to great variability between centers and between doctors. Several indices have been developed and validated to measure these parameters. Although there are some concerns about feasibility, the use of validated indices facilitates the collection of relevant data that otherwise may be overlooked. It is currently accepted

S. Sciascia
Center of Research of Immunopathology and Rare Diseases, Coordinating Center of the Network of Rare Diseases of Piedmont and Aosta Valley, Department of Rare, Immunologic, Hematologic and Immunohematologic Diseases, Giovanni Bosco Hospital, University of Turin, Piazza donatore di Sangue 3, Turin 10154, Italy

Lupus Research Unit, St. Thomas Hospital, Westminster Bridge, London Se17EH, UK
e-mail: savino.sciascia@unito.it

M.J. Cuadrado (✉)
Lupus Research Unit, St. Thomas Hospital, Westminster Bridge, London Se17EH, UK
e-mail: mjcuadrado@yahoo.com

D. Roccatello, L. Emmi (eds.), *Connective Tissue Disease: A Comprehensive Guide-Volume 1*, Rare Diseases of the Immune System 5,
DOI 10.1007/978-3-319-24535-5_4

that assessment of patients with SLE cannot be accomplished with a single index. Formal evaluation of three aspects of the disease, disease activity, disease damage, and patient-related quality of life is required.

No data are available in the literature to suggest an optimal frequency of clinical and laboratory assessment in patients with SLE. The European League Against Rheumatism (EULAR) made some recommendations for monitoring patients with SLE in clinical practice and in observational studies [1, 2]. The committee arbitrarily agreed on the need to assess patients with inactive disease, in the absence of organ damage and comorbidities, every 6–12 months. Patients with active disease should be assessed as often as necessary to evaluate the response to medication of clinical features as well as laboratory parameters.

Despite the heterogeneity of clinical presentation, a classification attempt can be done in order to establish some therapeutic approaches. Clinical features of SLE can be considered mild, moderate, or severe depending on the impact they can have in the patients' life.

This chapter aims to provide a critical overview on SLE clinical manifestations according to their severity. Specific features such as new insights into classification criteria and recent advances on cardiovascular risk, antiphospholipid syndrome, and QoL are also discussed.

4.2 Revised Classification Criteria

Recently, a major development has been the publication of the Systemic Lupus International Collaborating Clinics (SLICC) classification criteria [3]. This classification aimed to rationalize the clinical criteria and provided a modest expansion in recognized laboratory abnormalities (Table 4.1). One of the major differences when compared to the American College of Rheumatology Classification criteria is that biopsy-proven nephritis compatible with SLE in the presence of antinuclear or anti-double-stranded DNA antibodies in the absence of other lupus features is regarded as sufficient for a patient to be diagnosed as having SLE. The symptoms and laboratory abnormalities are cumulative and need not to be present concurrently.

4.3 Clinical Classification

4.3.1 Mild SLE

We can consider SLE mild when patients suffered with conditions that do not threaten their life and do not have a big impact in their health and quality of life. Mild skin involvement, arthralgia, fatigue, fibromyalgia, and mood disorders could be some of these symptoms. These manifestations are usually controlled with hydroxychloroquine. Skin and join involvements are discussed separately in this volume.

Table 4.1 Clinical and immunological criteria used in the Systemic Lupus International Collaborating Clinics (SLICC) classification system

Clinical criteria
1. Acute cutaneous lupus, including lupus malar rash, bullous lupus, toxic epidermal necrolysis variant of systemic lupus erythematosus, maculopapular lupus rash, photosensitive lupus rash, or subacute cutaneous lupus (psoriasiform or annular polycyclic lesions or both)
2. Chronic cutaneous lupus, including classic discoid rash (localized and generalized), hypertrophic lupus, lupus panniculitis, mucosal lupus, lupus erythematosus tumidus, chilblains lupus, and discoid lupus/lichen planus overlap
3. Oral ulcers or nasal ulcers
4. Non-scarring alopecia
5. Synovitis involving two or more joints and at least 30 min of morning stiffness
6. Serositis
7. Renal (urine protein-to-creatinine ratio [or 24-h urine protein]) representing 500 mg protein per 24-h or red blood cell casts
8. Neurological: seizures, psychosis, mononeuritis multiplex, myelitis, peripheral and cranial neuropathy, acute confusional state
9. Hemolytic anemia
10. Leukopenia (<4000 cells per μL at least once) or lymphopenia (<1000 cells per μL at least once)
11. Thrombocytopenia (<100,000 cells per μL) at least once
Immunological criteria
1. Antinuclear antibody concentration greater than laboratory reference range
2. Anti-double-stranded DNA antibody concentration greater than laboratory reference range (or twofold the reference range if tested by ELISA)
3. Anti-Sm: presence of antibody to Sm nuclear antigen
4. Antiphospholipid antibody positivity as determined by any of the following: positive test result for lupus anticoagulant, false-positive test result for rapid plasma reagin, medium-titer or high-titer anticardiolipin antibody concentration (IgA, IgG, or IgM), or positive test result for anti-2-glycoprotein I (IgA, IgG, or IgM)
5. Low complement C3, low C4, low CH50
6. Direct Coombs' test in the absence of hemolytic anemia

Fatigue is a common and often crippling symptom experienced by about 85–92 % of patients with SLE, with 50 % rating it as the most disabling symptom [4]. Indeed, it deeply impacts on QoL in SLE patients [5]. The pathophysiological mechanisms of SLE-related fatigue are probably multifactorial. Psychological domains such as mood disorders, poor sleep quality, anxiety, and chronic pain syndrome play a predominant role, and they have shown consistent associations with fatigue in SLE [6, 7]. Fatigue is usually poorly responsive to standard treatment for SLE and remains an unmet need. However, gentle exercise programs have been reported to have a positive impact on fatigue among SLE patients [8].

Fibromyalgia is a chronic pain disorder characterized by diffuse generalized pain, often associated with fatigue, anxiety, and sleep disturbances. The prevalence of fibromyalgia is much higher in autoimmune conditions to include SLE patients, when compared with the general population [9]. Fibromyalgia in SLE impacts QoL and correlates with psychosomatic and affective symptoms but not with disease activity or damage [9–11]. The widespread pain of concomitant fibromyalgia can represent a diagnostic challenge for the physician, leading to potential overtreatment if symptoms are mistaken for SLE disease activity.

Mood disturbances (mainly depression) are very common in patients with SLE [12, 13]. Depression may backside fatigue and cognitive dysfunction, contributing to a lower QoL in patients with SLE [14–16]. Although psychological effects of dealing with a chronic disease may contribute to the high prevalence of depression, disease-specific mechanisms probably can also play a significant role. Associations with specific antibodies and alterations in cerebral blood flow have been reported in depressed SLE patients [17, 18]. However, the data are not conclusive and depression in patients with SLE should be treated with conventional measures similar to the general population.

4.4 Moderate SLE

Previous symptoms if persists or are limiting patients' life in some way plus the presence of serositis, moderate lung involvement, and hematological involvement might be classified as moderate SLE. In details, moderate lung involvement includes pleuritis, abnormalities in diffusion as tested by diffusing capacity for carbon monoxide (DLCO), and mild fibrosis, while pulmonary hemorrhage and pulmonary hypertension severely impact on prognosis in patients with SLE. Similarly, from the cardiological perspective, patients with noncomplicated pericarditis and mild valve involvement may be classified as having moderate SLE; however, heart involvement can be life threatening when complicated pericarditis or myocarditis occurs.

4.4.1 Hematological Involvement

Hematological involvement is common in SLE and no specific treatment is necessary in mild asymptomatic cases, but close monitoring of cytopenia is warranted in most patients. Any significant changes in previous stable cell lineage parameters should be considered to be an indication of SLE flare and will need close investigation and monitoring. A detailed medical history for possible drug-induced myelosuppression should be part of the evaluation in order to identify all medications potentially interfering with bone marrow function.

There are various immune cytopenias associated with SLE. The most common is anemia. There are different etiologies for the anemia in SLE, to include chronic disease, renal insufficiency, hemorrhage, and drug-induced or autoimmune hemolysis. Red cell aplasia, aplastic anemia, and microangiopathic hemolytic anemia should be also mentioned.

Anemia of chronic disorder is the most common type of anemia in SLE, but autoimmune hemolytic anemia (AIHA) with high reticulocyte count is an SLE diagnostic criteria. Treatment of the anemia would be according to the cause. Glucocorticoids are the main treatment of AIHA, and about 96 % of patients have initial response to glucocorticoids, but rituximab, cyclosporine, IVIg, and cyclophosphamide have successfully been used in selective cases.

4.4.2 Leukopenia

Leukopenia is a well-known hematologic complication associated with SLE, and in majority of cases, no treatment is required. For classification purpose in SLE, leukopenia is defined as <4000/mm^3 on two or more occasions (according to the ACR and SLICC criteria). The pathogenic mechanisms of SLE itself, and several other factors to include immunosuppressive drugs, may contribute toward low white cell count in SLE patients. Leukopenia constitutes a paucity of granulocytes as well as lymphocytes, yet a greater absolute deficiency of granulocytes than lymphocytes is usually found [19].

Lymphopenia is common and T-cell lymphopenia is the most common type of lymphopenias, and absolute lymphopenia correlates with SLE activity and high DNA antibody titers. Lymphopenia per se can predispose to autoimmunity and can also be a consequence of disease activity in the setting of active SLE. Concomitant lymphopenia and thrombocytopenia are highly indicative of disease activity rather than as a cause for autoimmunity [19]. Lymphopenia is defined as $<1.5\times 109$ lymphocytes/L on two or more occasions according to current classification criteria. Low lymphocyte counts commonly occur in SLE with a prevalence ranging from 20 % to more than 90 % [19]. Lymphopenia is observed frequently in patients with active or severe disease [20, 21], and lymphocyte levels may fluctuate during the clinical course, irrespective of treatment [21].

Presence of lymphopenia may be clinically silent or associated with infections and/or active SLE. Data on the increased risk of infection are controversial and are complicated by the use of immunosuppressive therapies. Ethnicity may also play a role in explaining the heterogeneous results. However, glucocorticoids and immunosuppressive drugs may contribute to the lymphopenia in severe disease. In about 10 % of patients with SLE, lymphopenia can be quite striking with values $<0.5\times 109$/L. Lymphopenia usually occurs independently of neutropenia.

Neutropenia is usually defined as an absolute neutrophil count <1000 cells/mm^3. Although leukopenia occurs in about half of patients with SLE, WBC count <1000/mm is observed in about 15 % of the patients [22, 23]. The definition of a low WBC and/or low neutrophil count is complicated by the presence of benign ethnic neutropenia in many (25–50 %) persons of sub-Saharan African heritage [24]. In individuals with this condition, an abnormally low neutrophil count is not easily definable. Neutropenia is less common but may be associated with significant systemic infection when compared to lymphopenia. However, moderate/severe neutropenia (neutrophil count <1000/μL) is not a common hematologic finding in patients with SLE. Several mechanisms are responsible in inducing neutropenia, to include drug toxicity and disease activity.

4.4.3 Thrombocytopenia

Thrombocytopenia is a common and well-described manifestation of SLE directly related with morbidity and mortality. According to ACR classification criteria and the new SLICC criteria for SLE, the definition of thrombocytopenia is a platelet count <100,000/mm^3 (or 100 × 109/L) without any other identifiable cause. It is worth noting that distinguishing from thrombocytopenia as a result of pharmacological therapy may be especially difficult in patients with SLE. A careful examination of the peripheral blood smear looking for platelet aggregation and adherence to leukocytes may be helpful in recognizing pseudothrombocytopenia. Thrombocytopenia in patients with SLE can be thought of generally in two categories [25, 26]. One group of patients has thrombocytopenia as part of an SLE flare. In this setting, thrombocytopenia can be severe with the danger of life-threatening hemorrhage. The platelet count in these patients usually responds acutely to treatment with glucocorticoids. The other group of patients with SLE with low platelet count has a more chronic form that may present even when the disease is quiescent. In these patients, the glucocorticoid therapy may be less effective. However, they are also more likely to have only a modest decrease in the platelet count that may not require specific therapy.

There are growing evidences that thrombocytopenia in SLE is related to the presence of at least two types of autoantibodies, anti GPIIb/IIIa and anti-thrombopoietin receptor antibodies. Of importance of these two different autoantibodies is thrombocytopenia of patients with anti-thrombopoietin receptor antibody, which is less responsive to IVIg. It has been suggested that on the basis of presence of one of these autoantibodies or both, there are two different subsets of SLE patients with thrombocytopenia [26]. Corticosteroids are the first modality of treatment in SLE-associated thrombocytopenia, and about 20 % of patients have long-term remission. Intravenous pulse corticosteroid therapy is an alternative in unresponsive cases. Immunosuppressive drugs usually should be considered when initial treatment with steroids is not effective or if a dose higher that 10 m/daily of prednisone is required as maintenance therapy [27]. There are some emerging studies that show that rituximab and mycophenolate may be helpful in lupus-related thrombocytopenia.

4.5 Severe SLE

We can consider SLE severe when patients suffered with one or more major organ involvement potentially leading to life-threatening condition and/or having a big impact in their health and quality of life. Organ damage (due to both previous disease activity and/or drug toxicity) plays also a crucial role in this setting. Lupus nephritis (LN), neuropsychiatric SLE (NPSLE), cardiovascular involvement (myocarditis or events happening in the context of the antiphopsholipid syndrome (APS)), and infections are some of the conditions affecting patients with severe SLE. LN and NPSLE are discussed separately in this volume.

4.5.1 Lung Involvement

The involvement of the respiratory system is frequent, being pleuropulmonary manifestations present in almost half of the patients during the disease course. Pleurisy, coughing, and/or dyspnea are the most frequent symptoms. However, they are rarely the presenting symptoms of SLE. In some cases, however, abnormal pulmonary function tests (PFTs), including DLCO and/or abnormal chest radiographs, may present in asymptomatic patients. Pleuritis with or without pleural effusion and interstitial lung disease are usually mild to moderate symptoms in patients with SLE; conversely, lupus pneumonitis and alveolitis, pulmonary hemorrhage, pulmonary arterial hypertension, and pulmonary thromboembolic disease may severely impact on prognosis of patients with SLE as they can be life threatening. Complications due to secondary causes include pleuropulmonary manifestations of cardiac and renal failure, atelectasis due to diaphragmatic dysfunction, opportunistic pneumonia, and drug toxicity. The prevalence, clinical presentation, prognosis, and response to treatment vary, depending on the pattern of involvement. Pulmonary abnormalities usually do not correlate with makers of SLE activity (complement levels, or autoantibody levels such as anti-double-stranded DNA (dsDNA) and anti-Sm). Patients with SLE and lung involvement must always be evaluated for infection, particularly that due to bacteria or viruses. Given that many are immunocompromised, tuberculosis, fungal infections, and other opportunistic infections should also be considered.

4.5.2 Cardiac Involvement

Cardiac involvement is frequent in SLE, being as high as 50 % in some studies [28]. Any part of the heart can be affected, including the pericardium, myocardium, coronary arteries, valves, and the conduction system. In addition to pericarditis and myocarditis, a high incidence of CAD has become increasingly recognized as a cause of mortality.

In the past, cardiac manifestations were severe, often leading to death, and they were frequently found in postmortem examinations. Nowadays, thanks to early diagnosis, cardiac manifestations are often milder and asymptomatic, and they can be recognized by echocardiography and other noninvasive tests [29].

Pericarditis is a well-described cardiovascular manifestation of SLE, although often not evident clinically, and it is included in the ACR classification criteria for SLE. Pericarditis can be acute or chronic, and it appears more frequently at SLE onset or during SLE flares, although it can occur at any time of the disease [29]. Pericardial involvement usually occurs as an isolated attack or as recurrent episodes [30]. Clinical (symptomatic) pericarditis is estimated to occur in 25 % of SLE patients at some point in the course of their disease. Asymptomatic pericardial effusion is clearly more common than clinical pericarditis [31]. Coexistent pleurisy, effusion, or both are common [32]. Complications of pericarditis, such as cardiac tamponade, constrictive pericarditis, and purulent pericarditis, are rare.

Myocarditis is a potentially severe feature of myocardial involvement in SLE and myocardial involvement ranges from 3 % to 15 %, although it appears to be much more common in autopsy studies, suggesting the largely subclinical nature of lupus-associated myocarditis [33].

Signs and symptoms (including dyspnea, tachycardia, arrhythmias) do not differ from those of myocarditis due to other causes. A progression to ventricular dysfunction, dilated cardiomyopathy, and heart failure can occur. Cardiac enzymes may be normal and there are no typical findings on ECG.

Myocarditis is a potentially life-threatening condition and has to be treated immediately with high-dose steroids; in the most severe forms, it is necessary to use intravenous pulse corticosteroid followed by high oral doses. The addition of immunosuppressant such as azathioprine, cyclophosphamide, or intravenous immunoglobulines (IVIG) may be helpful in [34].

Heart valve abnormalities including vegetations and/or thickening are the most frequent cardiac manifestations of SLE, especially when associated to APS. These alterations were known as Libman–Sacks endocarditis, a verrucous endocarditis of valve leaflets, papillary muscles, and mural endocardium, originally described in SLE patients [28]. Valvular disease is usually mild and asymptomatic. Usually, less than 5 % of the patients with SLE, mainly those with antiphospholipid antibodies, develop valve disease severe enough to consider surgical treatment.

The valvular abnormalities resulting from Libman–Sacks lesions may predispose patients to bacterial endocarditis, so prophylactic antibiotics should be used for dental or surgical procedures with an increased risk of transient bacteremia.

4.5.3 Antiphospholipid Syndrome

APS can be an isolated disease or can be associated with SLE. It is characterized by recurrent venous or arterial thrombosis and/or pregnancy morbidity and persistent presence of antiphospholipid antibodies (aPL). Although 30–40 % of patients with lupus have aPL, the APS complicates only 10–15 % of cases of SLE. More than 40 aPL have been described so far, but only three are used currently for the confirmation of diagnosis [35]. Triple positivity for lupus anticoagulant, anticardiolipin antibodies, and anti-β2-glycoprotein 1 antibodies (at least one must be positive for the diagnosis of APS on two or more occasions 12 weeks apart) [36] has a strong association with the clinical symptoms of this syndrome.

APS has a broad range of clinical features, reflecting the site of thrombosis. The therapeutic approach to APS is mainly centered on modification of the general risk factors for thrombosis and use of antiplatelet and anticoagulant agents, notably heparin or warfarin [37]. However, the use of the new oral anticoagulants (namely, rivaroxaban, an inhibitor of factor Xa) is currently under investigation [38].

Statins are a very attractive addition to the drug regimen used for treatment of APS due to their anti-inflammatory/thrombotic effects [39].

4.6 Infection and Disease Activity

Infection is a common problem in SLE and is one of the main causes of mortality. Immunological dysfunction may play a critical role in the susceptibility to infections in patients with SLE [40]. Furthermore, immunosuppressive agents (mainly glucocorticoids) used in the treatment of moderate and severe lupus increase the risk of infections including opportunistic agents. Infections may mimic lupus flare, leading to confusion over the diagnosis and adequate treatment. It can be extremely difficult to distinguish between infection and disease exacerbation in some cases. Moreover, some infections may produce a systemic infection mimicking SLE, either superimposed or trigger a flare [41, 42].

Several studies evaluated characteristics of major infections in SLE patients requiring hospitalization [43–45]. According to these studies, acquired pneumonia, urinary tract infection, and vaginal infection are the most common infections in patients with SLE. Infections are usually attributed to the same pathogens as in the general population. Of note, some patients may develop tuberculosis. However, despite the pathogens often being the same as the general population, the clinical manifestations of the infections can be atypical, due to an abnormal immunological response or to ongoing treatment. Careful evaluation and timely collection of the specimens for bacterial culture are crucial to avoid misdiagnosis.

Viral, fungal, and protozoan infections can also occur. Rarely, multiple organisms can be detected [44].

In an outpatient setting, infections are usually non-life threatening and it has been reported that they are associated with disease activity only, independently of sociodemographic and therapeutic factors [42]. Infection in SLE can occasionally require hospitalization, especially when concomitant with a flare (mainly involving the kidney or central nervous system) or when therapy with steroids or immunosuppressive drugs is ongoing [46].

Infections are diagnosed by clinical features and positive cultures and/or response to antibiotic therapy. When cultures of bacterial isolates are negative or not available, diagnosis of infection relies on clinical findings, which can mimic a lupus flare. Physicians have to make treatment decisions based on clinical judgment as no laboratory parameters are totally reliable to distinguish between active disease and infection. In some patients, both situations can coexist making the diagnosis and therapeutic approach a real challenge.

References

1. Bertsias G, Ioannidis JP, Boletis J, Bombardieri S, Cervera R, Dostal C et al (2008) EULAR recommendations for the management of systemic lupus erythematosus. Report of a Task Force of the EULAR Standing Committee for International Clinical Studies Including Therapeutics. Ann Rheum Dis 67(2):195–205
2. Mosca M, Tani C, Aringer M, Bombardieri S, Boumpas D, Brey R et al (2010) European League Against Rheumatism recommendations for monitoring patients with systemic lupus erythematosus in clinical practice and in observational studies. Ann Rheum Dis 69(7):1269–1274

3. Petri M, Orbai AM, Alarcon GS, Gordon C, Merrill JT, Fortin PR et al (2012) Derivation and validation of the Systemic Lupus International Collaborating Clinics classification criteria for systemic lupus erythematosus. Arthritis Rheum 64(8):2677–2686
4. Zonana-Nacach A, Roseman JM, McGwin G Jr, Friedman AW, Baethge BA, Reveille JD et al (2000) Systemic lupus erythematosus in three ethnic groups. VI: factors associated with fatigue within 5 years of criteria diagnosis. LUMINA Study Group. LUpus in MInority populations: NAture vs nurture. Lupus 9(2):101–109
5. Pettersson S, Lovgren M, Eriksson LE, Moberg C, Svenungsson E, Gunnarsson I et al (2012) An exploration of patient-reported symptoms in systemic lupus erythematosus and the relationship to health-related quality of life. Scand J Rheumatol 41(5):383–390
6. Burgos PI, Alarcon GS, McGwin G Jr, Crews KQ, Reveille JD, Vila LM (2009) Disease activity and damage are not associated with increased levels of fatigue in systemic lupus erythematosus patients from a multiethnic cohort: LXVII. Arthritis Rheum 61(9):1179–1186
7. Jump RL, Robinson ME, Armstrong AE, Barnes EV, Kilbourn KM, Richards HB (2005) Fatigue in systemic lupus erythematosus: contributions of disease activity, pain, depression, and perceived social support. J Rheumatol 32(9):1699–1705
8. Tench CM, McCarthy J, McCurdie I, White PD, D'Cruz DP (2003) Fatigue in systemic lupus erythematosus: a randomized controlled trial of exercise. Rheumatology 42(9):1050–1054
9. Buskila D, Press J, Abu-Shakra M (2003) Fibromyalgia in systemic lupus erythematosus: prevalence and clinical implications. Clin Rev Allergy Immunol 25(1):25–28
10. Torrente-Segarra V, Carbonell-Abello J, Castro-Oreiro S, Manresa Dominguez JM (2010) Association between fibromyalgia and psychiatric disorders in systemic lupus erythematosus. Clin Exp Rheumatol 28(6 Suppl 63):S22–S26
11. Friedman AW, Tewi MB, Ahn C, McGwin G Jr, Fessler BJ, Bastian HM et al (2003) Systemic lupus erythematosus in three ethnic groups: XV. Prevalence and correlates of fibromyalgia. Lupus 12(4):274–279
12. Bachen EA, Chesney MA, Criswell LA (2009) Prevalence of mood and anxiety disorders in women with systemic lupus erythematosus. Arthritis Rheum 61(6):822–829
13. Meszaros ZS, Perl A, Faraone SV (2012) Psychiatric symptoms in systemic lupus erythematosus: a systematic review. J Clin Psychiatry 73(7):993–1001
14. Petri M, Naqibuddin M, Carson KA, Wallace DJ, Weisman MH, Holliday SL et al (2010) Depression and cognitive impairment in newly diagnosed systemic lupus erythematosus. J Rheumatol 37(10):2032–2038
15. Choi ST, Kang JI, Park IH, Lee YW, Song JS, Park YB et al (2012) Subscale analysis of quality of life in patients with systemic lupus erythematosus: association with depression, fatigue, disease activity and damage. Clin Exp Rheumatol 30(5):665–672
16. Moldovan I, Katsaros E, Carr FN, Cooray D, Torralba K, Shinada S et al (2011) The Patient Reported Outcomes in Lupus (PATROL) study: role of depression in health-related quality of life in a Southern California lupus cohort. Lupus 20(12):1285–1292
17. Lapteva L, Nowak M, Yarboro CH, Takada K, Roebuck-Spencer T, Weickert T et al (2006) Anti-N-methyl-D-aspartate receptor antibodies, cognitive dysfunction, and depression in systemic lupus erythematosus. Arthritis Rheum 54(8):2505–2514
18. Giovacchini G, Mosca M, Manca G, Della Porta M, Neri C, Bombardieri S et al (2010) Cerebral blood flow in depressed patients with systemic lupus erythematosus. J Rheumatol 37(9):1844–1851
19. Newman K, Owlia MB, El-Hemaidi I, Akhtari M (2013) Management of immune cytopenias in patients with systemic lupus erythematosus – old and new. Autoimmun Rev 12(7):784–791
20. Fayyaz A, Igoe A, Kurien BT, Danda D, James JA, Stafford HA et al (2015) Haematological manifestations of lupus. Lupus Sci Med 2(1):e000078
21. Rivero SJ, Diaz-Jouanen E, Alarcon-Segovia D (1978) Lymphopenia in systemic lupus erythematosus. Clinical, diagnostic, and prognostic significance. Arthritis Rheum 21(3):295–305
22. Harvey AM, Shulman LE, Tumulty PA, Conley CL, Schoenrich EH (1954) Systemic lupus erythematosus: review of the literature and clinical analysis of 138 cases. Medicine 33(4):291–437
23. Arenas M, Abad A, Valverde V, Ferriz P, Pascual R (1992) Selective inhibition of granulopoiesis with severe neutropenia in systemic lupus erythematosus. Arthritis Rheum 35(8):979–980

24. Haddy TB, Rana SR, Castro O (1999) Benign ethnic neutropenia: what is a normal absolute neutrophil count? J Lab Clin Med 133(1):15–22
25. He J, Guo JP, Ding Y, Li YN, Pan SS, Liu Y et al (2011) Diagnostic significance of measuring antibodies to cyclic type 3 muscarinic acetylcholine receptor peptides in primary Sjogren's syndrome. Rheumatology 50(5):879–884
26. Kuwana M, Kaburaki J, Okazaki Y, Miyazaki H, Ikeda Y (2006) Two types of autoantibody-mediated thrombocytopenia in patients with systemic lupus erythematosus. Rheumatology 45(7):851–854
27. Lurie DP, Kahaleh MB (1982) Pulse corticosteroid therapy for refractory thrombocytopenia in systemic lupus erythematosus. J Rheumatol 9(2):311–314
28. Tincani A, Biasini-Rebaioli C, Cattaneo R, Riboldi P (2005) Nonorgan specific autoantibodies and heart damage. Lupus 14(9):656–659
29. Sarzi-Puttini P, Atzeni F, Gerli R, Bartoloni E, Doria A, Barskova T et al (2010) Cardiac involvement in systemic rheumatic diseases: an update. Autoimmun Rev 9(12):849–852
30. Brigden W, Bywaters EG, Lessof MH, Ross IP (1960) The heart in systemic lupus erythematosus. Br Heart J 22:1–16
31. Kao AH, Manzi S (2002) How to manage patients with cardiopulmonary disease? Best Pract Res Clin Rheumatol 16(2):211–227
32. Godeau P, Guillevin L, Fechner J, Herreman G, Wechsler B (1981) Cardiac involvement in systemic lupus erythematosus. 103 cases (author's transl). Nouv Press Med 10(26):2175–2178
33. Tincani A, Rebaioli CB, Taglietti M, Shoenfeld Y (2006) Heart involvement in systemic lupus erythematosus, anti-phospholipid syndrome and neonatal lupus. Rheumatology 45(Suppl 4):iv8–iv13
34. Sherer Y, Levy Y, Shoenfeld Y (1999) Marked improvement of severe cardiac dysfunction after one course of intravenous immunoglobulin in a patient with systemic lupus erythematosus. Clin Rheumatol 18(3):238–240
35. Alessandri C, Conti F, Pendolino M, Mancini R, Valesini G (2011) New autoantigens in the antiphospholipid syndrome. Autoimmun Rev 10(10):609–616
36. Miyakis S, Lockshin MD, Atsumi T, Branch DW, Brey RL, Cervera R et al (2006) International consensus statement on an update of the classification criteria for definite antiphospholipid syndrome (APS). J Thromb Haemost: JTH 4(2):295–306
37. Ames PR, Antinolfi I, Scenna G, Gaeta G, Margaglione M, Margarita A (2009) Atherosclerosis in thrombotic primary antiphospholipid syndrome. J Thromb Haemost: JTH 7(4):537–542
38. Giles I, Khamashta M, D'Cruz D, Cohen H (2012) A new dawn of anticoagulation for patients with antiphospholipid syndrome? Lupus 21(12):1263–1265
39. Lopez-Pedrera C, Ruiz-Limon P, Aguirre MA, Rodriguez-Ariza A, Cuadrado MJ (2012) Potential use of statins in the treatment of antiphospholipid syndrome. Curr Rheumatol Rep 14(1):87–94
40. Mok CC, Kwok CL, Ho LY, Chan PT, Yip SF (2011) Life expectancy, standardized mortality ratios, and causes of death in six rheumatic diseases in Hong Kong, China. Arthritis Rheum 63(5):1182–1189
41. Souza DC, Santo AH, Sato EI (2012) Mortality profile related to systemic lupus erythematosus: a multiple cause-of-death analysis. J Rheumatol 39(3):496–503
42. Zonana-Nacach A, Camargo-Coronel A, Yanez P, Sanchez L, Jimenez-Balderas FJ, Fraga A (2001) Infections in outpatients with systemic lupus erythematosus: a prospective study. Lupus 10(7):505–510
43. Kang I, Park SH (2003) Infectious complications in SLE after immunosuppressive therapies. Curr Opin Rheumatol 15(5):528–534
44. Gladman DD, Hussain F, Ibanez D, Urowitz MB (2002) The nature and outcome of infection in systemic lupus erythematosus. Lupus 11(4):234–239
45. Pryor BD, Bologna SG, Kahl LE (1996) Risk factors for serious infection during treatment with cyclophosphamide and high-dose corticosteroids for systemic lupus erythematosus. Arthritis Rheum 39(9):1475–1482
46. Zandman-Goddard G, Shoenfeld Y (2005) Infections and SLE. Autoimmunity 38(7):473–485

Autoantibodies and Biomarkers: Diagnostic Aspects

5

Savino Sciascia and Maria Laura Bertolaccini

Autoantibodies, traditionally the hallmark of systemic lupus erythematosus (SLE), are typically present several years prior to diagnosis of SLE [1] and serve as markers for future disease development in otherwise normal individuals [2]. Autoantibodies frequently target intracellular antigens of the cell nucleus (double- and single-stranded DNA (dsDNA and ssDNA, respectively), histones, and extractable nuclear antigens (ENAs). These autoantibodies are usually polyclonal and heterogeneous in terms of isotype, affinity, and avidity. They have various specificities for SLE and might be produced nonspecifically as a result of polyclonal B-cell activation in other autoimmune conditions or during infections.

Autoantibody positivity is part of the 1982 American Rheumatism Association (ARA) [3] and the updated 1997 American College of Rheumatology [4] classification criteria for SLE.

The methods for detecting autoantibodies play a crucial role in the diagnosis of SLE, as the particular assay used remarkably influences the interpretation of the test. Gel precipitation assays, enzyme-linked immunosorbent assay (ELISA), *Crithidia luciliae* indirect immunofluorescence (CLIF), western blotting (WB) [5, 6], and the Farr immunoprecipitation assays are some of the common assays used in the detection of autoantibodies in lupus. All assays require careful validation to determine whether they perform adequately in detecting human autoantibodies.

An ideal diagnostic test should be sensitive (detects all those with SLE), specific (detects only those with SLE), and have high positive and negative predictive values. In addition, ideally, test results should reflect SLE disease activity, or predict

S. Savino (✉) • M.L. Bertolaccini
Center of Research of Immunopathology and Rare Diseases, Coordinating Center of the Network of Rare Diseases of Piedmont and Aosta Valley, Department of Rare, Immunologic, Hematologic and Immunohematologic Diseases, Giovanni Bosco Hospital, and University of Turin, Piazza del donatore di Sangue 3, Torino 10154, Italy
e-mail: savino.sciascia@unito.it

D. Roccatello, L. Emmi (eds.), *Connective Tissue Disease: A Comprehensive Guide-Volume 1*, Rare Diseases of the Immune System 5,
DOI 10.1007/978-3-319-24535-5_5

flare, thus allowing preemptive management. Currently, most of these tasks are not seen with any test.

Correct diagnosis requires an integration of the patient's symptoms, physical examination findings, and the results of multiple diagnostic testing.

In this chapter, we offer the reader an overview of the autoantibodies most commonly used in routine clinical practice.

5.1 Antinuclear Antibodies (ANA)

Antinuclear antibodies (ANA) are a diverse group of antibodies that target nuclear antigens. These antigens are present in all nucleated cells and have a role in transcription or translation, in the cell cycle, or as structural proteins. Most clinically relevant ANA are of the IgG subclass with the detection of IgM usually reducing the clinical utility of the test [7].

Nearly all patients with SLE have ANA while most ANA-positive individuals do not have SLE. The most common screening test is IIF on human epithelial (HEp-2) tissue [8], although IIF on rodent liver or ELISA tests are also available [9].

In brief, in the IIF ANA test, patient serum is placed on an HEp-2 cell slide. If ANA are present, the autoantibodies bind to the specific antigen in the nucleus of the cell. Subsequently, fluorescein-labeled antihuman IgG is added, and the cells are viewed under a microscope with ultraviolet light excitation.

In general, higher ANA titers are more meaningful, particularly in young patients. The precision and accuracy of the technique depends on several factors, including the assay configuration, the quality control procedures, and the experience of the reader [10].

5.1.1 Clinical Significance

Although ANA are very sensitive for SLE, positive ANAs are common, especially in elderly individuals [11, 12]. ANA positivity alone is not diagnostic for SLE as these antibodies have a low positive predictive value for SLE in unselected populations or when present in low titers. One in three healthy individuals have detectable ANA on HEp-2 cells at a screening dilution of 1/40, and 1 in 20 is positive at 1/160 [10]. Although a minority SLE patients were labeled as "ANA negative" [13] in the past, now this scenario is observed very rarely, and the absence of ANA at titers of 1/160 or less makes SLE very unlikely [7]. When a patient with high clinical suspicion for SLE is tested negative for ANA, ruling out the possibility of a technical artifact is mandatory (Fig. 5.1).

Drug-induced ANA is common and 10 % of SLE-like disease is drug induced and potentially reversible. Careful interpretation of the possible clinical relevance of an ANA in this context is needed.

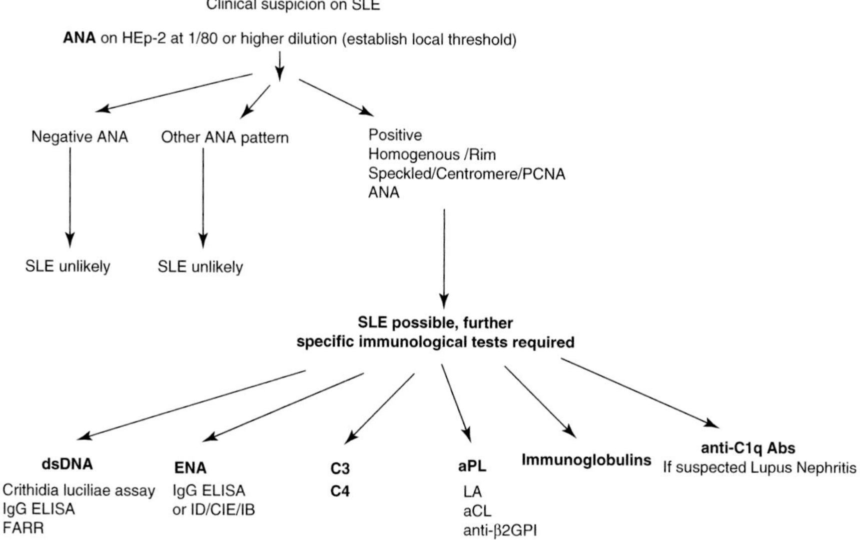

Fig. 5.1 Suggested diagnostic protocol for investigation of suspected SLE

Specific IIF patterns of ANA reflecting the types of antigens have been described. They include homogenous, speckled, rim, centromere, or nucleolar patterns. ANA showing an homogenous nuclear or a speckled nucleoplasmic staining pattern needs to be characterized further for specific individual antigens, known as extractable nuclear antigens or ENA (see ENA section below).

A nuclear homogeneous pattern is typically produced by anti-histone while anti-RNP, anti-Sm, anti-SS-A/Ro, and anti-SS-B/La most commonly produce a nuclear-speckled pattern. It is important to note that anti-SS-a/Ro and anti-SS-B/La can give a cytoplasmic or nucleolar pattern as well. Anti-dsDNA antibodies can give a rim pattern, also known as peripheral pattern, but this can also be an artifact. Anti-ribosomal P antibodies make a cytoplasmic pattern or a cytoplasmic and nucleolar pattern. Anti-centromere patterns are associated closely with Raynaud's phenomenon and limited scleroderma and are only seen when using Hep-2 as substrate for the assay.

In summary, when interpreting ANA test results, it would be useful to consider the following: (a) a positive IIF-ANA test result is virtually found in all SLE patients; (b) a positive IIF-ANA, especially at low titers (1:40 or 1:80) in the absence of clinical symptoms compatible with SLE is likely to be false positive; (c) SLE diagnosis can be made when IIF-ANA is positive at a reasonable titer always present within the appropriate clinical context (e.g., as swollen joints, pericarditis, or nephritis); and (d) other autoimmune conditions (i.e., Graves' disease or Hashimoto's thyroiditis) can cause a positive IIF-ANA. In addition, the false-positive rate increases with age.

5.2 Anti-DNA Antibodies

Anti-dsDNA antibodies are associated with SLE as a whole and more frequently within a specific clinical setting, such as nephritis. Indeed, the presence of anti-dsDNA and its titers has been correlated with SLE activity [14].

The best method for detecting anti-dsDNA is still a matter of debate. The most common used techniques are ELISA, *Crithidia luciliae* IIF (CLIF), and Farr immunoprecipitation assays.

Crithidia luciliae are hemoflagellates with a giant mitochondrion. The DNA in this mitochondrion, known as kinetoplast, serves as the substrate for the demonstration of antibodies to dsDNA by IIF [15].

The Farr assay is a quantitative radioimmuno method that detects high-avidity antibodies. The serum of the patient is mixed with isotope-labeled DNA. In presence of anti-DNA antibodies, the immune complex of immunoglobulin and the labeled DNA are detectable by precipitation with ammonium sulfate.

While the Farr assay shows the best correlation with disease activity and the highest specificity for SLE [10], both CLIF and Farr techniques have similar sensitivity. The IIF technique is easy to perform, does not require radiolabeled reagents, and permits to determine the Ig isotype of antibodies to DNA. In addition, IIF have be a minor rate of interference with antibodies to single-stranded DNA (ssDNA) when compared to Farr essays [10].

The anti-dsDNA ELISA is probably one of the most popular techniques for determining antibody reactivity toward dsDNA, since this assay system has proven high sensitivity and is easy to perform. However, this technique suffers from a poor specificity, and antibody reactivity toward dsDNA in an ELISA system should be confirmed in other anti-dsDNA assays [16].

5.2.1 Clinical Significance of Anti-dsDNA Antibodies

Anti-dsDNA are among the most specific antibodies in SLE. However, they are not particularly sensitive due to the fact that they may be present transiently, occurring in only half of the patients with SLE at some point in the course of their disease [10]. Anti-dsDNA autoantibodies can also be detected in other conditions, such as autoimmune hepatitis and infections, including syphilis, parasitic infections, and bacterial endocarditis. Increasing levels of anti-dsDNA antibody may herald lupus flares (e.g., lupus nephritis onset or exacerbations), and rises in anti-dsDNA may be used as clinical monitoring for relapse [17].

5.3 Antibodies to Extractable Nuclear Antigens (ENA)

Antibodies that produce speckled patterns in ANA IIF are commonly directed against extractable nuclear antigens (ENA) found in the cytoplasm of cultured human epithelial cells. Included in this group of ENA are ribonucleoproteins (RNP),

Smith (Sm), SS-A/Ro, SS-B/La, histidyl-sRNA synthetase (Jo-1), and topoisomerase (Scl70).

5.3.1 Anti-SS-A/Ro and SS-B/La Antibodies

Antibodies to SS-A/Ro and SS-B/La are frequently detected in connective tissue diseases, mainly SLE and Sjogren's syndrome (SS). ELISA or immunoblotting assays have replaced countercurrent immunoelectrophoresis assays for testing. Anti-60 kDa Ro occurs in 50 % of SLE patients, up to 90 % of SS and in about 60 % of patients with subcutaneous lupus. They have been associated with leucopenia (mainly neutropenia), lymphadenopathy, nephritis, and cutaneous manifestation [7]. These antibodies do not seem to fluctuate in time or with the activity of the disease [6].

While the role of anti-SS-A/Ro 60 kD and anti-SS-B/La antibodies in SLE pathogenesis remains controversial, neonatal lupus (NL) provides the strongest clinical evidence for a pathogenic role for these antibodies. NL is characterized by the presence of any combination of cytopenia, skin rash, cholestasis, or congenital heart block (CHB) occurring in children born to mothers positive for anti-SS-A/Ro antibodies. In anti-SS-A/Ro-positive pregnant women, the risk of developing CHB varies with the anti-SS-A/Ro specificity. CHB is associated with autoantibodies binding to Ro 52 kD antigen. These antibodies induce inflammation and fibrosis in fetal conduction tissues and lead to blockage of signal conduction at the atrioventricular node. Irreversible complete atrioventricular block is the main cardiac manifestation of CHB, although other severe cardiac complications, such as endocardial fibroelastosis or valvular insufficiency, even in the absence of cardiac block, have been reported [18].

5.3.2 Anti-Sm and Anti-RNP Antibodies

The presence of anti-Sm antibodies is considered pathognomonic of SLE and a criterion for the ACR classification for SLE [4]. However, low titer anti-Sm (by ELISA/immunoprecipitation assays) might also be detected in other autoimmune conditions [19].

The major targets are the so-called B and D polypeptides. Anti-Sm antibodies have been shown to be the most specific antibodies to lupus [20], and those reacting with synthetic SmD1-aa83-119 peptide are strongly associated with lupus nephritis [21]. Anti-Sm antibodies, although highly specific for SLE, do not correlate with disease activity.

Anti-RNP antibodies are associated with anti-Sm (virtually all anti-Sm sera are anti-nRNP positive [20]. Anti-Sm antibodies are highly specific, but relatively insensitive for SLE [22].

In SLE patients, myositis and Raynaud's phenomenon have been reported to be more strongly associated with antibodies to RNP rather than other clinical manifestations, such as lupus nephritis [23].

5.4 Anti-histone Antibodies

Up to 70 % of patients with SLE have IgG and/or IgM anti-histone antibodies (detected by immunoblotting or ELISA). Anti-histone antibodies may recognize total histones or some subfractions (H1, H2a, H2b, H3, and H4) as antigen. The clinical specificity is not well established for any subfraction. Anti-histone titers might reflect disease activity but are not specific for SLE. Anti-histone antibodies are found in 50–70 % of patients with SLE and in more than 95 % of patients with drug-induced lupus erythematosus. Nevertheless, their role in distinguishing between drug-induced SLE and idiopathic SLE is still under hot debate [24].

5.5 Anti-ribosomal P Antibodies

Anti-ribosomal antibodies target three ribosomal proteins (RP) P0, P1, and P2 (38, 19, and 17 kDa, respectively) located in the large ribosomal subunit. They have a high specificity for SLE and their association with other connective tissue diseases is only occasional [7]. It has been suggested that there is a preferential association of anti-RP with anti-Sm and/or anti-dsDNA antibodies, possibly due to partial cross-reactivity [25, 26]. Anti-RP antibodies have been associated with certain manifestations of neuropsychiatric SLE [26] (see section about NPSLE), but their predictive value is uncertain and available data controversial. Titers may rise in active SLE [27].

5.6 Anti-C1q Antibodies

The large number of different autoantibodies observed in SLE mostly target nuclear as well as cell surface antigens, but also serum molecules such as complement components. Among these, complement C1q is the most prominent target [28]. Complement C1q is the starter molecule of the classical pathway of the complement cascade and plays an important role in the clearance of immune complexes and apoptotic cell debris.

Anti-C1q antibodies are found in about 20–50 % of SLE patients. A number of cross-sectional studies on anti-C1q showed a significant association with renal involvement and general disease activity [29, 30], and these antibodies have been reported in up to 100 % of SLE patients with active proliferative lupus nephritis [31, 32]. Their value as a marker of disease activity in the follow-up of SLE patients has also been recently reported [33].

However, these findings are in contrast to other studies describing that anti-C1q antibodies were associated with SLE global disease activity but not specifically with active lupus nephritis [34].

5.7 Antiphospholipid Antibodies (aPL)

aPL are a family of immunoglobulins of IgG, IgM, IgA, or a combination of these isotypes, which were initially thought to recognize anionic phospholipids. Over the years, this concept has changed, and different specificities have been described for aPL. The presence of persistent aPL in a subject with recurrent arterial and venous thrombosis and/or pregnancy morbidity define the antiphospholipid syndrome (APS). Although initially described in patients with SLE, aPL were soon recognized to also occur in patients without any other underlying autoimmune disease.

aPL antibodies are present in 30–40 % of SLE patients, and 10–15 % of all SLE patients have clinical manifestations of APS.

aPL are detected by a variety of laboratory tests, the most useful for identifying SLE patients at higher risk for thrombosis or pregnancy morbidity being the lupus anticoagulant (LA) and the anticardiolipin antibody tests (aCL). These antibodies are distinct and separable immunoglobulins present alone or in combination [35].

5.7.1 The Lupus Anticoagulant (LA)

LA are heterogeneous aPL, which interfere with the phospholipid-dependent stages of blood coagulation in vitro and inhibit both the intrinsic and common pathways of coagulation [36]. LA has been reported in a wide variety of patient populations, ranging from autoimmune diseases (e.g., SLE, rheumatoid arthritis), drug exposure (e.g., chlorpromazine, procainamide, hydralazine), infections, and lymphoproliferative disorders to individuals with no apparent underlying disease [36]. The estimated prevalence in patients with SLE varies ranging from 6 to 65 % [37].

Their heterogeneous nature of the LA makes it necessary to perform more than one coagulation test to reach the diagnosis according to the classification criteria [38]. A number of features need to be demonstrated: (1) prolongation of a phospholipid-dependent clotting time, (2) evidence of inhibition shown by mixing studies, (3) evidence of phospholipid dependence, and (4) exclusion of specific inhibition of any one coagulation factor. In principle, the laboratory tests to detect the LA should use a sensitive screening test followed by a specific confirmation test [39]. The most commonly used is the activated partial thromboplastin time (aPTT), followed by the dilute Russell's viper venom time (dRVVT). The presence of LA should always be confirmed by performing the assays in the presence of excess of phospholipids, with a correction of the prolongation to normal times as a result [40]. In some subjects receiving oral anticoagulation, accurate detection of the LA might not be possible. In these particular cases, the kaolin cephalin time and the dRVVT performed on mixtures of control and patient plasmas or the Taipan and Textarin times might be useful [39].

In general, positive LA tests are more specific for the APS, whereas aCL antibodies are more sensitive.

5.7.2 Anticardiolipin Antibodies (aCL)

In 1983, Harris et al. developed a solid-phase radioimmunoassay to detect aCL using cardiolipin as antigen [41]. This assay proved to be more sensitive than the classical VDRL in detecting aPL. The specificity of aCL for APS increases with the titer and is higher for the IgG than for the IgM isotype. However, some patients may have only a positive IgM test, and a few are only IgA positive. However, in addition to detecting aCL, this assay also detects antibodies to serum or plasma proteins that bind to cardiolipin coated to the plate [42], in particular, antibodies to β2-glycoprotein I (anti-β2GPI).

Differences in the methods used to detect aPL have undoubtedly contributed to the wide range of reported frequencies. The prevalence of aCL in the normal population is low but measurable, between 2 and 4 % (depending on the assays applied). They are more common in elderly individuals. The estimated prevalence in patients with SLE varies ranging from around 20 % [43, 44] to 60 % [45–47]. In a meta-analysis of 21 studies [48], an average prevalence of 44 % for aCL was documented in patients with SLE, which may reflect the true occurrence. Despite several attempts, standardization of aCL testing is still much needed, and the availability of reference sera has greatly improved interlaboratory testing and quantification of aCL [35]. IgA aCL reference sera are now also available. Many clinical laboratories currently measure all three isotypes, and sensitive kits for this purpose are commercially available. While the pathogenic importance of IgG and IgM aCL is well established, the role of IgA aCL as an independent risk factor for thrombosis has not been clearly demonstrated [49].

5.7.3 Anti-β2-glycoprotein I Antibody

The observation that many aCL are directed to an epitope on β2GPI led to the development of the anti-β2GPI antibody (ab2GPI) immunoassay [50]. Anti-β2GPI antibodies are strongly associated with thrombosis and other features of the APS [51].

It is now well accepted that patients showing triple positivity for LA, aCL, and aβ2GPI are at the highest risk of thrombosis [52, 53]. However, in some patients with clinical features of APS, aβ2GPI antibodies are rarely the sole antibodies detected (ref).

5.7.4 Other aPL

The clinical utility of aPL assays for autoantibodies to phospholipids other than cardiolipin and to phospholipid-binding proteins other than β2GPI (i.e., prothrombin) is now under debate [54].

Antibodies to prothrombin can be detected by directly coating prothrombin on irradiated ELISA plates (aPT) or by using the phosphatidylserine/prothrombin complex as antigen (aPS/PT). They have been both related with the clinical manifestation of APS, and current evidence supports the concept that they belong to distinct populations of autoantibodies. Nevertheless, they can both be detected simultaneously in one patient [55].

aPS/PT (rather than aPT) have been shown to be helpful in the diagnosis of APS [56] and when assessing the associated risk for thrombosis or pregnancy morbidity [52].

5.7.5 aPL as Risk Factors

Recent evidence supports the concept that aPL antibody positivity in multiple tests is associated with an increase risk of thrombosis or pregnancy morbidity, both in SLE or in patients without any other underling connective tissue disease [52, 53]. As a consequence, the determination of antibody profiles and subclassification of patients, according to the number and the type of positive tests, are encouraged. Switching from the concept of aPL as diagnostic antibodies to aPL as risk factors for clinical events has enriched the clinical workup highlighting the need for assessing the risk linked to aPL.

5.8 Neuropsychiatric SLE (NPSLE) and Autoantibodies

NPSLE is one of the most important manifestations of SLE, and it includes a variety of focal or diffuse, central or peripheral, psychiatric, isolated, complex, simultaneous, and/or sequential symptoms and signs, representing both active and inactive disease states. Central nervous system disease predominates and may take the form of either diffuse (e.g., psychosis or depression) or focal disease (e.g., stroke or transverse myelitis) [57]. Available studies on the significance of different autoantibodies in NPSLE have shown controversial results [58]. The multitude of clinical manifestations related to NPSLE makes very unlikely that a single biomarker could reliably be associated with all neuropsychiatric events. We recently provided evidence that aPL, mainly LA, and anti-ribosomal P antibodies are significantly associated with specific manifestations of neuropsychiatric disease attributed to SLE, namely, cerebrovascular events and psychosis, respectively.

5.9 Lupus Nephritis

Lupus nephritis, which occurs in up to 50 % of all SLE patients [59], is a common and severe complication and considered to be a major cause of morbidity and mortality in SLE patients.

Most lupus nephritis patients have antichromatin/nucleosome antibodies (specificity 98 %; sensitivity 69 %) [60], and they may be positive when the anti-dsDNA antibodies are negative [61]. Similar findings were observed with anti-C1q antibodies [29], especially with nephritic flares (negative positive predictive value of 97–100 %) [31, 62], although their precise role has been debated.

Other specificities (e.g., anti-α actinin antibodies) have been described in patients with active lupus nephritis, and they may be more predictive of nephritis than anti-dsDNA antibodies, although larger studies are needed for confirmation [7]. Anti-Sc-70 (topoisomerase) antibodies have provided mixed results as well [7].

Conclusion

ANA IIF is an effective screening assay in patients with clinical features of SLE. False-positive results are common. The clinical importance cannot be extrapolated from the ANA titer or pattern, although higher titers (>1/160) are more likely to be important. HEp-2 cells are the most sensitive substrate for ANA detection, but this must be balanced against an increased incidence of insignificant positivity.

ANA-positive samples should be subjected to more specific assays for the diagnosis of SLE. A combination of ENA (Ro/La/Sm/RNP) and dsDNA assays will detect most patients with SLE.

A combination of anti-dsDNA, C3, C4, CRP, and ESR assays provides the most useful clinical information about SLE flares.

An appropriate management from both diagnostic and follow-up perspectives requires an integration of a patient's symptoms, physical examination findings, and the results of diagnostic multiple testing.

References

1. Arbuckle MR, McClain MT, Rubertone MV, Scofield RH, Dennis GJ, James JA et al (2003) Development of autoantibodies before the clinical onset of systemic lupus erythematosus. N Engl J Med 349(16):1526–1533
2. Scofield RH (2004) Autoantibodies as predictors of disease. Lancet 363(9420):1544–1546
3. Tan EM, Cohen AS, Fries JF, Masi AT, McShane DJ, Rothfield NF et al (1982) The 1982 revised criteria for the classification of systemic lupus erythematosus. Arthritis Rheum 25(11):1271–1277
4. Hochberg MC (1997) Updating the American College of Rheumatology revised criteria for the classification of systemic lupus erythematosus. Arthritis Rheum 40(9):1725
5. Kurien BT, Scofield RH (2003) Protein blotting: a review. J Immunol Methods 274(1–2):1–15
6. Kurien BT, Scofield RH (2006) Western blotting. Methods 38(4):283–293
7. Egner W (2000) The use of laboratory tests in the diagnosis of SLE. J Clin Pathol 53(6):424–432
8. van Venrooij WJ, Charles P, Maini RN (1991) The consensus workshops for the detection of autoantibodies to intracellular antigens in rheumatic diseases. J Immunol Methods 140(2):181–189
9. Yamamoto H, Sekiguchi T, Itagaki K, Saijo S, Iwakura Y (1993) Inflammatory polyarthritis in mice transgenic for human T cell leukemia virus type I. Arthritis Rheum 36(11):1612–1620
10. Kurien BT, Scofield RH (2006) Autoantibody determination in the diagnosis of systemic lupus erythematosus. Scand J Immunol 64(3):227–235
11. Emlen W, O'Neill L (1997) Clinical significance of antinuclear antibodies: comparison of detection with immunofluorescence and enzyme-linked immunosorbent assays. Arthritis Rheum 40(9):1612–1618

12. Froelich CJ, Wallman J, Skosey JL, Teodorescu M (1990) Clinical value of an integrated ELISA system for the detection of 6 autoantibodies (ssDNA, dsDNA, Sm, RNP/Sm, SSA, and SSB). J Rheumatol 17(2):192–200
13. Bohan A (1979) Seronegative systemic lupus erythematosus. J Rheumatol 6(5):534–540
14. Schur PH, Sandson J (1968) Immunologic factors and clinical activity in systemic lupus erythematosus. N Engl J Med 278(10):533–538
15. Aarden LA, de Groot ER, Feltkamp TE (1975) Immunology of DNA. III. Crithidia luciliae, a simple substrate for the determination of anti-dsDNA with the immunofluorescence technique. Ann N Y Acad Sci 254:505–515
16. Brinkman K, Termaat R, Van den Brink H, Berden J, Smeenk R (1991) The specificity of the anti-dsDNA ELISA. A closer look. J Immunol Methods 139(1):91–100
17. Pan N, Amigues I, Lyman S, Duculan R, Aziz F, Crow MK et al (2014) A surge in anti-dsDNA titer predicts a severe lupus flare within six months. Lupus 23(3):293–298
18. Brito-Zeron P, Izmirly PM, Ramos-Casals M, Buyon JP, Khamashta MA (2015) The clinical spectrum of autoimmune congenital heart block. Nat Rev Rheumatol 11(5):301–312
19. Maddison PJ, Skinner RP, Vlachoyiannopoulos P, Brennand DM, Hough D (1985) Antibodies to nRNP, Sm, Ro(SSA) and La(SSB) detected by ELISA: their specificity and inter-relations in connective tissue disease sera. Clin Exp Immunol 62(2):337–345
20. Hoch SO, Eisenberg RA, Sharp GC (1999) Diverse antibody recognition patterns of the multiple Sm-D antigen polypeptides. Clin Immunol 92(2):203–208
21. Jaekel HP, Klopsch T, Benkenstein B, Grobe N, Baldauf A, Schoessler W et al (2001) Reactivities to the Sm autoantigenic complex and the synthetic SmD1-aa83-119 peptide in systemic lupus erythematosus and other autoimmune diseases. J Autoimmun 17(4):347–354
22. Lyons R, Narain S, Nichols C, Satoh M, Reeves WH (2005) Effective use of autoantibody tests in the diagnosis of systemic autoimmune disease. Ann N Y Acad Sci 1050:217–228
23. Sawalha AH, Harley JB (2004) Antinuclear autoantibodies in systemic lupus erythematosus. Curr Opin Rheumatol 16(5):534–540
24. Xiao X, Chang C (2014) Diagnosis and classification of drug-induced autoimmunity (DIA). J Autoimmun 48–49:66–72
25. Gerli R, Caponi L (2005) Anti-ribosomal P protein antibodies. Autoimmunity 38(1):85–92
26. Sciascia S, Bertolaccini ML, Roccatello D, Khamashta MA, Sanna G (2014) Autoantibodies involved in neuropsychiatric manifestations associated with systemic lupus erythematosus: a systematic review. J Neurol 261(9):1706–1714
27. Sato T, Uchiumi T, Ozawa T, Kikuchi M, Nakano M, Kominami R et al (1991) Autoantibodies against ribosomal proteins found with high frequency in patients with systemic lupus erythematosus with active disease. J Rheumatol 18(11):1681–1684
28. Giles I, Putterman C (2008) Autoantibodies and other biomarkers – pathological consequences (1). Lupus 17(3):241–246
29. Marto N, Bertolaccini ML, Calabuig E, Hughes GR, Khamashta MA (2005) Anti-C1q antibodies in nephritis: correlation between titres and renal disease activity and positive predictive value in systemic lupus erythematosus. Ann Rheum Dis 64(3):444–448
30. Siegert C, Daha M, Westedt ML, van der Voort E, Breedveld F (1991) IgG autoantibodies against C1q are correlated with nephritis, hypocomplementemia, and dsDNA antibodies in systemic lupus erythematosus. J Rheumatol 18(2):230–234
31. Trendelenburg M, Lopez-Trascasa M, Potlukova E, Moll S, Regenass S, Fremeaux-Bacchi V et al (2006) High prevalence of anti-C1q antibodies in biopsy-proven active lupus nephritis. Nephrol Dial Transplant Off Publ Eur Dial Transplant Assoc Eur Renal Assoc 21(11):3115–3121
32. Trendelenburg M, Marfurt J, Gerber I, Tyndall A, Schifferli JA (1999) Lack of occurrence of severe lupus nephritis among anti-C1q autoantibody-negative patients. Arthritis Rheum 42(1):187–188
33. Bock M, Heijnen I, Trendelenburg M (2015) Anti-C1q antibodies as a follow-up marker in SLE patients. PLoS One 10(4):e0123572

34. Katsumata Y, Miyake K, Kawaguchi Y, Okamoto Y, Kawamoto M, Gono T et al (2011) Anti-C1q antibodies are associated with systemic lupus erythematosus global activity but not specifically with nephritis: a controlled study of 126 consecutive patients. Arthritis Rheum 63(8):2436–2444
35. Bertolaccini ML, Amengual O, Andreoli L, Atsumi T, Chighizola CB, Forastiero R et al (2014) 14th International Congress on Antiphospholipid Antibodies Task Force. Report on antiphospholipid syndrome laboratory diagnostics and trends. Autoimmun Rev 13(9):917–930
36. Court E (1997) Lupus anticoagulants: pathogenesis and laboratory diagnosis. Br J Biomed Sci 54:287–298
37. Worrall JG, Snaith ML, Batchelor JR, Isenberg DA (1990) SLE: a rheumatologic view. Analysis of the clinical features, serology, and immunogenetics in 100 SLE patients during long-term follow-up. Q J Med 74:319–330
38. Brandt JT, Triplett DA, Alving B, Scharrer I (1995) Criteria for the diagnosis of lupus anticoagulants: an update. On behalf of the Subcommittee on Lupus anticoagulant/Antiphospholipid Antibody of the Scientific and Standardisation Committee of the ISTH. Thromb Haemost 74:1185–1190
39. Greaves M, Cohen H, MacHin SJ, Mackie I (2000) Guidelines on the investigation and management of the antiphospholipid syndrome. Br J Haematol 109(4):704–715
40. Urbanus RT, Derksen RH, de Groot PG (2008) Current insight into diagnostics and pathophysiology of the antiphospolipid syndrome. Blood Rev 22:93–105
41. Harris EN, Gharavi AE, Boey ML, Patel BM, Mackworth-Young CG, Loizou S et al (1983) Anticardiolipin antibodies: detection by radioimmunoassay and association with thrombosis in systemic lupus erythematosus. Lancet ii(8361):1211–1214
42. Roubey RA (1994) Autoantibodies to phospholipid-binding plasma proteins: a new view of lupus anticoagulants and other antiphospholipid autoantibodies. Blood 84(9):2854–2867
43. Loizou S, McCrea JD, Rudge AC, Reynolds R, Boyle CC, Harris EN (1985) Measurement of anti-cardiolipin antibodies by an enzyme-linked immunosorbent assay (ELISA): standardization and quantitation of results. Clin Exp Immunol 62(3):738–745
44. Manoussakis MN, Gharavi AE, Drosos AA, Kitridou RC, Moutsopoulos HM (1987) Anticardiolipin antibodies in unselected autoimmune rheumatic disease patients. Clin Immunol Immunopathol 44(3):297–307
45. Weidmann CE, Wallace DJ, Peter JB, Knight PJ, Bear MB, Klinenberg JR (1988) Studies of IgG, IgM and IgA antiphospholipid antibody isotypes in systemic lupus erythematosus. J Rheumatol 15(1):74–79
46. Meyer O, Cyna L, Bourgeois P, Kahn MF, Ryckewaert A (1987) Profile and cross-reactivities of antiphospholipid antibodies in systemic lupus erythematosus and syphilis. Clin Rheumatol 6(3):369–377
47. Nahass GT (1997) Antiphospholipid antibodies and the antiphospholipid antibody syndrome. J Am Acad Dermatol 36(2 Pt 1):149–168; quiz 69–72
48. Love PE, Santoro SA (1990) Antiphospholipid antibodies: anticardiolipin and the lupus anticoagulant in systemic lupus erythematosus (SLE) and in non-SLE disorders. Prevalence and clinical significance. Ann Intern Med 112(9):682–698
49. Meijide H, Sciascia S, Sanna G, Khamashta MA, Bertolaccini ML (2013) The clinical relevance of IgA anticardiolipin and IgA anti-beta2 glycoprotein I antiphospholipid antibodies: a systematic review. Autoimmun Rev 12(3):421–425
50. Matsuura E, Igarashi Y, Yasuda T, Triplett DA, Koike T (1994) Anticardiolipin antibodies recognize beta 2-glycoprotein I structure altered by interacting with an oxygen modified solid phase surface. J Exp Med 179(2):457–462
51. Amengual O, Atsumi T, Khamashta MA, Koike T, Hughes GRV (1996) Specificity of ELISA for antibody to beta 2-glycoprotein I in patients with antiphospholipid syndrome. Br J Rheumatol 35(12):1239–1243

52. Sciascia S, Murru V, Sanna G, Roccatello D, Khamashta MA, Bertolaccini ML (2012) Clinical accuracy for diagnosis of antiphospholipid syndrome in systemic lupus erythematosus: evaluation of 23 possible combinations of antiphospholipid antibody specificities. J Thromb Haemost JTH 10(12):2512–2518
53. Pengo V, Ruffatti A, Legnani C, Gresele P, Barcellona D, Erba N et al (2010) Clinical course of high-risk patients diagnosed with antiphospholipid syndrome. J Thromb Haemost JTH 8(2):237–242
54. Giannakopoulos B, Krilis SA (2013) The pathogenesis of the antiphospholipid syndrome. N Engl J Med 368(11):1033–1044
55. Sciascia S, Bertolaccini ML (2014) Antibodies to phosphatidylserine/prothrombin complex and the antiphospholipid syndrome. Lupus 23(12):1309–1312
56. Sciascia S, Sanna G, Murru V, Roccatello D, Khamashta MA, Bertolaccini ML (2014) Anti-prothrombin (aPT) and anti-phosphatidylserine/prothrombin (aPS/PT) antibodies and the risk of thrombosis in the antiphospholipid syndrome. A systematic review. Thromb Haemost 111(2):354–364
57. Sciascia S, Bertolaccini ML, Baldovino S, Roccatello D, Khamashta MA, Sanna G (2013) Central nervous system involvement in systemic lupus erythematosus: overview on classification criteria. Autoimmun Rev 12(3):426–429
58. Greenwood DL, Gitlits VM, Alderuccio F, Sentry JW, Toh BH (2002) Autoantibodies in neuropsychiatric lupus. Autoimmunity 35(2):79–86
59. Cameron JS (1999) Lupus nephritis. J Am Soc Nephrol JASN 10(2):413–424
60. Cervera R, Vinas O, Ramos-Casals M, Font J, Garcia-Carrasco M, Siso A et al (2003) Anti-chromatin antibodies in systemic lupus erythematosus: a useful marker for lupus nephropathy. Ann Rheum Dis 62(5):431–434
61. Simon JA, Cabiedes J, Ortiz E, Alcocer-Varela J, Sanchez-Guerrero J (2004) Anti-nucleosome antibodies in patients with systemic lupus erythematosus of recent onset. Potential utility as a diagnostic tool and disease activity marker. Rheumatology 43(2):220–224
62. Moroni G, Trendelenburg M, Del Papa N, Quaglini S, Raschi E, Panzeri P et al (2001) Anti-C1q antibodies may help in diagnosing a renal flare in lupus nephritis. Am J Kidney Dis Off J Natl Kidney Found 37(3):490–498

Joint Involvement in Systemic Lupus Erythematosus

6

Daniela Rossi, Vittorio Modena, G. Bianchi,
Raffaele Pellerito, and Dario Roccatello

Systemic lupus erythematosus (SLE) is a chronic immune-mediated disease affecting multiple organs including skin, brain, peripheral nervous system, heart, gastrointestinal tract, kidney, and, almost invariably, joints. Clinical features in individual patients are highly variable, and arthritis and arthralgias in SLE deserve to be specifically addressed.

D. Rossi • V. Modena (✉)
CMID – Center of Research of Immunopathology and Rare Diseases, Coordinating Center of the Network of Rare Diseases of Piedmont and Aosta Valley, Department of Rare, Immunologic, Hematologic and Immunohematologic Diseases, Giovanni Bosco Hospital, University of Turin, Turin 10154, Italy
e-mail: daniela.rossi@unito.it; modenavittorio@libero.it

G. Bianchi
Division of Rheumatology, Department of Locomotor System, ASL3 Genovese, Genoa, Italy

R. Pellerito
Department of Rheumatology, Mauriziano Hospital, Turin 10128, Italy

D. Roccatello
CMID – Center of Research of Immunopathology and Rare Diseases, Coordinating Center of the Network of Rare Diseases of Piedmont and Aosta Valley, Department of Rare, Immunologic, Hematologic and Immunohematologic Diseases, Giovanni Bosco Hospital, and University of Turin, Turin 10154, Italy

SCDU Nephrology and Dialysis, Giovanni Bosco Hospital, and University of Turin, Turin, Italy
e-mail: dario.roccatello@unito.it

D. Roccatello, L. Emmi (eds.), *Connective Tissue Disease: A Comprehensive Guide-Volume 1*, Rare Diseases of the Immune System 5,
DOI 10.1007/978-3-319-24535-5_6

6.1 Arthritis and Arthralgias in SLE

Articular involvement is very frequent in SLE. In 34–50 % of patients with SLE, joint involvement is the first manifestation of the disease, whereas during the course of SLE, it is almost always present [1–4]. Joint involvement occurs more frequently in women, both at onset and during the course of the disease [5–7]. It is polymorphous and shows varying degrees of clinical severity, with increasing frequency depending on age at SLE onset, and it is more frequent in patients with onset of illness in adulthood [8, 9]. It represents one of the most frequent causes of difficulties in daily activities, job reduction, and abandonment [10–12].

Articular signs, such as arthralgia or arthritis, may be observed in the course of SLE. Arthralgia, which is defined as the presence of joint pain in the absence of clear synovitis, erosion, or deformities, is very frequent both at the onset and during the course of the disease [13]. Arthralgia is persistent, migrant, transient, and frequently associated with myalgia. It is often extremely intense and disproportionate to the finding at the physical examination [14]. In patients with arthralgia alone, the most recent imaging techniques, such as magnetic resonance imaging (MRI) and ultrasonography (US), may frequently reveal inflammatory articular changes which is undetectable by clinical evaluation [15–17].

Arthritis in the course of SLE can be acute, subacute, and/or chronic and is often detected (in 67–87 % of cases) (Table 6.1) at disease onset. The differences in prevalence reported in various studies may depend on the racial backgrounds of the cohorts, on the different age of the patients, and on the level of expertise of the enrolling center (e.g., nephrology centers or rheumatology centers).

Acute arthritis may occur as polyarthritis or oligoarthritis; it may be symmetric or asymmetric, with preferential involvement of the joints of the hands, wrists, and knees [18–26]. It is sensitive to anti-inflammatory treatment and usually does not recur during therapy [14]. It is frequently associated with visceral involvement and systemic signs; thus it can be a warning symptom of an SLE flare.

Subacute arthritis has a more prolonged course with milder inflammatory signs and it is frequently accompanied by morning stiffness. In older patients, the clinical picture may resemble rheumatic polymyalgia [14]. Lastly, arthritis in the course of SLE can occur as chronic arthritis without deformities and erosions, or as deforming, non-erosive, reversible arthropathy, or in some patients as erosive arthritis.

Examination of the synovial fluid shows some inflammatory liquid with a predominance of mononuclear cells and a decrease in complement levels with hypergammaglobulinemia. Antinuclear antibodies (ANA), lupus erythematosus (LE) cells, hematoxylin bodies, and ragocytes may be observed [14]. In a recent study, LE cells were present in 5/31 patients suffering from SLE and in 9/27 patients with the overlap syndrome (rheumatoid arthritis (RA)/SLE). In the same study, LE cells were observed in 2.6 % of 331 patients with RA and in none of 4 subjects with Still's disease, in 9 with systemic scleroderma, in 132 with ankylosing spondylitis, in 57 with Reiter's syndrome, and in 34 with psoriatic arthritis [27].

Common findings at synovial biopsy include synoviocyte hyperplasia, scarce inflammatory infiltrate, vascular proliferation, edema and congestion, fibrinoid

Table 6.1 Prevalence (%) of arthritis in different series of adult patients of SLE

Arthralgia or arthritis															
	Europe	**Brazil**	**Spain**	**Puerto Rico**	**Latin America**			**LUMINA (Hispanics)**		**Portugal**	**Brazil**	**Brazil**	**North America**	**Italy**
References	[18]	[19]	[20]	[21]	[2]			[22]		[23]	[24]	[4]	[25]	[17]
Year	1993	1995	1995	1999	2004			2004		2007	2012	2012	2014	2015
					European	**Mestizo**	**African**	**Tex**	**Puerto Rican**					
Number of patients	1,000	685	307	124	507	537	152	105	81	544	305	888	2,139	102
Arthritis %	84	82	83	67.5	93.5a	92.5a	94.1a	79.1	69.1	72	77.36a	87.4	70.8	94.1a

By Borba et al. [4], modified

necrosis and intimal fibrous hyperplasia of blood vessels, presence of fibrin on the synovial surface, and fibrin-like deposits in the chorion [28]. Indeed, some synovial alterations, ranging from simple hyperemia to synovitis, may mimic those found in RA [14]. Some studies have found differences in the synovium of patients with SLE and those suffering from RA and osteoarthritis (OA) from a gene expression profile perspective [29]. The synovium of patients with SLE suffering from arthritis shows a very distinct molecular signature as compared to what is observed in patients with OA and RA. It is characterized by the upregulation of interferon-inducible genes, as observed in the peripheral blood and kidney glomeruli of SLE patients [30], and downregulation of genes involved in extracellular matrix homeostasis. This might suggest the presence of different pathogenic mechanisms in SLE and RA, which would explain the lack of bone erosion observed in SLE patients with arthritis [29, 31].

6.2 Jaccoud's Arthropathy

The 1982 ACR classification criteria [32] modified the weight of joint involvement switching from "arthritis without deformity" of 1971 criteria [33] to "non-erosive arthritis." This change allowed to include patients with Jaccoud's arthropathy (JA) among those with SLE. In 2012, the SLICC criteria [34] proposed modifying the criterion to "synovitis ≥2 peripheral joints, characterized by pain, tenderness, swelling or morning stiffness ≥30 min," since new imaging techniques clearly show that some forms of SLE arthritis are in fact erosive [17].

In 1869, Jaccoud [35] first described deforming, non-erosive, reversible arthropathy associated with rheumatic fever. Later, this arthropathy was also observed in other rheumatic diseases and connective tissue diseases, as well as in sarcoidosis, infections, hypocomplementemic urticarial vasculitis, chronic pulmonary disease, inflammatory intestinal disease, pyrophosphate deposition disease, hypermobility syndrome, borreliosis, and neoplasia [36–41]. JA also occurs in an idiopathic form, in particular in the elderly, sometimes affecting several members of the same family [42, 43]. It was first described [44, 45] in patients suffering from SLE [24, 46–48] with a prevalence of up to 35 % [24, 26, 47–52].

The articular deformities of JA may be limited to the ulnar deviation at the metacarpal-phalangeal joint (MCP). Villaumey [53] and Alarcon-Segovia [46] considered this a diagnostic element for JA in the absence of erosions and rheumatoid factor (RF). JA may be widespread and can simulate evolved RA with lateral hyperlaxity of the distal interphalangeal articulations, swan neck deformities, boutonniere deformities, Z-shaped thumb, and carpal hyperlaxity. JA may also affect the feet [54, 55] and knees, sometimes in a disabling way, as well as the shoulders [14]. Deformities are usually reducible, even though some deformities may present elements of fixity [13].

In 1992, Spronk and coworkers [47] proposed a diagnostic index for JA (DIJA) based on the presence or absence of ulnar drift (>20′), swan neck deformities, boutonniere deformities, Z deformity, and limited MCP extension. Depending on the number of affected fingers, the first four items of the diagnostic index are graded from 2 to 3, whereas the fifth item is graded from 1 to 2, with a maximum total score of 23. JA was considered as being present if the index exceeded five points. This scoring method was frequently cited but never validated in well-designed studies [13, 56]. In 1998, van Vugt [57] introduced the term "mild deforming arthropathy" for patients who present DIJA with a score equal to or below 5 in the presence of deforming arthropathy without erosion. New imaging techniques led to the detection of erosive signs not previously detected by conventional radiology, thus leading to a new step in the differentiation between JA, mild deforming arthropathy, and erosive arthritis [26]. Recently, new criteria to differentiate between "idiopathic" and "senescent" JA were proposed by Santiago et al. [56], including: (1) typical joint deformities which are correctable in a passive position, (2) presence or history of articular inflammation in the deformed joints, regardless of its intensity or etiology (RA, SLE, etc.), (3) absence of similar deformities in other healthy members of the same family, and (4) no erosions on conventional radiology, magnetic resonance, or high-performance ultrasound examination.

The presence of JA in patients with SLE has been associated with older age [58] and disease duration [47, 59, 60]. However, these findings were not in agreement with the observations by Alarcon-Segovia et al. [46]. Besides it has been shown that the main determinant for JA was high disease activity in the absence of synovitis [61].

JA is positively associated with Sjogren's syndrome [46, 58] and frequent tendon rupture [62] and negatively associated with renal involvement [24, 51].

Some authors have pointed out an association with the presence of RF [46, 47], but this finding was not confirmed by other studies [51, 59]. JA was associated with higher levels of C-reactive protein (CRP) [47, 60, 63], with the presence of lupus anticoagulant and anticardiolipin antibodies [57], and with the presence of antibodies against U1 RNP [64], and inconstantly with anti SS-A/Ro and -B/La [47, 51, 58, 65, 66]. A correlation with the presence of antibodies to type II collagen [67], with higher levels of interleukin-6 (IL-6) [60] and with anti-double-stranded DNA antibodies [46], was observed. Interestingly, JA has never been associated with antipeptide citrulline (anti-CCP) antibodies [68, 69].

In general, the development of JA is correlated with abnormalities of soft tissues, with ligament and capsular laxity, relaxation, and subsequent deviation of tendons from their axis with the association of muscular dysfunction. Some authors have speculated that the laxity of the articular capsules and ligaments may be secondary to inflammation with fibrosis of the articular capsule [70, 71]. A role of synovial vasculitis [57] has been proposed. Besides, it has been also hypothesized a role in JA development for a synovial vasculitis [57], persistent inflammatory process of the synovium with inflammatory cells infiltrate and IL-1 and IL-6 production [47, 72]. These observations are in line with the high levels of CRP observed in patients with JA [47, 60, 63], but not in other patients with SLE even during disease flare [26].

The detection of high levels of RF in patients with JA is inconsistent [46, 47, 51, 59]. Thus, the presence of RF may act as a local inductor of the inflammatory process through the formation of immune complexes. However, it is worth noting that despite the documented presence of synovitis, this is not as aggressive as what is observed in RA [56]. JA can appear in other conditions as dermatomyositis, scleroderma, and chronic pulmonary disease without evidence of previous arthritis [40]. In 2006, Caznoch et al. [50] suggested a possible role of hyperparathyroidism linked to renal failure and the presence of an association between JA and the hypermobility syndrome, contrasting however with the previous observations by Klemp et al. [73]. A possible role for tenosynovitis has also been hypothesized [40], considering the reported association between JA and tendon ruptures [62]. As a matter of fact, 26 % of the 55 tendon ruptures in patients suffering from SLE were associated with the presence of JA [62]. Histological reports are very limited, though they led to the detection of mild synovitis without significant proliferation of the synovial membrane, light inflammatory infiltrates, microvascular alterations, fibrin precipitates, and hematoxylin corpuscles [47].

Based on a previous radiologic description, deforming chronic arthritis may present with swelling of the soft tissues; juxta-articular osteoporosis and joint space narrowing are rare, and exceptionally hook shaped erosions in the hands (and feet). All these features differ from what observed in RA (i.e., damage to the radial site of the metacarpal heads as well as a well-defined hook-shaped deformity with a sclerotic margin that is considered an adaptation to local stresses of persistent ulnar deviation) [74].

6.3 Rhupus

During the course of SLE, it is possible to observe, albeit rarely, an erosive arthritis similar to what is observed in RA. In 1971, Peter Schur [75] coined the term “rhupus” to describe patients with SLE who present arthritis and who also fulfill the classification criteria for RA [76]. Currently, the term rhupus is used by some to describe the coexistence of SLE and RA in the same patient [49, 57], while others use it to outline a subset of SLE patients with distinctive articular signs and typical clinical and radiological characteristics [3, 77]. However, the definition is still disputed since the immunopathological processes of SLE are considered to be exactly the opposite of the RA processes [78]. The real prevalence, the natural history and the clinical appearance are supported by few case series and small cohorts of patients, though with discrepancies in the definition of the cases and assessment methods [3, 77, 79–82]. It is however a very rare variant considering that until 2013, only 150 cases had been published [83]. Recently, the number of reports has been enriched by additional cohorts of patients [49, 84–86]. An epidemiological study showed a prevalence of about 0.09 % [79]. The prevalence of the more recent studies ranges from 1.30 to 5.8 % [49, 84, 85], which is surely higher than in previous reports [3, 79]. New imaging techniques for the study of the musculoskeletal system, like MRI and US [15–17, 70, 87, 88], have allowed to detect erosive alterations that would otherwise be undetectable by conventional radiology and to stress the higher prevalence of rhupus (9.7 %) [84].

Clinically, there are no statistically significant differences between the rhupus group and the control group regarding age and sex [49, 84, 85]. The signs of RA usually precede those of SLE [49, 84, 85] and these subjects have slower disease progression compared to patients with SLE without articular erosions [3, 49, 84, 89]. There were no significant differences in the prevalence of anti-double-stranded DNA, anti-Sm antibodies, anti- nuclear antibodies, and antiphospholipid antibodies between rhupus and SLE patients [49, 84]. On the other hand, patients suffering from rhupus present increased erythrocyte sediment rates and CRP levels [49, 84] and a greater presence of RF and antipeptide citrulline (anti-CCP) antibodies [49, 68, 84, 86, 90–94]. With regard to the presence of anti-CCP antibodies, a recent meta-analysis conducted on seven studies revealed 91.8 % and 47.8 % pooled specificity and sensitivity, respectively, in erosive arthropathy in SLE [92]. Comparatively in RA, a meta-analysis found the specificity and sensitivity of anti-CCP antibodies to be 95 % and 67 %, respectively [95]. The pooled specificity of anti-CCP antibodies in SLE patients with erosive disease is slightly lower than that of RA. It must be stressed that the studies by Qing et al. [93] and Zhao et al. [94] showed the highest sensitivity and lowest specificity, while Budhram et al. [92] hypothesized that these results can be explained by a threshold effect due to the low cutoff of anti-CCP antibody positivity that was used by the authors. Five studies reported anti-CCP antibody positivity in only 5 % or fewer patients with SLE and non-erosive arthritis [68, 91, 96–98]. The meta-analysis by Budhram suggests that the specificity of anti-CCP antibodies in SLE patients with erosive disease is comparable to that of RA when high cutoffs are used [92].

In rhupus, there is also a correlation between the severity of the articular involvement and positivity for anti-CCP antibodies [90–94]. A more recent study again confirms the association between anti-CCP antibodies and rhupus and highlights that the presence of these antibodies in patients suffering from SLE must make clinicians aware of the coexistence of RA [86], as confirmed by others Authors [69, 92].

Patients with rhupus have mild SLE activity and a lower incidence of visceral organ involvement compared to patients with SLE without RA and in particular with regard to renal and neurological involvement [49, 81, 84], although important clinical manifestations have also been reported [99, 100]. Patients with rhupus show a predominance of manifestations that are typical of RA, including clinical inflammation, deformities and erosions, and rheumatoid nodules, as well as a significantly high prevalence of RF and anti-CCP antibodies [3, 49, 69, 79, 81]. High titers of RF and anti-CCP antibodies are very often observed in patients meeting ACR criteria for RA and presenting articular erosions [69, 92]. Some authors believe that the appearance of rheumatoid nodules in patients with SLE represents a risk factor for rhupus [101].

A review of the medical literature on the correlation between anti-CCP antibodies and erosive arthritis in patients with SLE led Budhram et al. [92] to hypothesize the presence of two subgroups of patients with erosive arthritis. One subgroup presents a process that is pathologically different from that of RA, their anti-CCP antibodies are often negative, and these subjects likely do not meet the ACR criteria for RA. In the second subgroup, the pathogenesis of the erosions is the same as in RA, the anti-CCP antibodies are often positive, and these subjects likely meet the criteria for

RA. According to Budhram et al., patients in the two groups may present different erosive manifestations; in the former they may be similar to those described by Pastershank in JA [74], while the latter may show marginal erosions that are typical of RA. This theory should be investigated with specific imaging studies since the new imaging techniques, such as US and MRI, have shown an unexpectedly high prevalence of subclinical articular and periarticular involvement and, most importantly, a higher prevalence of bone erosions as compared to standard radiography, as well as an unexpectedly high prevalence of synovitis and tenosynovitis [15, 17, 102–104]. This hypothesis is supported by the observations that anti-CCP antibodies and RF show an additive effect on erosion and erosion size and number in RA [105].

Alongside the arthritic manifestations, tenosynovitis is frequently found in patients with SLE, mainly localized to the extensor tendons in the hands, with a prevalence ranging from 28 to 61 % [15, 17, 102–104].

6.4 Joint Involvment Management

There are some guidelines regarding the treatment of arthritis in the course of SLE [106]. An approach based on the type of arthritis has been proposed [107, 108]. First-line, short-term treatment with nonsteroidal anti-inflammatory drugs (NSAIDs) is frequent in the presence of acute or subacute arthritis, given the episodic and limited nature of articular flares in many patients with SLE [107, 108]. Clearly, administration of these drugs must include rigorous renal and hepatic monitoring; cardiovascular and skin photosensitivity risks must also be taken into consideration, as should reports on rare cases of aseptic meningitis [108]. Many patients cannot tolerate NSAIDs or may present contraindications to their use, while others show more persistent arthritic episodes that are refractory to these drugs. In these cases, antimalarial drugs are recommended, in particular hydroxychloroquine, usually at a dosage of 6 mg/kg/die [109]; if necessary, corticosteroids should be associated [107–110]. Low-dose corticosteroids (≤10 mg/day of prednisone equivalent) are usually administered, and if high doses are needed, corticoid-sparing agents should be used [108]. Direct injection of corticosteroids into joints can be useful, especially when involvement is limited to one or few joints or in tenosynovitis. In patients who do not respond to corticosteroids or antimalarial drugs, methotrexate or other immunosuppressants (azathioprine, leflunomide, mycophenolate mofetil) or non-conventional therapies must be taken into consideration [107, 111–113]. There is broad consensus on the use of methotrexate as a steroid-sparing agent [111] and its effectiveness in controlling articular manifestations [110, 111, 114–118]. Leflunomide proved to be effective in a controlled study of only 12 patients [119]; however, several cases of cutaneous lupus flare-up were reported [108]. Mycophenolate mofetil was also assumed to be effective [112, 120–122], even though evidence in the literature is limited [108]. Among the non-conventional drugs, some reports indicate the efficacy of rituximab [112, 122–124], even if there are no specific controlled studies on arthritic manifestations in SLE. With regard to belimumab, literature data [121, 126–128] suggest that it has potential for use in the treatment of severe joint symptoms in lupus that are resistant to corticosteroid treatment or refractory to conventional treatment [108, 113], whereas tocilizumab [129] is still being investigated.

Despite its reduced efficacy and frequently unfavorable effects [130], if all other therapies fail, abatacept may be taken into consideration (under strict control of a reference center or other experts) for patients in whom lupus manifests as a corticodependent joint disease [108], while the use of anti-TNF-alpha drugs is not recommended [108, 125].

Treatment of Jaccoud's arthropathy is the same as what is recommended for chronic arthritis in the course of SLE. However, despite their symptomatic effect, there are no guarantees that NSAIDs, low-dose steroids, antimalarial drugs, or methotrexate can inhibit the progression of deformities [56]. The benefits of physical therapy and the use of orthotic devices are yet to be demonstrated, and there are few reports on surgical procedures to correct JA [131–135] since the indications, the best modalities, and when to indicate them are still unknown [50].

There are several reports concerning the use of disease-modifying antirheumatic drugs (DMARDs), and in particular methotrexate, in rhupus [117, 136, 137], even in combination with other drugs [138]; however, many of them showed inadequate response [26]. There are small case series reporting the efficacy of mycophenolate mofetil [139] and cyclosporine [140]. Anti-TNF-alpha, which is effective in treating RA, seems to be less effective in treating rhupus and SLE. It can induce the production of autoantibodies, such as antinuclear antibodies and anti-DNA antibodies [141], and more rarely it may result in lupus manifestations in both RA [142, 143] and rhupus patients [144]. Thus, the use of anti-TNF-alpha is not recommended in SLE patients [125]. The use of rituximab shows more encouraging results, as demonstrated in small clinical series in open clinical studies [83, 145] as does abatacept [130, 146]. Finally, two of our patients benefited from the use of tocilizumab [147].

There is a need for further controlled studies and, consequently, specific guidelines for the various forms of arthritis during the course of SLE.

References

1. Cervera R, Kamasthta MA, Font J et al (1999) Morbidity and mortality in systemic lupus erythematosus during a 5 year period. A multicenter prospective study of 1000 patients. Medicine 78:167175
2. PonsEstel BA, Catoggio LJ, Cardiel MH et al (2004) The GLADEL multinational Latin American prospective inception cohort of 1,214 patients with systemic lupus erythematosus: ethnic and disease heterogeneity among "Hispanics". Medicine (Baltimore) 83:1–17
3. Fernandez A, Quintana G, Rondon F et al (2006) Lupus arthropathy: a case series of patients with rhupus. Clin Rheumatol 25:164–167
4. Borba EF, Araujo DB, Bonfa E, Shinjo SK (2013) Clinical and immunological features of 888 Brazilian systemic lupus patients from a monocentric cohort: comparison with other populations. Lupus 22:744–749
5. SchwartzmanMorris J, Putterman C (2012) Gender differences in the pathogenesis and outcome of lupus and of lupus nephritis. Clin Dev Immunol 1:9–18
6. Murphy G, Isenberg D (2013) Effect of gender on clinical presentation in systemic lupus erythematosus. Rheumatology 52:2108–2115

7. Faezi ST, Almodarresi MH, Akbarian M et al (2014) Clinical and immunological pattern of systemic lupus erythematosus in men in a cohort of 2355 patients. Int J Rheum Dis 17:394–399
8. Hoffman IEA, Lauwerys BR, De Keyser F et al (2009) Juvenile onset systemic lupus erythematosus: different clinical and serological pattern than adult onset systemic lupus erythematosus. Ann Rheum Dis 68:412–415
9. Feng X, Zou Y, Pan W, Wang X et al (2014) Associations of clinical features and prognosis with age at disease onset in patients with systemic lupus erythematosus. Lupus 23:327334
10. Malcus Johnsson P, Sandqvist G, Bengtsson A, Nived O (2008) Hand function and performance of daily activities in systemic lupus erythematosus. Arthritis Care Res 59:1432–1438
11. Yelin E et al (2012) A longitudinal study of the impact of incident organ manifestations and increased disease activity on work loss among persons with SLE. Arthritis Care Res (Hoboken) 64:169–175
12. Drenkard C, Bao G, Dennis G et al (2014) Burden of systemic lupus erythematosus on employment and work productivity: data from a large cohort in the southeastern United States. Arthritis Care Res 66:878–887
13. Ball EMA, Bell AL (2012) Lupus arthritis—do we have a clinically useful classification? Rheumatology 51:771779
14. Meyer, Kahn MF (2000) Lupus érithémateux Systémique. In: Kahn MF, Peltier AP, Meyer O, Piette JC (eds) Maladies et syndrome systemiques, vol 7. Médicines Sciences Flammarion, Paris, p 131396
15. Wright S, Filippucci E, Grassi W et al (2006) Hand arthritis in systemic lupus erythematosus: an ultrasound pictorial essay. Lupus 15:5016
16. Torrente Segarra V, Lisbona MP, RotésSala D et al (2013) Hand and wrist arthralgia in systemic lupus erythematosus is associated to ultrasonographic abnormalities. Joint Bone Spine 80:4026
17. Mosca M, Tani C, Carli L et al (2015) The role of imaging in the evaluation of joint involvement in 102 consecutive patients with systemic lupus erythematosus. Autoimmun Rev 14:10–15
18. Cervera R, Khamashta MA, Font J et al (1993) Systemic lupus erythematosus: clinical and immunologic patterns of disease expression in a cohort of 1000 patients. Medicine 72:113–124
19. Chahade WH, Sato EI, Moura JE Jr, Costallat LT, Andrade LE (1995) Systemic lupus erythematosus in Sa˜o Paulo/Brazil: a clinical and laboratory overview. Lupus 4:100–103
20. Blanco FJ, de la Mata J, Gòmez-Reino JJ et al (1995) Clinical and serological manifestations of 307 Spanish patients with systemic lupus erythematosus. Comparison with other ethnic groups [in Spanish]. Rev Clin Exp 195:534–540
21. Vilà LM, Mayor AM, Valentin AH, Garcia-Soberal M, Vilà S (1999) Clinical and immunological manifestations in 134 Puerto Rican patients with systemic lupus erythematosus. Lupus 8:279–286
22. Vilà LM, Alarcòn GS, McGwin G Jr et al (2004) LUMINA Study Group. Early clinical manifestations, disease activity and damage of systemic lupus erythematosus among two distinct US Hispanic subpopulations. Rheumatology (Oxford) 43:358–363
23. Santos MJ, Capela S, Figueira R et al (2007) Characterization of a Portuguese population with systemic lupus erythematosus. Acta Reumatol Port 32:153–161
24. Skare TL, Godoi Ade L, Ferreira VO (2012) Jaccoud arthropathy in systemic lupus erythematosus: clinical and serological findings. Rev Assoc Med Bras 58:48992
25. Somers EC, Marder W, Cagnoli P et al (2014) Population-based incidence and prevalence of systemic lupus erythematosus. The Michigan lupus epidemiology and surveillance program. Arthritis Rheumatol 66:369–378
26. Pipili C, Sfritzeri A, Cholongitas E (2008) Deforming arthropathy in systemic lupus erythematosus. Eur J Intern Med 19:4827
27. Puszczewicz M, Białkowska Puszczewicz G (2010) LE cells in synovial fluid: prevalence and diagnostic usefulness in rheumatic diseases. Ann Acad Med Stetin 56(Suppl 1):1058

28. Natour J, Montezzo LC, Moura LA, Atra E (1991) A study of synovial membrane of patients with systemic lupus erythematosus (SLE). Clin Exp Rheumatol 9:2215
29. Nzeusseu Toukap A, Galant C, Theate I, Maudoux AL et al (2007) Identification of distinct gene expression profiles in the synovium of patients with systemic lupus erythematosus. Arthritis Rheum 56:157988
30. Qing X, Putterman C (2004) Gene expression profiling in the study of the pathogenesis of systemic lupus erythematosus. Autoimmun Rev 3:5059
31. McInnes IB, Schett G (2011) The pathogenesis of rheumatoid arthritis. N Engl J Med 365:220519
32. Tan EM, Cohen AS, Fries JF, Masi AT, McShane DJ, Rothfield NF et al (1982) The 1982 revised criteria for the classification of systemic lupus erythematosus. Arthritis Rheum 25:1271–1277
33. Cohen AS, Reynolds WE, Franklin EC et al (1971) Preliminary criteria for the classification of systemic lupus erythematosus. Bull Rheum Dis 21:643–648
34. Petri M, Orbai AM, Alarcon GS et al (2012) Derivation and validation of the systemic lupus international collaborating clinics classification criteria for systemic lupus erythematosus. Arthritis Rheum 64:2677–2686
35. Jaccoud FS (1869) Sur une forme de rhumatisme chronique: lecions de clinique medicale faites a l'Hopital de la Charite. Paris, Delahaye, pp 598–616R
36. Bradley JD, Pinals RS (1984) Jaccoud's arthropathy in scleroderma. Clin Exp Rheumatol 2:337–340
37. Bradley JD (1986) Jaccoud's arthropathy in adult dermatomyositis. Clin Exp Rheumatol 4:273–276
38. Sturgess AS, Littlejohn GO (1988) Jaccoud's arthritis and panvasculitis in the hypocomplementemic urticarial vasculitis syndrome. J Rheumatol 15:858–861
39. Sukenik S, Hendler N, Yerushalmi B, Buskila D, Liberman N (1991) Jaccoud's type arthropathy: an association with sarcoidosis. Rheumatology 18:915–917
40. Santiago MB (2011) Miscellaneous noninflammatory musculoskeletal conditions. Jaccoud's arthropathy. Best Pract Res Clin Rheumatol 25:715725
41. Maher LV (2014) Jaccoud arthropathy. Am J Med Sci 348:81
42. Sivas F, Aydog S, Pekin Y, Ozoran K (2005) Idiopathic Jaccoud's arthropathy. APLAR J Rheumatol 8:60–62
43. Arlet JB, Pouchot J (2009) The senescent form of Jaccoud arthropathy. J Clin Rheumatol 15:151
44. Aptekar RG, Lawless OJ, Decker JL (1974) Deforming nonerosive arthritis of the hand in systemic lupus erythematosus. Clin Orthop Relat Res 100:120–124
45. Bywaters EGL (1975) Jaccoud's syndrome. A sequel to the joint involvement of systemic lupus erythematosus. Clin Rheum Dis 1:125148
46. AlarconSegovia D, AbudMendoza C, DiazJouanen E et al (1988) Deforming arthropathy of the hands in systemic lupus erythematosus. J Rheumatol 15:659
47. Spronk PE, ter Borg EJ, Kallenberg CG (1992) Patients with systemic lupus erythematosus and Jaccoud's arthropathy: a clinical subset with an increased C reactive protein response? Ann Rheum Dis 51:35861
48. Santiago MB, Galvão V (2008) Jaccoud arthropathy in systemic lupus erythematosus: analysis of clinical characteristics and review of the literature. Medicine (Baltimore) 87:3744
49. Li J, Honghua Wu H, Huang X et al (2014) Clinical analysis of 56 patients with rhupus syndrome: manifestations and comparisons with systemic lupus erythematosus a retrospective case–control study. Medicine 93:49–51
50. Caznoch CJ, Esmanhotto L, Silva MB et al (2006) Pattern of joint involvement in patients with systemic lupus erythematosus and its association with rheumatoid factor and hypermobility. Rev Bras Rheumatol 46:261–265
51. Molina JF, Molina J, Gutierrez S et al (1995) Deforming arthropathy of the hands (Jaccoud's) in systemic lupus erythematosus (SLE). An independent subset of SLE? Arthritis Rheum 38

52. AgmonLevin N, Mosca M, Petri M, Shoenfeld Y (2012) Systemic lupus erythematosus one disease or many? Autoimmun Rev 11:5935
53. Villaumey J, Arlet J, Avouac B (1986) Diagnostic criteria and new etiologic events in the arthropathy of jaccoud: a report of 10 cases. Clin Rheum Press 4:156–175
54. Morley KD, Leung A, Rynes RI (1982) Lupus foot. BMJ 284:557–558
55. Ribeiro DS, Santiago M (2011) Imaging of Jaccoud's arthropathy in systemic lupus erythematosus: not only hands but also knees and feet. Rheumatol Int 3:34–38
56. Santiago MB (2013) Jaccoud's arthropathy: proper classification criteria and treatment are still needed. Rheumatol Int 33:2953–2954
57. van Vugt RM, Derksen RH, Kater L, Bijlsma JW (1998) Deforming arthropathy or lupus and rhupus hands in systemic lupus erythematosus. Ann Rheum Dis 57:540
58. Takeishi M, Mimori A, Suzuki T (2001) Clinical and immunological features of systemic lupus erythematosus complicated by Jaccoud's arthropathy. Mod Rheumatol 11:47–51
59. Esdaile JM, Danoff D, Rosenthall L et al (1981) Deforming arthritis in systemic lupus erythematosus. Ann Rheum Dis 40:124–126
60. Atta AM, Oliveira RC, Oliveira IS et al (2015) Higher level of IL6 in Jaccoud's arthropathy secondary to systemic lupus erythematosus: a perspective for its treatment? Reumatol Int 35:167–170
61. Bleifeld CJ, Inglis AE (1974) The hand in systemic lupus erythematosus. J Bone Joint Surg Am 56:1207–1215
62. Alves EM, Macieira JC, Borba E, Chiuchetta FA, Santiago MB (2010) Spontaneous tendon rupture in systemic lupus erythematosus: association with Jaccoud's arthropathy. Lupus 19:247–254
63. Manthorpe R, Bendixed G, Schioler H, Viderbal A (1980) Jaccoud's syndrome: a nasographic entity associated with SLE. J Rheumatol 7:169–177
64. Reilly PA, Evison G, McHugh NJ et al (1990) Arthropathy of hands and feet in systemic lupus erythematosus. J Rheumatol 17:777–784
65. Franchescini F, Cretti L, Quinzanini M, Rizzini FL, Cattaneo R (1994) Deforming arthropathy of the hands in systemic lupus erythematosus is associated with antibodies to SSA/Ro and to SSB/La. Lupus 3:419–422
66. Paredes JG, Lazaro MA, Citera G, Da Representacao S, Maldonado Cocco JA (1997) Jaccoud's arthropathy of the hands in overlap syndrome. Clin Rheumatol 16:65–69
67. Choi EK, Gatenby PA, Bateman JF, Cole WG (1990) Antibodies to type II collagen in SLE: a role in the pathogenesis of deforming arthritis? Immunol Cell Biol 68:27–31
68. DamiánAbrego GN, Cabiedes J, Cabral AR (2008) Anticitrullinated peptide antibodies in lupus patients with or without deforming arthropathy. Lupus 17:300–304
69. Kakumanu P, Sobel ES, Narain S et al (2009) Citrulline dependence of anti cyclic citrullinated peptide antibodies in systemic lupus erythematosus as a marker of deforming/erosive. Arthritis J Rheumatol 36:2682–2690
70. Ostendorf B, Scherer A, Specker C, Modder U, Schneider M (2003) Jaccoud's arthropathy in systemic lupus erythematosus: differentiation of deforming and erosive patterns by magnetic resonance imaging. Arthritis Rheum 48:157–165
71. Martini A, Ravelli A, Viola S, Burgio RG (1987) Systemic lupus erythematosus with Jaccoud's arthropathy mimicking juvenile rheumatoid arthritis. Arthritis Rheum 30:1062–1064
72. Eilertsen G, Nikolaisen C, BeckerMerok A, Nossent JC (2011) Interleukin6 promotes arthritis and joint deformation in patients with systemic lupus erythematosus. Lupus 20:60713
73. Klemp P, Majoos FL, Chalton D (1987) Articular mobility in systemic lupus erythematosus (SLE). Clin Rheumatol 6:202–207
74. Pastershank SP, Resnick D (1980) 'Hook' erosions in Jaccoud's arthropathy. J Can Assoc Radiol 31:1745
75. Schur PH (1971) Systemic lupus erythematosus. In: Beeson PB, McDermott W (eds) Cecilloeb textbook of medicine, 13th edn. WB Saunders, Philadelphia, p 821

76. Arnett F, Edworthy S, Bloch D et al (1988) The American Rheumatism Association 1987 revised criteria for the classification of rheumatoid arthritis. Arthritis Rheum 31:315–332
77. AmezcuaGuerra LM (2009) Overlap between systemic lupus erythematosus and rhematoid arthritis: is real or just an illusion? J Rheumatol 36:4–6
78. Hayakawa S, KomineAizawa S, Osaka S et al (2007) Rembrandt's Maria Bockenolle has a butterfly rash and digital deformities: overlapping syndrome of rheumatoid arthritis and systemic lupus erythematosus. Med Hypotheses 68:906–909
79. Panush RS, Edwards NL, Longley S, Webester E (1988) Rhupus syndrome. Arch Intern Med 148:1633–1636
80. Brand CA, Rowley MJ, Tait BD, Muirden KD, Whittingham SF (1992) Coexistent rheumatoid arthritis and systemic lupus erythematosus; clinical, serological, and phenotypic features. Ann Rheum Dis 51:17–36
81. Simon JA, Seeded J, Cabiedes J, Ruiz Morals J, Alcocer J (2002) Clinical and immunogenetic characterization of Mexican patients with 'rhupus'. Lupus 11:287–292
82. Satoh M, Ajmani AK, Akizuki M (1994) What is the definition for coexistent rheumatoid arthritis and systemic lupus erythematosus? Lupus 3:1378
83. Andrade-Ortega L, Irazoque-Palazuelos F, Mu˜nóz-López S, Rosales-Don Pablo VM (2013) Efficacy and tolerability of rituximab in patients with rhupus. Reumatol Clin 9:201–205
84. Tani C, D'Aniello D, Delle Sedie A et al (2013) Rhupus syndrome: assessment of its prevalence and its clinical and instrumental characteristics in a prospective cohort of 103 SLE patients. Autoimmun Rev 12:537–541
85. Liu T, Li G, Mu R, Ye H, Li W (2014) Clinical and laboratory profiles of rhupus syndrome in a Chinese population: a single centre study of 51 patients. Lupus 23:958963
86. Amaya A, MolanoGonzàlez N, Franco JS, RodrıguezJiménez M, RojasVillarraga A, Anaya JM (2015) AntiCCP antibodies as a marker of rhupus. Lupus 0:1–3
87. Delle Sedie A, Riente L, Scirè CA, Iagnocco A, Filippucci E, Meenagh G (2009) Ultrasound imaging for the rheumatologist XXIV. Sonographic evaluation of wrist and hand joint and tendon involvement in systemic lupus erythematosus. Clin Exp Rheumatol 27:897–901
88. Boutry N, Hachulla E, Flipo RM, Cortet B, Cotten A (2005) MR imaging findings in hands in early rheumatoid arthritis: comparison with those in systemic lupus erythematosus and primary Sjögren syndrome. Radiology 236:593–600
89. Prete M, Racanelli V, Digiglio L et al (2011) Extraarticular manifestations of rheumatoid arthritis: an update. Autoimmun Rev 11:123–131
90. Martinez JB, Valero AJ, Restrepo JF (2007) Erosive arthropathy: clinical variance in lupus erythematosus and association with anti-CCP case series an review of the literature. Clin Exp Rheumatol 25:47–51
91. Chan M, Owen P, Dumpy J, Cox B, Carmichael C, Korendowych E et al (2008) Associations of erosive arthritis with anticyclic citrullinated peptide antibodies and MHC class II alleles in systemic lupus erythematosus. J Rheumatol 35:77–83
92. Budhram A, Chu R, RustaSalleh S, Ioannidi G, Denbur JA, Adachi JD, Haaland DA (2014) Anti cyclic citrullinated peptide antibody as a marker of erosive arthritis in patients with systemic lupus erythematosus: a systematic review and meta-analysis. Lupus 23:1156–1163
93. Qing YF, Zhang QB, Zhou JG et al (2009) The detecting and clinical value of anticyclic citrullinated peptide antibodies in patients with systemic lupus erythematosus. Lupus 18:713–717
94. Zhao Y, Li J, Li XX, Li C, Li L, Li ZG (2009) What can we learn from the presence of anticyclic citrullinated peptide antibodies in systemic lupus erythematosus? Joint Bone Spine 76:501–507
95. Nishimura K, Sugiyama D, Kogata Y et al (2007) Metaanalysis: diagnostic accuracy of anticyclic citrullinated peptide antibody and rheumatoid factor for rheumatoid arthritis. Ann Intern Med 146:797–808
96. Mediwake R, Isenberg DA, Schellekens GA, van Venrooij WJ (2001) Use of anticitrullinated peptide and antiRA33 antibodies in distinguishing erosive arthritis in patients with systemic lupus erythematosus and rheumatoid arthritis. Ann Rheum Dis 60:67–68

97. Amezcua-Guerra LM, Márquez-Velasco R, Bojalil R (2008) Erosive arthritis in systemic lupus erythematosus is associated with high serum C-reactive protein and anti-cyclic citrullinated peptide antibodies. Inflamm Res 57:555–557
98. Taraborelli M, Inverardi F, Fredi M et al (2012) Anticyclic citrullinated peptide antibodies in systemic lupus erythematosus patients with articular involvement: a predictive marker for erosive disease? Reumatismo 64:321–325
99. Wang JG, Tang HH, Tan CY, Liu Y, Lin H, Chen YT (2010) Diffuse lupus encephalopathy in a case of rhupus syndrome. Rheumatology 30:9613
100. Sciascia S, Roccatello D, Rossi D, Russo A, Mereuta MO, Cavallo R (2012) High-titer anti-aquaporin4 IgG-associated myelitis in rhupus syndrome. J Rheumatol 39:8713
101. Richter Cohen M, Steiner G, Smolen JS et al (1998) Erosive arthritis in systemic lupus erythematosus: analysis of a distinct clinical and serological subset. Br J Rheumatol 37:421–424
102. Gabba A, Piga M, Vacca A, Porru G, Garau P, Cauli A et al (2012) Joint and tendon involvement in systemic lupus erythematosus: an ultrasound study of hands and wrists in 108 patients. Rheumatology 51:2278–2285
103. Iagnocco A, Ossandon A, Coari G, Conti F, Priori R, Alessandri C et al (2004) Wrist joint involvement in systemic lupus erythematosus. An ultrasonographic study. Clin Exp Rheumatol 22:621–624
104. Iagnocco A, Ceccarelli F, Rizzo C, Truglia S, Massaro L, Spinelli FR et al (2013) Ultrasound evaluation of hand, wrist and foot joint synovitis in systemic lupus erythematosus. Rheumatology 2:34–41
105. Hecht C, Englbrecht M, Rech J et al (2014) Additive effect of anti-citrullinated protein antibodies and rheumatoid factor on bone erosions in patients with RA. Ann Rheum Dis 2:34–55
106. Tunnicliffe DJ, Singh-Grewal D, Kim S, Craig JC, Tong A (2015) Diagnosis, monitoring and treatment of systemic lupus erythematosus: a systematic review of clinical practice guidelines. Arthritis Care Res (Hoboken). doi:10.1002/acr.22591 [Epub ahead of print]
107. Grossman JM (2009) Lupus arthritis. Best Pract Res Clin Rheumatol 23:495–506
108. Artifoni M, Puéchala X (2012) How to treat refractory arthritis in lupus? Joint Bone Spine 79:347–350
109. Nikpour M, Bridge JA, Richter S (2014) A systematic review of prevalence, disease characteristics and management of systemic lupus erythematosus in Australia: identifying areas of unmet need. Intern Med J 44:1170–1179
110. Islam MN, Hossain M, Haq SA et al (2012) Efficacy and safety of methotrexate in articular and cutaneous manifestations of systemic lupus erythematosus. Int J Rheum Dis 15:62–68
111. Sakthiswary R, Suresh E (2014) Methotrexate in systemic lupus erythematosus: a systematic review of its efficacy. Lupus 23:225–235
112. Calvo-Alen J, Silva-Fernandez L, Ucar-Angulo E, Pego-Reigosa JM, Olive A, Martinez-Fernandez C et al (2013) SER consensus statement on the use of biologic therapy for systemic lupus erythematosus. Reumatol Clin 09:281–296
113. Muangchan C, van Vollenhoven RF, Bernatsky SR et al (2015) Treatment algorithms in systemic lupus erythematosus. Arthritis Care Res (Hoboken). doi:10.1002/acr.22589 [Epub ahead of print]
114. Miescher P, Riethmueller D (1965) Diagnosis and treatment of systemic lupus erythematosus. Semin Hematol 2:1–28
115. Gansauge S, Breitbart A, Rinaldi N, Schwarz-Eywill M (1997) Methotrexate in patients with moderate systemic lupus erythematosus (exclusion of renal and central nervous system disease). Ann Rheum Dis 56:382–385
116. Rahman P, Humphrey-Murto S, Gladman DD, Urowitz MB (1998) Efficacy and tolerability of methotrexate in antimalarial resistant lupus arthritis. J Rheumatol 25:243–246
117. Carneiro JR, Sato EI (1999) Double blind, randomized, placebo controlled clinical trial of methotrexate in systemic lupus erythematosus. J Rheumatol 26:1275–1279

118. Pego-Reigosa JM, Cobo-Ibáñez T, Calvo-Alén J et al (2013) Efficacy and safety of nonbiologic immunosuppressants in the treatment of nonrenal systemic lupus erythematosus: a systematic review. Arthritis Care Res (Hoboken) 65:1775–1785
119. Tam LS, Li EK, Wong CK et al (2004) Double-blind, randomized, placebo controlled pilot study of leflunomide in systemic lupus erythematosus. Lupus 13:601–604
120. Karim MY, Alba P, Cuadrado MJ et al (2002) Mycophenolate mofetil for systemic lupus erythematosus refractory to other immunosuppressive agents. Rheumatology (Oxford) 41:876–882
121. Ginzler EM, Wofsy D, Isenberg D et al (2010) Nonrenal disease activity following mycophenolate mofetil or intravenous cyclophosphamide as induction treatment for lupus nephritis: findings in a multicenter, prospective, randomized, open-label, parallel-group clinical trial. Arthritis Rheum 62:211–221
122. Aringer M, Burkhardt H, Burmester GR et al (2011) Current state of evidence on "off label" therapeutic options for systemic lupus erythematosus, including biological immunosuppressive agents, in Germany, Austria, and Switzerland – a consensus report. Lupus 3:34–41
123. Terrier B, Amoura Z, Ravaud P et al (2010) Safety and efficacy of rituximab in systemic lupus erythematosus: results from 136 patients from the French autoimmunity and rituximab registry. Arthritis Rheum 62:2458–2466
124. Bang SY, Lee CK, Kang YM et al (2012) Multicenter retrospective analysis of the effectiveness and safety of rituximab in Korean patients with refractory systemic lupus erythematosus. Autoimmune Dis 5:65039
125. Aringer M, Smolen JS (2015) Safety of off-label biologicals in systemic lupus erythematosus. Expert Opin Drug Saf 14:243–251
126. Manzi S, Sanchez-Guerrero J, Merrill JT et al (2010) Belimumab, a BLyS-specific inhibitor, reduced disease activity across multiple organ domains: combined efficacy results from the phase 3 BLISS-52 and -76 studies (abstract). Arthritis Rheum 62:S607–S608
127. Navarra SV, Guzmán RM, Gallacher AE et al (2011) Efficacy and safety of belimumab in patients with active systemic lupus erythematosus: a randomised, placebo-controlled, phase 3 trial. Lancet 377:721–731
128. Furie R, Petri M, Zamani O, for the BLISS-76 Study Group et al (2011) A phase III, randomized, placebo-controlled study of belimumab, a monoclonal antibody that inhibits B lymphocyte stimulator, in patients with systemic lupus erythematosus. Arthritis Rheum 63:3918–3930
129. Illei GG, Shirota Y, Yarboro CH et al (2010) Tocilizumab in systemic lupus erythematosus: data on safety, preliminary efficacy, and impact on circulating plasma cells from an open-label phase I dosage-escalation study. Arthritis Rheum 62:542–552
130. Merrill JT, Burgos-Vargas R, Westhovens R et al (2010) The efficacy and safety of abatacept in patients with non-life-threatening manifestations of systemic lupus erythematosus: results of a twelve-month, multicenter, exploratory, phase IIb, randomized, double-blind, placebo-controlled trial. Arthritis Rheum 62:3077–3087
131. Evans JA, Hastings DE, Urowitz MB (1977) The fixed lupus hand deformity and its surgical correction. J Rheumatol 4:170–175
132. Schumacher HR, Zweiman B, Bora FW Jr (1976) Corrective surgery for the deforming hand arthropathy of systemic lupus erythematosus. Clin Orthop Relat Res 17:292–295
133. Dray GJ, Millender LH, Nalebuff EA, Philips C (1981) The surgical treatment of hand deformities in systemic lupus erythematosus. J Hand Surg [Am] 6:339–345
134. Alnot JY, Liverneaux P, Welby F (2004) Jaccoud's arthropathy. Surgical results of 41 hands. Chir Main 23:229–236
135. Oda R, Fujiwara H, Tokunaga D et al (2014) Spontaneous flexor tendon rupture in systemic lupus erythematosus: a case report. Mod Rheumatol 20:1–4
136. Fortin PR, Abrahamowicz M, Ferland D et al (2008) Steroid-sparing effects of methotrexate in systemic lupus erythematosus: a double-blind, randomized, placebo-controlled trial. Arthritis Rheum 59:1796–1804

137. Winzer M, Aringer M (2010) Use of methotrexate in patients with systemic lupus erythematosus and primary Sjogren's syndrome. Clin Exp Rheumatol 28(5 Suppl 61):S156–S159
138. Li J, Wu H, Huang X et al (2014) Clinical analysis of 56 patients with rhupus syndrome: manifestations and comparisons with systemic lupus erythematosus a retrospective case–control study. Medicine (Baltimore) 93:e49
139. Benavente EP, Paira SO (2011) Rhupus: report of 4 cases. Reumatol Clin 7:333–335
140. Seo SR, Lee SJ, Park DJ et al (2011) Successful treatment using cyclosporine in a patient with rhupus complicated by aplastic anemia: a case report and review of the literature. Clin Exp Rheumatol 29:708–711
141. Eriksson C, Engstrand S, Sundqvist K-G et al (2005) Autoantibody formation in patients with rheumatoid arthritis treated with anti-TNF α . Ann Rheum Dis 3:403–407
142. Charles PJ, Smeenk RJ, De Jong J et al (2000) Assessment of antibodies to double-stranded DNA induced in rheumatoid arthritis patients following treatment with infliximab, a monoclonal antibody to tumor necrosis factor alpha: findings in open-label and randomized placebo-controlled trials. Arthritis Rheumatol 43:2383–2390
143. De Bandt M, Sibilia J, Le Loet X et al (2005) Systemic lupus erythematosus induced by antitumour necrosis factor alpha therapy: a French national survey. Arthritis Res Ther 3:R545–R551
144. Chogle AR, Shah CV, Murthy AK et al (2011) Role of anti-tumor necrosis factor-α blockers in inducing lupus erythematosus tumidus in 'rhupus syndrome'. J Rheumatol 38:1218–1219
145. Piga M, Gabba A, Cauli A, Garau P, Vacca A, Mathieu A (2013) Rituximab treatment for 'rhupus syndrome': clinical and power-Doppler ultrasonographic monitoring of response. A longitudinal pilot study. Lupus 22:624–628
146. Ikeda K, Sanayama Y, Makita S et al (2013) Efficacy of abatacept for arthritis in patients with an overlap syndrome between rheumatoid arthritis and systemic lupus erythematosus. Clin Dev Immunol 2013:697525
147. Rossi D, Sciascia S, Manna E, Binello G, Modena V, Roccatello D (2013) Tocilizumab as a therapeutic option for Rhupus patients who do not respond to conventional therapy. Ann Rheum Dis 72(Suppl3):1004

7 The Spectrum of Cutaneous Manifestations in Systemic Lupus Erythematosus and Novel Classification

Simone Ribero, Dan Lipsker, and Luca Borradori

7.1 Introduction

Systemic lupus erythematosus (SLE) is a complex autoimmune syndrome showing a broad and protean spectrum of clinical and immunological features. Cutaneous involvement is frequently found in SLE. Affected patients may show a variety of different "specific" and "nonspecific" cutaneous manifestations as either an initial leading sign of the disease or as complication in its course. Hence, knowledge of the typical and more unusual cutaneous features associated with SLE is important for the proper diagnosis and management of affected patients [1–4].

After articular involvement, the skin represents the second most frequently affected organ in SLE [1]. In fact, approximately 80 % of patients will display skin manifestations during the course of the disease [2, 3].

Cutaneous manifestations may constitute the first sign of SLE in up to 25 % of cases. Therefore, in all patients with newly diagnosed cutaneous lupus erythematosus (CLE), the clinician is invariably faced with the dilemma of whether the observed cutaneous lesions constitute the first sign of SLE or not.

The estimated risk of experiencing a transition from CLE to SLE has been differently estimated with rates up to 25 % [4]. Durosaro et al. reported that in patients with newly diagnosed CLE, the cumulative incidence of SLE among patients was 5 % at

S. Ribero (✉)
Section of Dermatology, Department of Medical Sciences, University of Turin, Turin, Italy

Department of Twin Research and Genetic Epidemiology, King's College London, London, UK
e-mail: simone.ribero@unito.it

D. Lipsker
Dermatologic Clinic, University of Strasbourg, Strasbourg, France

L. Borradori
Department of Dermatology, University of Bern, Inselspital, Berne, Switzerland

D. Roccatello, L. Emmi (eds.), *Connective Tissue Disease: A Comprehensive Guide-Volume 1*, Rare Diseases of the Immune System 5,
DOI 10.1007/978-3-319-24535-5_7

5 years, 10 % at 10 years, 15 % at 15 years, 19 % at 20 years, and 23 % at 25 years after diagnosis, respectively [5]. In a population-based Swedish cohort study, Grönhagen et al. showed that the probabilities of developing SLE in the first and third year after CLE diagnosis are 12.1 % and 20.0 %, respectively. Vice versa, in 24 % of patients with newly diagnosed CLE, there is a current history of SLE [6]. However, the risk of developing SLE differs between subjects with acute CLE and those with localized discoid cutaneous lupus erythematosus (DLE). Therefore, the majority of patients with CLE will never develop any evidence for internal organ involvement.

The *Systemic Lupus International Collaborating Clinics* (SLICC) group recently revised the ACR-SLE classification criteria to improve their relevance. In the new classification, mucocutaneous signs again constituted 4 of 11 criteria used for SLE classification [7]. Among the SLE-specific skin manifestations, DLE is the most common, followed by subacute CLE (SCLE) and acute CLE (ACLE). The SLE nonspecific skin manifestations include Raynaud's phenomenon and, more rarely, non-scarring alopecia and cutaneous "vasculitis" [8].

7.2 Epidemiology of Cutaneous Involvement

Two recent population-based studies reported an incidence of 4 new cases of CLE per 100,000 inhabitants per year in Sweden and the USA [4]. Prevalence of CLE is about 70 cases per 100,000 persons. Discoid chronic CLE (CCLE), the most common subset of CLE, is found in 80 % of cases [5]. Fifteen percent of cases have SCLE, while less than 5 % of cases display other types of CLE, such as lupus profundus. DLE seems to be more common among African Americans [5, 9], whereas SCLE is found more frequently in Caucasians. Finally, there is good evidence indicating that SLE is more common in Asians and African Americans than in Caucasians [10, 11].

7.3 Pathogenesis

SLE is regarded as heterogeneous group of diseases that develop in genetically susceptible individuals. In those, environmental triggers are thought to lead to the activation of both innate and adaptive immune responses with a loss of tolerance to self-antigens. Development of autoantibodies, activation of the complement system, deficiency in the removal of immune complexes, and other inflammatory processes ultimately lead to cell and tissue injury [12]. Environmental factors include ultraviolet rays, viral infections, or chemicals. Sexual hormones as well as emotional neuroimmunomodulatory factors also contribute to the development of SLE.

CLE shares genetic abnormalities with SLE. Genome-wide association studies (GWASs) have provided evidence for the presence of distinct gene polymorphisms conferring disease susceptibility and which are associated with specific target organ damage [13].

Aberrant clearance of nucleic-acid-containing debris and immune complexes, excessive innate immune activation involving Toll-like receptors (TLRs) and type I interferons (IFNs), and abnormal T- and B-lymphocyte activation constitute pathways involved in disease pathogenesis [14]. For example, patients with SCLE, DLE, and SLE have distinct polymorphisms in the IFN-regulatory factor 5 (IRF5) gene. The latter appears to modulate pathways that mediate production of IFN-1 and the cellular response to IFN-1. In family studies, increased IFN-1 production was found to represent a genetic risk of developing SLE [15]. Type I IFN exerts many biologic effects, including activation of dendritic cells, promotion of the differentiation of monocytes into antigen-presenting cells and B cells into plasma cells, respectively, stimulation of the Th1 pathway, prevention of apoptosis of activated cytotoxic T cells, and suppression of regulatory T cells [16].

Failure to degrade genomic dsDNA represents another major pathway of immune activation as illustrated by TREX1-mediated autoimmune disease [17]. TREX1 contributes to the regulation of PARP1, a nuclear DNA repair enzyme involved in the DNA damage response. Hence, alterations in the function of TREX1 affecting PARP1 activity appear to favor either the development or the progression of autoimmune diseases [18].

UV irradiation (UVR) represents another important trigger for CLE. Patients with DLE, lupus erythematosus tumidus (LET), or SCLE are often photosensitive. Approximately half of CLE patients develop lesions upon exposure to UV light [19]. UV irradiation can result in altered keratinocyte morphology, expression of autoantigens on cell membranes, and cell apoptosis. UV radiation is able to trigger the release of cytokines and chemokines, such as IFN, TNF-α, IL-1, IL-10, and IL-17 from keratinocytes and other cells. The latter contribute to the initiation and amplification of the inflammatory process. In the early phase of UVR-induced CLE skin lesions, there is an accumulation of CD4+ T cells at the dermal-epidermal junction area, whereas in the late phase CD8+ T cells predominate [20]. CCR5 expression is increased, while CCR3 expression is decreased [21]. This shift to Th1-associated chemokine receptor profile might be a marker for the activity of CLE.

7.4 Classification of Cutaneous Involvement

The spectrum of cutaneous features occurring in the course of SLE is broad and heterogeneous. In a fundamental work of 1981, Gilliam and Sontheimer proposed a classification based on grouping together patients with similar clinical features and similar response to treatment [22]. This classification constituted a progress by identifying cutaneous lesions, which were specific for lupus erythematosus (LE). Specific LE lesions were defined by the presence of interface dermatitis, characterized histopathologically by the presence of vacuolization and necrosis of basal keratinocytes, basal basement membrane thickening, pigment incontinence, and a lymphocytic infiltrate at the dermo-epidermal junction. These specific lesions were classified in acute, subacute, or chronic lesions and were either localized, disseminated, or generalized [23]. This terminology turned out to be misleading and confusing and provided nightmares to generations of medical students, generalists, and specialists for several reasons. First, histologically, the lesions of CLE can often not be classified in one of the three acute, subacute, or chronic subsets. Second, interface dermatitis is also observed in other conditions, such as dermatomyositis, drug reactions, or graft-versus-host disease [24]. Third, entities potentially observed in SLE, such as papulonodular mucinosis of LE and Jessner's lymphocytic infiltrate of the skin/lupus tumidus or lupus panniculitis, cannot be classified histopathologically as specific LE lesions since they are lacking interface dermatitis. Finally, adjectives referring to *chronology* such as acute, subacute, or chronic are used to describe *morphologic* variants and are mixed with ill-defined extent scores such as localized or disseminated referring to *topography*. Ackerman regarded at the cutaneous changes associated with ACLE, SCLE, and CCLE as the result of the same pathological process [25]. The observed tissue damage may indeed vary according to the intensity of the process and its duration [26]. In this context, we recently proposed a novel classification of lesions of cutaneous signs in patients with LE [26]. This new simple classification is essentially based on findings clinical and from light microscopy studies (Table 7.1). The lesions are

Table 7.1 Classification of cutaneous signs in patients with lupus erythematosus (LE) [26]

I. "Specific" signs of LE	
Dermo-epidermal LE	Acute
	Subacute
	Chronic
	Indeterminate
	LE-specific vesiculobullous disease
Dermal LE	Jessner's lymphocytic infiltrate of the skin, tumid LE
	Reticular erythematous mucinosis (REM syndrome)
	Papulonodular mucinosis (of LE)
Hypodermal (subcutaneous) LE	Lupus panniculitis
II. Signs indicative of a thrombotic vasculopathy	Livedo (racemosa-like)
	Degos-like papules
	Atrophie blanche
	Non-infiltrated acrally located stellar purpura; splinter hemorrhage
	Cutaneous necrosis
	Anetoderma
	Thrombophlebitis
III. Neutrophilic cutaneous LE	Amicrobial pustulosis of skin folds
	Bullous LE
	Neutrophilic dermatosis of (occurring in) patients with LE
	Urticarial vasculitis of LE
IV. Others, of yet uncertain pathogenetic significance	

classified according to the level of the cellular infiltrate and tissue damage in the epidermis, dermis, and/or subcutis. Furthermore, we highlighted in this classification the clinical very relevant lesions, pointing to the presence of a thrombotic vasculopathy and to distinct inflammatory, neutrophilic-mediated reaction pattern. By taking into consideration these variables, all cutaneous lesions in LE can be easily classified in clinical practice.

7.4.1 Specific Signs of LE

7.4.1.1 Dermo-epidermal LE

Dermo-epidermal LE encompasses the classic acute, subacute, chronic, indeterminate, and vesiculobullous forms of LE.

Acute Cutaneous Lupus Erythematosus (ACLE)

ACLE presents most commonly as the classic "malar" or "butterfly" rash. The latter, which may occur transiently, can precede the onset of SLE by weeks or months and persist for months without evidence of systemic disease. There are typically small, discrete erythematous macules and papules in the central areas of the face, such as on the nose, chin, front, and then cheeks and malar regions (Fig. 7.1). Earlobes, scalp, and neck may also be involved. In contrast to dermatomyositis, nasolabial folds and periorbital regions are often spared. Lesions may become confluent, with scaling, erosions, and crusting. Severe facial edema may be observed, mimicking dermatomyositis [3, 27]. Erosions and ulcerations of the oral and/or nasal mucosa may complicate ACLE.

In generalized ACLE there are widespread erythematous macular and papular lesions, which are found on the lateral aspect of the arms, elbows, shoulders, knees, and trunk. Lesions predominate on UV-exposed areas. In contrast to

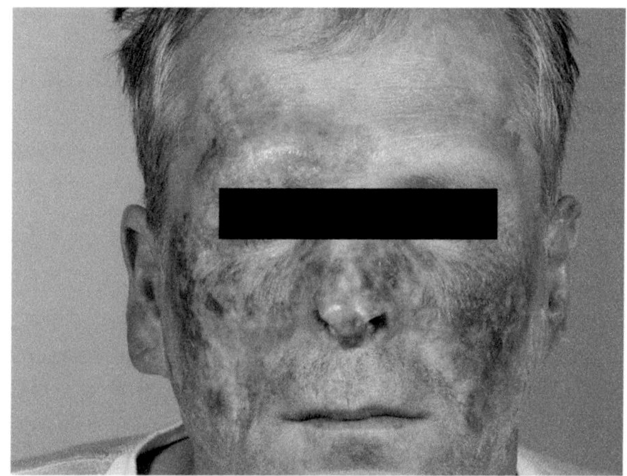

Fig. 7.1 Cutaneous lupus erythematosus. Patient with lesions on the cheeks and on the front. The butterfly distribution is typical for acute cutaneous lupus erythematosus. Nevertheless, the intensity and chronicity of the process already resulted in scarring and pigmentary and localized hyperkeratotic changes characteristic for chronic cutaneous lupus erythematosus

dermatomyositis, erythematous lesions are found between the metacarpophalyngeal joints and interphalangeal joints, whereas the knuckles are typically spared. Palms and soles may also be affected.

As ACLE lesions generally occur in the setting of evolving SLE, patients are often treated with steroids and/or immunosuppressors for other reasons such as nephropathy or cytopenia. ACLE then usually regresses without any sequel or leaving transient pigmentary changes, especially in dark-skin people.

Subacute Cutaneous Lupus Erythematosus (SCLE)

The lesions of SCLE are typically symmetrically distributed on the upper trunk, shoulders, V area of the neck, and arms. There are erythematous macules or papules which evolve into either scaly papulosquamous psoriasiform lesions or annular patches and plaques in, respectively, half of the patients (Fig. 7.2a). Annular lesions may enlarge and give rise to large polycyclic lesions. Mixed form with both annular and psoriasiform lesions is observed. Healing leads to postinflammatory hyper- and/or hypopigmentation, atrophic scarring grayish, and telangiectasias.

Discoid Chronic Cutaneous Lupus Erythematosus (DLE)

DLE is the most common form of CCLE. Lesions affect the face, the scalp, and/or the neck. In disseminated DLE, which occurs in less than 20 % of the cases, lesions spread below the neck. Significant involvement of the back of the hands mainly appears in smokers with a complement deficiency [28]. Patients with disseminated lesions of DLE are considered at increased risk for progression to SLE [29]. DLE is characterized by the presence of a coin-shaped, erythematous plaque of variable size associated with an adherent follicular hyperkeratosis (Fig. 7.3a). There is first an erythema with follicular hyperkeratosis, which then progress to atrophy, pigmentary changes, and scarring. The latter are persistent, contrarily to what is observed in ACLE and SCLE. On the scalp, depending on the severity and duration of the lesions, DLE can lead to scarring alopecia (Fig. 7.3b).

Indeterminant LE

Sontheimer used the term of indeterminant LE to describe long-lasting erythematous lesions and plaques without surface alteration, which however shows a LE typical interface dermatitis (Fig. 7.4) on histopathological evaluation. This type of lesions does not fit into the description of any of the classic subsets originally described.

LE-Specific Vesiculobullous Disease

Blistering may be a secondary phenomenon in severe CLE. If the interface changes at the dermo-epidermal junction are extensive, the epidermis detaches from the dermis. If the damage involves the entire epidermis and is widespread, the changes may clinically mimic Stevens-Johnson syndrome or toxic epidermal necrolysis.

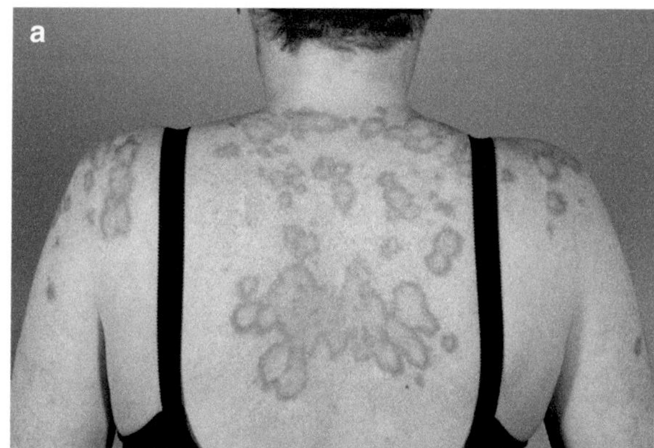

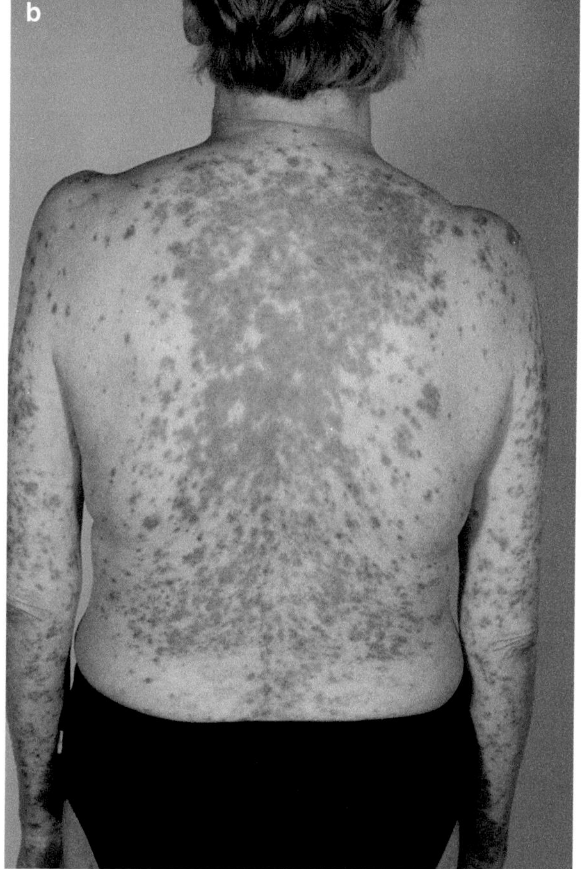

Fig. 7.2 (**a**) Typical lesions of subacute cutaneous lupus erythematosus with annular and polycyclic configuration. Note the more erythematous and scaly infiltrated borders with central clearing and pigmentary changes. (**b**) Drug-triggered subacute cutaneous lupus erythematosus. Widespread and confluent erythematous plaques on the neck, shoulders, back, and upper limbs. The lesions are very inflammatory and may result in blistering and erosions

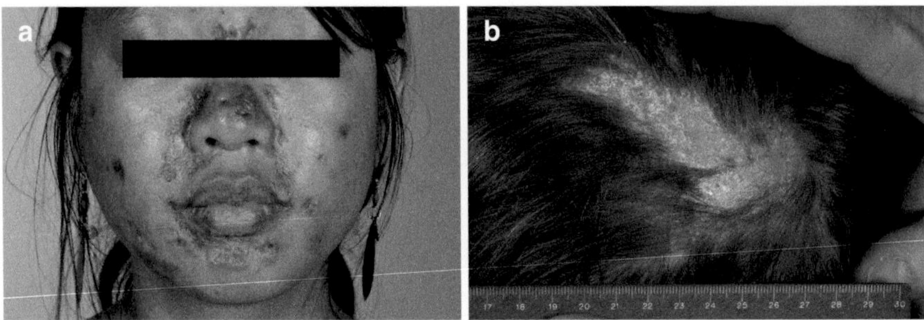

Fig. 7.3 (**a**) Discoid cutaneous lupus erythematosus. There are erythematous plaques with follicular hyperkeratosis, which have resulted in scarring and pigmentary changes. Certain lesions are still active and show an erythematous inflammatory rim. Note specific involvement of the lips and vermillion. (**b**) Discoid cutaneous lupus erythematosus of the scalp leading to scarring alopecia

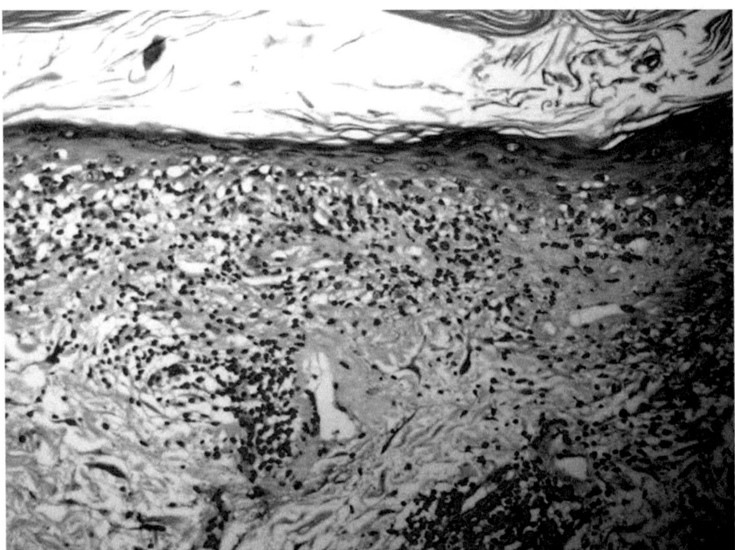

Fig. 7.4 Histopathology of a LE sample reveals under an interface dermatits a perivascular and periadnexal infitrate in the dermis. The epidermidis shows atrophy and a vacuolar basal cell degeneration with apoptotic keratinocytes and a marked thickening of the basement membrane. Dermis is interested by an edema with mucin deposition

7.4.1.2 Dermal LE

Dermal LE includes lupus tumidus and Jessner's lymphocytic infiltrate, as well as reticular erythematous mucinosis and the papulonodular mucinosis of LE. From a pathological point of view, these entities are characterized by a lymphocytic infiltrate and mucin deposition, respectively.

Lupus Erythematosus Tumidus and Jessner-Kanof Lymphocytic Infiltrate of the Skin

Lupus erythematosus tumidus (LET) differs from other variants of CLE. LET has been anecdotally associated with other types of CLE or even SLE. The distinction of LET from benign lymphocytic infiltrate of Jessner-Kanof is virtually impossible and often debated: they most likely represent the same condition [30]. LET is characterized by the development of papular lesions and plaques. The lesions may have a succulent, urticaria-like appearance, with reddish or violaceous smooth surface. The lesions, which may have an arc-shaped and annular appearance, are located on sun-exposed areas, such as the face, upper back, V area of the neck, and extensor aspects of the arms and shoulders [31].

Papulonodular Mucinosis

The cutaneous mucinoses are a heterogeneous group of disorders characterized by aberrant accumulation of glycosaminoglycans between collagen in the dermis [32]. The presence of mucin deposition is a relatively common histological finding in connective tissue diseases, such as LE and dermatomyositis [33]. However, mucin accumulation is rarely so abundant to produce clinically visible lesions. The latter appear as skin-colored or slightly red papules and nodules without epidermal changes. Since the first description by Gold [34], several cases of papulonodular mucinosis have been reported in combination with either SLE or DLE. It typically involves the trunk and upper extremities, while face and other areas of the body may also be affected [34].

7.4.1.3 Lupus Panniculitits (Lupus Profundus)

Lupus panniculitis (LEP) is another relatively rare but typical form of CLE characterized by the development of painful indurated dermo-hypodermal nodules or plaques that result in scarring and skin depression. It typically affects the thighs, the upper arms, or the cheek area of the face. LEP may occur either alone, in association with other forms of CLE, or in the course of SLE. The histological findings include lobular panniculitis with prominent lymphocytic infiltrate and mucin deposition between collagen bundles. Lymphocytic nuclear dust is observed. Differentiation of LEP from a panniculitis-like T-cell lymphoma is sometimes challenging.

7.4.2 Signs Indicative of a Thrombotic Vasculopathy

The spectrum of cutaneous lesions related and potentially reflecting a thrombotic vasculopathy is wide. It includes Degos' like papules, atrophie blanche, livedo (racemosa type), non-infiltrated acrally located stellar purpura, splinter hemorrhage, cutaneous necrosis, anetoderma, and thrombophlebitis.

Thrombotic vasculopathy represents an important and prognostic significant sign in SLE, since it may lead to devastating complications. In fact 5 years after initial diagnosis of SLE, thrombotic and ischemic events represent the main cause of morbidity and mortality [35]. Degos' disease, stellar purpura, splinter hemorrhage, and cutaneous necrosis with retiform purpura may constitute the initial presentation of an antiphospholipid syndrome. Its diagnosis has relevant prognostic and therapeutic implications [26]: affected patients may develop strokes, ischemic attacks, heart valve abnormalities, and hypertension [36, 37]. In these cases, the search and management of additional cardiovascular risk factors are essential.

7.4.2.1 Livedo Racemosa

Livedo racemosa is one of the most frequent dermatological manifestations in SLE-related antiphospholipid syndrome and is found in approximately 20 % of affected patients [38]. It is characterized by a bluish netlike non-infiltrated discoloration of the skin, which is usually observed in a suspended localization (the buttocks, thighs, trunk, or even face). In some cases, the livedo first affects the hands and feet and then spreads centripetally. In contrast to cutis marmorata, the fishnet has an *irregular* reticular patter with "*broken*" circles. In anti-phospholipid antibody-negative patients with Sneddon syndrome, the fishnet is larger and clinically more obvious. In SLE patients with livedo racemosa, additional causes have to be considered, including cholesterol thrombi and calciphylaxis.

7.4.2.2 Degos-Like Papules

Malignant atrophic papulosis (also called papulosis maligna or Köhlmeier-Degos' disease) presents with porcelain-white atrophic lesions surrounded by an erythematous rim of less than 1 cm in diameter [39]. Less than 200 cases have been described. The lesions occur on the trunk and upper extremities [40]. The palms, soles, scalp, and face are rarely involved. The early lesion is an erythematous papule, which becomes porcelain white, atrophic, and depressed in the center, while it is surrounded by a slightly elevated red, sometimes telangiectatic border. Histologically, there is a typical wedge-shaped connective tissue necrosis related to the thrombotic occlusion of the small arteries [41]. Patients with generalized disease develop severe neurologic, gastrointestinal, and ocular involvement related to ischemia and infarction. Lesions similar to those observed in Degos' disease may be found in a subset of SLE and are often located acrally.

7.4.2.3 Thrombophlebitis

SLE patients who have antiphospholipid antibodies have an increased risk of developing venous thromboembolism [42]. Thrombophlebitis usually occurs within 1 year after the onset of systemic disease, but may also antedate the diagnosis of SLE by several years. Several factors account for the occurrence of thrombophlebitis, such as slow chronic, disseminated intravascular coagulation, vasculitis-triggered platelet activation and aggregation, and prolonged immobility.

7.4.2.4 Anetoderma

Anetoderma is a relatively uncommon disorder characterized by a focal decrease or loss of elastic tissue in the dermis. Anetoderma presents as a localized herniated or punched-out skin lesions [43]. In practice, after exclusion of an infectious etiology, such as syphilis and tuberculosis, the diagnosis of anetoderma should prompt the exclusion of either a systemic immune-mediated disease, such as antiphospholipid syndrome, or another hypercoagulable state.

7.4.2.5 Vasculitis of the Skin

Based on a new revised international nomenclature, vasculitis associated with a systemic disease is defined using a prefix specifying the association [41]. The denomination of *lupus vasculitis* is nevertheless somehow confusing. First, it does not specify the type of vessels or of organs involved. Skin manifestations may be highly variable with palpable purpura, urticarial vasculitis, panarteritis nodosa-like dermo-hypodermal nodules, or ulcerations. Second, the vasculitis may be due to factors independent from SLE, such as drugs and infections [2]. It should be noted that ischemic microinfarcts of the fingertips and splinter hemorrhages are usually not related to vasculitis, but to coagulation defects. In the latter case, anticoagulation therapy may be effective.

7.4.3 Neutrophilic Cutaneous LE

In patients with SLE and other inflammatory and immune-mediated disorders, a significant infiltration of the skin by neutrophils may be occasionally observed. In addition to bullous LE and urticarial vasculitis, neutrophilic dermatoses such as amicrobial pustulosis of the skin folds, Sweet syndrome, and pyoderma gangrenosum may occur in patients with SLE [44, 45]. The striking accumulation of neutrophils in the skin reflects the activation of the innate immune response in SLE [46].

7.4.3.1 Amicrobial Pustulosis of Skin Folds

Amicrobial pustulosis of skin folds is characterized by the development of papules and pustules [47], with formation of erosive macerated areas and crusts. The lesions are symmetrically distributed and localized in large body folds such as the axilla and groins. Isolated pustules over the trunk and limbs also occur. External auditory meatus, nares, retroauricular flexures, and interdigital spaces can also be affected as well as the scalp. Histologically, there is spongiform subcorneal pustule formation together with a superficial and deep dermal infiltrate of neutrophils and lymphocytes [48].

7.4.3.2 Bullous LE

Bullous LE most often occurs in young African Americans with SLE [49]. Vesicles and bullae, which arise on clinically normal-appearing or inflamed skin, occur on sun-exposed areas or are widespread. Lesions may have an arciform or figurate distribution pattern and are accompanied by a burning sensation rather than pruritus [50]. In contrast to epidermolysis bullosa acquisita (EBA), in the vast majority of BSLE patients, scarring and milia formation do not occur and there is further a striking therapeutic response to dapsone [51]. Histologically, subepidermal vesicles, neutrophil microabscesses, nuclear "dust," and fibrin at the tips of dermal papillae are found. Direct immunofluorescence shows linear deposits of IgG and C3 along the epidermal basement membrane. Affected patients have circulating autoantibodies directed against type VII collagen [51]. Despite its classification as "neutrophilic cutaneous LE" [26], bullous LEs show thus the same immunopathological features of epidermolysis bullosa acquisita, an acquired autoimmune subepidermal bullous disease.

7.4.3.3 Neutrophilic Urticarial Dermatosis

Neutrophilic urticarial dermatosis (NUD) was recently delineated as a new entity within the spectrum of the neutrophilic dermatoses [52]. NUD is characterized by the development of widespread rose or red macules or slightly elevated papules vanishing within 24 h, associated with fever and joint pain. The histopathological findings consist of a dense perivascular and interstitial infiltrate of neutrophils with leukocytoclasia but without vasculitis. The development of NUD in a patient with known SLE is often mistaken as exacerbation of LE. The therapy of choice of NUD is either dapsone or colchicine rather than increasing immunosuppression [46].

7.4.4 Other Signs of Yet Uncertain Pathogenesis

There are number of conditions which are (or at least seem to be) epidemiologically more frequent in SLE. These include neurovascular conditions, such as Raynaud's syndrome, erythromelalgia, as well as granulomatous tissue reactions, such as interstitial granulomatous diseases and rheumatoid nodules. Other lesions such as eruptive fibromas may occur. Their significance in the context of SLE needs to be better assessed.

7.5 Drug Induced Cutaneous LE

Approximately 10 % of SLE cases can be related to drugs [53]. Drug-induced SLE usually occurs after several months or years of continuous therapy. Compared to "idiopathic" SLE, drug-induced SLE occurs in older people [54]. Arthralgias, myalgias, arthritis, fever, and serositis are often milder than in SLE, whereas malar rash, photosensitivity, and oral ulcers are less common [55]. Drugs involved in drug-induced SLE include typically procainamide, hydralazine, isoniazid, diltiazem, and minocycline [56].

It is important to distinguish drug-induced SLE from a relatively common form of CLE, drug-induced SCLE [57], in which the cutaneous involvement is the leading manifestation. Drug-induced SCLE presents with non-scarring annular or papulosquamous eruptions (Fig. 7.3b). Rarely, pityriasiform, bullous, erythrodermic, poikilodermatous, toxic epidermal necrolysis-like, and erythema multiforme-like presentations have been described [58]. Anti-Ro/SSA antibodies are often detectable [59].

Drug-induced SCLE has been associated with several drugs, including most frequently hydrochlorothiazide, antihypertensive agents, proton pomp inhibitors, and terbinafine. TNF-alpha antagonists are potential triggers of both drug-induced SCLE and DIL. Drug-triggered CLE is rare and typically reported in association with the intake of fluorouracil agents.

It has been proposed to divide drug-induced LE into systemic (DI-SLE) with or without cutaneous manifestations and DI-LE with predominant skin involvement. The latter comprises drug-induced SCLE (DI-SCLE) and drug-induced CCLE (DI-CCLE) [60].

In all cases, when a specific drug is considered as potential trigger for the development or aggravation of cutaneous or systemic manifestations of LE, it should be discontinued whenever possible [61].

7.6 Photosensitivity

The original SLE classification of the ACR included also photosensitivity as criterion [62]. "Photosensitivity" was defined as a "skin rash as a result of unusual reaction to sunlight by patient history or physician observation." Unfortunately, this definition is not precise enough. A variety of other benign conditions are associated with light sensitivity, such as polymorphous light eruption, photoallergic contact dermatitis, solar urticaria, or porphyrias. The latter, according to the clinical context, may be wrongly classified as SLE. Furthermore, in patients with CLE, inaccurate assessment of photosensitivity results in an overestimation of SLE [63]. Some authors defined photosensitivity as an induction of skin lesions following sun exposure, while others also considered sunburn and aggravation of the disease in the spring and summer times [64]. Moreover, UV light exposure is not only able to induce and exacerbate lesions of almost all subtypes of CLE [65], but can also trigger significant organ involvement in SLE, including lupus nephritis [66].

The frequency of photosensitivity in the different subtypes of CLE has been variably estimated. This is also due to the lack of well-defined criteria for photosensitivity. Photosensitivity has been reported in 27–100 % of patients with SCLE and in 25–90 % of patients with DLE [67].

Photoprovocation tests with different wavelengths are useful to assess the photosensitivity in patients with CLE. UVB, UVA2, and UVA1 can induce de novo or exacerbate skin manifestations. When compared to other photodermatoses, such as polymorphous light eruption or porphyrias, UV-induced LE-specific lesions usually do not develop immediately, but after 1 week, and persist up to 2 months. For this reason, a number of LE patients do not recognize the association between UV exposure and the induction of skin lesions.

7.7 CLASI, a Useful Instrument to Assess Cutaneous Activity

The Cutaneous Lupus Erythematosus Disease Area and Severity Index (CLASI) is a relatively novel tool that quantifies disease activity and damage in CLE. The activity score is based on the degree of erythema, scale, mucous membrane lesions, and non-scarring alopecia. Unlike other outcome measures, CLASI scores are not based solely on the area of involved skin. Instead, parts of the body that are most visible are weighted more heavily than those that are usually covered [68]. The CLASI has been shown to have good content validity, addressing the most relevant aspects of CLE [69].

CLASI has been found to correlate with the "physicians" and "patients" global assessment of disease activity on a 0–10 visual analog scale [69]. Although the CLASI was firstly designed as an instrument useful in therapeutic trials, it can easily and rapidly be employed in clinical practise.

7.8 Treatment of Cutaneous Lupus Erythematosus: Basic Principles

The treatment of LE is covered in depth in Chaps. 17 and 18. The basic principles of treating cutaneous LE can be summarized as follows. All patients should use broad-spectrum UVA/UVB sunscreen with SPF > 30. Furthermore, the patients should be informed about appropriate protective measures (sun avoidance, clothing, use of hats or wigs). The first-line treatment of CLE lesions includes antimalarials (mainly hydroxychloroquine and less frequently chloroquine) [4, 70, 71]. Topical steroids or calcineurin inhibitors can be used for isolated lesions in patients without any signs of systemic disease as well as in combination with antimalarials or other drugs. The choice of the second-line treatment varies throughout Europe. Patients who are refractory to antimalarials are usually treated with either methotrexate, azathioprine, or mycophenolate mofetil [71]. Other options include dapsone, acitretin, or thalidomide [71]. Oral steroids and other immunosuppressants are usually not used to treat specific LE lesions, except in severe cases with widespread lesions and risk of significant scarring in specific situations. Photopheresis, belimumab, and rituximab should only be used by very experienced clinicians in exceptional situations [71]. Cessation of cigarette smoking should always be recommended [72].

Conclusions

The spectrum of cutaneous manifestations occurring in SLE is broad. Since they can constitute the initial manifestation of the disease, its prompt recognition is important for proper management and workup of affected patients. Furthermore, the development of distinct cutaneous signs, such as thombo-occlusive and vascular complications, has significant prognostic and therapeutic implications. In practice, the first step is to clinically and histologically differentiate between LE-specific and LE-nonspecific lesions [22]. If CLE is diagnosed, activity and damage should be assessed using the CLASI. Appropriate clinical and laboratory exams should be performed to exclude extracutaneous involvement. The patient should be correctly informed about the cutaneous disease and the potential development of SLE – even in the absence of extracutaneous findings. It is important to systematically consider the possibility of drug triggers, which should be eliminated. The patient should be aware of the aggravating factors, such as smoking and sun exposure, and be systematically instructed about sun protective measures, such as use of sunscreens, sun avoidance, and use of appropriate clothing and hats.

References

1. Obermoser G, Sontheimer RD, Zelger B (2010) Overview of common, rare and atypical manifestations of cutaneous lupus erythematosus and histopathological correlates. Lupus 19(9):1050–1070
2. Rothfield N, Sontheimer RD, Bernstein M (2006) Lupus erythematosus: systemic and cutaneous manifestations. Clin Dermatol 24(5):348–362
3. Werth VP (2005) Clinical manifestations of cutaneous lupus erythematosus. Autoimmun Rev 4(5):296–302
4. Kuhn A, Ruland V, Bonsmann G (2011) Cutaneous lupus erythematosus: update of therapeutic options part I. J Am Acad Dermatol 65(6):179–193
5. Durosaro O, Davis MD, Reed KB, Rohlinger AL (2009) Incidence of cutaneous lupus erythematosus, 1965–2005: a population-based study. Arch Dermatol 145(3):249–253
6. Gronhagen CM, Fored CM, Granath F, Nyberg F (2011) Cutaneous lupus erythematosus and the association with systemic lupus erythematosus: a population-based cohort of 1088 patients in Sweden. Br J Dermatol 164(6):1335–1341
7. Petri M, Orbai A-M, Alarcón GS, Gordon C, Merrill JT, Fortin PR, Bruce IN, Isenberg D, Wallace DJ, Nived O, Sturfelt G, Ramsey-Goldman R, Bae SC, Hanly JG, Sánchez-Guerrero J, Clarke A, Aranow C, Manzi S, Urowitz M, Gladman D, Kalunian K, Costner M, Werth VP, Zoma A, Bernatsky S, Ruiz-Irastorza G, Khamashta MA, Jacobsen S, Buyon JP, Maddison P, Dooley MA, van Vollenhoven RF, Ginzler E, Stoll T, Peschken C, Jorizzo JL, Callen JP, Lim SS, Fessler BJ, Inanc M, Kamen DL, Rahman A, Steinsson K, Franks AG Jr, Sigler L, Hameed S, Fang H, Pham N, Brey R, Weisman MH, McGwin G Jr, Magder LS et al (2012) Derivation and validation of the Systemic Lupus International Collaborating Clinics classification criteria for systemic lupus erythematosus. Arthritis Rheum 64(8):2677–2686
8. Grönhagen CM, Gunnarsson I, Svenungsson E, Nyberg F (2010) Cutaneous manifestations and serological findings in 260 patients with systemic lupus erythematosus. Lupus 19(10):1187–1194
9. Fernández M, Alarcón GS, Calvo-Alén J, Andrade R, McGwin G Jr, Vilá LM, Reveille JD, LUMINA Study Group (2007) A multiethnic, multicenter cohort of patients with systemic lupus erythematosus (SLE) as a model for the study of ethnic disparities in SLE. Arthritis Rheum 57(4):576–584
10. Chiu Y-M, Lai C-H (2010) Nationwide population-based epidemiologic study of systemic lupus erythematosus in Taiwan. Lupus 19(10):1250–1255
11. Lee HJ, Sinha AA (2006) Cutaneous lupus erythematosus: understanding of clinical features, genetic basis, and pathobiology of disease guides therapeutic strategies. Autoimmunity 39(6):433–444
12. Freire EAM, Souto LM, Ciconelli RM (2011) Medidas de avaliação em lúpus eritematoso sistêmico (Assessment measures in systemic lupus erythematosus). Rev Bras Reumatol 51:75–80
13. Liu Z, Davidson A (2012) Taming lupus-a new understanding of pathogenesis is leading to clinical advances. Nat Med 18(6):871–882
14. Deng y, Tsao BP (2010) Genetic susceptibility to systemic lupus erythematosus in the genomic era. Nat Rev Rheumatol 6(12):683–692

15. Niewold TB, Hua J, Lehman TJ, Harley JB, Crow MK (2007) High serum IFN-alpha activity is a heritable risk factor for systemic lupus erythematosus. Genes Immun 8:492–502
16. Jacob N, Stohl W (2011) Cytokine disturbances in systemic lupus erythematosus. Arthritis Res Ther 13:228
17. Tüngler V, Silver RM, Walkenhorst H, Günther C, Lee-Kirsch MA (2012) Inherited or de novo mutation affecting aspartate 18 of TREX1 results in either familial chilblain lupus or Aicardi-Goutières syndrome. Br J Dermatol 167:212–214
18. Miyazaki T, Kim YS, Yoon J, Wang H, Suzuki T, Morse H (2014) The 3′-5′ DNA exonuclease TREX1 directly interacts with poly(ADP-ribose) polymerase-1 (PARP1) during the DNA damage response. J Biol Chem 289(47):32548–32558
19. Kuhn A, Wozniacka A, Szepietowski J, Gläser R, Lehmann P, Haust M, Sysa-Jedrzejowska A, Reich A, Oke V, Hügel R, Calderon C, de Vries DE, Nyberg F et al (2011) Photoprovocation in cutaneous lupus erythematosus: a multicenter study evaluating a standardized protocol. J Invest Dermatol 131:1622–1630
20. Kind P, Lehmann P, Plewig G (1993) Phototesting in lupus erythematosus. J Invest Dermatol 100:53S–57S
21. Freutel S, Gaffal E, Zahn S, Bieber T, Tüting T, Wenzel J (2011) Enhanced CCR5+/CCR3+ T helper cell ratio in patients with active cutaneous lupus erythematosus. Lupus 20(12):1300–1304
22. Gilliam JN, Sontheimer RD (1981) Distinctive cutaneous subsets in the spectrum of lupus erythematosus. J Am Acad Dermatol 4(4):471–475
23. Gilliam JN, Sontheimer RD (1982) Skin manifestations of SLE. Clin Rheum Dis 8(1):207–218
24. Sontheimer RD (2009) Lichenoid tissue reaction/interface dermatitis: clinical and histological perspectives. J Invest Dermatol 129(5):1088–1099
25. Ackerman AB, Boer A, Benin B, Gottlieb GJ (2005) Histopathological diagnosis of inflammatory skin diseases, 3rd edn. Ardor Scribendi, New York
26. Lipsker D (2010) The need to revisit the nosology of cutaneous lupus erythematosus: the current terminology and morphologic classification of cutaneous LE: difficult, incomplete and not always applicable. Lupus 19(9):1047–1049
27. Kuhn A, Lehmann P, Ruzicka T (2004) Clinical manifestations of cutaneous lupus erythematosus. In: Kuhn A, Lehmann P, Ruzicka T (eds) Cutaneous lupus erythematosus. Springer, Heidelberg, pp 59–92
28. Boeckler P, Milea M, Meyer A, Uring-Lambert B, Heid E, Hauptmann G, Cribier B, Lipsker D (2005) The combination of complement deficiency and cigarette smoking as risk factor for cutaneous lupus erythematosus in men; a focus on combined C2/C4 deficiency. Br J Dermatol 152(2):265–270
29. Tebbe B, Mansmann U, Wollina U, Auer-Grumbach P, Licht-Mbalyohere A, Arsenmeier M, Orfanos CE (1997) Markers in cutaneous lupus erythematosus indicating systemic involvement. A multicenter study on 296 patients. Acta Derm Venereol 77:305–308
30. Rémy-Leroux V, Léonard F, Lambert D, Wechsler J, Cribier B, Thomas P, Adamski H, Marguery MC, Aubin F, Leroy D, Bernard P (2008) Comparison of histopathologic-clinical characteristics of Jessner's lymphocytic infiltration of the skin and lupus erythematosus tumidus: multicenter study of 46 cases. J Am Acad Dermatol 58(2):217–223
31. Kuhn A, Richter-Hintz D, Oslislo C, Ruzicka T, Megahed M, Lehmann P (2000) Lupus erythematosus tumidus e a neglected subset of cutaneous lupus erythematosus: report of 40 cases. Arch Dermatol 136:1033–1041
32. Rongioletti F, Rebora A (1991) The new cutaneous mucinoses. A review with an up-to-date classification of cutaneous mucinoses. J Am Acad Dermatol 24:265–270
33. Ortize VG, Krishnan RS, Chen LL, Hsu S (2004) Papulonodular mucinosis in systemic lupus erythematosus. Dermatol Online J 10:16
34. Gold SC (1954) An unusual papular eruption associated with lupus erythematosus. Br J Dermatol 66:429–433

35. Cervera R, Khamashta MA, Font J, Sebastiani GD, Gil A, Lavilla P, Mejía JC, Aydintug AO, Chwalinska-Sadowska H, de Ramón E, Fernández-Nebro A, Galeazzi M, Valen M, Mathieu A, Houssiau F, Caro N, Alba P, Ramos-Casals M, Ingelmo M, Hughes GR, European Working Party on Systemic Lupus Erythematosus (2003) Morbidity and mortality in systemic lupus erythematosus during a 10-year period: a comparison of early and late manifestations in a cohort of 1,000 patients. Medicine (Baltimore) 82(5):299–308
36. Francès C, Piette JC (2000) The mystery of Sneddon syndrome: relationship with antiphospholipid syndrome and systemic lupus erythematosus. J Autoimmun 15(2):139–143
37. Englert HJ, Loizou S, Derue GG, Walport MJ, Hughes GR (1989) Clinical and immunologic features of livedo reticularis in lupus: a case-control study. Am J Med 87:408–410
38. Francès C, Niang S, Laffitte E, Pelletier F, Costedoat N, Piette JC (2005) Dermatologic manifestations of the antiphospholipid syndrome: two hundred consecutive cases. Arthritis Rheum 52(6):1785–1793
39. Ball E, Newburger A, Ackerman AB (2003) Degos' disease: a distinctive pattern of disease, chiefly of lupus erythematosus, and not a specific disease per se. Am J Dermatopathol 25(4):308–320
40. Theodoridis A, Makrantonaki E, Zouboulis CC (2013) Malignant atrophic papulosis (Köhlmeier-Degos disease) – a review. Orphanet J Rare Dis 8:10
41. Lipsker D (2012) In: Goldsmith L, Katz S, Gilchrest B, Paller A, Leffell D, Wolff K (eds) Fitzpatrick's dermatology in general medicine. McGraw-Hill, New York, pp 2072–2076, Malignant atrophic papulosis (Degos disease)
42. Wahl DG, Guillemin F, de Maistre E, Perret-Guillaume C, Lecompte T, Thibaut G (1998) Meta-analysis of the risk of venous thrombosis in individuals with antiphospholipid antibodies without underlying autoimmune disease or previous thrombosis. Lupus 7(1):15–22
43. Venencie PY, Winkelmann RK (1985) Monoclonal antibody studies in the skin lesions of patients with anetoderma. Arch Dermatol 121:747–749
44. Gusdorf L, Bessis D, Lipsker D (2014) Lupus erythematosus and neutrophilic urticarial dermatosis: a retrospective study of 7 patients. Medicine (Baltimore) 93(29):e351
45. Mitsias DI, Kapsogeorgou EK, Moutsopoulos HM (2006) Sjögren's syndrome: why autoimmune epithelitis? Oral Dis 12:523–532
46. Lipsker D, Saurat JH (2008) Neutrophilic cutaneous lupus erythematosus. At the edge between innate and acquired immunity? Dermatology 216(4):283–286
47. Marzano AV, Ramoni S, Caputo R (2008) Amicrobial pustulosis of the folds. Report of 6 cases and a literature review. Dermatology 216(4):305–311
48. Lee HY, Pelivani N, Beltraminelli H, Hegyi I, Yawalkar N, Borradori L (2011) Amicrobial pustulosis-like rash in a patient with Crohn's disease under anti-TNF-alpha blocker. Dermatology 222:304–310
49. Fujimoto W, Hamada T, Yamada J, Matsuura H, Iwatsuki K (2005) Bullous systemic lupus erythematosus as an initial manifestation of SLE. J Dermatol 32:1021–1027
50. Camisa C, Sharma HM (1983) Vesiculobullous systemic lupus erythematosus. J Am Acad Dermatol 9:924–933
51. Hall RP, Lawley TJ, Smith HR, Katz SI (1982) Bullous eruption of systemic lupus erythematosus. Dramatic response to dapsone therapy. Ann Intern Med 197:165–170
52. Kieffer C, Cribier B, Lipsker D (2009) Neutrophilic urticarial dermatosis; a variant of neutrophilic urticaria strongly associated with systemic disease. Report of 9 new cases and review of the literature. Medicine (Baltimore) 88:23–31
53. Vedove CD, Del Giglio M, Schena D, Girolomoni G (2009) Drug-induced lupus erythematosus. Arch Dermatol Res 301:99–105
54. Xiao X, Chang C (2014) Diagnosis and classification of drug-induced autoimmunity (DIA). J Autoimmun 48–49:66–72
55. Katz U, Zandman-Goddard G (2010) Drug-induced lupus: an update. Autoimmun Rev 10:46–50
56. Fritzler MJ (1994) Drugs recently associated with lupus syndromes. Lupus 3(6):455–459

57. Chlebus E, Wolska H, Blaszczyk M, Jablonska S (1998) Subacute cutaneous lupus erythematosus versus systemic lupus erythematosus: diagnostic criteria and therapeutic implications. J Am Acad Dermatol 38(3):405–412
58. Marzano AV, Lazzari R, Polloni I, Crosti C, Fabbri P, Cugno M (2011) Drug-induced subacute cutaneous lupus erythematosus: evidence for differences from its idiopathic counterpart. Br J Dermatol 165(2):335–341
59. Sontheimer RD, Maddison PJ, Reichlin M, Jordon RE, Stastny P, Gilliam JN (1982) Serologic and HLA associations in subacute cutaneous lupus erythematosus, a clinical subset of lupus erythematosus. Ann Intern Med 97:664–667
60. Marzano AV, Vezzoli P, Crosti C (2009) Drug-induced lupus: an update on its dermatologic aspects. Lupus 18:935–940
61. Rubin RL (2015) Drug-induced lupus. Expert Opin Drug Saf 2:1–18
62. Hochberg MC (1997) Updating the American College of Rheumatology revised criteria for the classification of systemic lupus erythematosus. Arthritis Rheum 40(9):1725
63. Kuhn A, Wenzel J, Weyd H (2014) Photosensitivity, apoptosis, and cytokines in the pathogenesis of lupus erythematosus: a critical review. Clin Rev Allergy Immunol 47(2):148–162
64. Nyberg F, Hasan T, Puska P, Stephansson E, Häkkinen M, Ranki A, Ros AM (1997) Occurrence of polymorphous light eruption in lupus erythematosus. Br J Dermatol 136(2):217–221
65. Kim A, Chong BF (2013) Photosensitivity in cutaneous lupus erythematosus. Photodermatol Photoimmunol Photomed 29(1):4–11
66. Schmidt E, Tony H-P, Bröcker E-B, Kneitz C (2007) Sun-induced life-threatening lupus nephritis. Ann N Y Acad Sci 1108:35–40
67. Kuhn A, Ruland V, Bonsmann G (2010) Photosensitivity, phototesting, and photoprotection in cutaneous lupus erythematosus. Lupus 19(9):1036–1046
68. Klein R, Moghadam-Kia S, LoMonico J, Okawa J, Coley C, Taylor L, Troxel AB, Werth VP (2011) Development of the CLASI as a tool to measure disease severity and responsiveness to therapy in cutaneous lupus erythematosus. Arch Dermatol 147(2):203–208
69. Bonilla-Martinez ZL, Albrecht J, Troxel AB, Taylor L, Okawa J, Dulay S, Werth VP (2008) The cutaneous lupus erythematosus disease area and severity index: a responsive instrument to measure activity and damage in patients with cutaneous lupus erythematosus. Arch Dermatol 144(2):173–180
70. Okon LG, Werth VP (2013) Cutaneous lupus erythematosus: diagnosis and treatment. Best Pract Res Clin Rheumatol 27(3):391–404
71. Kuhn A, Ruland V, Bonsmann G (2011) Cutaneous lupus erythematosus: update of therapeutic options part II. J Am Acad Dermatol 65(6):e195–e213
72. Kuhn A, Sigges J, Biazar C, Ruland V, Landmann A, Amler S, Bonsmann G, WUSCLE coauthors (2014) Influence of smoking on disease severity and antimalarian therapy in cutaneous lupus erythematosus: analysis of 1002 patients from the EUSCLE database. Br J Dermatol 171:571–579

8 Lupus Nephritis

Antonello Pani, Andrea Angioi, and Franco Ferrario

Systemic lupus erythematosus (SLE) is a chronic autoimmune disease defined, as suggested by J.S. Cameron, by "its clinical picture" typically dominated by proteiform signs and symptoms, together with autoantibodies directed against one or more nuclear components, in particular, double-stranded DNA Ab (dsDNA). Lupus nephritis (LN) consists in kidney involvement in SLE. Glomerular inflammation dominates the histological picture, but any renal structure may be involved to different degrees.

8.1 Epidemiology of Kidney Involvement

After more than 40 years of investigation, and despite the huge amount of available data on the epidemiology of SLE (and LN), no firm conclusions have been reached, and results from different studies are heterogeneous, thus leading to a certain degree of confusion. Several variables should be considered when predicting the individual and collective risk of developing LN and SLE, in particular age, sex, geographic location, income, ethnicity, comorbidities, and genetics.

The incidence of SLE is now at least threefold higher as compared to estimates made in the 1950s [1]; the reasons underlying this phenomenon are still not fully understood. Similarly, the incidence of LN in the United States has progressively

A. Pani • A. Angioi
Division of Nephrology and Dialysis, Azienda Ospedaliera Giuseppe Brotzu, Piazzale Ricchi n 1, Cagliari 09131, Italy
e-mail: antonellopani@aob.it; andrea.angioi@gmail.com

F. Ferrario (✉)
Department of Pathology, University Milano-Bicocca, San Gerardo Hospital, Via Pergolesi 33, Monza 20900, Italy
e-mail: f.ferrario@hsgerardo.org

D. Roccatello, L. Emmi (eds.), *Connective Tissue Disease: A Comprehensive Guide-Volume 1*, Rare Diseases of the Immune System 5, DOI 10.1007/978-3-319-24535-5_8

increased to 6.9 per 100,000 adults with a prevalence of 30.9 per 100,000 [2]. When subclinical LN is excluded, LN is clinically detectable in 3.1–76.1 % of individuals with a diagnosis of SLE [3, 4].

Until the 1970s, the overall survival rates of SLE with LN were comparable to those of patients with some solid tumors and ranged from 10 to 50 % 5 years after diagnosis. Overall survival in SLE has now progressively improved and has been reported to be as high as 91.4 % in recent studies [5, 6]. These data are probably influenced by the progressive inclusion of subjects with benign disease (previously not recognized or not identified by applied diagnostic tests). However, despite the recent decrease in overall mortality rate (estimated at 1.4 % and 1.6 % at 5 and 10 years, respectively), the annual incidence of patients that progress to end-stage renal disease (ESRD) because of LN is still high, i.e., 4.9 patients per million/year [7]. Indeed, even an early therapeutic approach is often not sufficient to prevent the decline of renal function in some patients with SLE.

8.1.1 Risk factors and development of LN

Increasing use of oral contraception and estrogen replacement therapy and exposure to ultraviolet radiation, pollution, and smoke are some of the potential factors underlying the increased prevalence of LN. Female gender is an independent risk factor for SLE, since women are six times more likely to be affected than men [2]; women are also more prone to show renal involvement. However, males are likely to develop more aggressive disease, leading to increased rates of ESRD [2]. Ethnicity is an important factor that weighs on incidence rates and prognosis and thus on the response of LN treatment. The LUMINA study, a multiethnic cohort of American individuals affected with SLE, showed that Hispanic and African-American individuals were more likely to develop LN (60.6 and 68.9 %, respectively) [8] compared to other ethnicities. In 2004, the GLADEL cohort confirmed these observations, showing that the cumulative incidence of renal involvement in SLE patients was 43.6 % in Caucasians, 58.3 % in Mestizos, and 55.3 % in African-Latin Americans 32 months after diagnosis [9]. Socioeconomic factors have been found to impact on the onset of LN [10]. The LUMINA analysis showed that the risk of developing LN in individuals having the same ethnic roots but with relevant sociopolitical differences, such as Puerto Rican Hispanics (US citizens) and Texan Hispanics (recent immigrants), was higher for those in low income groups [10]. Notably, alcohol intake, smoking, and recreational drug use do not appear to affect the onset of LN [8].

8.2 Clinical Features of LN

8.2.1 Clinical Renal Syndrome at Presentation

LN is the first manifestation in 20–25 % of patients with SLE. In general, LN develops within 5 years of SLE diagnosis. Clinical manifestations may be identified by six patterns: (1) urinary abnormalities, (2) nephritic syndrome, (3) nephrotic syndrome, (4) acute renal failure, (5) chronic renal failure, and (6) rapidly progressive renal failure.

These six patterns may be concurrent, and together they define four main clinical presentations:

(a) Mild urinary abnormalities (microscopic hematuria, inflammatory casts, sterile leukocyturia) with or without mild to moderate proteinuria. These patients may have normal urine sediment most of the time; therefore, to avoid missing this subtle presentation of LN, urine analysis should be performed every 6–12 months in all SLE patients.
(b) Nephrotic (proteinuria >3.5 g/day, serum albumin <2.5 g/dl) or nephritic syndrome (sometimes together) and reduced renal function. They are often concomitant with systemic flares and suggest proliferative ± class V LN.
(c) Acute renal failure may be the first manifestation of the disease. Although infrequent, diffuse glomerular thrombosis induced by antiphospholipid antibodies may be observed. Acute interstitial nephritis should be considered, as should bilateral renal vein thrombosis in patients with nephrotic syndrome.
(d) Rapidly progressive renal failure may be an expression of focal segmental or, more frequently, diffuse proliferative LN with segmental necrosis and extracapillary proliferation.

8.2.2 Clinical Renal Course During Follow-Up

The clinical picture during follow-up can be addressed and classified into three groups:

1. New onset or persistence of mild urinary abnormalities after induction therapy. Despite mild or silent clinical activity, ESRD may occur because of the persistence of smoldering immunological activity.
2. Moderate to severe proteinuria with or without nephrotic syndrome, paired with active urinary sediment. Hypertension is usually concomitant. This pattern has poor prognostic value, and ESRD is observed in 50 % of individuals after 10 years. Similarly as in the previous pattern, mild to moderate serological activity and systemic disease are usually observed, but with more aggressive features of systemic involvement, nephrotic syndrome, hypertension, and renal failure. These individuals have poor overall and renal survival rates after 2 years of follow-up due to the challenges related to controlling the systemic and renal disease.
3. The last group has an aggressive clinical course defined by resistant hypertension with malignant features (papilledema), encephalopathy, heart failure, and rapidly progressive renal failure. Thrombotic microangiopathy (TMA) is the most worrisome event [11–13].

8.3 Morphological Features

Approximately 50 % of patients with SLE develop LN, which increases the risk of renal failure, cardiovascular disease, and death. EULAR (European League Against Rheumatism), ACR (American College of Rheumatology), and ECS (European consensus statement on the terminology for the management of LN) have issued guidelines to optimize the management of LN [14–17].

8.3.1 Indications for Renal Biopsy in SLE

Any sign of renal involvement – in particular, urinary findings such as reproducible proteinuria ≥0.5 g/24 h, especially with glomerular hematuria and/or cellular casts – should be an indication for renal biopsy. Renal biopsy is indispensable as clinical, serological, or laboratory tests cannot accurately predict renal biopsy findings.

8.3.2 Pathological Assessment of Kidney Biopsy

The use of the International Society of Nephrology/Renal Pathology Society (ISN/RPS) classification (2003) is recommended, including an assessment of active and chronic glomerular and tubulointerstitial changes and of vascular lesions associated with antiphospholipid antibodies/syndrome [18]. The classification of LN has evolved over the past 40 years.

The current classification, which was proposed in 1982 and revised in 1995, reflects the understanding of the pathogenesis of the various forms of renal injury in SLE nephritis. The ISN/RPS classification introduces several important modifications, mainly concerning quantitative and qualitative differences in order to distinguish between class III and IV lesions. Glomerular immune deposits attributable to LN, as detected by immunofluorescence (IF), almost always contain dominant polyclonal IgG, as well as C3 and, in most instances, C1q, with variable co-deposits of IgA and IgM. The role of electron microscopy (EM) in the diagnosis and classification of LN cannot be underestimated and may be essential in some cases [19].

Class I

Class I (Fig. 8.1) is defined as mesangial immune deposits identified by IF and/or EM (Fig. 8.2), without glomerular alterations seen by light microscopy.

Class II

Class II (Fig. 8.3) is defined as mesangial proliferative LN characterized by any degree of mesangial hypercellularity (i.e., three or more mesangial cells per mesangial area in a 3 μm thick section) associated with mesangial immune deposits. IF or EM may show rare, isolated small immune deposits involving the peripheral capillary walls in some class II samples.

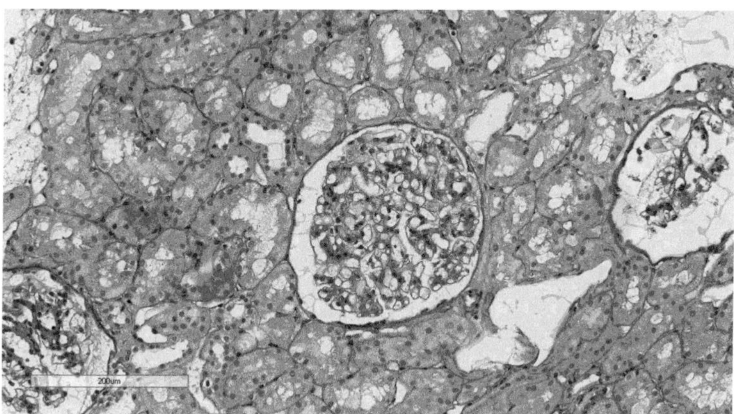

Fig. 8.1 Minimal mesangial LN (class I)

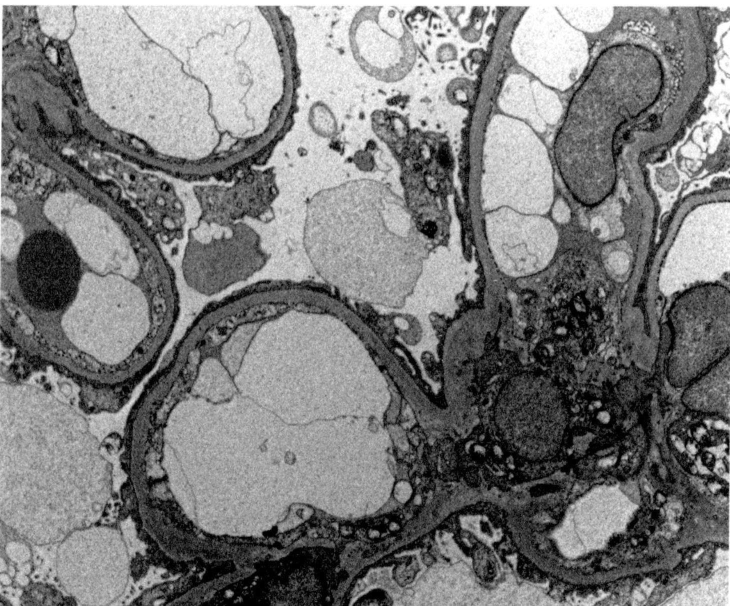

Fig. 8.2 Mesangial immune deposits identified by EM

Class III

Class III (Fig. 8.4) is defined as focal LN involving <50 % of all glomeruli. Affected glomeruli usually display segmental endocapillary proliferative lesions or inactive glomerular scars, with or without capillary wall necrosis and crescents, with subendothelial deposits. A specific diagnosis of combined class III and class V LN requires membranous involvement of at least 50 % of the glomerular capillary surface area in at least 50 % of glomeruli, as shown by light microscopy or IF.

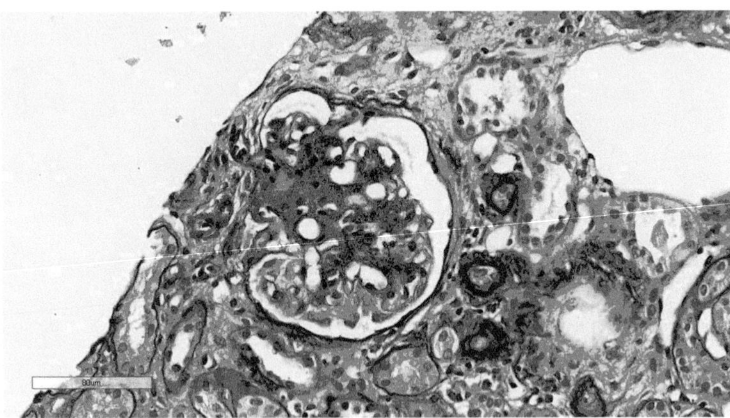

Fig. 8.3 Mesangial proliferative LN (class II)

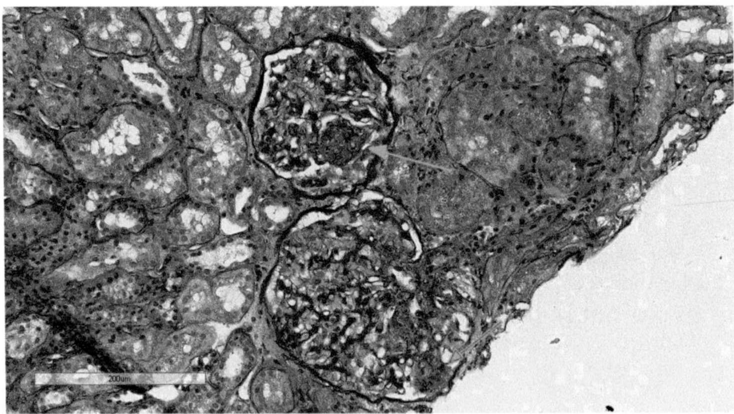

Fig. 8.4 Focal and segmental proliferative glomerulonephritis (class III)

Class IV

Class IV is defined as diffuse LN involving 50 % or more of glomeruli in the biopsy sample. In the affected glomeruli, the lesions as described below may be segmental, defined as sparing at least half of the glomerular tuft, or global, defined as involving more than half of the glomerular tuft. This class is subdivided into diffuse segmental LN (class IV-S) (Fig. 8.5) when <50 % of the involved glomeruli have segmental lesions and diffuse global LN (class IV-G) (Fig. 8.6) when >50 % of the involved glomeruli show global lesions. Class IV-S typically shows segmental endocapillary proliferation encroaching upon capillary lumen with or without necrosis and may be superimposed upon similarly distributed glomerular scars. Class IV-G is characterized by diffuse and global endocapillary, extracapillary, or mesangiocapillary proliferation or widespread wire loops. A diagnosis of combined class IV and class V is warranted only if subepithelial

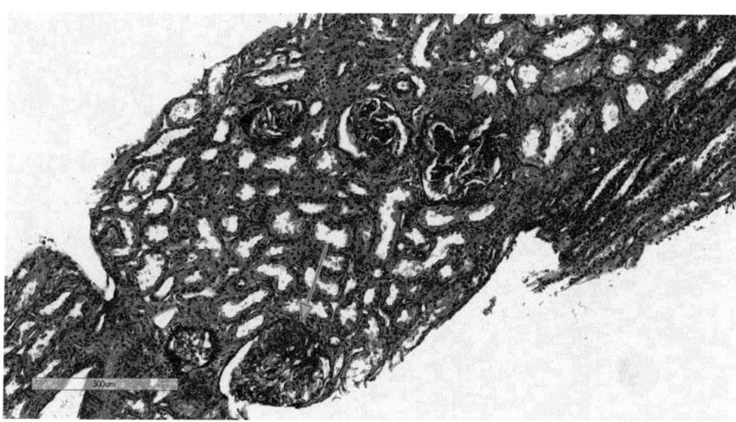

Fig. 8.5 Diffuse segmental LN (class IV-S)

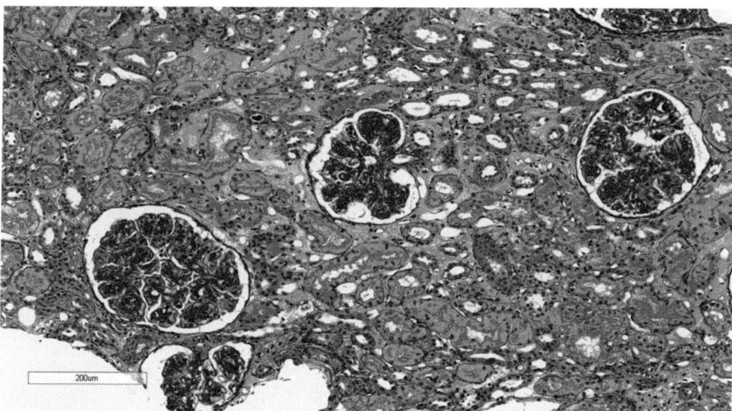

Fig. 8.6 Diffuse global LN (class IV-G) with >50 % of the involved glomeruli showing global lesions

deposits involve at least 50 % of the glomerular capillary surface area in at least 50 % of glomeruli as shown by light microscopy or IF. In assessing the extent of the lesions, both active and sclerotic lesions should be taken into account.

Class V

Class V (Fig. 8.7) is defined as membranous LN with global or segmental continuous granular subepithelial immune deposits, often with concomitant mesangial immune deposits. Any degree of mesangial hypercellularity may occur in class V. When a diffusely distributed membranous lesion is associated with an active lesion of class III or IV, both diagnoses are to be reported in the diagnostic line (Fig. 8.8).

Class VI

Class VI (Fig. 8.9) designates biopsies with >90 % global glomerulosclerosis, in which there is clinical or pathologic evidence that the sclerosis is attributable to LN.

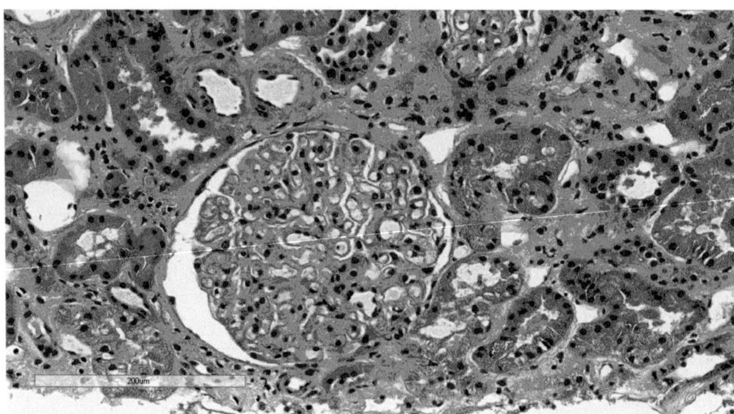

Fig. 8.7 Membranous LN with global or segmental continuous granular subepithelial immune deposits

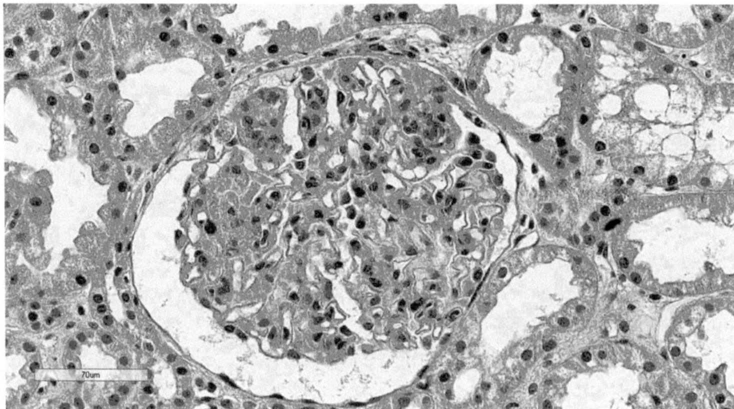

Fig. 8.8 Diffusely distributed membranous lesion associated with an active lesion of class III/IV

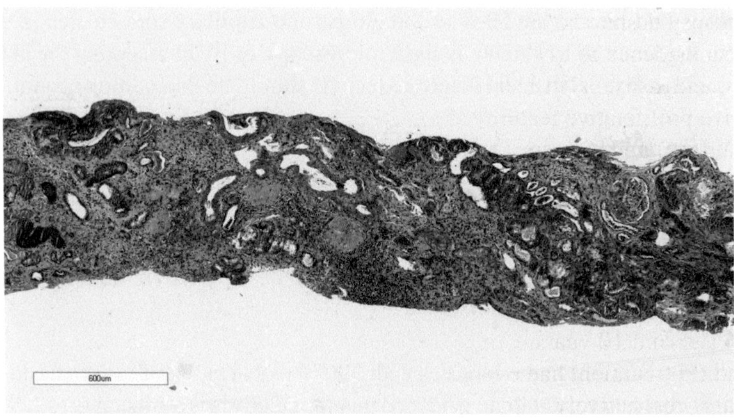

Fig. 8.9 Global glomerulosclerosis (class VI)

8.3.3 Histological Follow-Up

Histological transformation among different classes of LN has been reported in some studies [20]. However, those studies were mainly retrospective and included small cohorts of patients. Moreover, they were based on the previous WHO classification and therefore not comparable with the new criteria of ISN/RPS classification. They concluded that a single biopsy may not be sufficient to manage LN throughout the course of the disease. EULAR/ERA-EDTA guidelines support repeating the renal biopsy for the management of adult and pediatric LN. This may be the "gold standard" for the therapeutic follow-up in selected cases, such as individuals with persistent proteinuria lasting more than 1 year and/or worsening GFR, or at relapse. However, repeating kidney biopsy may also be considered in other clinical patterns, since a considerable percentage of patients are switched to different therapeutic strategies based on the results of their second biopsy [20]. Therefore, we suggest that complete remission should be declared only if no immunological activity is documented in the renal biopsy.

8.3.4 Clinical risk factors and prognosis

Caucasian race, low baseline proteinuria, early LN diagnosis, low serum creatinine (sCr) at diagnosis, stable sCr after 4 weeks of treatment, and class IV±V LN (WHO) are predictive of favorable outcomes. Conversely, African race, circulating anti-Ro antibodies, class III±V LN (WHO) with ≥50 % severe segmental glomerulonephritis, and refractory disease with the standard of care approach predict poorer outcomes [21]. These patients need closer follow-up and, if necessary, more aggressive therapeutic regimens. Further predictors of poor outcome that are generally identified at diagnosis include elevated sCr (≥2.4 mg/dl) and low hematocrit (<26 %) [22].

The previously mentioned clinical variables have to be considered when LN is overt; however, LN may occur in a subclinical manner called "silent LN." Although difficult to diagnose, the prognosis is encouraging. In 1996, a meta-analysis by Gonzales-Crespo et al. considered 193 patients affected with SLE who underwent renal biopsy despite no clinical signs of renal disease; 12 % of patients had no histological evidence of LN, 49 % had class II, 21 % had class III, 15 % had class IV lesions, and lastly, 3/191 had class V [23]. Although some histological classes with extensive proliferative features were included, outcomes were excellent, i.e., 98 % renal survival after 5 years.

As with other proliferative renal diseases, the first objective for clinicians is to obtain quick and complete remission of immunological activity and an early drop in proteinuria [24]. This approach is exhaustively discussed by Korbet et al. who reported a retrospective analysis that demonstrated how patients who were fully responsive to induction therapy had outstanding overall survival rates (95 %) at 5 and 10 years. Conversely, patients who were classified as refractory to standard treatment had overall survival rates between 65 % and 60 % at 5 and 10 years, respectively. Clearly, renal survival rates were influenced as well, being as high as 94 % after 5 and 10 years of treatment in responders and 46 and 31 % in patients with resistant diseases [25]. Interestingly, individuals who achieved partial remission were more likely to evolve to ESRD as compared to those with complete remission: after 10 years of follow-up, those with evidence of class IV LN and partial renal response showed overall survival rates of 76 % compared to 94 % of complete responders and 19 % of nonresponders, while overall renal survival rate was 45 % (92 % complete responders, 13 % nonresponders) [26].

8.4 Diagnostic Approach

Early diagnosis should be obtained since it improves prognosis and supports clinical remission [27]. Therefore, a complete diagnostic approach should include the following:

- *Urine sediment*: direct observation should always be considered in order to investigate the presence of inflammatory casts, leukocytes, crystals or lipid droplets, and structural alterations of red cells. This latter finding is strikingly important: these cells are called "acanthocytes" (from the Greek word "akanthos" = spike) and define inflammation and blood leaking from glomeruli when ≥5 acanthocytes among 100 excreted erythrocytes are found in the urine (acanthocyturia). Red cells lose their ring shape and acquire round processes in the cellular membrane due to mechanical stress when they pass through inflamed capillary loops. Urine casts are frequently observed, especially granular ones, and are composed of red and/or white cells. Hyaline casts are not specific indicators of tubular injury and may be observed during remission phases. Positive hemoglobin reaction in the urine should be considered as an indirect sign of urinary hemolysis; this pattern should raise the suspicion of a concurrent TMA if it is associated with renal failure, anemia, and positive intravascular markers of hemolysis.
- *Proteinuria*: it is mainly an expression of glomerular involvement and should be accurately dosed. If 24 h proteinuria cannot be obtained due to technical limits, the proteinuria/creatininuria ratio (uPCR) is a useful tool.
- *Serum creatinine and estimation of glomerular filtration rate*: we suggest using sCr only for a gross evaluation of renal function. The real glomerular filtration rate (GFR) should be considered as the main parameter of renal function. GFR can be estimated (eGFR) by equations: in particular, the CKD-EPI equation is the most accurate. GFR can also be measured with expensive and less practical analyses that use inert substances filtered by glomeruli and that are not influenced by tubular input and output (e.g., iothalamate). No equations can precisely provide eGFR in individuals with ongoing acute kidney injury.

8.5 LN Treatment

8.5.1 General Principles

General SLE treatment is described elsewhere in this textbook.
Herewith, there are some general principles for LN therapy.
Three different therapeutic approaches are generally considered:

- General strategies against the progression to ESRD
  - Antihypertensive therapy with angiotensin-converting enzyme inhibitors (ACEIs) and angiotensin II receptor antagonists (ARBs), in an effort to reduce proteinuria to below 1 g/day and blood pressure <130/80 mmHg
  - Lipid control with diet and/or drugs
  - Low-sodium diet (<4 g/day)
  - Low-protein diet, depending on the degree of proteinuria
  - Avoiding nephrotoxic drugs (e.g., NSAIDs)
  - BMI control
- Immunomodulating agents, especially in class III/IV LN with A or A/C activity indexes with or without class V, and class V alone (see below)
- Other immunomodulating agents that influence clinical response (e.g., hydroxychloroquine), but that do not achieve remission alone.

8.5.2 Outcome Measures in LN

No single parameter has high diagnostic accuracy in terms of both sensitivity and specificity in predicting a LN flare. Several composite measures to assess clinical response have been used in the past. In general, most clinicians define the clinical response of LN on the basis of the following criteria:

- *Complete response*:
  - sCr returns to previous baseline
  - Evidence of a declining uPCR (<500 mg/g)
- *Partial response*:
  - Stabilization (±25 %) or reduction of sCr without complete recovery
  - ≥50 % decrease in uPCR
  - If nephrotic-range proteinuria is present (uPCR ≥3000 mg/g), a ≥50 % reduction in uPCR and a uPCR <3000 mg/g may be expected.

Moreover, reduced immunological activity is empirically proven by the normalization of urine sediment. In particular, pyuria disappears (≤5 leukocytes per high-power field (HPF)) together with inflammatory casts and hematuria (≤5 dysmorphic red cells per high-field magnification, negative red cell casts, and hemoglobin in stick urine test); C3 and C4 levels become nearly or completely normal, and the anti-DNA antibody titer decreases. These markers should especially be taken into account considering that chronic scarring may definitively alter the amount of proteinuria and renal function.

Another clinical problem lies in defining treatment failure. Some authors propose "*clinical deterioration*" as the criteria to switch to other therapeutic strategies. It is defined by a worsening of renal function, in particular of sCr, by more than 25 % from the beginning of the induction therapy. Other parameters, such as worsening proteinuria and renal biopsy after 3 months of therapy, have not yet been validated.

Minimal mesangial LN (class I)

No specific treatment is usually required in patients with class I LN. In general, this histological class is identified when investigating a suspicion of renal involvement in the context of a systemic flare or because of confounding variables (e.g., lower urinary tract hematuria and leukocyturia for infections).

Mesangial proliferative LN (class II)

As discussed for class I, it is an infrequent finding because most of the time it is clinically silent. Conversely, if a podocytopathy is concomitant with a high degree of proteinuria, therapy with steroids may be beneficial as is the case for minimal change disease.

Focal and segmental proliferative glomerulonephritis (class III) and diffuse proliferative glomerulonephritis (class IV)

In the last 10 years, the therapeutic approach to proliferative LN has progressively changed: cyclophosphamide (CYC)-based regimens that have dominated clinical practice despite being sustained by small randomized trials carried out in the 1980s are now shifting to less toxic solutions with proven equal efficacy. An aggressive approach is needed because unlike class I and II LN, class III and IV may evolve to ESRD. Renal biopsy is mandatory to plan the therapeutic approach which is mainly based on a two-step process: induction and maintenance therapy.

8.5.3 Induction and Maintenance Therapy of Proliferative LN

The role of the induction therapy is to provide a rapid resolution of the inflammatory state before permanent fibrotic changes replace the functional parenchyma. Induction therapy in LN bases on conventional and innovative agents.

Glucocorticoids (GCs) GCs alone are not effective at inducing remission of class III and IV LN, but they should be associated with almost every immunomodulating regimen (see below) [28].

- i.v. methylprednisolone 500–1000 mg/day for 1–3 days followed by prednisone 1 mg/kg/day, progressively tapered over 6–12 months

Cyclophosphamide-Based Regimens Before considering CYC-based regimens, a risk and benefit assessment is mandatory. Infections, infertility, and malignancies are the most worrisome short- and long-term side effects. CYC should be titrated based on renal function and cumulative dose (max. 36 g/lifetime) [29].

Two CYC-based regimens have been proposed:

- NIH regimen: i.v. CYC 500–1000 mg/m^2 monthly for 6 months + GCs as described above. Mean total cumulative dose: 8 g
- Euro-Lupus regimen (low CYC dose): i.v. CYC 500 mg + GCs as above, every 2 weeks for 3 months. Mean total cumulative dose: 3 g

In the 1990s, the need to reduce the incidence of CYC-related side effects, especially in patients with less aggressive forms of LN, prompted clinicians to modify the standard NIH regimen in favor of low-dose CYC regimens. The Euro-Lupus trial [30] was the response to this interest, demonstrating that after a median of 41 months, low-dose and high-dose groups had similar remission rates (71 % vs. 54 %, respectively) and renal flare rates (27 % vs. 29 %), while the high-dose group had an increased infection rate. The "quality" of remission (risk of ESRD and malignancy rate) was assessed in 2009 by the same authors after long-term follow-up (>73 months): only 7 % reached ESRD and the risk of malignancy was equal [24].

Although strongly debated, these promising response rates in class III and IV LN, especially in severe cases with necrosis and crescents, make CYC-based regimens the preferred approach by some authors when compared to mycophenolate mofetil (MMF). The low prevalence of ESRD in the Euro-Lupus trial may be explained by the persistence of GCs and/or immunomodulatory therapy for years in both groups. Based on clinical practice, some authors suggest that high-risk ethnicities, in particular non-Caucasian and non-Asian races, may benefit from prolonged high-dose CYC regimens, although MMF may be a valid alternative as shown in the post-hoc analysis of the ALMS trial [31].

However, in everyday clinical practice, LN is mostly diagnosed in young individuals in whom gonadal function should be preserved. We feel that in these cases, MMF should be preferred to CYC as a first approach.

Mycophenolate Mofetil Interest in MMF rose at the end of the 1990s, with the intent to apply the new knowledge on immunomodulating therapy in kidney transplant to native kidney diseases [32].

In 2005, for the first time, MMF proved to be better than i.v. CYC in inducing complete remission (22.5 % vs. 5.8 %), and considering combined partial and complete remission rates (52.1 % vs. 30.4 %), it was found to be better even in the short term (24 weeks) [33]. However, the trial was statistically underpowered to demonstrate the actual superiority of MMF compared to CYC. Later on, in 2009, the ALMS study, which included several ethnicities, showed that MMF was equal, but not superior to the NIH protocol (88 % and 83 % clinical response, respectively). Adverse events, including death and infection rates, did not differ significantly between the two regimens [31]. Similar findings were documented in Chinese patients in the short- and long term [34, 35].

In crescentic LN, MMF seems to be as effective as CYC, though with higher complete remission rates (54 % vs. 27 %). In a study by Tang et al., MMF performed remarkably well considering that about 25 % of patients had sCr >3 mg/dlat baseline [36].

In summary, MMF may be used as an alternative to i.v. CYC, although some authors still have concerns regarding patients with severe proliferative LN. MMF is well tolerated by patients, especially after 1–2 weeks of intake. Unlike CYC, gonadal toxicity or bladder cancers are not observed [37].

Azathioprine (AZA) AZA is well tolerated and shows fewer side effects compared to CYC, but it has never been shown to be superior to MMF. Azathioprine preserves remission in pregnancy and has no fetal toxicity. AZA is as effective as CYC at inducing remission in proliferative LN and at reducing the incidence of ESRD. However, after 5 years, more relapses and short-term infections are observed in patients on AZA [38]. It is still under debate whether AZA may suffice to control a smoldering renal inflammation and if it is associated with an increased rate of progression to ESRD.

Cyclosporine A (CSA) The CYCLOFA-LUNE trial compared the use of CSA to a modified NIH regimen. Differences between arms were not significant after 9 and 18 months of follow-up [39]. The safety profile was similar, and as expected, CSA was more likely to result in a transient increase in creatinine, in hypertension, and in relapses after tapering. Like AZA, CSA is safe in pregnancy.

Multi-target therapy (MTT) MTT is defined as the association of tacrolimus (TAC), MMF, and GCs. MTT was superior to i.v. CYC in a Chinese study and showed a similar safety profile [40, 41]. MMT proved to be safe and effective in patients with both class IV and V LN and in those refractory to standard MMF regimens. MMT may be considered in individuals with relative or absolute contraindications to CYC.

Rituximab (RTX) RTX is a promising treatment for LN. However, the LUNAR study [42] showed that RTX in addition to standard of care therapy (MMF and GCs) failed to provide further benefits. Although RTX is not recommended as induction therapy by KDIGO guidelines, we suggest using RTX in class III and IV LN, with or without CYC in selected cases including young patients with pregnancy perspectives and subjects with relative/absolute contraindications or intolerance to CYC [43].

A RTX-based protocol (RA schedule) has been recently proposed as a steroid-sparing regimen including methylprednisolone (500 mg on days 1 and 15) in the induction phase and MMF as a long-term maintenance treatment (Rituxilup trial) [43].

A different approach, initially employed as a rescue therapy in refractory LN, has been proposed in order to minimize the long-term effects of both corticosteroids and the immunosuppressive agents used for remission maintenance. It was based on an intensified B-lymphocyte depletion consisting of "four (weekly) plus two (monthly) doses" of rituximab (375 mg/sm), associated with two i.v administrations of 10 mg/kg cyclophosphamide and three pulses of 15 mg/kg methylprednisolone, followed by oral prednisone tapered to 5 mg/day in 10 weeks, without further immunosuppressive maintenance therapy [44].

Maintenance Therapy The maintenance phase aims to avoid relapses once remission is achieved. The length of treatment is not predetermined and it is based on clinical status and history. The goal is to progressively titrate the immunomodulating agents until discontinuation or to reach the lowest possible dose needed to prevent relapses. Several drugs can be used to maintain remission in LN.

MMF is currently preferred. The maintenance phase of the ALMS trial [45] demonstrated that MMF is superior to AZA (16 % vs. 32 %) in reducing the clinical endpoints (death, ESRD, relapse, sustained doubling of sCr, need for rescue therapy). Conversely, the MAINTAIN [46] trial showed no differences between MMF and AZA in obtaining the primary endpoint, which includes time to renal flare, and safety profile. However, more relapses were observed in the AZA group. These data were confirmed in the long-term follow-up (5 years) [47].

CSA has a good safety profile and is as effective as AZA [48]. Therefore, CSA may be considered as an option in patients who do not tolerate AZA and MMF.

8.5.4 Therapy of Membranous LN (Class V)

Patients with pure class V LN should be aggressively treated if nephrotic-range proteinuria (>3.5 g/day) and increased sCr are present.

There is no clear consensus on the best strategy for pure class V. CSA achieved remission in 83 % of patients, followed by CYC (60 %) and GCs alone (27 %) in one study [48]. Conversely, as expected, relapse rates were more frequent in the CSA arm (60 % after 36 months) as compared to CYC (20 % after 50 months) [49]. Based on the ALMS cohort, MMF and CYC were equally effective after 24 weeks of treatment.

Patients with class V LN associated with proliferative changes should be treated according to the concomitant presence of class III and IV LN (see above) [50–52].

References

1. Uramoto KM et al (1999) Trends in the incidence and mortality of systemic lupus erythematosus, 1950–1992. Arthritis Rheum 42(1):46–50
2. Feldman CH et al (2013) Epidemiology and sociodemographics of systemic lupus erythematosus and lupus nephritis among US adults with Medicaid coverage, 2000–2004. Arthritis Rheum 65(3):753–763

3. Wang F et al (1997) Systemic lupus erythematosus in Malaysia: a study of 539 patients and comparison of prevalence and disease expression in different racial and gender groups. Lupus 6(3):248–253
4. Iseki K, Morita O, Fukiyama K (1996) Seasonal variation in the incidence of end-stage renal disease. Am J Nephrol 16(5):375–381
5. Pollak VE et al (1973) The clinical course of lupus nephritis: relationship to the renal histologic findings. Perspect Nephrol Hypertens 1 Pt 2(0):1167–1181
6. Mak A et al (2012) Global trend of survival and damage of systemic lupus erythematosus: meta-analysis and meta-regression of observational studies from the 1950s to 2000s. Semin Arthritis Rheum 41(6):830–839
7. Ward MM (2010) Access to care and the incidence of endstage renal disease due to systemic lupus erythematosus. J Rheumatol 37(6):1158–1163
8. Bastian HM et al (2002) Systemic lupus erythematosus in three ethnic groups. XII. Risk factors for lupus nephritis after diagnosis. Lupus 11(3):152–160
9. Pons-Estel BA et al (2004) The GLADEL multinational Latin American prospective inception cohort of 1,214 patients with systemic lupus erythematosus: ethnic and disease heterogeneity among "Hispanics". Medicine (Baltimore) 83(1):1–17
10. Alarcon GS et al (2006) Systemic lupus erythematosus in a multiethnic cohort: LUMINA XXXV. Predictive factors of high disease activity over time. Ann Rheum Dis 65(9):1168–1174
11. Cameron J (2001) Clinical manifestations of lupus nephritis. In: Rheumatology and the kidney. Oxford University Press, Oxford, pp 16–32
12. Pollak VE, Pirani CL, Schwartz FD (1964) The natural history of the renal manifestations of systemic lupus erythematosus. J Lab Clin Med 63:537–550
13. Ponticelli C (2005) Systemic lupus erythematosus (clinical). In: The kidney in systemic disease. Oxford University Press, Oxford, pp 824–842
14. Bertsias G et al (2008) EULAR recommendations for the management of systemic lupus erythematosus. Report of a Task Force of the EULAR Standing Committee for International Clinical Studies Including Therapeutics. Ann Rheum Dis 67(2):195–205
15. Dooley MA, Aranow C, Ginzler EM (2004) Review of ACR renal criteria in systemic lupus erythematosus. Lupus 13(11):857–860
16. Bertsias GK et al (2012) Joint European League Against Rheumatism and European Renal Association-European Dialysis and Transplant Association (EULAR/ERA-EDTA) recommendations for the management of adult and paediatric lupus nephritis. Ann Rheum Dis 71(11):1771–1782
17. Gordon C et al (2009) European consensus statement on the terminology used in the management of lupus glomerulonephritis. Lupus 18(3):257–263
18. Weening JJ et al (2004) The classification of glomerulonephritis in systemic lupus erythematosus revisited. J Am Soc Nephrol 15(2):241–250
19. Herrera GA (1999) The value of electron microscopy in the diagnosis and clinical management of lupus nephritis. Ultrastruct Pathol 23(2):63–77
20. Alsuwaida A et al (2012) Strategy for second kidney biopsy in patients with lupus nephritis. Nephrol Dial Transplant 27(4):1472–1478
21. Korbet SM et al (2007) Severe lupus nephritis: racial differences in presentation and outcome. J Am Soc Nephrol 18(1):244–254
22. Austin HA 3rd et al (1994) Predicting renal outcomes in severe lupus nephritis: contributions of clinical and histologic data. Kidney Int 45(2):544–550
23. Gonzalez-Crespo MR et al (1996) Outcome of silent lupus nephritis. Semin Arthritis Rheum 26(1):468–476
24. Houssiau FA et al (2010) The 10-year follow-up data of the Euro-Lupus Nephritis Trial comparing low-dose and high-dose intravenous cyclophosphamide. Ann Rheum Dis 69(1):61–64
25. Korbet SM et al (2000) Factors predictive of outcome in severe lupus nephritis. Lupus Nephritis Collaborative Study Group. Am J Kidney Dis 35(5):904–914

26. Chen YE et al (2008) Value of a complete or partial remission in severe lupus nephritis. Clin J Am Soc Nephrol 3(1):46–53
27. Faurschou M et al (2006) Prognostic factors in lupus nephritis: diagnostic and therapeutic delay increases the risk of terminal renal failure. J Rheumatol 33(8):1563–1569
28. Donadio JV Jr et al (1978) Treatment of diffuse proliferative lupus nephritis with prednisone and combined prednisone and cyclophosphamide. N Engl J Med 299(21):1151–1155
29. Philibert D, Cattran D (2008) Remission of proteinuria in primary glomerulonephritis: we know the goal but do we know the price? Nat Clin Pract Nephrol 4(10):550–559
30. Houssiau FA et al (2002) Immunosuppressive therapy in lupus nephritis: the Euro-Lupus Nephritis Trial, a randomized trial of low-dose versus high-dose intravenous cyclophosphamide. Arthritis Rheum 46(8):2121–2131
31. Appel GB et al (2009) Mycophenolate mofetil versus cyclophosphamide for induction treatment of lupus nephritis. J Am Soc Nephrol 20(5):1103–1112
32. Dooley MA et al (1999) Mycophenolate mofetil therapy in lupus nephritis: clinical observations. J Am Soc Nephrol 10(4):833–839
33. Ginzler EM et al (2005) Mycophenolate mofetil or intravenous cyclophosphamide for lupus nephritis. N Engl J Med 353(21):2219–2228
34. Chan TM et al (2000) Efficacy of mycophenolate mofetil in patients with diffuse proliferative lupus nephritis. Hong Kong-Guangzhou Nephrology Study Group. N Engl J Med 343(16):1156–1162
35. Chan TM et al (2005) Long-term study of mycophenolate mofetil as continuous induction and maintenance treatment for diffuse proliferative lupus nephritis. J Am Soc Nephrol 16(4):1076–1084
36. Tang Z et al (2008) Effects of mycophenolate mofetil for patients with crescentic lupus nephritis. Nephrology (Carlton) 13(8):702–707
37. Kuiper-Geertsma DG, Derksen RH (2003) Newer drugs for the treatment of lupus nephritis. Drugs 63(2):167–180
38. Grootscholten C et al (2006) Azathioprine/methylprednisolone versus cyclophosphamide in proliferative lupus nephritis. A randomized controlled trial. Kidney Int 70(4):732–742
39. Zavada J et al (2010) Cyclosporine A or intravenous cyclophosphamide for lupus nephritis: the Cyclofa-Lune study. Lupus 19(11):1281–1289
40. Bao H et al (2008) Successful treatment of class V+IV lupus nephritis with multitarget therapy. J Am Soc Nephrol 19(10):2001–2010
41. Liu Z et al (2015) Multitarget therapy for induction treatment of lupus nephritis: a randomized trial. Ann Intern Med 162(1):18–26
42. Rovin BH et al (2012) Efficacy and safety of rituximab in patients with active proliferative lupus nephritis: the Lupus Nephritis Assessment with Rituximab study. Arthritis Rheum 64(4):1215–1226
43. Condon MB et al (2013) Prospective observational single-centre cohort study to evaluate the effectiveness of treating lupus nephritis with rituximab and mycophenolate mofetil but no oral steroids. Ann Rheum Dis 72(8):1280–1286
44. Roccatello D, Sciascia S, Rossi D et al (2011) Intensive short-term treatment with rituximab, cyclophosphamide and methylprednisolone pulses induces remission in severe cases of SLE with nephritis and avoids further immunosuppressive maintenance therapy. Nephrol Dial Transplant 26:3987–3992
45. Dooley MA et al (2011) Mycophenolate versus azathioprine as maintenance therapy for lupus nephritis. N Engl J Med 365(20):1886–1895
46. Houssiau FA et al (2010) Azathioprine versus mycophenolate mofetil for long-term immunosuppression in lupus nephritis: results from the MAINTAIN Nephritis Trial. Ann Rheum Dis 69(12):2083–2089
47. Tamirou F et al (2015) Long-term follow-up of the MAINTAIN Nephritis Trial, comparing azathioprine and mycophenolate mofetil as maintenance therapy of lupus nephritis. Ann Rheum Dis. [Epub ahead of print]

48. Moroni G et al (2006) A randomized pilot trial comparing cyclosporine and azathioprine for maintenance therapy in diffuse lupus nephritis over four years. Clin J Am Soc Nephrol 1(5):925–932
49. Austin HA 3rd et al (2009) Randomized, controlled trial of prednisone, cyclophosphamide, and cyclosporine in lupus membranous nephropathy. J Am Soc Nephrol 20(4):901–911
50. Dooley MA et al (2013) Effect of belimumab treatment on renal outcomes: results from the phase 3 belimumab clinical trials in patients with SLE. Lupus 22(1):63–72
51. Group AT (2014) Treatment of lupus nephritis with abatacept: the Abatacept and Cyclophosphamide Combination Efficacy and Safety Study. Arthritis Rheumatol 66(11):3096–3104
52. Schwartz MM et al (1987) The prognosis of segmental glomerulonephritis in systemic lupus erythematosus. Kidney Int 32(2):274–279

Neuropsychiatric Systemic Lupus Erythematosus

9

Karen Schreiber and Soren Jacobsen

9.1 Introduction

Systemic lupus erythematosus (SLE) is a chronic autoimmune disorder, which can present itself with a wide spectrum of clinical and immunological manifestations. Treatment advances in SLE have resulted in an increased survival of patients with SLE, and clinicians have become more aware of neuropsychiatric SLE (NPSLE) as an important manifestation of SLE [1]. NPSLE is defined as the neurological syndromes of the central, peripheral, and autonomic nervous system and the psychiatric syndromes observed in patients with SLE in whom other causes have been excluded [2]. It is the current understanding that the underlying pathology of NPSLE is a result of multifactorial sources including the presence of autoantibodies, changes in the microvasculature, and the intracranial production of inflammatory mediators, either alone or in combination [3].

NPSLE involvement is associated with different degrees of morbidity, varies in presentation and severity, may overlap, and can be of particular challenge for the clinician as symptoms may be difficult to distinguish from other neuropsychiatric conditions with different etiologies.

K. Schreiber
Lupus Research Unit, Division of Women's Health, The Rayne Institute, King's College London, London SE17EH, UK

Department of Rheumatology, Rigshospitalet, Blegdamsvej 9, Copenhagen DL-2100, Denmark
e-mail: Karen.schreiber@gstt.nhs.uk

S. Jacobsen (✉)
Department of Rheumatology, Rigshospitalet, Blegdamsvej 9, Copenhagen DL-2100, Denmark
e-mail: sj@dadlnet.dk

D. Roccatello, L. Emmi (eds.), *Connective Tissue Disease: A Comprehensive Guide-Volume 1*, Rare Diseases of the Immune System 5,
DOI 10.1007/978-3-319-24535-5_9

The major challenge with regard to diagnosis, treatment, and research within the field of NPSLE has been the lack of consensus in classifying the disease, due to the fact that the vast majority of the available literature on NPSLE long has been based on individual clinical interpretations. With the view of improving the definition and classification of NPSLE, the American College of Rheumatology agreed in 1999 on case definitions for 19 different central, peripheral, and autonomic nervous system syndromes in patients with SLE for which other causes have been excluded [4].

The central nervous system (CNS) symptoms, as defined by the ACR include focal neurological manifestations (cerebrovascular disease, seizures, myelopathy, aseptic meningitis, movement disorder, and demyelinating syndrome) or diffuse psychiatric/neuropsychological syndromes such as cognitive dysfunction, mood and anxiety disorders, psychosis, acute confusional state, and headaches. Peripheral neurologic conditions include cranial neuropathy, polyneuropathy, mononeuropathy, acute inflammatory demyelinating polyradiculoneuropathy (Guillain–Barré syndrome), myasthenia gravis, plexopathy, and autonomic disorders as summarized in Table 9.1.

This chapter provides an overview of NPSLE including aspects of the ACR classification and the current understanding of the various manifestations of NPSLE with a special emphasis on practical aspects of the diagnosis and management of neurological manifestations based on the EULAR management guidelines for the treatment guidelines for NPSLE [5]. The chapter focuses on the central nervous system manifestations of NPSLE, and peripheral nervous system manifestations will not be discussed in detail.

9.2 Epidemiology of NPSLE

SLE is an autoimmune disorder, which potentially can affect any organ and present itself with a wide spectrum of clinical and immunological manifestations. Specific classification criteria for SLE were updated by the American College of Rheumatology (ACR) in 1997 and include the serial or simultaneous presence of 4 of 11 defined criteria as shown in Table 9.2 [6]. The Systemic Lupus International Collaborating Clinics (SLICC) group has recently revised and validated a new set of classification criteria. The SLICC criteria require at least four of the proposed criteria, including at least one clinical and one immunological criterion for an SLE classification (Table 9.2) resulting in fewer misclassifications compared to the ACR criteria (Table 9.3) [7].

The annual incidence (per 100,000) of SLE in Europe ranges between 3.3 per year in Iceland and 4.7 in Sweden, compared to 21.9 in the Afro-Caribbeans. The prevalence varies according to the studied population, but studies suggest ranges between 26 per 100,000 in the UK (including all races) and 42 per 100,000 in Sweden, whereas the overall prevalence in the USA is reported lying between 14.6 and 50 cases per 100,000 persons [8].

NPSLE consists of a heterogeneous variety of neurological and psychiatric syndromes, none of which are exclusive or specific for SLE. The reported prevalence of NPSLE varies from 12 to 95 % between studies in which NPSLE criteria were

Table 9.1 Neuropsychiatric syndromes observed in systemic lupus erythematosus

Central nervous system	ACR criteria (1999)	Revision of the ACR criteria by Ainiala et al. (2001)[a]
	Aseptic meningitis	Aseptic meningitis
	Cerebrovascular disease	Cerebrovascular disease
	Demyelinating syndrome	Demyelinating syndrome
	Myelopathy	Myelopathy
	Seizure disorders	Seizure disorders
	Acute confusional state	Acute confusional state
	Cognitive dysfunction	Cognitive dysfunction (moderate or severe)
	Movement disorder (chorea)	Movement disorder (chorea)
	Psychosis	Psychosis
	Mood disorder	Severe depression
	Anxiety disorder	
	Headache (including migraine and benign intracranial hypertension)	
Peripheral nervous system	Acute inflammatory demyelinating polyradiculoneuropathy (Guillain–Barré syndrome)	Acute inflammatory demyelinating polyradiculoneuropathy (Guillain–Barré syndrome)
	Neuropathy, cranial	Neuropathy, cranial
	Mononeuropathy, single/multiplex	Mononeuropathy, single/multiplex
	Plexopathy	Plexopathy
	Myasthenia gravis	Myasthenia gravis
	Autonomic neuropathy	Autonomic disorder
	Polyneuropathy	Polyneuropathy with electroneuromyographic confirmation

Abbreviations: *ACR* American College of Rheumatology, *SLE* systemic lupus erythematosus

[a]Ainiala et al. performed a cross-sectional validation study on the 1999 ACR criteria, and it was shown to have a specificity of only 46 %; however, exclusion of the syndromes without evidence for neuronal damage (headache, mild cognitive dysfunction, and mild mood and anxiety disorders), as well as polyneuropathy without electrophysiological confirmation, halved the frequency of NPSLE diagnosis and increased the specificity of the 1999 ACR criteria to 91 % [47]

applied to SLE patients. The wide range has been suggested to indirectly reflect the variation in study design, definition of neurological involvement, and ethnicity or geography, but may also be attributable to the availability of neurological expertise and investigations [9–11].

At least half of NPSLE manifestations occur at disease onset or within the first year after SLE onset, mainly in the presence of generalized disease activity [12].

Manifestations such as headache, mood disorders, anxiety, and mild cognitive dysfunction are common, but do not usually reflect overt CNS lupus activity [12]. Cognitive dysfunction and cerebrovascular events correlate with advancing age based on data from the general population, but this question has yet to be answered for patients with underlying SLE [13].

Table 9.2 1997 update on 1982 ACR classification criteria for SLE

Criterion	Definition
Malar rash	Fixed erythema, flat or raised, over the malar eminences, tending to spare the nasolabial folds
Discoid rash	Erythematous raised patches with adherent keratotic scaling and follicular plugging; atrophic scarring may occur in older lesions
Photosensitivity	Skin rash as a result of unusual reaction to sunlight, by patient history or physician observation
Oral ulcers	Oral or nasopharyngeal ulceration, usually painless, observed by physician
Non-erosive arthritis	Involving two or more peripheral joints, characterized by tenderness, swelling, or effusion
Pleural or pericarditis	Pleuritis, convincing history of pleuritic pain or rubbing heard by a physician or evidence of pleural effusion; *OR* pericarditis, documented by electrocardiogram or rub or evidence of pericardial effusion
Renal disorder	Persistent proteinuria >0.5 g/day or > than 3+ if quantitation not performed, *OR*
	Cellular casts – may be red cell, hemoglobin, granular, tubular, or mixed
Neurologic disorder	Seizures – in the absence of offending drugs or known metabolic derangements, e.g., uremia, ketoacidosis, or electrolyte imbalance, *OR*
	Psychosis – in the absence of offending drugs or known metabolic derangements, e.g., uremia, ketoacidosis, or electrolyte imbalance
Hematologic disorder	Hemolytic anemia – with reticulocytosis, *OR* leukopenia $<4,000/mm^3$ on ≥ 2 occasions, *OR*
	Lymphopenia $<1,500/mm^3$ on ≥ 2 occasions, *OR* thrombocytopenia $<100,000/\ mm^3$ in the absence of offending drugs
Immunologic disorder	Anti-DNA: antibody to native DNA in abnormal titer, *OR* anti-Sm: presence of antibody to Sm nuclear antigen, *OR* positive finding of antiphospholipid antibodies on:
	1. An abnormal serum level of IgG or IgM anticardiolipin antibodies
	2. A positive test result for lupus anticoagulant using a standard method
	3. A false-positive test result for at least 6 months confirmed by *Treponema pallidum* immobilization or fluorescent treponemal antibody absorption test
Positive antinuclear antibody	An abnormal titer of antinuclear antibody by immunofluorescence or an equivalent assay at any point in time and in the absence of drugs

Any combination of 4 or more of 11 criteria, well-documented at any time during a patient's history, makes it likely that the patient has SLE (specificity and sensitivity are 95 % and 75 %, respectively)

Table 9.3 2012 published SLICC criteria for SLE classification

Clinical criteria
1. Acute or subacute lupus
2. Chronic cutaneous lupus
3. Oral/nasal ulcers
4. Non-scarring alopecia
5. Inflammatory synovitis with physician-observed swelling of two or more joints *OR* tender joints with morning stiffness
6. Serositis
7. Renal: urine protein/creatinine (or 24 h urine protein) representing at least 500 mg of protein/24 h or red blood cell casts
8. Neurologic: seizures, psychosis, mononeuritis multiplex, myelitis, peripheral or cranial neuropathy, cerebritis (acute confusional state)
9. Hemolytic anemia
10. Leukopenia (<4,000/mm^3 at least once) OR lymphopenia (<1,000/mm^3 at least once)
11. Thrombocytopenia (<100,000/mm^3) at least once
Immunological criteria
1. ANA above laboratory reference range
2. Anti-dsDNA above laboratory reference range (except ELISA: twice above laboratory reference range)
3. Anti-Sm
4. Antiphospholipid antibody, lupus anticoagulant, false-positive test for syphilis, anticardiolipin – at least twice normal or medium-high-titer anti-b2 glycoprotein 1
5. Low complement (low C3, low C4, low CH50)
6. Direct Coombs test in absence of hemolytic anemia

After Petri et al. [7]
Biopsy-proven lupus nephritis with ANA or anti-dsDNA

9.3 Pathogenic Mechanisms of NPSLE

The current understanding of the underlying pathological mechanisms which result in the multifaceted clinical presentations of NPSLE is suggested to be caused by a variety of mechanisms, including vascular injury mediated by mainly antiphospholipid antibodies (aPL) and immune complexes (mainly leading to transient ischemic attacks or strokes and seizures) and diffuse neuropsychiatric manifestations (such as cognitive impairment) in combination or alone [14].

With regard to thrombotic ischemic cerebral events, aPL have in the past been associated with focal neurological syndromes due to their ability to cause thrombotic events within vessels of different calibers leading to tissue ischemia [15]. In particular, the role of anticardiolipin (aCL) and lupus anticoagulant (LAC) has been investigated in NPSLE. A strong correlation between aPL and the overall frequency of neuropsychiatric manifestations was reported in a range of studies [16–19], but was questioned in other studies [20–23].

Menon et al. found the persistent presence of aPL to be associated with cognitive impairment [24]. aCL has been found to be associated with an overall NPSLE involvement more often than LAC [17, 19, 25]; however, on investigating cerebrovascular disease, predominantly stroke, LAC has been proved to be the most strongly associated aPL [26–30]. Despite the fact that most data have demonstrated an association between aCL and/or LAC and NPSLE, the role of anti-β2 glycoprotein I (anti-b2GPI) is less clear.

In vitro studies have also suggested a direct modulatory effect of aPL on neuronal cell function [31] and a pathogenic effect on neuronal cells [32].

Anti-ribosomal P protein antibodies (aRP) have a high specificity for SLE and have been found to be present in 6–46 % of subjects with SLE [33]. Elevated titers of aRP have been found in patients during SLE flares and may be associated with particular clinical manifestations including NPSLE [34]. Data from the Systemic Lupus International Collaborating Clinics (SLICC) inception cohort on 1,710 patients confirmed the association between elevated titers of aRP and psychosis [29]. However, a meta-analysis evaluating the diagnostic accuracy of anti-RP for NPSLE for psychosis, mood disorders, or both and for other diffuse manifestations did not confirm an association between aRP and any manifestation of NPSLE. Karassa et al. reported a sensitivity and specificity for the diagnosis of NPSLE of 26 % and 80 %, respectively. For psychosis, mood disorder, or both, the sensitivity and specificity were 27 % and 80 %, respectively. For other diffuse manifestations, the sensitivity was 24 % and the specificity 80 % [35]. Consequently, aRP testing does not discriminate between patients with NPLSE manifestations compared to those without NPSLE, and a role in clinical practice is yet to be fully defined. However, high titers of aRP are suggested to play a role in patients with suspected SLE psychosis [36].

Other autoantibodies of interest in the setting of NPSLE are antineuronal antibodies [37]. This subset of antibodies has been identified in the cerebrospinal fluid (CSF) and postmortem neuronal tissues of patients with NPSLE [38, 39]. Circulating anti-NR2 antibodies have been associated with NPSLE; however, studies on circulating anti-NR2 antibodies are inconsistent [40], whereas their presence in the CSF seem to be more consistent [14, 41, 42]. Subsets of the commonly occurring anti-dsDNA antibodies in SLE patients have also been suggested to be able to cross react with NMDA receptors in the CNS causing diffuse neuropsychiatric manifestations [37].

9.4 Classification of NPSLE

The first description of neuropsychiatric involvement in a patient with SLE (NPSLE) goes back to the nineteenth century [43]. In details, NPSLE was first described in the nineteenth century by Kaposi and Osler in a patient with pleurisy, pneumonia, *disturbed neurologic function*, and rapid progression to death [43]. As the neurological symptoms of NPSLE can present focally, diffusely, centrally, peripherally, and psychiatric, in isolation or simultaneously, they remain a challenge for the treating clinician. Due to this complexity, it is therefore not surprising that the definition of a uniform terminology and classification long has kept clinicians' and scientists' minds busy. Prior to 1999, several classifications had been proposed to describe the diverse clinical presentations of CNS involvement in SLE, and discrepancies existed among recommended methods of evaluation [36, 44, 45].

In 1985, How et al. established a range of neurological and psychiatric manifestations to support a diagnosis of NPSLE. Accordingly, a classification of NPSLE required the presence of one major criterion alone or one minor criterion (such as an abnormal finding on electroencephalography, nuclear brain scanning, CSF examination, or cerebral angiography). It was, however, recommended to rule out other causes such as infection, drugs, metabolic causes (such as uremia), or hypertension [45].

Two years later, Singer et al. published a consensus document with the aim to ascertain the level of agreement on neuropsychiatric SLE manifestations among a group of international experts in autoimmune diseases [46]. The majority of the participating experts felt that the ACR criteria for SLE were "insufficient for clinical usage" in the setting of NPSLE. Starting from a list of more than 50 possible clinical, laboratory findings and imaging manifestations of neuropsychiatric SLE, only four items were selected. These included atypical psychosis, several categories of seizures, transverse myelitis, and global cognitive dysfunction. This approach would have represented the basis for further studies and could have possibly expanded the ACR classification criteria for SLE; however, subsequent validation studies were never performed [14].

In 1997, the ACR Research Committee convened an ad hoc multidisciplinary committee consisting of 35 members across specialties, such as rheumatology, neurology, psychiatry, neuropsychiatry, and hematology, with the aim of developing a standard nomenclature for neuropsychiatric SLE. The ACR committee developed neuropsychiatric SLE case definitions with diagnostic criteria, exclusions, associations, and ascertainment. The implementation of standards and recommendations for essential laboratory evaluations and imaging techniques was a main advancement in the attempts to classify NPSLE [36]. The ACR NPSLE case definitions include 12 central nervous system syndromes and 7 syndromes of the peripheral nervous system compatible with the disease (Table 9.1). According to the ACR definition, the central nervous system symptoms are relatively common in patients with NPSLE, accounting for around 93 % of cases [9].

The defined clinical ACR manifestations can be divided in neurological manifestations affecting the CNS (focal or diffuse) and the peripheral syndromes. The first group includes aseptic meningitis, cerebrovascular disease, myelopathy, seizures, acute confusional state, cognitive dysfunction, movement disorders (chorea), psychosis, mood and anxiety disorders, and headaches. The peripheral syndromes encompass the remaining 7 % of NPSLE cases and include acute inflammatory demyelinizing polyradiculoneuropathy (Guillain–Barré syndrome), cranial neuropathy, mono- or polyneuropathy (single/multiplex), myasthenia gravis, autonomic disorders, and plexopathy (Table 9.1). NPSLE classification criteria provide an operational framework for the study of NP manifestations in SLE; however, when applied to the general population, their specificity is low due to the occurrence of such manifestations in the general population [47].

The European League against Rheumatism (EULAR) has recently published a guideline for the diagnosis and management of NPSLE manifestations [12]. One of the core statements of the EULAR consensus document is the recommendation, that the initial management of these patients should not differ to those without SLE. The treatment recommendations will be mentioned in each subsection of this chapter [12].

9.5 Clinical Manifestations, Diagnosis, and Management of NPSLE

9.5.1 Aseptic Meningitis

Aseptic meningitis refers to patients who have clinical and laboratory evidence for meningeal inflammation with negative routine bacterial cultures. The most common cause is enterovirus. Additional etiologies include other infections, medications, and malignancy. Aseptic meningitis is a rare finding in SLE patients. If meningitis is suspected, any underlying infectious cause must be ruled out. In patients receiving immunosuppressive therapy, opportunistic pathogens, such as *Listeria monocytogenes*, reactive tuberculosis, and *Cryptococcus neoformans*, should be considered. Kim et al. reported from a retrospective cohort of 1,420 SLE patients that 20 (1.4 %) were identified with meningitis. In over half of these patients, microorganisms were identified, and the most common organism was *Cryptococcus neoformans*, and a diagnosis of aseptic meningitis was made in nine patients [48]. Thus, a lumbar puncture and analysis of the cerebrospinal fluid (CSF) are generally indicated if meningitis is suspected. CSF results with a white cell count of less than 500 cells/mm^3, over 50 % CSF lymphocytes, total protein less than 80–100 mg/dL, and normal glucose, and a negative Gram stain may suggest aseptic meningitis.

A variety of drugs can induce aseptic meningitis which therefore may be considered if a patient presents with a clinical picture suggesting aseptic meningitis. In patients with connective tissue disease, the use of nonsteroidal anti-inflammatory drugs (especially ibuprofen) has in the past been linked to aseptic meningitis [49, 50]. The treatment of aseptic meningitis is based on supportive management [12].

9.5.2 Cerebrovascular Disease

Cerebrovascular disease in SLE is in over 80 % of the cases attributable to transient ischemic attacks (TIA) or ischemic strokes. The main risk factors are high and persistent SLE activity, cumulative corticosteroid dosage, the persistent presence of moderate-to-high titers of aPL, heart valve disease, systemic hypertension, and age in itself [12]. The less commonly seen are hemorrhagic strokes (7–12 %), subarachnoid hemorrhage (3–5 %), and sinus thrombosis (2 %) [12, 51].

In comparison to the acute onset of focal neurological disease, the mechanisms underlying diffuse, multifocal CNS manifestations are less defined and less clear in presentation and may develop slowly over time not necessarily in association with

SLE disease activity [52]. Magnetic resonance imaging and CT angiography can be useful to rule out cerebral hemorrhage, may inform on the localization and the extent of the ischemic brain injury, and help to characterize the brain lesion [12].

The acute management of a stroke in patients with SLE is not different to the management in the general population. Stroke teams are available in most centers and should be made aware of any patient with a suspected stroke according as, for example, described in the UK National Institute of Clinical Excellence (NICE) guideline on stroke management [53]. Thrombolysis may subsequently be considered in eligible patients, and therapy is otherwise based on anti-aggregation. A full work-up for secondary stroke prevention includes the modification of cardiovascular risk factors (such as hypertension, hypercholesterolemia, diabetes mellitus, etc). An electrocardiogram (ECG) and ultrasound of the carotid arteries with or without carotid endarterectomy should be performed as part of the work-up. In case of underlying SLE activity, this may be managed with steroids and/or immunosuppressive therapy [12].

In patients with persistent aPL and stroke fulfilling the classification criteria for APS [54], long-term anticoagulation should be initiated [55]. The dosage of anticoagulation is an ongoing subject of debate. Two randomized controlled trials have compared the standard anticoagulant treatment (target INR 2–3) with high-intensity treatment (target INR 3.5), and both studies did not show an advantage of high-intensity vitamin K antagonist (VKA) for the prevention of recurrent thrombotic events. However, in both studies, patients randomized to the high-intensity group frequently did not achieve adequate anticoagulation targets. In one of these studies, patients were only in target 43 % of the time and included a relatively low number of patients with arterial events [56]. However, in a systematic review of sixteen studies, Ruiz-Irastorza et al. recommended high-intensity warfarin therapy for patients with recurrent events while on VKA (target 2–3) [57]. The role of new oral anticoagulants such as direct factor Xa and thrombin inhibitors still remains to be determined in this setting awaiting results from randomized controlled trials.

9.5.3 Myelopathy

Myelopathy in NPSLE is defined as a disorder of the spinal cord characterized by rapidly evolving paraparesis and/or sensory loss, with a demonstrable motor and/or sensory cord level (to include transverse) and/or sphincter involvement. Usually, the myelopathy has rapid onset (hours or days) of one or more of the following diagnostic manifestations: (1) bilateral weakness of legs with or without arms (paraplegia/quadriplegia), which may be asymmetric, and (2) sensory impairment with cord level similar to that of motor weakness, with or without bowel and bladder dysfunction [58]. The underlying pathomechanism may be caused by ischemia/thrombosis and/or inflammation, and patients may present with signs of grey matter dysfunction (which includes flaccidity and hyporeflexia) or white matter dysfunction (such as spasticity and hyperreflexia) [52, 59].

Neuromyelitis optica (NMO), also known as Devic syndrome, is a severe demyelinating disorder of the central nervous system causing longitudinal transverse myelitis of at least three vertebral segments, recurrent optic neuritis, and normal brain MRI. NMO has been reported in patients with SLE and is associated with the presence of anti-aquaporin antibodies (IgG subtype) [14].

Myelitis is estimated to affect 1–2 % of patients with SLE which is more than 1,000 times greater than the prevalence of idiopathic myelitis in the general population [60, 61].

Transverse myelitis has also been associated with aPL and, in atypical presentations, an important differential diagnosis remains multiple sclerosis [62]. Anecdotal reports of transverse myelitis associated with aPL have been described since 1985 when Harris et al. reported it in a 45-year-old woman with a lupus-like illness and high-titer aCL of the IgM isotype [63].

Current views suggest that underlying prothrombotic mechanisms related to aPL play a key role in the development of acute transverse myelitis in patients with SLE [64–66]. D'Cruz et al. described a series of 15 patients with transverse myelitis as the presenting manifestation of SLE. Seventy percent of the patients were aPL positive, supporting the view of a strong association of transverse myelitis with aPL [67].

Contrast-enhanced MRI is the imaging method of choice [12]. A CSF analysis is useful to rule out underlying infection. Immunosuppressive therapy with intravenous methylprednisolone and intravenous cyclophosphamide can be effective in SLE myelitis, particularly when instituted within the first few hours of presentation. More than half of the patients have relapses; steroids should therefore be tapered cautiously and maintenance immunosuppression may be indicated. Plasma exchange therapy has been used in severe refractory cases. In case of persistent aPL, anticoagulation may be indicated [68, 69].

9.5.4 Seizures

Generalized primary seizures and partial seizures are a common neurological manifestation found in up to 20 % of patients with SLE (compared with 0.5–1.0 % in the general population). Seizures have been described among the early CNS manifestations and may precede a diagnosis of SLE [51, 70, 71]. Cerebrospinal fluid (CSF) pleocytosis is common, suggesting that a low-grade lupus-related encephalopathy may be a possible underlying cause. Cerebral atrophy has also been described in patients with SLE and may predispose to seizures [52, 72].

Results from the Systemic Lupus International Collaborating Clinics (SLICC group) prospective inception cohort of 1,631 SLE patients showed that 4.6 % of patients had at least one seizure, most of which occurred around the time of their SLE diagnosis. This finding is in conjunction with our own findings [71].

Interestingly, there was some indication that the regular use of antimalarial drugs reduced the risk of seizures. A higher risk of seizure was seen within three groups, patients with lower education status forslag, patients with more organ damage since the diagnosis of SLE, and lupus patients of African ethnicity forslag. There was an association with disease activity but not with autoantibodies [70]. The group also found that seizures due to SLE frequently got better without long-term seizure medication and without decreasing quality of life.

The treatment is based on anticonvulsive therapy, which may be considered in patients with high recurrence risk, brain MRI structural abnormalities causally linked to seizures, focal neurological signs, partial seizure, and epileptiform EEG [12]. Seizures secondary to SLE disease activity may be treated with glucocorticoids and immunosuppression, and in case of refractory seizures, cyclophosphamide has been used in anecdotal cases [73].

9.5.5 Acute Confusional State

Acute confusional state (delirium) has been described in up to 7 % of patients with SLE in whom other underlying pathology has been excluded. Characterized by an acute-onset variation (or fluctuation) of the level of consciousness, acute confusional states may at worse progress to a coma [12]. Milder forms of acute confusional state include the reduced ability to focus attention, mood disturbances, and impaired cognition.

The initial acute management requires exploration of underlying causes. CSF examination is required to exclude any underlying infection. The imaging of choice is SPECT; however, possible limitations in expertise and availability may restrict clinical practice to CT or MRI in order to rule out ischemic events, underlying hemorrhage or malignancy [13]. Benzodiazepines or antipsychotics may be required in the acute setting. Glucocorticoid and immunosuppression play some role and may in selected cases have to be escalated to plasma exchange and cyclophosphamide. Rituximab has been used in refractory cases [68, 69].

9.5.6 Cognitive Dysfunction

Cognitive dysfunction ranges from mild to moderate or severe impairment and manifests itself by reduced cognitive function (such as memory problems or the reduced ability of abstract thinking) and is a common finding among patients with SLE. In up to 80 % of SLE patients, mild to moderate cognitive dysfunction has been reported [51, 74], whereas severe cognitive dysfunction is a rare complication found in up to 5 % of patients with SLE [12]. It has been reported to occur in the absence of SLE disease activity and fluctuates over the course of the disease, often independently of depression or anxiety [14]. In patients with persistently aPL, anecdotal evidence suggest cognitive impairment to improve on anticoagulation [55].

A major challenge in diagnosing cognitive impairment remains the fact that other common manifestations of SLE, such as fatigue, widespread pain, and depression are associated with cognitive impairment [14]. A study of SLE outpatients showed that SLE patients complaining of cognitive dysfunction generally performed normally on neuropsychological tests but had traits of depression whereas actual poor neuropsychological performance not always was noticed by the patient [75].

The management of cognitive dysfunction is supportive, and exacerbating factors such as anxiety and depression should be managed accordingly. Bertsias et al. have recommended psychoeducational group interventions as being useful. Equally may steroids and/or immunosuppressive therapy be considered to control concurrent SLE or other NPSLE activity [76].

9.5.7 Movement Disorders (Chorea)

Movement disorders, such as chorea, ataxia, choreoathetosis, dystonia, and hemiballismus, occur in roughly 1 % patients with SLE [29]. The existing literature mainly consists of anecdotal reports, case reports, and small case series and has been described as juvenile SLE onset, associated with the use of contraceptives and in patients with aPL [77–79]. Chorea has in the past been associated with the persistent presence of aPL [80]. The underlying pathological mechanisms have been suggested as multifactorial; there does not seem to be an exclusive ischemic underlying pathology [77].

In addition to symptomatic therapy for persistent symptoms (dopamine antagonists), antiplatelet agents may be considered in SLE patients with aPL according to the recent EULAR guidelines. Glucocorticoids and immunosuppressive and/or anticoagulation therapy may be considered in severe cases when generalized disease activity and/or thrombotic manifestations are present [12].

9.5.8 Psychosis

In the context of severe psychiatric manifestations, the WHO has defined acute psychosis as an "acute psychotic disorder in which 'hallucinations, delusions, and perceptual disturbances are obvious but markedly variable, changing from day to day or even from hour to hour. Emotional turmoil, with intense transient feelings of happiness and ecstasy or anxieties and irritability, is also frequently present" [81]. According to the EULAR task force report, any patient presenting with possible NPSLE should receive the standard of care to rule out underlying causes organic systemic disease, metabolic abnormalities, etc. in case of a presentation of any NPSLE manifestation, such as acute psychosis. Corticosteroid-induced psychiatric disease occurs in 10 % of patients treated with prednisone 1 mg/kg (or more) and manifests itself primarily as mood disorder rather than psychosis but remains an important differential diagnosis [82]. NPSLE has been reported to present with paranoia with visual and auditory hallucinations [83]. Recovery is usually complete, but relapses are not rare, and the treatment may include antidepressive agents, steroids, and/or immunosuppressive agents if SLE activity is suspected. In a subgroup analysis from a large single-center study on 751 patients, cyclophosphamide followed by azathioprine maintenance therapy has shown a significant effect [84].

9.5.9 Mood and Anxiety Disorders

Despite epidemiological controversies, anxiety and depression consistently are one of the most commonly reported NPSLE manifestations. The most common psychological symptom in patients with SLE is depression [85–88]. Depressive symptoms may begin acutely accordingly with disease onset [89], possibly reflecting the patient's reaction to chronic illness and the associated lifestyle limitations, including fatigue, limited sun exposure, and chronic medication use [87, 90].

Some studies have postulated an organic cause. An association has been reported between severe depression and aRP antibodies, and antibodies to NMDA receptors, but not with other antibodies [89, 91–93]. Elevated levels of aRP antibodies have been found up to 88 % of these patients [91, 92].

As reported for depression, following the initial diagnosis of SLE, or after an acute exacerbation, some patients display symptoms of anxiety, either instead of or in addition to depression. The patient may become anxious about a variety of possible consequences of their illness, including disfigurement, disability, dependency, loss of a job, social isolation, or death. Ishikura et al. showed that prevalence and intensity of anxiety in the course of SLE positively correlated with insufficient knowledge about disease and its therapy, perceived by the patient at the beginning of disease, and did not correlate with SLE activity [94]. Furthermore, Hawro et al. reported a shorter SLE duration in patients with anxiety disorder [95]. Thus, one may speculate that patients anxiety may be caused by inadequate knowledge about their chronic illness and its treatment options.

9.5.10 Headaches

The term "lupus headache" is used for a particular type of headache directly attributable to SLE and is a stand-alone variable with comparable definitions in at least two composite indices of global SLE disease activity: firstly, the British Isles Lupus Assessment Group (BILAG) 2004 index [96], which defines lupus headache as a disabling headache that is unresponsive to narcotic analgesia and lasts >3 days, and secondly, the SLEDAI-2K [97], which defines lupus headache as a severe, persistent headache (which may be migrainous, but must be nonresponsive to narcotic analgesia).

However, the specificity of this term is under debate as headaches are common in SLE patients but probably not more frequent than in the general population of similar age and gender.

In a review of 50 studies and 115,000 participants in 17 European countries [32], Stovner and Andree reported that the 1-year prevalence of headache in the general population was 55 % (62 % in women and 45 % in men) and the lifetime prevalence of headache was 77 %. In addition, Stovner et al. reported a 1-year prevalence of migraine of 15 % (19 % in women and 8 % in men), and the lifetime prevalence rates were 16 % overall (20 % in women and 11 % in men) [98]. The 1-year prevalence of tension headache was 80 %. Data from the SLICC cohort showed that the frequency of headache at the enrollment visit was comparable to the 1-year prevalence rates in the general population [99]. In the SLICC cohort of a total of 308 patients, 17.8 % had some type of headache. The specific headache types were migraine in 187 patients (60.7 %), tension in 119 (38.6 %), intractable nonspecific in 22 (7.1 %), cluster in 8 (2.6 %), and intracranial hypertension in 3 (1.0 %) [99]. The occurrence of headache is not related to overall SLE disease activity and is not associated with changes in lupus medications. The majority of headaches in SLE patients are unlikely caused by a direct effect of SLE. Regardless of the cause, SLE patients with headaches report a lower quality of life. Most headaches in SLE patients get better and resolve over time.

Conclusions

Neuropsychiatric symptoms affect up to half of the patients with SLE. The effect on disease severity, quality of life, and prognosis is extremely heterogeneous. Symptoms of NPSLE range from mild diffuse conditions to acute life-threatening events. Although the underlying mechanisms are still largely unraveled, several pathogenic pathways have been identified, such as antibody-mediated neurotoxicity, vasculopathy due aPL, and cytokine-induced neurotoxicity.

A diagnosis of NPSLE requires the exclusion of other conditions, and clinical assessment directs the selection of appropriate investigations, including neuroimaging to evaluate brain structure and function, analysis of CSF, electrophysiological studies, and neuropsychological assessment. Treatment includes the use of symptomatic therapies and specific interventions with either anticoagulation or immunosuppressive agents, according to the underlying pathogenetic mechanism. The management of comorbidities contributing to the neuropsychiatric event is also crucial.

References

1. Ginzler EM, Dvorkina O (2005) Newer therapeutic approaches for systemic lupus erythematosus. Rheum Dis Clin North Am 31(2):315–328
2. Nived O, Sturfelt G, Liang MH, De Pablo P (2003) The ACR nomenclature for CNS lupus revisited. Lupus 12(12):872–876
3. Hanly JG (2005) Neuropsychiatric lupus. Rheum Dis Clin North Am 31(2):273–298, vi
4. The American College of Rheumatology nomenclature and case definitions for neuropsychiatric lupus syndromes (1999) Arthritis Rheum. 42(4):599–608
5. Bertsias G, Ioannidis JP, Boletis J, Bombardieri S, Cervera R, Dostal C et al (2008) EULAR recommendations for the management of systemic lupus erythematosus. Report of a Task Force of the EULAR Standing Committee for International Clinical Studies Including Therapeutics. Ann Rheum Dis 67(2):195–205
6. Tan EM, Cohen AS, Fries JF, Masi AT, McShane DJ, Rothfield NF, et al. (1982) The 1982 revised criteria for the classification of systemic lupus erythematosus. Arthritis Rheum 25(11):1271–1277
7. Petri M, Orbai AM, Alarcon GS, Gordon C, Merrill JT, Fortin PR, et al. (2012) Derivation and validation of the Systemic Lupus International Collaborating Clinics classification criteria for systemic lupus erythematosus. Arthritis Rheum 64(8):2677–2686.

8. D'Cruz DP, Khamashta MA, Hughes GR (2007) Systemic lupus erythematosus. Lancet 369(9561):587–596
9. Hanly JG, Su L, Farewell V, McCurdy G, Fougere L, Thompson K (2009) Prospective study of neuropsychiatric events in systemic lupus erythematosus. J Rheumatol 36(7):1449–1459
10. Mok CC, To CH, Mak A (2006) Neuropsychiatric damage in Southern Chinese patients with systemic lupus erythematosus. Medicine (Baltimore) 85(4):221–228
11. Sanna G, Bertolaccini ML, Cuadrado MJ, Laing H, Khamashta MA, Mathieu A et al (2003) Neuropsychiatric manifestations in systemic lupus erythematosus: prevalence and association with antiphospholipid antibodies. J Rheumatol 30(5):985–992
12. Bertsias GK, Ioannidis JP, Aringer M, Bollen E, Bombardieri S, Bruce IN et al (2010) EULAR recommendations for the management of systemic lupus erythematosus with neuropsychiatric manifestations: report of a task force of the EULAR standing committee for clinical affairs. Ann Rheum Dis 69(12):2074–2082
13. Kelly-Hayes M (2010) Influence of age and health behaviors on stroke risk: lessons from longitudinal studies. J Am Geriatr Soc 58(Suppl 2):S325–S328
14. Hanly JG (2014) Diagnosis and management of neuropsychiatric SLE. Nat Rev Rheumatol 10(6):338–347
15. Meroni PL, Borghi MO, Raschi E, Tedesco F (2011) Pathogenesis of antiphospholipid syndrome: understanding the antibodies. Nat Rev Rheumatol 7(6):330–339
16. Mok CC, Lau CS, Wong RW (2001) Neuropsychiatric manifestations and their clinical associations in southern Chinese patients with systemic lupus erythematosus. J Rheumatol 28(4):766–771
17. Afeltra A, Garzia P, Mitterhofer AP, Vadacca M, Galluzzo S, Del Porto F et al (2003) Neuropsychiatric lupus syndromes: relationship with antiphospholipid antibodies. Neurology 61(1):108–110
18. Yu HH, Lee JH, Wang LC, Yang YH, Chiang BL (2006) Neuropsychiatric manifestations in pediatric systemic lupus erythematosus: a 20-year study. Lupus 15(10):651–657
19. Borowoy AM, Pope JE, Silverman E, Fortin PR, Pineau C, Smith CD et al (2012) Neuropsychiatric lupus: the prevalence and autoantibody associations depend on the definition: results from the 1000 faces of lupus cohort. Semin Arthritis Rheum 42(2):179–185
20. Houman MH, Smiti-Khanfir M, Ben Ghorbell I, Miled M (2004) Systemic lupus erythematosus in Tunisia: demographic and clinical analysis of 100 patients. Lupus 13(3):204–211
21. Kamen DL, Barron M, Parker TM, Shaftman SR, Bruner GR, Aberle T et al (2008) Autoantibody prevalence and lupus characteristics in a unique African American population. Arthritis Rheum 58(5):1237–1247
22. Singh S, Gupta MK, Ahluwalia J, Singh P, Malhi P (2009) Neuropsychiatric manifestations and antiphospholipid antibodies in pediatric onset lupus: 14 years of experience from a tertiary center of North India. Rheumatol Int 29(12):1455–1461
23. Kozora E, Filley CM, Zhang L, Brown MS, Miller DE, Arciniegas DB et al (2012) Immune function and brain abnormalities in patients with systemic lupus erythematosus without overt neuropsychiatric manifestations. Lupus 21(4):402–411
24. Menon S, Jameson-Shortall E, Newman SP, Hall-Craggs MR, Chinn R, Isenberg DA (1999) A longitudinal study of anticardiolipin antibody levels and cognitive functioning in systemic lupus erythematosus. Arthritis Rheum 42(4):735–741
25. Mikdashi J, Handwerger B (2004) Predictors of neuropsychiatric damage in systemic lupus erythematosus: data from the Maryland lupus cohort. Rheumatology 43(12):1555–1560
26. Brey RL, Holliday SL, Saklad AR, Navarrete MG, Hermosillo-Romo D, Stallworth CL et al (2002) Neuropsychiatric syndromes in lupus: prevalence using standardized definitions. Neurology 58(8):1214–1220
27. Hanly JG, Urowitz MB, Siannis F, Farewell V, Gordon C, Bae SC et al (2008) Autoantibodies and neuropsychiatric events at the time of systemic lupus erythematosus diagnosis: results from an international inception cohort study. Arthritis Rheum 58(3):843–853
28. Hanly JG, Urowitz MB, Jackson D, Bae SC, Gordon C, Wallace DJ et al (2011) SF-36 summary and subscale scores are reliable outcomes of neuropsychiatric events in systemic lupus erythematosus. Ann Rheum Dis 70(6):961–967

29. Hanly JG, Urowitz MB, Su L, Bae SC, Gordon C, Clarke A et al (2011) Autoantibodies as biomarkers for the prediction of neuropsychiatric events in systemic lupus erythematosus. Ann Rheum Dis 70(10):1726–1732
30. Sciascia S, Bertolaccini ML, Roccatello D, Khamashta MA, Sanna G (2014) Autoantibodies involved in neuropsychiatric manifestations associated with systemic lupus erythematosus: a systematic review. J Neurol 261(9):1706–1714
31. Chapman J, Cohen-Armon M, Shoenfeld Y, Korczyn AD (1999) Antiphospholipid antibodies permeabilize and depolarize brain synaptoneurosomes. Lupus 8(2):127–133
32. Martinez-Cordero E, Rivera Garcia BE, Aguilar Leon DE (1997) Anticardiolipin antibodies in serum and cerebrospinal fluid from patients with systemic lupus erythematosus. J Investig Allergol Clin Immunol 7(6):596–601
33. Eber T, Chapman J, Shoenfeld Y (2005) Anti-ribosomal P-protein and its role in psychiatric manifestations of systemic lupus erythematosus: myth or reality? Lupus 14(8):571–575
34. Zandman-Goddard G, Chapman J, Shoenfeld Y (2007) Autoantibodies involved in neuropsychiatric SLE and antiphospholipid syndrome. Semin Arthritis Rheum 36(5):297–315
35. Karassa FB, Afeltra A, Ambrozic A, Chang DM, De Keyser F, Doria A et al (2006) Accuracy of anti-ribosomal P protein antibody testing for the diagnosis of neuropsychiatric systemic lupus erythematosus: an international meta-analysis. Arthritis Rheum 54(1):312–324
36. Sciascia S, Bertolaccini ML, Baldovino S, Roccatello D, Khamashta MA, Sanna G (2013) Central nervous system involvement in systemic lupus erythematosus: overview on classification criteria. Autoimmun Rev 12(3):426–429
37. Weiner SM, Klein R, Berg PA (2000) A longitudinal study of autoantibodies against central nervous system tissue and gangliosides in connective tissue diseases. Rheumatol Int 19(3):83–88
38. Bluestein HG, Williams GW, Steinberg AD (1981) Cerebrospinal fluid antibodies to neuronal cells: association with neuropsychiatric manifestations of systemic lupus erythematosus. Am J Med 70(2):240–246
39. Zvaifler NJ, Bluestein HG (1982) The pathogenesis of central nervous system manifestations of systemic lupus erythematosus. Arthritis Rheum 25(7):862–866
40. Lauvsnes MB, Omdal R (2012) Systemic lupus erythematosus, the brain, and anti-NR2 antibodies. J Neurol 259(4):622–629
41. Yoshio T, Onda K, Nara H, Minota S (2006) Association of IgG anti-NR2 glutamate receptor antibodies in cerebrospinal fluid with neuropsychiatric systemic lupus erythematosus. Arthritis Rheum 54(2):675–678
42. Arinuma Y, Yanagida T, Hirohata S (2008) Association of cerebrospinal fluid anti-NR2 glutamate receptor antibodies with diffuse neuropsychiatric systemic lupus erythematosus. Arthritis Rheum 58(4):1130–1135
43. Osler W (1895) On the visceral complications of the erythema exudativum multiforme. Am J Med Sci 110:629–646
44. Kassan SS, Lockshin MD (1979) Central nervous system lupus erythematosus. The need for classification. Arthritis Rheum 22(12):1382–1385
45. How A, Dent PB, Liao SK, Denburg JA (1985) Antineuronal antibodies in neuropsychiatric systemic lupus erythematosus. Arthritis Rheum 28(7):789–795
46. Singer J, Denburg JA (1990) Diagnostic criteria for neuropsychiatric systemic lupus erythematosus: the results of a consensus meeting. The Ad Hoc Neuropsychiatric Lupus Workshop Group. J Rheumatol 17(10):1397–1402
47. Ainiala H, Hietaharju A, Loukkola J, Peltola J, Korpela M, Metsanoja R et al (2001) Validity of the new American College of Rheumatology criteria for neuropsychiatric lupus syndromes: a population-based evaluation. Arthritis Rheum 45(5):419–423
48. Kim JM, Kim KJ, Yoon HS, Kwok SK, Ju JH, Park KS et al (2011) Meningitis in Korean patients with systemic lupus erythematosus: analysis of demographics, clinical features and outcomes; experience from affiliated hospitals of the Catholic University of Korea. Lupus 20(5):531–536
49. Bernstein RF (1980) Ibuprofen-related meningitis in mixed connective tissue disease. Ann Intern Med 92(2 Pt 1):206–207

50. Karmacharya P, Mainali NR, Aryal MR, Lloyd B (2013) Recurrent case of ibuprofen-induced aseptic meningitis in mixed connective tissue disease. BMJ Case Rep pii: bcr2013009571
51. Hanly JG, Harrison MJ (2005) Management of neuropsychiatric lupus. Best Pract Res Clin Rheumatol 19(5):799–821
52. Jeltsch-David H, Muller S (2014) Neuropsychiatric systemic lupus erythematosus: pathogenesis and biomarkers. Nat Rev Neurol 10(10):579–596
53. Swain S, Turner C, Tyrrell P, Rudd A, Guideline DG (2008) Diagnosis and initial management of acute stroke and transient ischaemic attack: summary of NICE guidance. BMJ 337:a786
54. Miyakis S, Lockshin MD, Atsumi T, Branch DW, Brey RL, Cervera R et al (2006) International consensus statement on an update of the classification criteria for definite antiphospholipid syndrome (APS). J Thromb Haemost 4(2):295–306
55. Khamashta MA, Cuadrado MJ, Mujic F, Taub NA, Hunt BJ, Hughes GR (1995) The management of thrombosis in the antiphospholipid-antibody syndrome. N Engl J Med 332(15):993–997
56. Crowther M, Crowther MA (2010) Intensity of warfarin coagulation in the antiphospholipid syndrome. Curr Rheumatol Rep 12(1):64–69
57. Ruiz-Irastorza G, Crowther M, Branch W, Khamashta MA (2010) Antiphospholipid syndrome. Lancet 376(9751):1498–1509
58. Cikes N, Bosnic D, Sentic M (2008) Non-MS autoimmune demyelination. Clin Neurol Neurosurg 110(9):905–912
59. Birnbaum J, Petri M, Thompson R, Izbudak I, Kerr D (2009) Distinct subtypes of myelitis in systemic lupus erythematosus. Arthritis Rheum 60(11):3378–3387
60. Theodoridou A, Settas L (2006) Demyelination in rheumatic diseases. J Neurol Neurosurg Psychiatry 77(3):290–295
61. Kaplin AI, Krishnan C, Deshpande DM, Pardo CA, Kerr DA (2005) Diagnosis and management of acute myelopathies. Neurologist 11(1):2–18
62. Karussis D, Leker RR, Ashkenazi A, Abramsky O (1998) A subgroup of multiple sclerosis patients with anticardiolipin antibodies and unusual clinical manifestations: do they represent a new nosological entity? Ann Neurol 44(4):629–634
63. Harris EN, Gharavi AE, Mackworth-Young CG, Patel BM, Derue G, Hughes GR (1985) Lupoid sclerosis: a possible pathogenetic role for antiphospholipid antibodies. Ann Rheum Dis 44(4):281–283
64. Alarcon-Segovia D, Deleze M, Oria CV, Sanchez-Guerrero J, Gomez-Pacheco L, Cabiedes J et al (1989) Antiphospholipid antibodies and the antiphospholipid syndrome in systemic lupus erythematosus. A prospective analysis of 500 consecutive patients. Medicine (Baltimore) 68(6):353–365
65. Lavalle C, Pizarro S, Drenkard C, Sanchez-Guerrero J, Alarcon-Segovia D (1990) Transverse myelitis: a manifestation of systemic lupus erythematosus strongly associated with antiphospholipid antibodies. J Rheumatol 17(1):34–37
66. Ruiz-Arguelles GJ, Guzman-Ramos J, Flores-Flores J, Garay-Martinez J (1998) Refractory hiccough heralding transverse myelitis in the primary antiphospholipid syndrome. Lupus 7(1):49–50
67. D'Cruz DP, Mellor-Pita S, Joven B, Sanna G, Allanson J, Taylor J et al (2004) Transverse myelitis as the first manifestation of systemic lupus erythematosus or lupus-like disease: good functional outcome and relevance of antiphospholipid antibodies. J Rheumatol 31(2):280–285
68. Neuwelt CM (2003) The role of plasmapheresis in the treatment of severe central nervous system neuropsychiatric systemic lupus erythematosus. Ther Apher Dial Off Peer-Rev J Int Soc Apher Jpn Soc Apher Jpn Soc Dial Ther 7(2):173–182
69. Bartolucci P, Brechignac S, Cohen P, Le Guern V, Guillevin L (2007) Adjunctive plasma exchanges to treat neuropsychiatric lupus: a retrospective study on 10 patients. Lupus 16(10):817–822
70. Hanly JG, Urowitz MB, Su L, Gordon C, Bae SC, Sanchez-Guerrero J et al (2012) Seizure disorders in systemic lupus erythematosus results from an international, prospective, inception cohort study. Ann Rheum Dis 71(9):1502–1509

71. Jacobsen S, Petersen J, Ullman S, Junker P, Voss A, Rasmussen JM et al (1998) A multicentre study of 513 Danish patients with systemic lupus erythematosus. I. Disease manifestations and analyses of clinical subsets. Clin Rheumatol 17(6):468–477
72. Joseph FG, Scolding NJ (2010) Neurolupus. Pract Neurol 10(1):4–15
73. Barile-Fabris LA (2005) Treatment of neuropsychiatric manifestations of systemic lupus erythematosus. Reumatol Clin 1(Suppl 2):S42–S45
74. Ainiala H, Loukkola J, Peltola J, Korpela M, Hietaharju A (2001) The prevalence of neuropsychiatric syndromes in systemic lupus erythematosus. Neurology 57(3):496–500
75. Vogel A, Bhattacharya S, Larsen JL, Jacobsen S (2011) Do subjective cognitive complaints correlate with cognitive impairment in systemic lupus erythematosus? A Danish outpatient study. Lupus 20(1):35–43
76. Hanly JG, Cassell K, Fisk JD (1997) Cognitive function in systemic lupus erythematosus: results of a 5-year prospective study. Arthritis Rheum 40(8):1542–1543
77. Baizabal-Carvallo JF, Alonso-Juarez M, Koslowski M (2011) Chorea in systemic lupus erythematosus. J Clin Rheumatol 17(2):69–72
78. Caramelli P, Toledo SM, Marchiori PE, Barbosa ER, Scaff M (1993) Chorea as a sign of systemic lupus erythematosus activity. Case report. Arq Neuropsiquiatr 51(2):267–269
79. Mathur AK, Gatter RA (1988) Chorea as the initial presentation of oral contraceptive induced systemic lupus erythematosus. J Rheumatol 15(6):1042–1043
80. Orzechowski NM, Wolanskyj AP, Ahlskog JE, Kumar N, Moder KG (2008) Antiphospholipid antibody-associated chorea. J Rheumatol 35(11):2165–2170
81. World Health Organization (1993) The ICD-10 classification of mental and behavioural disorders: diagnostic criteria for research. Geneva: World Health Organization: 263 p
82. Chau SY, Mok CC (2003) Factors predictive of corticosteroid psychosis in patients with systemic lupus erythematosus. Neurology 61(1):104–107
83. Segui J, Ramos-Casals M, Garcia-Carrasco M, de Flores T, Cervera R, Valdes M et al (2000) Psychiatric and psychosocial disorders in patients with systemic lupus erythematosus: a longitudinal study of active and inactive stages of the disease. Lupus 9(8):584–588
84. Rahman P, Humphrey-Murto S, Gladman DD, Urowitz MB (1997) Cytotoxic therapy in systemic lupus erythematosus. Experience from a single center. Medicine 76(6):432–437
85. Kozora E, Ellison MC, West S (2006) Depression, fatigue, and pain in systemic lupus erythematosus (SLE): relationship to the American College of Rheumatology SLE neuropsychological battery. Arthritis Rheum 55(4):628–635
86. Goodwin JM, Goodwin JS, Kellner R (1979) Psychiatric symptoms in disliked medical patients. Jama 241(11):1117–1120
87. Kozora E, Ellison MC, Waxmonsky JA, Wamboldt FS, Patterson TL (2005) Major life stress, coping styles, and social support in relation to psychological distress in patients with systemic lupus erythematosus. Lupus 14(5):363–372
88. Stoll T, Kauer Y, Buchi S, Klaghofer R, Sensky T, Villiger PM (2001) Prediction of depression in systemic lupus erythematosus patients using SF-36 Mental Health scores. Rheumatology 40(6):695–698
89. Shortall E, Isenberg D, Newman SP (1995) Factors associated with mood and mood disorders in SLE. Lupus 4(4):272–279
90. Jump RL, Robinson ME, Armstrong AE, Barnes EV, Kilbourn KM, Richards HB (2005) Fatigue in systemic lupus erythematosus: contributions of disease activity, pain, depression, and perceived social support. J Rheumatol 32(9):1699–1705
91. West SG, Emlen W, Wener MH, Kotzin BL (1995) Neuropsychiatric lupus erythematosus: a 10-year prospective study on the value of diagnostic tests. Am J Med 99(2):153–163
92. Schneebaum AB, Singleton JD, West SG, Blodgett JK, Allen LG, Cheronis JC et al (1991) Association of psychiatric manifestations with antibodies to ribosomal P proteins in systemic lupus erythematosus. Am J Med 90(1):54–62

93. Lapteva L, Nowak M, Yarboro CH, Takada K, Roebuck-Spencer T, Weickert T et al (2006) Anti-N-methyl-D-aspartate receptor antibodies, cognitive dysfunction, and depression in systemic lupus erythematosus. Arthritis Rheum 54(8):2505–2514
94. Ishikura R, Morimoto N, Tanaka K, Kinukawa N, Yoshizawa S, Horiuchi T et al (2001) Factors associated with anxiety, depression and suicide ideation in female outpatients with SLE in Japan. Clin Rheumatol 20(6):394–400
95. Hawro T, Krupinska-Kun M, Rabe-Jablonska J, Sysa-Jedrzejowska A, Robak E, Bogaczewicz J et al (2011) Psychiatric disorders in patients with systemic lupus erythematosus: association of anxiety disorder with shorter disease duration. Rheumatol Int 31(10):1387–1391
96. Isenberg DA, Rahman A, Allen E, Farewell V, Akil M, Bruce IN et al (2005) BILAG 2004. Development and initial validation of an updated version of the British Isles Lupus Assessment Group's disease activity index for patients with systemic lupus erythematosus. Rheumatology 44(7):902–906
97. Romero-Diaz J, Isenberg D, Ramsey-Goldman R (2011) Measures of adult systemic lupus erythematosus: updated version of British Isles Lupus Assessment Group (BILAG 2004), European Consensus Lupus Activity Measurements (ECLAM), Systemic Lupus Activity Measure, Revised (SLAM-R), Systemic Lupus Activity Questionnaire for Population Studies (SLAQ), Systemic Lupus Erythematosus Disease Activity Index 2000 (SLEDAI-2 K), and Systemic Lupus International Collaborating Clinics/American College of Rheumatology Damage Index (SDI). Arthritis Care Res 63(Suppl 11):S37–S46
98. Stovner LJ, Andree C (2010) Prevalence of headache in Europe: a review for the Eurolight project. J Headache Pain 11(4):289–299
99. Hanly JG, Urowitz MB, O'Keeffe AG, Gordon C, Bae SC, Sanchez-Guerrero J et al (2013) Headache in systemic lupus erythematosus: results from a prospective, international inception cohort study. Arthritis Rheum 65(11):2887–2897

Cardiovascular Issues in SLE

10

Maria Gerosa, Mara Taraborelli, Pier Luigi Meroni,
and Angela Tincani

10.1 Introduction

Systemic lupus erythematosus (SLE) is a systemic autoimmune disease affecting different organs and systems. Heart and vessels are a direct target of the autoimmune process, but cardiovascular involvement can be also an indirect consequence of the accelerated atherosclerosis associated to the inflammatory cascade or to the disease treatment. Cardiovascular disease (CVD) is a significant cause of morbidity and mortality in SLE patients.

10.2 Cardiovascular Risk in Systemic Lupus Erythematosus

10.2.1 Epidemiology

Urowitz et al. [1] first described how mortality in SLE follows a bimodal pattern with an early peak (first year) related to active disease and a late peak (more than 5 years after diagnosis) due to premature CVD. Although the overall mortality in SLE has significantly reduced over the last decades, mortality due to CVD has not significantly improved and CVD still remains one of the leading causes of death in those patients [2].

M. Gerosa (✉) • P.L. Meroni
Department of Clinical Sciences and Community Health and Division of Rheumatology, University of Milan, Istituto Ortopedico Gaetano Pini, Milan, Italy
e-mail: maria.gerosa@unimi.it; pierluigi.meroni@unimi.it

M. Taraborelli • A. Tincani
Department of Rheumatology and Clinical Immunology, University of Brescia, Spedali Civili of Brescia, Brescia, Italy
e-mail: mara.taraborelli@gmail.com; angela.tincani@unibs.it

D. Roccatello, L. Emmi (eds.), *Connective Tissue Disease: A Comprehensive Guide-Volume 1*, Rare Diseases of the Immune System 5,
DOI 10.1007/978-3-319-24535-5_10

The CVD risk is at least doubled in SLE patients compared to the general population [3]. The increased prevalence of CVD is particularly striking in young premenopausal women, who generally are a low-risk category [4]. Nevertheless, the absolute risk of CVD remains higher in older SLE patients [3].

Accelerated atherosclerosis is responsible for premature CVD in SLE patients and has been estimated to develop or progress in 10 % of patients each year [5]. Vascular abnormalities have been observed in SLE patients even close to disease diagnosis [6]. Subclinical atherosclerosis is more prevalent than clinical events and was first observed in autopsy studies that showed that up to 50 % of young SLE patients had significant coronary artery narrowing [7, 8]. More recent noninvasive techniques have confirmed that observation in living asymptomatic patients. Electron beam computed tomography [9, 10] showed coronary artery calcifications in 30–40 % of SLE patients, and a similar prevalence of carotid artery plaques was detected by carotid ultrasound [11, 12] in different studies. More than half of SLE subjects have an endothelial dysfunction measured by flow-mediated dilation [13].

Clinical events include coronary artery disease (CAD), heart failure (CHF), cerebrovascular disease (CVA), and peripheral vascular disease.

Most studies reported a two- to tenfold increase of CAD risk in SLE patients compared to the general population [3], but a 50-fold increase has been described in young patients aged 35–44 [14]. Fatal myocardial infarction (MI) has been reported to be three times more frequent in SLE patients than controls [15]. A prolonged hospitalization for acute MI [16] and a worse outcome after coronary revascularization procedures defined as higher risk of MI or repeated revascularization [17] have been observed in SLE compared to non-SLE patients. The risk of CHF and related hospitalization/mortality is also significantly increased in SLE patients compared to controls [16, 18].

Similarly to MI, SLE patients have an approximately twofold increase of CVA risk compared to controls, and this risk is particular evident in young patients [19–21].

Although no studies reported the relative risk of peripheral vascular disease in SLE patients, this complication has been shown to affect very young patients (mean age 36.5 years) and to be associated to a higher risk of death in a large cohort [22].

10.2.2 Risk Factors

Hypercholesterolemia, hypertension, diabetes, and metabolic syndrome have been shown to be more prevalent in SLE than in the general population and to be independent risk factors for CVD in those patients [3]. Male sex, older age, and smoking, even if not more prevalent, can contribute to increase that risk. Anyway traditional risk factors do not fully explain the premature atherosclerosis and the increased incidence of CVD observed in SLE patients [23].

SLE-related inflammation is now recognized, as other rheumatic conditions, as an independent factor for the development of atherosclerosis. SLE disease activity, measured by validated indexes, has been found to be a predictor of CVD in most of the studies [21, 24], with renal [25] and neuropsychiatric [26] involvement recognized as the most relevant-related factors. No consensus exists about the correlation between disease duration and CVD [14, 27]. Antiphospholipid antibodies (aPL) have been associated to a fourfold increase risk of CVD in SLE patients [27].

10.3 Pathogenesis of Cardiovascular Involvement

Different mechanisms have been recognized as possibly involved in the pathogenesis of accelerated atherosclerosis in SLE patients. Recent studies showed that vascular damage is increased (as demonstrated by higher levels of circulating apoptotic endothelial cells) and vascular repair is compromised (as shown by lower levels of circulating endothelial progenitor cells and myelomonocytic angiogenic cells) in SLE [28]. Interferon alfa (IFN-α), a cytokine that is known to be increased in SLE, plays a major role in that altered vasculogenesis by inhibiting proangiogenetic factors (interleukin 1β and vascular endothelial growth factor) and by upregulating antiangiogenetic factors (interleukin 1 receptor antagonist) [29]. Interferon alfa also induces tumor necrosis factor-related apoptosis inducing ligand expression by CD4+ T cells, which can increase the risk of plaque rupture [30].

Tumor necrosis factor α, whose levels are increased in SLE patients and even more in those with CVD compared to those without CVD, increases the expression of adhesion molecules on the endothelial surface and the production of chemotactic proteins with a consequent promoting effect on inflammation of the atherosclerotic plaque [31].

aPL can contribute to accelerated atherosclerosis by interacting with endothelial cells and inducing a proinflammatory endothelial phenotype [32]. Other aPL-related mechanisms include the upregulation of tissue factor expression on endothelial cells and blood monocytes and the promotion of endothelial leukocyte adhesion, cytokine secretion, and prostaglandin E2 synthesis [32].

Complement can interact with immune complexes and promote the expression of endothelial adhesion molecules [33].

At last an abnormal chylomicron processing has been observed in SLE, with resulting higher levels of proinflammatory high-density lipoproteins that can promote accelerated atherosclerosis as they are not effective in preventing low-density lipoprotein oxidation [34].

10.4 Prevention

Traditional risk factor identification and aggressive reduction in all SLE patients are clearly an essential step of CVD prevention; the awareness of patients and physicians about those risk factors is increasing over time but is not optimal also in academic centers [35, 36]. According to the European League Against Rheumatism (EULAR) recommendations for the management of SLE, lifestyle modifications (smoking cessation, weight control, exercise) should be encouraged, and depending on the individual medication and the clinical situation, other agents (low-dose aspirin, calcium/

vitamin D, biphosphonates, statins, anti-hypertensives in particular angiotensin receptor blockers) should be considered [37]. Some authors suggested that SLE, as diabetes, should be considered as a previous CAD event and that targets for blood pressure (<130/80 mmHg) and lipid levels (low-density cholesterol <100 mg/dL) should be lower than those recommended for the general population [38].

Reducing SLE disease activity is the other way to prevent CVD, as demonstrated, for example, by the fact that aortic atherosclerosis risk is lower in patients who have been treated with cyclophosphamide compared to those who have not received it [39]. Although corticosteroids have anti-inflammatory effects, they are associated with an increase of traditional risk factors (hypertension, diabetes, hypercholesterolemia). The lowest possible dose for the shortest time should be used to minimize those risks.

An increasing interest for specific drugs used to treat SLE has come to light for their potential cardiovascular protective effects in SLE patients. Hydroxychloroquine has a cardio- and vasculoprotective effect (by blocking toll-like receptor 7- and 9-related interferon α release), prevents thrombotic events (by reverting platelet aggregation and reducing aPL exposure), and reduces hypercholesterolemia and hyperglycemia (by increasing insulin response) [40]. This drug has been associated with an improved survival in SLE patients [41]. Mycophenolate mofetil has several potential antiatherogenic effects including the inhibition oxidative stress, the reduction of the recruitment of T cells in the plaque, and possibly the improvement of high-density lipoprotein activity [42]. The effect of new biologic drugs in CVD prevention in SLE needs to be investigated.

Other medications used to treat hypercholesterolemia and diabetes could have a role in CVD prevention in SLE. Statins lower lipid levels but also have anti-inflammatory properties that could help to prevent atherosclerosis, like inhibition of inflammatory cytokines/T-cell activation/reactive oxygen species formation and nitric oxide synthesis upregulation [43]. Those medications have been shown to reduce atherosclerotic lesions in murine models [44], but effects described in SLE patients are inconsistent (improved endothelium-dependent flow-mediated dilation versus no significant reduction of coronary calcium/intima media thickness/prevention of cardiovascular events) [45, 46]. Thiazolidinediones have also shown promising effects in murine models (reduced atherosclerosis) [47] and in SLE patients (improved high-density lipoprotein levels, insulin resistance, and reduced C reactive protein) [48]. Both these medication effects should be further investigated, and their use in SLE patients remains based on standard CVD guidelines.

10.5 Cardiac Manifestations in Systemic Lupus Erythematosus

In addition to cardiovascular disease, several other cardiac manifestations can occur in SLE patients. The reported prevalence of heart involvement is very variable, ranging from 14 to more than 50 % [49–51]. This inconsistency can be ascribed to several reasons, including the heterogeneity of patient populations, the timing of assessment during the course of the disease, but also the differences of the definition of heart disease and the methodology of evaluation. Moreover, prognosis and survival rates in SLE patients have dramatically changed over time together with the improvement of the diagnostic and therapeutic armamentarium, leading to important modifications of the clinical characteristics of the disease [52]. Postmortem studies report a very high rate of silent pericardial, myocardial, or endocardial involvement, while clinically evident heart disease is much less common [49, 51, 53].

10.5.1 Pericarditis

Pericarditis is the most common cardiac abnormality and is the only cardiac manifestation included both in the "historical" 1997 American College of Rheumatology and the "new" 2012 Systemic Lupus International Collaborating Clinics classification criteria for SLE [54, 55]. The prevalence of symptomatic pericarditis is extremely variable among studies, ranging from 5 % to more than 50 % [51, 56]. However, subclinical pericardial involvement, such as pericardial thickening or mild pericardial effusion, has been detected in a higher proportion of patients (up to 80 %) in echocardiographic and postmortem evaluations [49–51, 56, 57].

Acute pericarditis can represent the first manifestation of SLE or manifest during disease relapses. It can be isolated or occur as part of a generalized serositis with ascites and pleural effusions. Positional precordial chest pain, typically associated with fatigue, fever, tachycardia, and friction rubs, characterizes the clinical picture of the disease. Pericardial effusion is inconstantly present and mild in most cases, while cardiac tamponade is very rare [49–51]. Complement depletion and increase of acute-phase proteins are usually observed in the serum. Notably, while C reactive protein (CRP) does not significantly change during SLE flares, pericarditis is one of the few SLE manifestations that can induce a rise of this serological marker [57, 58].

Pericardial inflammation in SLE is sustained by immune complex deposition and subsequent activation of the complement cascade [51, 59]. Accordingly, immunopathological studies have demonstrated the presence of granular deposits of C1q, C3, and class G immunoglobulins (IgG) by indirect immunofluorescence, and increased levels of complement split products have been detected in the pericardial fluid [59]. The pericardial fluid examination may also demonstrate antinuclear and anti-DNA antibodies, leukocytosis, and low glucose levels [51, 59].

Recently, an association between common variants in TRAF3IP2 gene and susceptibility to SLE has been reported. In this study, the variant allele of all the single nucleotide polymorphisms (SNPs) of this gene was significantly associated with development of pericarditis, accounting for an odds ratio ranging from 2.38 to 2.59 [60].

Nonsteroidal anti-inflammatory drugs (NSAIDs) are the first choice for the treatment of idiopathic and viral pericarditis, but are usually unhelpful in SLE patients. Colchicine has been successfully used in cases refractory to NSAIDs; however, data in connective tissue diseases are too limited to draw any definite conclusion [61, 62]. In SLE patients, intermediate doses of oral prednisone (0.5–1 mg per kilogram of body weight daily) are usually effective in mild disease, while high-dose intravenous corticosteroids (2–5 mg per kilogram of body weight daily) are requested to control more severe pericardial involvement [51]. In the last years, some authors have reported the effectiveness of tocilizumab for the treatment of severe pericarditis in SLE patients not responding to high-dose steroids [63–65]. For long-term treatment of refractory cases, immunosuppression with azathioprine, methotrexate, or mycophenolate mofetil can be beneficial for the prevention of recurrence [51]. There are no available data regarding the potential use of belimumab in this particular SLE manifestation; however, a beneficial effect of the drug can be hypothesized [66].

10.5.2 Myocardial Involvement

Since its first description in 1954, lupus carditis has been addressed as a very severe manifestation of the disease, contributing to morbidity and mortality of SLE [67]. However, the prevalence of clinically evident inflammatory myocardial involvement has dramatically decreased from the 55 % of Harvey et al. to less than 10 % of the latest publications [51, 67]. A very recent study exploring the occurrence of primary cardiac disease in a large cohort of SLE patients reports an incidence of myocarditis of 3.5 % [50]. Such a decrease is likely ascribable to the more aggressive treatment of SLE and its major complications in the last decades, based on high-dose steroids and immunosuppression. Moreover, the introduction of very sensible imaging techniques, such as echocardiography, scintigraphy, and magnetic resonance imaging (MRI), has allowed an earlier diagnosis and a prompt intervention, thus preventing severe complications.

The clinical symptoms of SLE myocarditis are similar to that of other types of myocardial inflammation and include fever, tachycardia, and signs of ventricular dysfunction, leading to dilated cardiomyopathy and CHF [51]. Typical laboratory findings are represented by high erythrocyte sedimentation rate (ESR) and acute-phase proteins (including CRP), low C3 and C4, leukocytosis, and increases in the cardiac fraction of creatine kinase (CK-MB), troponin T, and troponin I.

Histopathological examination of the myocardium can reveal interstitial edema, focal necrosis or fibrosis, and focal or diffuse lymphocyte and plasma cell infiltrations. Indirect immunofluorescence shows deposition of IgG and complement fragments, suggesting an immune complex-mediated inflammation [59]. Recently, high expression of TNF-α and interleukin (IL) 8 and IL 10, together with abundant deposits of C3a, was demonstrated in the postmortem examination of the myocardium of an SLE patient who died for severe pancarditis [68].

In addition to acute myocarditis, several studies based on noninvasive diagnostic techniques have revealed the presence of subtle, asymptomatic myocardial involvement in a substantial proportion of SLE patients [51, 56, 57, 69–72]. Reduced left ventricular ejection fraction (LVEF), diastolic dysfunction, prolonged isovolumic relaxation time, left atrial dilation, and increased right ventricular systolic pressure have been reported in a very variable percentage in echocardiographic studies [51, 56, 57]. In the last decade, a growing interest has been committed to cardiac magnetic resonance (CMR) as a sensitive tool in the evaluation of the structure and function of the myocardium because of its ability to detect early subtle tissue changes [70]. This technique has been suggested to be useful for the detection of myocarditis and/or signs of previous myocardial ischemia such as myocardial fibrosis even in asymptomatic patients [69–71].

Given that even mild myocarditis can lead to CHF, it has to be promptly and aggressively treated. High-dose intravenous pulse corticosteroids are usually used in the acute phase, but intravenous immunoglobulin can be required in refractory cases. Maintenance of remission is usually obtained with immunosuppressants, namely, cyclophosphamide or azathioprine.

10.5.3 Valvular Abnormalities

Libman-Sacks endocarditis represents the first cardiac manifestation described in SLE in 1924 [73]. It is characterized by sterile, verrucous vegetations or masses, mainly affecting the left-side valves. The posterior mitral leaflet is the preferential localization, but any of the four valves can be involved. Similar lesions have rarely been described on the chordae tendineae, the papillary muscles, and the endocardial surface [74].

Valve thickening, stenosis, and regurgitation have also been reported in SLE patients, with a higher frequency than verrucous endocarditis [53, 74, 75]. The prevalence of anatomical or functional valvular abnormalities ranges from 11 to 74 % in different studies and has increased in the last decades in parallel with the improvement of imaging techniques and the prolonged survival of SLE patients [53, 74]. Valvular abnormalities can change over time in SLE patients, and prospective studies have demonstrated that they can disappear or occur de novo during the course of the disease, independently of the disease activity [76]. Several studies have demonstrated that transesophageal is significantly superior to transthoracic echocardiography for the diagnosis of valve involvement, and more recently CMR has been shown to be another sensitive technique [71, 77].

Libman-Sacks endocarditis is asymptomatic in most cases, even if it can occasionally manifest with fever, splinter hemorrhages, new murmur, and arthralgias or arthritis, mimicking signs and symptoms of infective endocarditis [74, 77].

Overlying infection, insufficiency, and thromboembolism represent the most important complications of valvular involvement. Infective endocarditis can superimpose verrucous lesions, especially in the presence of strong immunosuppression [74, 77]. Thus, antibiotic prophylaxis should be recommended in all SLE patients with valvular involvement in case of increased risk, such as dental surgical treatment. Thromboembolic events, usually involving the cerebral circulation, can also occur and can be independently related to the presence of antiphospholipid antibodies [74, 75]. The presence of valvular vegetations has been recently associated with a three- to fivefold risk of cerebromicroembolism and/or brain lesions [78]. Valvular insufficiency and stenosis are rare, but should be taken into account as they can lead to symptomatic heart failure and surgical valve replacement [74].

The association of valvular involvement with aPL has been frequently advocated and has been recently confirmed by a wide meta-analysis including 23 primary studies for a total of 1,656 SLE patients, 508 of whom with valvular disease [75]. This meta-analysis concluded that the overall pooled odds ratio for valvular involvement in aPL-positive patients, in comparison with aPL-negative SLE patients, was 3.51 and that lupus anticoagulant (LA) displayed the strongest risk (odds ratio 5.88), followed by anticardiolipin IgG (odds ratio 5.63) [75].

In line with these findings, histopathological studies have demonstrated aPL and complement deposits on specimens of altered valve leaflets from aPL-positive patients with or without SLE [79]. Several authors have hypothesized a direct pathogenetic role of these autoantibodies, which could eventually enhance thrombus formation on valves already deformed by inflammation and/or complement deposition.

The management of asymptomatic valvular involvement is still controversial. Steroids have been suggested to be effective in the treatment of Libman-Sacks endocarditis, but their use is still controversial, because they can accelerate healing of valve vegetations, with fibrosis and valve deformity [74]. Anticoagulant therapy should be recommended to patients with a previous cardioembolic event or in those with large valvular lesions. However, several studies report persistent valvular disease in aPL-positive patients despite oral anticoagulation suggesting that this therapy is not always effective in inducing valve involvement regression [74].

10.5.4 Rhythm and Conduction System Disorders

Electrocardiographic abnormalities, including conduction and rhythm disturbances, have been poorly evaluated in adult SLE patients.

Sinus tachycardia is very frequent and can be related to the systemic symptoms of the disease, such as fever or anemia, or be associated with other types of cardiac involvement, generally pericarditis and/or myocarditis [51, 80].

Atrioventricular blocks, intraventricular conduction defects, and sinus node dysfunction have been rarely reported and can appear as a consequence of myocarditis, myocardial ischemia, or fibrosis involving the conduction system [80].

An increased incidence of prolonged corrected QT (QTc) interval has also been reported in SLE patients. As sinus bradycardia and QTc interval prolongation have been described, in addition to congenital heart block, in neonatal lupus syndrome (NLS), several authors have advocated a possible association of prolonged QTc with anti-Ro/SSA antibodies in SLE patients [81–85]. However, data from the literature are not univocal. Lazzerini et al. have reported a statistically significant prolongation of QTc in anti-Ro-/SSA-positive adult patients suffering from various systemic autoimmune diseases including SLE [86, 87], while Gordon et al. did not confirm this finding in a population of selected anti-Ro-/SSA-positive SLE patients [88]. More recently, Bourré-Tessier et al. showed an increased risk of prolonged QTc in anti-Ro-/SSA-positive SLE patients, with an adjusted odds ratio ranging from 5.1 to 12.6 [84]. However, the importance of these data in the clinical practice is uncertain and the actual risk of severe complications such as ventricular arrhythmias and sudden death in SLE patients with this conduction abnormality has not been established up to now.

Conclusion

The cardiovascular system is commonly affected in SLE patients. A careful clinical and instrumental monitoring together with a strict control of modifiable cardiovascular risk factors is essential to reduce the impact of the disease and to increase survival in these patients.

References

1. Urowitz MB, Bookman AA, Koheler BE et al (1976) The bimodal mortality pattern of systemic lupus erythematosus. Am J Med 60:221–225
2. Yurkovich M, Vostretsova K, Chen W et al (2014) Overall and cause-specific mortality in patients with systemic lupus erythematosus: a meta-analysis of observational studies. Arthritis Care Res (Hoboken) 66:608–616
3. Schoenfeld SR, Kasturi S, Costenbader KH (2013) The epidemiology of atherosclerotic cardiovascular disease among patients with SLE: a systematic review. Semin Arthritis Rheum 43:77–95
4. Manzi S, Selzer F, Sutton-Tyrrell K et al (1999) Prevalence and risk factors of carotid plaque in women with systemic lupus erythematosus. Arthritis Rheum 42:51–60
5. Roman MJ, Crow MK, Lockshin MD et al (2007) Rate and determinants of progression of atherosclerosis in systemic lupus erythematosus. Arthritis Rheum 56:3412–3419
6. Rajagopalan S, Somers EC, Brook RD et al (2004) Endothelial cell apoptosis in systemic lupus erythematosus: a common pathway for abnormal vascular function and thrombosis propensity. Blood 103:3677–3683
7. Haider YS, Roberts WC (1981) Coronary arterial disease in systemic lupus erythematosus; quantification of degrees of narrowing in 22 necropsy patients (21 women) aged 16 to 37 years. Am J Med 70:775–781
8. Bulkley BH, Roberts WC (1975) The heart in systemic lupus erythematosus and the changes induced in it by corticosteroid therapy. A study of 36 necropsy patients. Am J Med 58:243
9. Manger K, Kusus M, Forster C et al (2003) Factors associated with coronary artery calcification in young female patients with SLE. Ann Rheum Dis 62:846
10. Kao AH, Wasko MC, Krishnaswami S et al (2008) C-reactive protein and coronary artery calcium in asymptomatic women with systemic lupus erythematosus or rheumatoid arthritis. Am J Cardiol 102:755
11. Roman MJ, Shanker BA, Davis A et al (2003) Prevalence and correlates of accelerated atherosclerosis in systemic lupus erythematosus. N Engl J Med 349:2399
12. Thompson T, Sutton-Tyrrell K, Wildman RP et al (2008) Progression of carotid intima-media thickness and plaque in women with systemic lupus erythematosus. Arthritis Rheum 58:835
13. Recio-Mayoral A, Mason JC, Kaski JC et al (2009) Chronic inflammation and coronary microvascular dysfunction in patients without risk factors for coronary artery disease. Eur Heart J 30:1837–1843
14. Manzi S, Meilahn EN, Rairie JE et al (1997) Age-specific incidence rates of myocardial infarction and angina in women with systemic lupus erythematosus: comparison with the Framingham study. Am J Epidemiol 145:408–415
15. Zeller CB, Appenzeller S (2008) Cardiovascular disease in systemic lupus erythematosus: the role of traditional and lupus related risk factors. Curr Cardiol Rev 4:116–122
16. Shah MA, Shah AM, Krishnan E (2009) Poor outcomes after acute myocardial infarction in systemic lupus erythematosus. J Rheumatol 36:570–575
17. Maksimowic-Mckinnon K, Selzer F, Manzi S et al (2008) Poor 1-year outcomes after percutaneous coronary interventions in systemic lupus erythematosus: report from the National Heart, Lung, and Blood Institute Dynamic Registry. Circ Cardiovasc Interv 1:201–208

18. Van der Laan-Baalbergen NE (2009) Heart failure as presenting manifestations of cardiac involvement in systemic lupus erythematosus. Neth J Med 67:295–301
19. Hak AE, Karlson EW, Feskanich D et al (2009) Systemic lupus erythematosus and the risk of cardiovascular disease: results from the nurses' health study. Arthritis Rheum 61:1396–1402
20. Mok CC, Ho LY, To CH (2009) Annual incidence and standardized incidence ratio of cerebrovascular accidents in patients with systemic lupus erythematosus. Scand J Rheumatol 38:362–368
21. Bengtsson C, Ohman ML, Nived O (2012) Cardiovascular event in systemic lupus erythematosus in northern Sweden: incidence and predictors in a 7-year follow-up study. Lupus 21:452–459
22. Burgos PI, Vila LM, Reveille JD et al (2009) Peripheral vascular damage in systemic lupus erythematosus: data from LUMINA, a large multi-ethnic U.S. cohort (LXIX). Lupus 18:1303–1308
23. Esdaile JM, Abrahamowicz M, Grodzicky T et al (2001) Traditional Framingham risk factors fail to fully account for accelerated atherosclerosis in systemic lupus erythematosus. Arthritis Rheum 44:2331–2337
24. Mikdashi J, Handwerger B, Langenberg P et al (2007) Baseline disease activity, hyperlipidemia, and hypertension are predictive factors for ischemic stroke and stroke severity in systemic lupus erythematosus. Stroke 382:281–285
25. Mak A, Mok CC, Chu WP et al (2007) Renal damage in systemic lupus erythematosus: a comparative analysis of different age groups. Lupus 16:28–34
26. Urowitz MB, Gladman D, Ibanez D et al (2007) Clinical manifestations and coronary artery disease risk factors at diagnosis of systemic lupus erythematosus: data from an international inception cohort. Lupus 169:731–735
27. Toloza SM, Uribe AG, McGwin G Jr et al (2004) Systemic lupus erythematosus in a multiethnic US cohort (LUMINA). XXIII. Baseline predictors of vascular events. Arthritis Rheum 50:3947–3957
28. Kahlenberg JM, Kaplan MJ (2011) The interplay of inflammation and cardiovascular disease in systemic lupus erythematosus. Arthritis Res Ther 13:203
29. Denny MF, Thacker S, Mehta H et al (2007) Interferon-alpha promotes abnormal vasculogenesis in lupus: a potential pathway for premature atherosclerosis. Blood 110:2907–2915
30. Niessner A, Weyand CM (2010) Dendritic cells in atherosclerotic disease. Clin Immunol 134:25–32
31. Svenungsson E, Fei GZ, Jensen-Urstad K et al (2003) TNF-alpha: a link between hypertriglyceridaemia and inflammation in SLE patients with cardiovascular disease. Lupus 12:454–461
32. Meroni PL, Borghi MO, Raschi E et al (2011) Pathogenesis of antiphospholipid syndrome: understanding the antibodies. Nat Rev Rheumatol 7:330–339
33. Clancy RM (2000) Circulating endothelial cells and vascular injury in systemic lupus erythematosus. Curr Rheumatol Rep 2:39–43
34. McMahon M, Grossman J, Skaggs B et al (2009) Dysfunctional proinflammatory high-density lipoproteins confer increased risk of atherosclerosis in women with systemic lupus erythematosus. Arthritis Rheum 60:2428–2437
35. Petri M, Spence D, Bone LR et al (1992) Coronary artery disease risk factors in the Johns Hopkins Lupus Cohort: prevalence, recognition by patients, and preventive practices. Medicine (Baltimore) 71:291
36. Costenbader KH, Wright E, Liang MH et al (2004) Cardiac risk factor awareness and management in patients with systemic lupus erythematosus. Arthritis Rheum 51:983–988
37. Bertsias G, Ioannidis JP, Boletis J et al (2008) EULAR recommendations for the management of systemic lupus erythematosus. Report of a task force of the EULAR standing committee for international clinical studies including therapeutics. Ann Rheum Dis 67:195–205
38. Bruce IN (2005) 'Not only…but also': factors that contribute to accelerated atherosclerosis and premature coronary heart disease in systemic lupus erythematosus. Rheumatology (Oxford) 44:1492–1502

39. Roldan C, Joson J, Sharrar J et al (2010) Premature aortic atherosclerosis in systemic lupus erythematosus: a controlled transesophageal echocardiographic study. J Rheumatol 37:71–78
40. Costedoat-Chalumeau N, Dunogué B, Morel N et al (2014) Hydroxychloroquine: a multifaceted treatment in lupus. Presse Med 43:e167–e180
41. Alarcón GS, McGwin G Jr, Bastian HM et al (2001) Systemic lupus erythematosus in three ethnic groups. VII [correction of VIII]. Predictors of early mortality in the LUMINA cohort. LUMINA study group. Arthritis Rheum 45:191–202
42. Skaggs BJ, Hahn BH, McMahon M (2012) Accelerated atherosclerosis in patients with SLE – mechanisms and management. Nat Rev Rheumatol 8:214–223
43. Forrester JS, Libby P (2007) The inflammation hypothesis and its potential relevance to statin therapy. Am J Cardiol 99:732–738
44. Aprahamian T, Bonegio R, Rizzo J et al (2006) Simvastatin treatment ameliorates autoimmune disease associated with accelerated atherosclerosis in a murine lupus model. J Immunol 177:3028–3034
45. Ferreira GA, Navarro TP, Telles RW, Andrade LE, Sato EI et al (2007) Atorvastatin therapy improves endothelial-dependent vasodilation in patients with systemic lupus erythematosus: an 8 weeks controlled trial. Rheumatology (Oxford) 46:1560–1565
46. Petri M, Kiani A, Post W et al (2006) Lupus atherosclerosis prevention study (LAPS): a randomized double blind placebo controlled trial of atorvastatin versus placebo. Arthritis Rheum 54:S520
47. Aprahamian T, Bonegio RG, Richez C et al (2009) The peroxisome proliferator-activated receptor gamma agonist rosiglitazone ameliorates murine lupus by induction of adiponectin. J Immunol 182:340–346
48. Juarez-Rojas JG, Medina-Urrutia AX, Jorge-Galarza E et al (2012) Pioglitazone improves the cardiovascular profile in patients with uncomplicated systemic lupus erythematosus: a double-blind randomized clinical trial. Lupus 21:27–35
49. Riboldi P, Gerosa M, Luzzana C et al (2002) Cardiac involvement in systemic autoimmune diseases. Clin Rev Allergy Immunol 23:247–261
50. Garcia MA, Alarcon GS, Boggio G et al (2014) Primary cardiac disease in systemic lupus erythematosus patients: protective and risk factors – data from a multi-ethnic Latin American cohort. Rheumatology 53:1431–1438
51. Doria A, Iaccarino L, Sarzi-Puttini P et al (2005) Cardiac involvement in systemic lupus erythematosus. Lupus 14:683–686
52. Urowitz MB, Gladman DD, Tom BD et al (2008) Changing patterns in mortality and disease outcomes for patients with systemic lupus erythematosus. J Rheumatol 35:2152–2158
53. Miner JJ, Kim AHJ (2014) Cardiac manifestations of systemic lupus erythematosus. Rheum Dis Clin N Am 40:51–60
54. Hochberg MC, Diagnostic and Therapeutic Criteria Committee of the American College of Rheumatology (1997) Updating the American College of Rheumatology revised criteria for the classification of systemic lupus erythematosus. Arthritis Rheum 40:1725
55. Petri M, Orbai AM, Alarcon GS et al (2012) Derivation and validation of the systemic lupus international collaborating clinics classification criteria for systemic lupus erythematosus. Arthritis Rheum 64:2677–2686
56. Bourré-Tessier J, Huynh T, Clarke AE et al (2011) Features associated with cardiac abnormalities in systemic lupus erythematosus. Lupus 20:1518–1525
57. Plazak W, Gryga K, Milewski M et al (2011) Association of heart structure and function abnormalities with laboratory findings in patients with systemic lupus erythematosus. Lupus 20:936–944
58. Mok CC, Birmingham DJ, Ho LY et al (2013) High-sensitivity C-reactive protein, disease activity, and cardiovascular risk factors in systemic lupus erythematosus. Arthritis Care Res 65:441–447
59. Jain D, Halushka MK (2009) Cardiac pathology of systemic lupus erythematosus. J Clin Pathol 62:584–592

60. Perricone C, Ciccacci C, Ceccarelli F et al (2013) TRAF3IP2 gene and systemic lupus erythematosus: association with disease susceptibility and pericarditis development. Immunogenetics 65:703–709
61. Imazio M, Bobbio M, Cecchi E et al (2005) Colchicine in addition to conventional therapy for acute pericarditis: results of the COlchicine for acute PEricarditis (COPE) trial. Circulation 112:2012–2016
62. Imazio M, Brucato A, Cemin R et al (2013) A randomized trial of colchicine for acute pericarditis. N Engl J Med 369:1522–1528
63. Iwai A, Naniwa T, Tamechika S et al (2014) Short-term add-on tocilizumab and intravenous cyclophosphamide exhibited a remission-inducing effect in a patient with systemic lupus erythematosus with refractory multiorgan involvements including massive pericarditis and glomerulonephritis. Mod Rheumatol 30:1–4 [Epub ahead of print]
64. Kamata Y, Minota S (2012) Successful treatment of massive intractable pericardial effusion in a patient with systemic lupus erythematosus with tocilizumab. BMJ Case Rep. pii: bcr2012007834
65. Maeshima K, Ishii K, Torigoe M et al (2012) Successful tocilizumab and tacrolimus treatment in a patient with rheumatoid arthritis complicated by systemic lupus erythematosus. Lupus 21:1003–1006
66. Ginzler EM, Wallace DJ, Merrill JT et al (2014) Disease control and safety of belimumab plus standard therapy over 7 years in patients with systemic lupus erythematosus. J Rheumatol 41:300–309
67. Harvey AM, Shulman LE, Tumulty PA et al (1954) Systemic lupus erythematosus: review of the literature and clinical analysis of 138 cases. Medicine 33:291–437
68. Pomara C, Neri M, Bello S et al (2010) C3a, TNF-a and interleukin myocardial expression in a case of fatal sudden cardiac failure during clinic reactivation of systemic lupus erythematosus. Lupus 19:1246–1249
69. Abdel-Aty H, Siegle N, Natusch A et al (2008) Myocardial tissue characterization in systemic lupus erythematosus: value of a comprehensive cardiovascular magnetic resonance approach. Lupus 17:561–567
70. Mavrogeni S, Bratis K, Markussis V et al (2013) The diagnostic role of cardiac magnetic resonance imaging in detecting myocardial inflammation in systemic lupus erythematosus. Differentiation from viral myocarditis. Lupus 22:34–43
71. O'Neill AG, Woldman S, Bailliard F et al (2009) Cardiac magnetic resonance imaging in patients with systemic lupus erythematosus. Ann Rheum Dis 68:1478–1481
72. Edwards NC, Ferro CJ, Townend JN et al (2007) Myocardial disease in systemic vasculitis and autoimmune disease detected by cardiovascular magnetic resonance. Rheumatology 46:1208–1209
73. Libman E, Sacks B (1924) A hitherto undescribed form of valvular and mural endocarditis. Arch Intern Med 33:701–737
74. Lee JL, Naguwa SM, Cheema GS et al (2009) Revisiting Libman-Sacks endocarditis: a historical review and update. Clin Rev Allergy Immunol 36:126–130
75. Zuily S, Regnault V, Selton-Suty C et al (2011) Increased risk for heart valve disease associated with antiphospholipid antibodies in patients with systemic lupus erythematosus. Circulation 124:215–224
76. Roldan CA, Shively BK, Crawford MH (1996) An echocardiographic study of valvular heart disease associated with systemic lupus erythematosus. N Engl J Med 335:1424–1430
77. Roldan CA, Qualls CR, Sopko KS et al (2008) Transthoracic versus transesophageal echocardiography for detection of Libman–Sacks endocarditis: a randomized controlled study. J Rheumatol 35:224–229
78. Roldan CA, Sibbitt WL, Qualls CR et al (2013) Libman-Sacks endocarditis and embolic cerebrovascular disease. J Am Coll Cardiol Img 6:973–983
79. Ziporen L, Goldberg I, Arad M et al (1996) Libman-Sacks endocarditis in the antiphospholipid syndrome: immunopathologic findings in deformed heart valves. Lupus 5:196–205

80. Seferovic' PM, Ristic' AD, Maksimovic R (2006) Cardiac arrhythmias and conduction disturbances in autoimmune rheumatic diseases. Rheumatology 45:iv39–iv42
81. Brucato A, Cimaz R, Catelli L et al (2000) Anti-Ro-associated sinus bradycardia in newborns. Circulation 102:E88–E89
82. Costedoat-Chalumeau N, Amoura Z, Lupoglazoff JM et al (2004) Outcome of pregnancies in patients with anti-SSA/Ro antibodies: a study of 165 pregnancies, with special focus on electrocardiographic variations in the children and comparison with a control group. Arthritis Rheum 50:3187–3194
83. Gerosa M, Cimaz R, Stramba-Badiale M et al (2007) Electrocardiographic abnormalities in infants born from mothers with autoimmune diseases: a multicenter prospective study. Rheumatology 46:1285–1289
84. Bourré-Tessier J, Clarke AE, Huynh T et al (2011) Prolonged corrected QT interval in anti-Ro/SSA-positive adults with systemic lupus erythematosus. Arthritis Care Res 63:1031–1037
85. Lazzerini PE, Capecchi PL, Laghi-Pasini F (2010) Anti-Ro/SSA antibodies in cardiac arrhythmias in the adults: facts and hypothesis. Scand J Immunol 72:213–222
86. Lazzerini PE, Acampa M, Guideri F et al (2004) Prolongation of the corrected QT interval in adult patients with anti-Ro/SSA–positive connective tissue diseases. Arthritis Rheum 50:1248–1252
87. Lazzerini PE, Capecchi PL, Guideri F et al (2007) Comparison of frequency of complex ventricular arrhythmias in patients with positive versus negative anti-Ro/SSA and connective tissue disease. Am J Cardiol 100:1029–1034
88. Gordon PA, Rosenthal E, Khamashta MA et al (2001) Absence of conduction defects in the electrocardiograms [correction of echocardiograms] of mothers with children with congenital complete heart block. J Rheumatol 28:366–369

Systemic Lupus Erythematosus and Pregnancy

11

Paula Alba and Munther Khamashta

Systemic lupus erythematosus (SLE) is a multisystem autoimmune disease that affects predominantly women during their reproductive years. As expected, pregnancy is a common event in these women. Pregnancy was not recommended in women with lupus in the past because of maternal and fetal complications [1, 2]. A better understanding of the disease, the advances of the treatment, and creation of specialized multidisciplinary groups with experience in autoimmune diseases (involving physicians, obstetricians, pediatricians, and midwives) have led to dramatic improvement in disease management and pregnancy outcome over the last 20 years [3, 4]. However, maternal and fetal complications are still present. Risk factors for fetal and obstetric complications are disease activity at the conception and during pregnancy, lupus nephritis (LN), arterial hypertension, positive antiphospholipid antibodies (APLs), and anti-Ro/SSA antibodies [3].

11.1 Preconception Counseling

Fertility in women with SLE seems to be similar to women in the general population, although patients with chronic renal failure, amenorrhea due to previous high cumulative dose of cyclophosphamide (Cyc), and active disease may present reduced fertility. The risk of ovarian failure due to Cyc treatment is related to the cumulative dose of the drug and the administration in women older than 35 years old [5].

P. Alba (✉)
Rheumatology Department, Hospital Córdoba, Cátedra de Medicina I. UHMI N 3, Universidad Nacional de Córdoba, Córdoba, Argentina
e-mail: paulaalba@yahoo.com

M. Khamashta
The Lupus Research Unit, St. Thomas Hospital, London, UK
e-mail: munther.khamashta@kcl.ac.uk

D. Roccatello, L. Emmi (eds.), *Connective Tissue Disease: A Comprehensive Guide-Volume 1*, Rare Diseases of the Immune System 5,
DOI 10.1007/978-3-319-24535-5_11

The management of pregnancy in women with SLE should be started before the conception. The preconceptional visit should include a detailed summary of previous obstetric history and chronic organ damage, recent serologic profile, current disease activity and last flare date, medical history and risk factors of interest, and baseline blood pressure and renal function. Main risks for the mother and the baby should be discussed accordingly. High risk factors in lupus pregnancy are adverse obstetrical history, cardiac and renal involvement, pulmonary hypertension, interstitial lung disease, disease activity, high dose of steroid treatment, positivity of APLs and Ro and La antibodies, and multiparity [6]. Women with active lupus should postpone conception until stable disease remission is achieved at least 6 months before conception [7]. Presence of APL and/or APS is associated with maternal thrombosis and fetal mortality and the presence of Ro and La antibodies with congenital heart block (CHB) in 2 % of the babies [7–9, 11]. Severe chronic renal impairment is associated with obstetric complications as preeclampsia and miscarriages [10].

Pregnancy should be contraindicated in some clinical situations (Table 11.1: pregnancy contraindications in SLE). Women with the following conditions should avoid to get pregnant: severe lupus flare or stroke over the last 6 months, pulmonary hypertension, moderate to severe heart failure (ejection fraction of left ventricle <40 %), severe restrictive lung disease (FVC <1 l), severe chronic renal impairment (GFR <35 mil/min), uncontrolled hypertension, and previous severe preeclampsia despite therapy with aspirin plus heparin [7, 9–11, 13]. However, the principal contraindication of pregnancy must be symptomatic pulmonary hypertension because of 30 % of maternal mortality during pregnancy and puerperium [14, 15].

All the medications that patients received to control the disease should be carefully reviewed. Steroids, hydroxychloroquine (HCQ), azathioprine (AZA), and calcineurin inhibitors are considered safe during pregnancy. HCQ is a fundamental treatment in SLE because of their protective properties on activity, damage, long-term survival, and thrombosis. HCQ has been used successfully in pregnancy as steroid-sparing agent, and the discontinuation has been associated with flares of the disease [16–22]. Moreover, its safety profile for both mother and the baby has been widely addressed [16–22]. Methotrexate (MTX), mycophenolate mofetil, and Cyc are teratogenic drugs and they should be avoided and stopped 3 months before the

Table 11.1 Contraindications of pregnancy in SLE

Severe pulmonary hypertension
Severe restrictive lung disease
Heart failure
Uncontrolled hypertension
Severe chronic renal impairment
Severe preeclampsia despite therapy with aspirin plus heparin
Recent stroke (6 months)
Recent lupus flare (6 months)

conception and they should be replaced by AZA to avoid a lupus flare (Table 11.2) [16, 17, 74, 75]. A recent observational study showed that among patients with previous LN, replacing MMF with AZA in women with quiescent LN for pregnancy planning rarely leads to renal flares [75].

Belimumab (BM) and rituximab (RTX) are the most used biological drugs in lupus. The experience of BM in pregnancy is scarce; hence, the current recommendation is to withdraw it at least 4 months before conception. Animal studies showed that BM crossed the placenta, but there is not definitive relationship between BM and congenital abnormalities [76–78]. In the case of RTX, given the maternal indications for its use and the heterogenicity of the reports, until more robust data are available, women should be counseled against pregnancy for 6–12 months after RTX exposure due to the risk of neonatal B cell depletion.

The nonsteroidal anti-inflammatory drugs (NSAIDs) are generally safe in pregnancy if they are used for short limited courses. Their use should be withheld toward the end of pregnancy (>30–32 weeks) due to increased risk of premature closure of baby's ductus arteriosus. At present, there are not reliable data on selective COX-2 inhibitors and they should be avoided [16]. The drugs of choice for managing hypertension in pregnancy are labetalol, methyldopa, and nifedipine and less frequently hydralazine and doxazosin. Angiotensin converting enzyme (ACE) inhibitors, angiotensin II receptor blockers (ARBs), and diuretics are generally contraindicated during pregnancy due to fetal renal impairment and oligohydramnios and increased risk of miscarriages.

Table 11.2 Medications during pregnancy and breastfeeding

	Pregnancy	Breastfeeding
NSAIDs	Yes**	Yes
Hydroxychloroquine	Yes	Yes
Steroids	Yes	Yes
Cyclosporine	Yes	Yes
Azathioprine	Yes	Yes
Mycophenolate mofetil	No	No
Methotrexate	No	No
Cyclophosphamide	No	No
Warfarin	No*	Yes
Heparin	Yes	Yes
Aspirin (low dose)	Yes	Yes
Anti-TNFα	Yes	Yes
Rituximab	No	No
Abatacept	No	No
Belimumab	No	No

NAIDs Nonsteroidal anti-inflammatory drugs, *TNFα* tumor necrosis factor alpha, **(avoid after 32 weeks), warfarin* (could be given after 1st trimester)

11.2 Activity Disease in Pregnancy

Pregnancy is considered a high-risk time for lupus patients, as flares during pregnancy have been described. However, whether or not pregnancy increases the risk of lupus flare is still an unsolved question. Several prospective controlled studies have shown an increase in lupus flares during pregnancy [22–24], while other studies showed opposite results [25–28]. However, the lupus flare rate during pregnancy was around 50 % in all the studies. The risk of flare appears to be dependent on the disease activity 6–12 months prior to conception and previous treatment with HCQ [18, 24, 29]. However, recent studies have shown a reduced frequency of lupus flares when compared to old studies [30, 31].

Distinguishing pregnancy-related signs and symptoms from certain lupus features may sometimes be difficult, as they can mimic each other. Assessment by experienced physicians is of great importance in order to ensure a correct clinical judgment. Fatigue, arthralgia, hair loss, dyspnea, headaches, malar and palmar erythema, edema, anemia, and thrombocytopenia represent some of the most ambiguous manifestations.

In pregnancy, erythrocyte sedimentation rate (ESR) is usually raised; hence it may not be valid as an activity marker. Serum C3 and C4 levels also rise in pregnancy due to increased liver production, so even in women with active lupus, they may remain within normal range. Relative variation rather than absolute levels of C3 and C4 should be taken into consideration. A drop of 25 % or more in serum complement levels should be taken into consideration [32]. Several activity indexes for pregnancy have been used for research purposes; however, physicians should take therapeutic decisions by clinical judgment [33, 34].

Lupus flares during pregnancy and postpartum are normally non-severe, characterized by articular, dermatological, and mild hematological involvement and are usually well controlled with HCQ and short-term introduction or increase in steroids. Nonetheless, severe flares with major organ involvement may occur, and the patients may require high doses of steroids, pulses of steroids, and early treatment with AZA to spare steroids [3, 16, 32].

11.3 Lupus Nephritis and Pregnancy

Active LN at conception confers a higher risk of flare during pregnancy, and even women with LN in remission have an increased risk of flare [33–44]. In contrast, patients with no previous renal involvement are at the lowest risk. Arterial hypertension and renal impairment are important prognostic factors in LN. As a result of increased renal blood flow in pregnancy, glomerular filtration rate (GFR) increases by more than 50 %, leading to reduce creatinine level. Increased tubular flow may increase urine protein leakage; thus levels up to 300 mg/day are considered normal in pregnancy. In patients with permanent significant protein loss due to previous LN, proteinuria may elevate throughout pregnancy with or without being indicative of active nephritis. This phenomenon could explain the variable incidence of renal flares (8–64 %) in different studies, while the renal flares with renal impairment are between 0 % and 23 % [33–41]. Moreover, different definitions of lupus flare could also explain it. Moroni et al. defined nephritic flare as an increase more than 30 % of serum creatinine plus pathologic urine sediment and proteinuric flare as an increase in proteinuria level (more than 2 g/day if the basal level was less than 3.5 g/day and the double value if the basal level was in nephrotic range) without creatinine serum modification. The authors identify a rate of 25 % of lupus flares with this definition [40]. Moderate and severe renal insufficiency at the conception increases the risk to develop maternal hypertension and premature delivery. In patients with mild and stable renal impairment and control of blood pressure, the risk of progression to end-stage renal failure is low. On the other hand, if the patients have moderate renal impairment (serum creatinine between 1.4 and 3.0 mg/dl), the prognosis of renal function is worse. Patients with severe renal insufficiency have a bad maternal and fetal prognosis [45, 46]. A recent meta-analysis evaluated 37 studies in 2,751 pregnancies with LN and they found the presence of APL and the LN increased the risk of maternal hypertension and premature delivery [47]. However, another retrospective study analyzed patients with and without LN, and they found an increased number of renal lupus flares but the same outcome in terms of fetal survival, premature delivery, preeclampsia, and weight of birth [86].

The early diagnosis of lupus flare is very important for the treatment and prognosis. The irreversible renal insufficiency has been reported between 0 % and 10 % and persistent hypertension in around 13 % of patients [35, 36, 40].

Preeclampsia is defined as the presence of arterial hypertension plus proteinuria after 20 weeks of pregnancy. Patients with SLE, LN, and/or APL present higher risk to develop preeclampsia compared with the general population [48, 49]. Differentiating preeclampsia from LN may not be straightforward, as both may include hypertension, raising proteinuria, edema, renal function impairment, and thrombocytopenia, and sometimes both may overlap. Table 11.3 shows useful findings to differentiate preeclampsia from LN. Active urine sediment, the increase in serum creatinine level, and the positivity of anti-dsDNA antibodies and lower levels of complement could suggest a renal flare [50].

Table 11.3 Differential diagnosis of preeclampsia and lupus nephritis

	Preeclampsia	Lupus nephritis
Blood pressure	High	Normal/high
Platelets	Low/normal	Low/normal
Complement	Normal	Low
Anti-dsDNA	Normal	High
Uric acid	High	Normal
Creatinine level	Normal/high	Normal/high
Hematuria	Present (+/–)	Present
Active urine sediment	No	Yes
Extrarenal SLE activity	No	Yes
Steroid response	No	Yes

Lupus flare treatment includes steroids, pulses of steroids, and AZA. Cyc and MMF are contraindicated during pregnancy and they should be avoided [16, 17]. Tacrolimus is a calcineurin inhibitor and prevents the activation of T cells and the transcription of IL-2, and it can be used during pregnancy [74]. Webster et al. reported the use of tacrolimus in 9 LN patients for renal flares or maintenance treatment [79].

Low-dose aspirin started before 16 weeks of gestation reduces the risk of preeclampsia and its complications [51]. Taking into account its low side effects and recent data suggesting its benefit, antiplatelet therapy for the prevention of preeclampsia is recommended in patients with SLE with or without APL. Some studies have evaluated the use of low-dose aspirin plus heparin in patients with severe preeclampsia in previous pregnancies with positive results [52–54]. However, heparin is not recommended for prevention of preeclampsia, and prospective studies should be done to confirm these results.

11.4 Antiphospholipid Syndrome and Pregnancy

APLs are found more frequently in patients with SLE (30–40 %) than in the background of population (1–5 %) and represent the major risk factor for poor obstetric outcome [55, 56]. Several studies have identified APL carrier women at increased risk of developing preeclampsia, IUGR, prematurity, and fetal loss during pregnancy [8, 11, 57]. Recurrent pregnancy loss occurs in more than 50 % of women with high titers of APL [11]. A meta-analysis studied the relationship between different APLs (LA, ACL IgG, ACL IgM, and anti-B2 glycoprotein I antibodies) and recurrent pregnancy loss. LA, ACL IgG, and ACL IgM had a strong association with recurrent pregnancy loss before 24 weeks of pregnancy and ACL IgG with early miscarriages (before 13 weeks of pregnancy) [58].

Treatment of women with obstetric APS is still the subject of controversy and should be individualized, as most of the evidence is based on observational studies. Current recommendations include low-dose aspirin alone or in association with prophylactic low-molecular-weight heparin (LMWH) for women with recurrent early miscarriages (<10 weeks of gestation) and low-dose aspirin plus prophylactic LMWH for women with previous fetal death (>10 weeks of gestation) and/or preterm delivery (<34 weeks of gestation) [11, 59–64] (Table 11.4). All women with APL positivity should receive low-dose aspirin before the conception to decrease the risk of miscarriages and preeclampsia [49, 51, 64].

All women should be assessed regarding risk factors of venous thromboembolism prior to conception and periodically throughout pregnancy and should receive thromboprophylaxis accordingly. Anticoagulation doses of LMWH are indicated for patients with history of thrombosis, as warfarin is contraindicated in the first trimester of pregnancy because of its fetal effects [65]. All women with APL should receive at least prophylactic LMWH for 7 days after delivery in the absence of other risk factors. Some experts recommend extending this treatment for 4–8 weeks postpartum [65]. In all the patients under treatment with heparin, calcium and vitamin D

Table 11.4 APS treatment in pregnancy

Clinical manifestation	Recommendations
APL(+) without thrombosis or obstetric morbidity	Low-dose aspirin (no evidence)
APS: early recurrent miscarriages	Low-dose aspirin or aspirin + heparin
APS with history of fetal death, preeclampsia, IUGR	Low-dose aspirin + LMWH prophylactic dose during pregnancy and puerperium
APS with venous thrombosis	Warfarin is avoided in the 1st trimester
	Low-dose aspirin + LMWH (anticoagulation dose after 16 weeks)
APS with arterial thrombosis	Warfarin is avoided in the 1st trimester
	Low-dose aspirin + LMWH anticoagulation dose during pregnancy and puerperium
APS recurrent pregnancy loss in spite of aspirin + LMWH	Steroids, HCQ

for prevention of osteoporosis should be considered [65, 66]. On the other hand, warfarin and heparin can be used during breastfeeding.

11.5 Neonatal Lupus

Neonatal lupus (NL) is associated with the presence of maternal anti-Ro and anti-La antibodies that are present in 30 % of lupus patients and in Sjogren's syndrome. Congenital heart block (CHB) is the most severe complication of NL and happens in around 2 % of babies born to anti-Ro/La-positive mothers. This risk increases up to 18 % if the mother has already had a child affected by CHB and up to 50 % if she has had two children affected [12, 67, 68]. The risk of perinatal death among affected children is approximately 10–20 %, and most of the surviving children need a permanent pacemaker.

CHB normally develops between 16 and 24 weeks of gestation and can be detected by fetal low heart rate (<60 beats per minute). Early diagnosis is crucial for correct management in CHB. Ultrasound is the accepted technique for fetal CHB diagnoses. Current recommendations include serial fetal echocardiograms between 18 and 28 weeks of gestation for pregnant women with anti-Ro/La antibodies. When the complete CHB is detected, it is not reversible. Some authors suggest dexamethasone treatment as effective in second-degree CHB [69].

The PR Interval and Dexamethasone Evaluation (PRIDE) study was designed to evaluate the efficacy of dexamethasone treatment to prevent or revert the recently diagnosed CHB. This study also evaluated if first-degree heart block was a predictor factor to progress to complete heart block. They found the prolongation of PR interval did not predict complete CHB. The presence of echodensities and tricuspid regurgitation were early signs of heart damage [70].

In a murine model, treatment with intravenous immunoglobulins (IVIGs) was proved to inhibit anti-Ro/La antibody placental transfer and their consequent fetal heart damage. Nevertheless, two multicenter prospective studies failed to reduce the risk of CBH in women, with a previously affected baby, treated with IVIG during pregnancy [71, 72]. A recent multicenter case-control study suggested that, in mothers with anti-Ro/La, exposure to HCQ during pregnancy may decrease the risk of fetal development of CHB [73]. Recently, two other studies showed a decrease in recurrences of CHB in mothers who were exposed to HCQ [80, 81, 87]. These results should be evaluated in future studies.

11.6 Pregnancy Management

Prepregnancy counseling; risk assessment; multidisciplinary approach; antenatal and postnatal management plan, together with experienced team; and early recognition of signs related to SLE complications are essential cornerstones for both maternal and fetal successful outcomes. The preconceptional visit should include a summary of previous obstetric history and chronic organ damage, recent serology profile (APL, anti-Ro/La, anti-dsDNA, complement), current disease activity and last flare date, medical history and risk factors of interest (diabetes, hypertension, cardiac and cardiovascular problems, nephropathy, thyroid function, detrimental habits, and their complications), and baseline blood pressure, urine analysis, and renal function [82]. Anomaly scan and uterine arterial Doppler are recommended around 20 weeks of gestation, and the latter should be repeated around the 24th week if abnormal. Abnormal wave forms are good predictors of preeclampsia, whereas normal results are related to good obstetric outcomes. Ultrasound scans (including biophysical profile and amniotic fluid volume assessment) around 28–30 weeks and 32–34 are recommended. Regular umbilical artery Doppler should be performed with the previous scans, as their abnormal values are predictors of mortality and risk of fetal compromise. Additional scans may be indicated depending on previous obstetric history and the progress of pregnancy [83–85].

Every visit should include urine analysis and maternal assessment with special attention to hypertension and other features of preeclampsia. Women with previous renal and/or hypertensive diseases should have more frequent regular blood pressure checks. Confirmation by protein/creatinine ratio is mandatory in case of positive urine dipstick. Regular blood tests including full blood count, liver function tests, renal profile, anti-dsDNA and complement every 4–8 weeks are recommended. All women on steroids and those with high risk factors of diabetes should have a glucose tolerance test around 24–28 weeks of gestation in order to exclude gestational diabetes and avoid further obstetric risk. All women should ideally take folic acid 12 weeks before the conception and calcium and vitamin D supplements for women on steroids and heparin treatment to prevent osteoporosis [82].

Conclusions

SLE is no longer considered an obstacle to pregnancy. Some fetal and obstetric complications can be predicted and in some cases prevented. A tight control of patients should be performed before and after conception. These patients should be managed by a multidisciplinary team, including at least a rheumatologist and an obstetrician, thus allowing an improvement of maternal and fetal prognosis.

References

1. Donaldson LB, De Alvarez RR (1962) Further observations on lupus erythematosus associated with pregnancy. Am J Obstet Gynecol 83:1461–1473
2. Ellis FA, Bereston ES (1952) Lupus erythematosus associated with pregnancy and menopause. AMA Arch Derm Syphilol 65:170–176
3. Khamashta MA (2006) Systemic lupus erythematosus and pregnancy. Best Pract Res Clin Rheumatol 20:685–694
4. Cervera R, Font J, Carmona F, Balasch J (2002) Pregnancy outcome in systemic lupus erythematosus: good news for the new millennium. Autoimmun Rev 1:354–359
5. Boumpas DT, Austin HA, Vaughan EM et al (1993) Risk for sustained amenorrhea in patients with systemic lupus erythematosus receiving intermittent pulse cyclophosphamide therapy. Ann Intern Med 119:366–369
6. Ruiz-Irastorza G, Khamashta MA (2008) Lupus and pregnancy: ten questions and some answers. Lupus 17:416–420
7. Clowse MEB, Magder LS, Petri M (2005) The impact of increased lupus activity on obstetric outcomes. Arthritis Rheum 52:514–521
8. Lima F, Khamashta MA, Buchanan NMM et al (1996) A study of sixty pregnancies in patients with antiphospholipid syndrome. Clin Exp Rheumatol 14:131–136
9. Ramsey-Goldman R, Kutzer JE, Kuller LH et al (1993) Pregnancy outcome and anti-anticardiolipin antibody in women with systemic lupus erythematosus. Am J Epidemiol 138:1057–1069
10. Germain S, Nelson-Piercy C (2006) Lupus nephritis and renal disease in pregnancy. Lupus 15:148–155
11. Branch DW, Khamashta MA (2003) Antiphospholipid syndrome: obstetric diagnosis, management and controversies. Obstet Gynecol 101:1333–1344
12. Brucato A, Frassi M, Franceschini F et al (2001) Risk of congenital complete heart block in newborns of mothers with anti-Ro/SSA antibodies detected by counterimmunoelectrophoresis: a prospective study of 100 women. Arthritis Rheum 44:1832–1835
13. Cuadrado MJ, Mendonca LLF, Khamashta MA et al (1999) Maternal and fetal outcome in antiphospholipid syndrome pregnancies with a history of previous cerebral ischemia. Arthritis Rheum 42:S265
14. Bonnin M, Mercier FJ, Sitbon O et al (2005) Severe pulmonary hypertension during pregnancy. Mode of delivery and anesthetic management of 15 consecutive cases. Anesthesiology 102:1133–1137
15. Mc Millan E, Martin WL, Waugh J et al (2002) Management of pregnancy in women with pulmonary hypertension secondary to SLE and antiphospholipid syndrome. Lupus 11:392–398
16. Ostensen M, Khamashta MA, Lockshin M et al (2006) Anti-inflammatory and immunosuppressive drugs and reproduction. Arthritis Res Ther 8:209–227
17. Ostensen M, Lockshin M, Doria A et al (2008) Update on safety during pregnancy of biological agents and some immunosuppressive antirheumatic drugs. Rheumatology 47:28–31
18. Clowse MEB, Magder L, Witter F et al (2006) Hydroxycloroquine in lupus pregnancy. Arthritis Rheum 54:3640–3647
19. Ruiz-Irastorza G, Ramos-Casals M, Brito-Zeron P, Khamashta MA (2010) Clinical efficacy of antimalarials in systemic lupus erythematosus: a systematic review. Ann Rheum Dis 69:20–28
20. Buchanan NM, Toubi E, Khamashta MA et al (1996) Hydroxicloroquine and lupus pregnancy: review of a series of 36 cases. Ann Rheum Dis 55:486–488

21. Costedoat-Chalumeau N, Amoura Z, Duhaut P et al (2003) Safety of hydroxycloroquine in pregnant patients with connective tissue diseases: a study of one hundred thirty-three cases compared with a control group. Arthritis Rheum 48:3207–3211
22. Mintz G, Nitz J, Gutierrez G et al (1986) Prospective study of pregnancy in systemic lupus erythematosus: results of a multi-disciplinary approach. J Rheumatol 13:732–739
23. Lockshin MD, Reinitz E, Druzin ML et al (1984) Lupus pregnancy: case-control prospective study demonstrating absence of lupus exacerbation during or after pregnancy. Am J Med 77:893–898
24. Urowitz MB, Gladman DD, Farewell VT et al (1993) Lupus and pregnancy studies. Arthritis Rheum 36:1392–1397
25. Petri M, Howard D, Repke J (1991) Frequency of lupus flare in pregnancy: the Hopkins lupus pregnancy center experience. Arthritis Rheum 34:1538–1545
26. Ruiz-Irastorza G, Lima F, Alves J et al (1996) Increased rate of lupus flare during pregnancy and puerperium. Br J Rheumatol 35:133–138
27. Wong KL, Chan FY, Lee XP (1991) Outcome of pregnancy in patients with systemic lupus erythematosus. A prospective study. Arch Intern Med 151:269–273
28. Tandon A, Ibanez D, Gladman DD et al (2004) The effect of pregnancy on lupus nephritis. Arthritis Rheum 50:3941–3946
29. Levy RA, Vilela VS, Cataldo MJ et al (2001) Hydroxycloroquine in lupus pregnancy: double-blind and placebo -controlled study. Lupus 10:401–404
30. Cortes-Hernandez J, Ordi-Ros J, Paredes F et al (2002) Clinical predictors of fetal and maternal outcome in systemic lupus erythematosus: a prospective study of 103 pregnancies. Rheumatology 41:643–650
31. Khamashta MA, Ruiz-Irastorza G, Hughes GRV (1997) Systemic lupus erythematosus flares during pregnancy. Rheum Dis Clin North Am 23:15–30
32. Petri M (2007) The Hopkins Lupus Pregnancy Center: ten key issues in management. Rheum Dis Clin N Am 33:27–35
33. Hayslett JP, Lynn RI (1980) Effect of pregnancy in patients with lupus nephropathy. Kidney Int 18:207–220
34. Jungers P, Dougados M, Pelissler C et al (1982) Lupus nephropathy and pregnancy. Report of 104 cases in 36 patients. Arch Intern Med 142:771–776
35. Imbasciati E, Surian M, Bottino S et al (1984) Lupus nephropathy and pregnancy. A study of 26 pregnancies in patients with systemic lupus erythematosus and nephritis. Nephron 36:46–51
36. Packham DK, Lam SS, Nicholls K et al (1992) Lupus nephritis and pregnancy. Q J Med 83:315–324
37. Julkunem H (1998) Renal lupus in pregnancy. Scand J Rheumatol 27:80–83
38. Huong DT, Wechsler B, Vauther-Brouzes D et al (1994) Pregnancy and its outcome in systemic lupus erythematosus. Q J Med 87:721–729
39. Oviasu E, Hicks J, Cameron JS (1991) The outcome of pregnancy in women with lupus nephritis. Lupus 1:19–25
40. Moroni G, Quaglini S, Banfi G et al (2002) Pregnancy in lupus nephritis. Am J Kidney Dis 40:713–720
41. Imbasciati E, Tincani A, Gregorini G et al (2009) Pregnancy in women with pre-existing lupus nephritis: predictors of fetal and maternal outcome. Nephrol Dial Transplant 24(2):344–347
42. Zulman J, Tala N, Hoffman GS et al (1980) Problems associated with the management of pregnancies in patients with systemic lupus erythematosus. J Rheumatol 7:37–49
43. Bobrie G, Liote F, Houiller P et al (1987) Pregnancy in lupus nephritis and related disorders. Am J Kidney Dis 9:339–343
44. Carmona F, Font J, Moga I et al (2005) Class III-IV proliferative lupus nephritis and pregnancy: a study of 42 cases. Am J Reprod Immunol 53:182
45. Moroni G, Ponticelli C (2005) Pregnancy after lupus nephritis. Lupus 14:89–94
46. Day CJ, Lipkin GW, Savage COS (2009) Lupus nephritis and pregnancy in the 21 st century. Nephrol Dial Transplant 24:344–347

47. Smyth A, Oliveira GH, Lahr BD et al (2010) A systematic review and meta-analysis of pregnancy outcomes in patients with systemic lupus erythematosus and lupus nephritis. Clin J Am Soc Nephrol 5:2060–2068
48. Milne F, Redman C, Walker J et al (2005) The preeclampsia community guideline (PRECOG): how to screen for and detect onset of preeclampsia in the community. Br Med J 330:576–580
49. Barton JR, Sibai BM (2008) Prediction and prevention of recurrent preeclampsia. Obstet Gynecol 112:359–372
50. Mackillop LH, Germain SJ, Nelson-Piercy C, Hughes GRV (2002) Effects of lupus and antiphospholipid syndrome on pregnancy. Yearb Obstet Gynecol 10:105–119
51. Askie LM, Duley L, Henderson-Smart DJ, PARIS Collaborative Group et al (2007) Antiplatelet agents for prevention of preeclampsia: a meta-analysis of individual patient data. Lancet 369:1791–1798
52. North RA, Ferrier C, Gamble C et al (1995) Prevention of preeclampsia with heparin and antiplatelet drugs in women with renal disease. Aust N Z J Obstet Gynaecol 35:357–362
53. Sergio F, Maria Clara D, Gabriella F et al (2006) Prophylaxis of recurrent preeclampsia: low molecular weight heparin plus low dose aspirin versus low dose aspirin alone. Hypertens Pregnancy 25:115–127
54. Mecacci F, Bianchi B, Pieralli A et al (2009) Pregnancy outcome in systemic lupus erythematosus complicated by antiphospholipid antibodies. Rheumatology 48(3):246–249
55. Love PE, Santoro SA (1990) Antiphospholipid antibodies: anticardiolipin and the lupus anticoagulant in SLE and in non-SLE disorders. Ann Intern Med 112:682–698
56. Miyakis S, Lockshin MD, Atsumi T, Branch DW, Brey RL, Cervera R et al (2006) International consensus statement on an update of the classification criteria for definitive antiphospholipid syndrome. J Thromb Haemost 4:295–306
57. Lima F, Buchanan NM, Khamashta MA et al (1995) Obstetric outcome in systemic lupus erythematosus. Semin Arhtritis Rheum 25:184–192
58. Opatrny L, David M, Kahn SR et al (2006) Association between antiphospholipid antibodies and recurrent fetal loss in women without autoimmune disease: a metaanalysis. J Rheumatol 33:2214–2221
59. Derksen RH, Khamashta MA, Branch DW (2004) Management of the obstetric antiphospholipid syndrome. Arthritis Rheum 50:1028–1039
60. Empson M, Lassere M, Craig J et al (2005) Prevention of recurrent miscarriages for women with antiphospholipid antibody or lupus anticoagulant. Cochrane Database Syst Rev 18(2), CD002859
61. Petri M, Qazi U (2006) Management of the antiphospholipid syndrome in pregnancy. Rheum Dis Clin N Am 32:591–607
62. Ruiz Irastorza G, Khamashta MA (2007) Antiphospholipid syndrome in pregnancy. Rheum Dis Clin N Am 33:287–297
63. Carmona F, Font J, Azulay M et al (2001) Risk factors associated with fetal losses in treated antiphospholipid syndrome pregnancies: a multivariate análisis. Am J Reprod Immunol 46:274–279
64. Ruiz Irastorza G, Khamashta MA, Hughes GRV (2002) Treatment of pregnancy loss in Hughes syndrome: a critical update. Autoimmun Rev 1:298–304
65. Ruiz Irastorza G, Khamashta MA (2005) Management of thrombosis in antiphospholipid syndrome and systemic lupus erythematosus in pregnancy. Am N Y Acad Sci 1051:606–612
66. Ruiz Irastorza G, Khamashta MA, Nelson-Piercy C et al (2001) Lupus pregnancy: is heparin a risk factor for osteoporosis? Lupus 10:597–600
67. Gordon P, Khamashta MA, Rosenthal E et al (2004) Anti-52 kDa Ro, anti-60 kDa Ro and anti La antibody profiles in neonatal lupus. J Rheumatol 31:2480–2487
68. Buyon JP, Hiebert R, Copel J et al (1998) Autoimmune associated congenital heart block: demographics, mortality, morbidity, and recurrence rates obtained from a national neonatal lupus registry. J Am Coll Cardiol 31:1658–1666
69. Saleeb S, Copel J, Friedman D et al (1999) Comparison of treatment with fluorinated glucocorticoids to the national history of autoantibody-associated congenital heart block: retrospective review of the research registry for neonatal lupus. Arthritis Rheum 42:2335–2345

70. Friedman D, Kim MY, Copel JA et al (2008) Utility of cardiac monitoring in fetuses at risk for congenital heart block (PRIDE) prospective study. Circulation 117:485–493
71. Pisoni CN, Brucato A, Ruffatti A et al (2010) Intravenous immunoglobulin to prevent congenital heart block: findings of a multicenter, prospective, observational study. Arthritis Rheum 62:1147–1152
72. Friedman DM, Llanos C, Izmirly PM et al (2010) Evaluation of fetuses in a study of intravenous immunoglobulin as preventive therapy for congenital heart block: results of a multicenter, prospective, open-label clinical trial. Arthritis Rheum 62:1138–1146
73. Izmirly PM, Kim MY, Llanos C, Le PU et al (2010) Evaluation of the risk of anti-SSA/Ro-SSB/La antibody-associated cardiac manifestations of neonatal lupus in fetuses of mothers with systemic lupus erythematosus exposed to hydroxycloroquine. Ann Rheum Dis 69:1827–1830
74. Ostensen M, Forger F (2013) How safe are anti-rheumatic drugs during pregnancy? Curr Opin Pharmacol 13:1–6
75. Fischer-Betz R, Specker C, Brinks R et al (2013) Low risk of renal flares and negative outcomes in women with lupus nephritis conceiving after switching from mycophenolate mofetil to azathioprine. Rheumatology (Oxford) 52(6):1070–1076
76. Auyeung-Kim DJ, Devalaraja MN, Migone TS et al (2009) Development and peri postnatal study in cynomolgus monkeys with belimumab, a monoclonal antibody directed against B lymphocyte stimulator. Reprod Toxicol 28:443–455
77. GlaxoSmithKline (2013) Use of intravenous (IV) benlysta in pregnant patients with systemic lupus erythematosus (SLE)
78. Peart E, Clowse MEB (2014) Systemic lupus erythematosus and pregnancy outcomes: an update and review of the literature. Curr Opin Rheumatol 26:118–123
79. Webster P, Wardle A, Bramham K et al (2014) Tacrolimus is an effective treatment for lupus nephritis in pregnancy. Lupus 0:1–5
80. Izmirly PM, Costedoat-Chalumeau N, Pisoni CN et al (2012) Maternal use of hydroxychloroquine is associated with a reduced risk of recurrent anti-SSA/Ro-antibody-associated cardiac manifestations of neonatal lupus. Circulation 126(1):76–82
81. Barsalou J, Jaeggi E, Tian SY et al (2014) A149: does prenatal exposure to antimalarial decrease the risk of neonatal lupus: a Bayesian perspective. Arthritis Rheumatol 66(Suppl 11):S193
82. Ateka-Barrutia O, Khamashta MA (2013) The challenge of pregnancy for patients with SLE. Lupus 22:1295–1308
83. Cnossen JS, Morris RK, ter Riet G et al (2008) Use of uterine artery Doppler ultrasonography to predict pre-eclampsia and intrauterine growth restriction: a systematic review and bivariable metaanalysis. CMAJ 178:701–711
84. Madazli R, Yuksel MA, Oncul M et al (2014) Obstetric outcomes and prognostic factors of lupus pregnancies. Arch Gynecol Obstet 289(1):49–53
85. Morris RK, Malin G, Robson SC et al (2011) Fetal umbilical artery Doppler to predict compromise of fetal/neonatal wellbeing in a high risk population: systematic review and bivariate meta-analysis. Ultrasound Obstet Gynecol 37:135–142
86. Saavedra MA, Cruz-Reyes C, Vera Lastra O et al (2012) Impact of previous lupus nephritis on maternal and fetal outcomes during pregnancy. Clin Rheumatol 31:813–819
87. Brito-Zeron P, Izmirly PM, Ramos-Casals M, Buyon JP, Khamashta MA. Nat Rev Rheumatol 2015;11(5):301–12.

Vitamin D, Autoimmune Diseases, and Systemic Lupus Erythematosus

12

Sabrina Paolino, Vanessa Smith, Carmen Pizzorni, Bruno Seriolo, Alberto Sulli, and Maurizio Cutolo

12.1 Introduction

Vitamin D is a steroid hormone (calcitriol – 1,25(OH)D3, D-hormone) that regulates not only bone metabolism, but like other steroid hormones such as glucocorticoids (GCs) and gonadal hormones, it also interferes with the immune system and estrogen-modulated cells. This occurs by reducing the aromatase activity and limiting the negative effects related to the increased peripheral estrogens (including B cell proliferation and overactivity). Consequently, serum vitamin D deficiency [25(OH)D] is considered a risk factor for several chronic/inflammatory or autoimmune conditions [1, 2].

The primary source of vitamin D is the synthesis of vitamin D3 in the skin upon exposure to UVB radiation. Any condition that potentially reduces sun exposure could further contribute to decreased serum levels of vitamin D, as observed in patients with systemic lupus erythematosus (SLE) [3–5].

Calcitriol (1,25(OH)D3, D-hormone) is the peripherally active endogenous metabolite of vitamin D originating from cholesterol. It is considered a true steroid hormone affecting the regulation of bone metabolism. Recently, the role of vitamin D has been investigated in several chronic pathological conditions including infectious diseases, type 1 diabetes, multiple sclerosis, and autoimmune rheumatic diseases (ARDs). In ARD such as rheumatoid arthritis (RA) or systemic lupus erythematosus (SLE), the D-hormone seems to exert numerous immunomodulatory activities [6, 7].

S. Paolino • C. Pizzorni • B. Seriolo • A. Sulli • M. Cutolo (✉)
Research Laboratory and Academic Division of Clinical Rheumatology, Department of Internal Medicine, University of Genova, Viale Benedetto XV 6, Genoa 16132, Italy
e-mail: mcutolo@unige.it

V. Smith
Department of Rheumatology, Ghent University Hospital, Ghent University, Ghent, Belgium

D. Roccatello, L. Emmi (eds.), *Connective Tissue Disease: A Comprehensive Guide-Volume 1*, Rare Diseases of the Immune System 5,
DOI 10.1007/978-3-319-24535-5_12

Eighty to 90 % of vitamin D synthesis is regulated by sunlight [8]. The hypothesis that vitamin D is linked to autoimmune disorders originally arose from the observation that people living near the equator are at decreased risk of developing common autoimmune diseases, as well as by the fact that there is a greater prevalence of RA in northern European countries as compared to the southern ones [9].

Patients with RA and SLE have multiple risk factors for vitamin D deficiency that seem to influence disease severity and, at least in RA, disease activity that shows a yearly rhythm (being more severe in winter) [10–13].

These observations suggest a pathophysiological and possibly therapeutic role for 1,25(OH)2D3 in clinical practice as a modulator of the immune system [14–16]. A recent study on vitamin D status in SLE patients analyzed the potential benefits of 2 years of supplementation and showed the results of different types of cholecalciferol regimens. It indicated that supplementation with an intensive dosage (300,000 IU initial bolus followed by 50,000 IU monthly for the first year) and then switching to the standard regimen (25,000 IU monthly, immediately after patient enrollment, throughout the study) in the second year is safe, and it allows to obtain a sufficient level of vitamin D. However, such a regimen does not seem to influence disease activity as compared to the standard regimen [17].
All these aspects will be discussed in this chapter.

12.2 Immune-Modulating Activities of Vitamin D

Vitamin D status influences the risk of developing several chronic/inflammatory conditions and immune-mediated rheumatic diseases. It exerts modulating effects on dendritic cells (DCs) and B cell and T cell functions, including regulatory T lymphocytes (T^{regs}) and Th17 cells, and acts on the self-tolerance and immune responses [5, 18–20].

In normal conditions, 1,25(OH)D3 regulates both innate and adaptive immunity, potentiating the innate response (antimicrobial activity of macrophages) but suppressing the adaptive immunity by acting on B lymphocytes and on Ig production [1, 2, 21, 22] (Fig. 12.1). In addition, 1,25(OH)2D3 has also been shown to inhibit the maturation of monocyte-derived DCs [1, 2, 21].

In previous studies, 1,25(OH)D3 was shown to inhibit the production of tumor necrosis factor (TNF)-alpha, interleukin-17 (IL-17), and interferon gamma (IFN-gamma). Conversely, it stimulates IL-4, IL-5, and IL-10 expression in peripheral blood mononuclear cells (PBMCs) and in CD4 T cells from healthy volunteers [23, 24].

Recently, 1,25(OH)D3 was found to reduce *in vitro* interleukin-17A (IL-17A) and IFN-gamma and to increase IL-4 levels in stimulated PBMCs from treatment-naive patients with early RA (Fig. 12.1) [12, 25].

Higher percentages of IL-17A- and IL-22-expressing CD4 T cells and IL-17A-expressing memory T cells were observed in PBMCs from treatment-naive patients with early RA as compared to healthy controls. Interestingly, recent studies showed that TNF-alpha blockade alone does not suppress IL-17A and IL-22 and that the

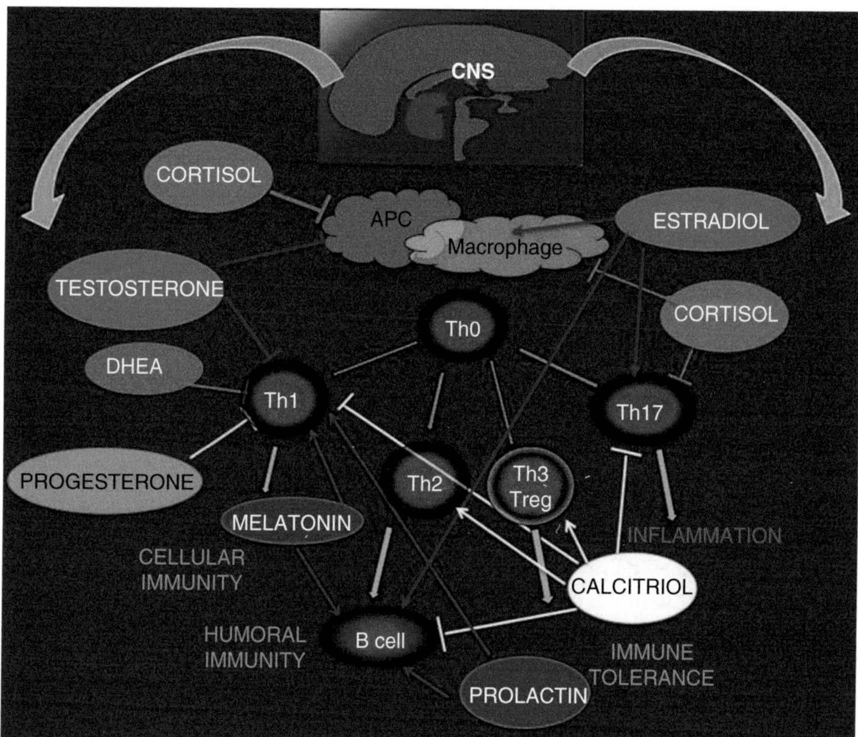

Fig. 12.1 Effects of 1,25(OH)D3 on immune response in normal conditions. Vitamin D (1,25(OH) D3) interferes with the neuroendocrine immune network which includes interactions between the central nervous system, the endocrine system, and the immune system. 1,25(OH)D3 regulates both innate and adaptive immunity, potentiating the innate response (antimicrobial activity of macrophages), decreasing antigen presentation and suppressing the adaptive immunity (B lymphocyte and selected T lymphocyte functions). However, in normal conditions, 1,25(OH)D3 increases the Th2 cytokines (i.e., IL-10) and the efficiency of regulatory T lymphocytes (Tregs). *CNS* central nervous system, *APC* antigen-presenting cell, *DHEA* dehydroepiandrosterone, *Th* helper T lymphocytes (Th0, Th1, Th2, Th3/reg, Th17)

addition of 1,25(OH)D3 on cultured synovial cells from early RA patients is needed to suppress cytokine production [26]. The combination of TNF-alpha blockade and 1,25(OH)D3 seems to control human Th17 activity and inhibit synovial inflammation. These observations might suggest a synergic effect of activating vitamin D receptor signaling and TNF neutralization strategies in patients with RA [24].

Severe serum 25(OH)D deficiency (<10 ng/ml) appears to be involved in the generation of characteristic symptoms of immune/inflammatory rheumatic diseases (i.e., with a negative correlation between 1,25(OH)2D3 and disease activity in RA), though supplementation seems to result in partial improvement [27–29].

Interestingly, it was found that a deficiency of vitamin D (less than 20 ng/ml) is not only present in patients with autoimmune diseases but is also observed in healthy subjects with a yearly rhythm, with lower levels in winter/spring [2, 19].

12.3 Synergic Effects of Vitamin D and Glucocorticoids

Literature dealing with vitamin D and glucosteroids suggests a synergic effect, supported by the observation that the combination of dexamethasone (DEX) and 1,25(OH)D3 is able to inhibit Th1 cytokine production and lymphocyte proliferation, thereby indicating immunosuppressive properties [28].

More specifically, IFN-gamma production in lymphocyte cultures was significantly decreased with either DEX or 1,25(OH)D3 when compared with control culture media. Moreover, when both agents were added to the same culture, IFN-gamma production was further decreased compared to either agent alone [30]. In contrast, 1,25(OH)D3 significantly increased IL-5 and IL-13, whereas DEX significantly decreased these two cytokines. When 1,25(OH)D3 was combined with DEX, IL-5 and IL-13 production increased as compared to DEX alone [30].

Another study showed that the combination of 1,25(OH)D3 with DEX enhanced cell cycle arrest and apoptosis, at least on cultured carcinoma cells, and that vitamin D receptor (VDR) protein levels were higher due to the additive effect of 1,25(OH)D3 and DEX compared with 1,25(OH)D3 treatment alone [19]. Conversely, glucocorticoid receptor (GR) protein levels and ligand binding increased with 1,25(OH)D3 alone, but not with the combination with DEX [31].

The antiproliferative action of 1,25(OH)D3 on cell cycle and induction of apoptosis varies among cell types, and the effect depends on the levels of the VDR, a member of the steroid receptor superfamily that includes GR receptors, in which VDR acts as a ligand-inducible transcription factor [32].

The VDR-1,25(OH)D3 complex regulates transcription by binding the so-called vitamin D response elements/genes (VDREs) [32, 33].

1,25(OH)D3 is an important regulator of VDR both at the transcriptional and posttranscriptional levels [34, 35].

Recent data suggest vitamin D to stimulate GC-mediated anti-inflammatory effects in human monocytes [36]. Lower 25(OH)D serum levels in asthmatic children have been associated with increased GC use [37].

Lastly, in psoriatic patients, the combined use of calcipotriol, a vitamin D analog, and betamethasone has shown a combined effect on keratinocyte proliferation and differentiation, with clinical improvement and inflammation control [38, 39].

12.4 Deficit of Vitamin D and Autoantibody Production

Significant vitamin D deficiency has been reported in several immune-mediated or idiopathic inflammatory myopathies, like polymyositis, dermatomyositis, and inclusion body myositis, supporting the concept that low levels of vitamin D might be a risk factor for autoimmunity [20, 40]. Lower levels of serum 25(OH)D, as well as a higher frequency of anti-Jo-1 autoantibodies, were observed in patients with inflammatory myopathies as compared to controls [22].

The role of 25(OH)D as a risk factor for autoimmune diseases is also supported by the observation that vitamin D levels are lower in ANA-positive healthy controls as compared to ANA-negative subjects. Furthermore, vitamin D may prevent autoimmune diseases by stimulating naturally occurring regulatory T cells [41].

Vitamin D deficiency plays a role in increased autoantibody production and in B cell autoimmunity [42, 43] (Fig. 12.1).

These observations may explain the potential role of vitamin D in B cell-related disorders such as SLE. In fact, the vitamin D concentration in the serum of SLE patients shows a negative correlation with clinical disease activity and anti-dsDNA titer. Besides, a reduction in the serum 25(OH)D levels has been found to be associated with the presence of autoimmune response, and a significant negative correlation between the titers of ANA and serum levels of 25(OH)D was observed [44].

12.5 Vitamin D Deficiency and Peripheral Metabolism of Estrogens in Autoimmunity

The role of vitamin D on estrogen-mediated cell proliferative activity has been shown, especially in cancer tissues where 1,25(OH)D3 decreases the expression of aromatase, the enzyme that catalyzes the peripheral synthesis of estrogens from androgens [45].

Notably, this effect is very important in breast and prostate cancer where aromatase and its intracrine activity are overexpressed [27].

In clinical practice, aromatase inhibitors, which are used in breast cancer treatment, inhibit enzymatic activity, while 1,25(OH)D3 reduces aromatase expression, inhibits estrogen synthesis and signaling and its anti-inflammatory action (see below), and consequently plays an important role in inhibiting estrogen receptor-positive breast cancer [46, 47].

Consequently, the inhibitory effect of 1,25(OH)D3 on aromatase and cytokine synthesis on cultures of human macrophages has also been observed [48, 49]. More specifically, 1,25(OH)D3 exerts its action by direct repression of aromatase transcription via promoter II and at the same time also by an indirect effect due to a reduction in the levels and biological activity of prostaglandins (especially PGE2), which are considered the main stimulators of aromatase transcription through promoter II [50].

Interestingly, inflammatory cytokines (tumor necrosis factor alpha, interleukins 6 and 1) act as enhancers of aromatase activity, as observed in chronic inflammatory conditions such as RA synovitis or cutaneous lupus erythematosus [51, 52].

The higher incidence of autoimmune rheumatic diseases in women might be favored by possible links between 1,25(OH)D3 deficiency (with reduced aromatase downregulation) and the increase in the synthesis of peripheral estrogens [46, 53].

12.6 Vitamin D and Systemic Lupus Erythematosus (SLE)

Vitamin D has several effects on growth, proliferation, apoptosis, and cell functions. It shows pleiotropic action on various tissues as well as on the immune system on which it exerts an anti-inflammatory effect through the modulation of both cellular proliferation and differentiation via the nuclear vitamin D receptor (also expressed on antigen-presenting cells) [1, 54].

In particular, vitamin D inhibits Th1 and Th17 cell proliferation, and it promotes Th2 response on T lymphocytes, thus influencing the transcription of several key cytokines and inhibiting the production of IFN-γ and IL-2.

Several studies have further suggested that vitamin D deficiency may play a role in the pathogenesis of systemic autoimmune diseases [24, 25, 55].

SLE is a chronic multisystem inflammatory autoimmune disease characterized by the presence of autoantibodies against intracellular antigens, by increased T cell activation and likely by an alteration of regulatory T cells [56].

Hypovitaminosis D is highly prevalent in SLE as a result of reduced exposure to sunshine caused by photosensitivity, use of photoprotection, alterations of the renal vitamin D metabolism, or the use of medications such as glucocorticoids or antimalarials [2].

A number of cross-sectional studies have examined the association of vitamin D deficiency with SLE disease activity in recent years. Most, but not all, have shown an association of 25(OH)D deficiency with increased SLE disease activity [57].

In addition, it is well established that seasonal variations in sun exposure influence 25(OH)D serum levels. Moreover, several data show the influence exerted by vitamin D levels on SLE activity, thereby supporting the notion that vitamin D deficiency in winter can be a risk factor for disease flares [10, 58].

Of note, low vitamin D concentrations have also been associated with complications of the disease such as osteoporosis, fatigue, and certain cardiovascular risk factors [55].

Therefore, since the active vitamin D metabolite 1,25(OH)D3 has been shown to modulate immunological pathways, its administration might affect SLE development and progression.

In this context, pharmacological supplementation of vitamin D results in a decrease in memory B cells and anti-DNA antibodies and an increase in naive CD4+ T cells and regulatory T cells together with a decrease in effector Th1 and Th17 cells [22].

A very recent study analyzed the effects of different monthly regimens of vitamin D supplementation on the circulating numbers of T cells and on cytokine production in SLE patients [59]. This study concluded that increasing vitamin D serum levels through long-term monthly cholecalciferol treatment increases Treg cells and promotes Th2 response [59].

Another recent 2-year study of SLE patients proposes supplementation with cholecalciferol using two different regimens: standard, 25,000 IU monthly, and intensive, 300,000 IU initial bolus followed by 50,000 IU monthly for the first year, switching to the standard regimen in the second year. The study shows that intensive vitamin D supplementation is needed to reach optimal vitamin D status. Notably, no effects were observed on SLE disease activity or laboratory parameters such as anti-DNA and complement levels [17].

Studies correlating low vitamin D serum levels with higher SLE activity reported controversial results [10, 60, 61]. However, it is generally accepted that vitamin D insufficiency represents a predisposing factor for the onset and perpetuation of autoimmune processes [1].

Conclusions

Calcitriol (1,25(OH)D3) is recognized as a true steroid hormone that exerts several biological activities, including regulation of the immune system, and that supports pathophysiological mechanisms for the development/risk of chronic/inflammatory autoimmune diseases [20, 62–64].

A possible synergism between 1,25(OH)D3 and glucocorticoids could represent a new approach for the management of chronic autoimmune diseases.

Supplementation with immediate-release cholecalciferol (especially in SLE patients) appears to induce sufficient serum levels of vitamin D in most subjects; however, it does not seem to influence disease activity, at least in short- to medium-term trials.

Conflicts of Interest The authors declare no conflicts of interest with the contents of the present manuscript.

References

1. Cutolo M, Pizzorni C, Sulli A (2011) Vitamin D endocrine system involvement in autoimmune rheumatic diseases. Autoimmun Rev 11:84–87
2. Cutolo M, Plebani M, Shoenfeld Y et al (2011) Vitamin D endocrine system and the immune response in rheumatic diseases. Vitam Horm 86:327–351
3. Ruiz-Irastorza G, Egurbide MV, Olivares N et al (2008) Vitamin D deficiency in systemic lupus erythematosus: prevalence, predictors and clinical consequences. Rheumatology 47:920–923
4. Cusack C, Danby C, Fallon JC et al (2008) Photoprotective behaviour and sunscreen use: impact on vitamin D levels in cutaneous lupus erythematosus. Photodermatol Photoimmunol Photomed 24:260–267
5. Agmon-Levin N, Theodor E, Segal RM et al (2013) Vitamin D in systemic and organ-specific autoimmune diseases. Clin Rev Allergy Immunol 45:256–266
6. Adorini L, Penna G (2008) Control of autoimmune diseases by the vitamin D endocrine system. Nat Clin Pract Rheumatol 4:404–412
7. Pludowski P, Holick MF, Pilz S et al (2013) Vitamin D effects on musculoskeletal health, immunity, autoimmunity, cardiovascular disease, cancer, fertility, pregnancy, dementia and mortality-a review of recent evidence. Autoimmun Rev 12:976–989
8. Holick MF (2003) Vitamin D: a millennium perspective. J Cell Biochem 88:296–307
9. Cutolo M, Otsa K, Laas K et al (2006) Circannual vitamin D serum levels and disease activity in rheumatoid arthritis: Northern versus Southern Europe. Clin Exp Rheumatol 24:702–704
10. Dall'Ara F, Andreoli L, Piva N et al (2015) Winter lupus flares are associated with low vitamin D levels in a retrospective longitudinal study of Italian adult patients. Clin Exp Rheumatol 33:153–158
11. Cutolo M (2009) Vitamin D involvement in rheumatoid arthritis and systemic lupus erythaematosus. Ann Rheum Dis 68(3):446–447
12. Cutolo M, Otsa K, Uprus M et al (2007) Vitamin D in rheumatoid arthritis. Autoimmun Rev 7:59–64
13. Schoindre Y, Jallouli M, Tanguy ML et al (2014) Lower vitamin D levels are associated with higher systemic lupus erythematosus activity, but not predictive of disease flare-up. Lupus Sci Med 1(1), e000027
14. Wang J, Nuite M, McAlindon TE (2010) Association of estrogen and aromatase gene polymorphisms with systemic lupus erythematosus. Lupus 19:734–744

15. Cutolo M (2010) Hormone therapy in rheumatic diseases. Curr Opin Rheumatol 22:257–263
16. Souberbielle JC, Body JJ, Lappe JM et al (2010) Vitamin D and musculoskeletal health, cardiovascular disease, autoimmunity and cancer: recommendations for clinical practice. Autoimmun Rev 9:709–715
17. Andreoli L, Dall'Ara F, Piantoni S et al (2015) A 24 months, prospective study on the efficacy and safety of two different monthly regimens of vitamin D supplementation in pre-menopausal women with systemic lupus erythematosus. Lupus 24:499–506
18. Olliver M, Spelmink L, Hiew J et al (2013) Immunomodulatory effects of vitamin D on innate and adaptive immune responses to Streptococcus pneumoniae. J Infect Dis 208:1474–1481
19. Cantorna MT, Mahon BD (2004) Mounting evidence for vitamin D as an environmental factor affecting autoimmune disease prevalence. Exp Biol Med (Maywood) 229:1136–1142
20. Gatenby P, Lucas R, Swaminathan A (2013) Vitamin D deficiency and risk for rheumatic diseases: an update. Curr Opin Rheumatol 25:184–191
21. Tiosano D, Wildbaum G, Gepstein V et al (2013) The role of vitamin D receptor in innate and adaptive immunity: a study in hereditary vitamin D-resistant rickets patients. J Clin Endocrinol Metab 98:1685–1693
22. Terrier B, Derian N, Schoindre Y et al (2012) Restoration of regulatory and effector T cell balance and B cell homeostasis in systemic lupus erythematosus patients through vitamin D supplementation. Arthritis Res Ther 14:R221
23. Borgogni E, Sarchielli E, Sottili M et al (2008) Elocalcitol inhibits inflammatory responses in human thyroid cells and T cells. Endocrinology 149:3626–3634
24. Rausch-Fan X, Leutmezer F, Willheim M et al (2002) Regulation of cytokine production in human peripheral blood mononuclear cells and allergen-specific th cell clones by 1alpha,25-dihydroxyvitamin D3. Int Arch Allergy Immunol 128:33–41
25. Colin EM et al (2010) 1,25-dihydroxyvitamin D3 modulates Th17 polarization and interleukin-22 expression by memory T cells from patients with early rheumatoid arthritis. Arthritis Rheum 62:132–142
26. van Hamburg JP, Asmawidjaja PS, Davelaar N et al (2012) TNF blockade requires 1,25(OH)2D3 to control human Th17-mediated synovial inflammation. Ann Rheum Dis 71:606–612
27. Sasano H, Miki Y, Nagasaki S, Suzuki T (2009) *In situ* estrogen production and its regulation in human breast carcinoma: from endocrinology to intracrinology. Pathol Int 59:777–789
28. Haque UJ, Bartlett SJ (2010) Relationships among vitamin D, disease activity, pain and disability in rheumatoid arthritis. Clin Exp Rheumatol 28:745–747
29. Gopinath K, Danda D (2011) Supplementation of 1,25 dihydroxy vitamin D3 in patients with treatment naive early rheumatoid arthritis: a randomised controlled trial. Int J Rheum Dis 14:332–339
30. Jirapongsananuruk O, Melamed I, Leung DY (2000) Additive immunosuppressive effects of 1,25-dihydroxyvitamin D3 and corticosteroids on TH1, but not TH2, responses. J Allergy Clin Immunol 106:981–985
31. Hidalgo AA, Deeb KK, Pike JW et al (2011) Dexamethasone enhances 1,25-dihydroxyvitamin D3 effects by increasing vitamin D receptor transcription. J Biol Chem 286:36228–36237
32. Deeb KK, Trump DL, Johnson CS (2007) Vitamin D signalling pathways in cancer: potential for anticancer therapeutics. Nat Rev Cancer 7:684–700
33. Mangelsdorf DJ, Thummel C, Beato M et al (1995) The nuclear receptor superfamily: the second decade. Cell 83:835–839
34. Kallay E, Pietschmann P, Toyokuni S et al (2001) Characterization of a vitamin D receptor knockout mouse as a model of colorectal hyperproliferation and DNA damage. Carcinogenesis 22:1429–1435
35. Yu WD, McElwain MC, Madzelewski RA et al (1998) Enhancement of 1,25-dihydroxyvitamin D3-mediated antitumor activity with dexamethasone. J Natl Cancer Inst 90:134–141
36. Zhang Y, Leung DY, Goleva E (2013) Vitamin D enhances glucocorticoid action in human monocytes: involvement of granulocyte-macrophage colony-stimulating factor and mediator complex subunit 14. J Biol Chem 288:14544–14553

37. Searing DA, Zhang Y, Murphy JR et al (2010) Decreased serum vitamin D levels in children with asthma are associated with increased corticosteroid use. J Allergy Clin Immunol 125:995–1000
38. Menter A, Gold S, Bukualo M et al (2013) Calcipotriene plus betamethasone dipropionate topical suspension for the treatment of mild to moderate psoriasis vulgaris on the body: a randomized, double-blind, vehicle-controlled trial. J Drugs Dermatol 12:92–98
39. Kragballe K, Austad J, Barnes L et al (2008) A 52-week randomized safety study of a calcipotriol/betamethasone dipropionate two-compound product (Dovobet/Daivobet/Taclonex) in the treatment of psoriasis vulgaris. Br J Dermatol 154:1155–1160
40. Azali P, Barbasso Helmers S, Kockum I et al (2013) Low serum levels of vitamin D in idiopathic inflammatory myopathies. Ann Rheum Dis 72:512–516
41. Prietl B, Pilz S, Wolf M et al (2010) Vitamin D supplementation and regulatory T cells in apparently healthy subjects: vitamin D treatment for autoimmune diseases? Isr Med Assoc J 12:136–139
42. Ritterhouse LL, Crowe SR, Niewold TB et al (2011) Vitamin D deficiency is associated with an increased autoimmune response in healthy individuals and in patients with systemic lupus erythematosus. Ann Rheum Dis 70:1569–1574
43. Mok CC, Birmingham DJ, Ho LY et al (2012) Vitamin D deficiency as marker for disease activity and damage in systemic lupus erythematosus: a comparison with anti-dsDNA and anti-C1q. Lupus 21:36–42
44. Li W, Zhang R, Zhang K et al (2012) Reduced vitamin D levels are associated with autoimmune response in tuberculosis patients. Ann Rheum Dis 71:790–794
45. Cutolo M, Sulli A, Straub RH (2013) Estrogen's effects in chronic autoimmune/inflammatory diseases and progression to cancer. Expert Rev Clin Immunol 10(1):31–39
46. Krishnan AV, Swami S, Peng L et al (2010) Tissue-selective regulation of aromatase expression by calcitriol: implications for breast cancer therapy. Endocrinology 5:32–34
47. Krishnan AV, Swami S, Feldman D (2012) The potential therapeutic benefits of vitamin D in the treatment of estrogen receptor positive breast cancer. Steroids 77:1107–1112
48. Villaggio B, Soldano S, Cutolo M (2012) Vitamin D modulates aromatase expression in human macrophages and downregulates proinflammatory cytokine production via ERK/MAPK signaling. Ann Rheum Dis 71(supl1):A75
49. Villaggio B, Soldano S, Cutolo M (2012) 1,25-dihydroxyvitamin D3 downregulates aromatase expression and inflammatory cytokines in human macrophages. Clin Exp Rheumatol 30:934–938
50. Cutolo M (2012) The challenges of using vitamin D in cancer prevention and prognosis. Isr Med Assoc J 14:637–639
51. Cutolo M, Sulli A, Straub RH (2012) Estrogen metabolism and autoimmunity. Autoimmun Rev 11:A460–A464
52. Capellino S, Montagna P, Villaggio B et al (2008) Hydroxylated estrogen metabolites influence the proliferation of cultured human monocytes: possible role in synovial tissue hyperplasia. Clin Exp Rheumatol 26:903–909
53. Bosland MC, Mahmoud AM (2011) Hormones and prostate carcinogenesis: androgens and estrogens. J Carcinog 10:33–37
54. Correale J, Ysrraelit MC, Gaitán MI (2009) Immunomodulatory effects of Vitamin D in multiple sclerosis. Brain 132:1146–1160
55. Mok CC (2013) Vitamin D and systemic lupus erythematosus: an update. Expert Rev Clin Immunol 9:453–463
56. Rahman A, Isenberg DA (2008) Systemiclupuserythematosus. N Engl J Med 358:929–939
57. Yap K, Morand E (2015) Vitamin D and systemic lupus erythematosus: continued evolution. Int J Rheum Dis 18(2):242–249
58. Birmingham DJ, Hebert LA, Song H et al (2012) Evidence that abnormally large seasonal declines in vitamin D status may trigger SLE flare in non-African Americans. Lupus 21(8):855–864

59. Piantoni S, Andreoli L, Zanola A et al (2015) Phenotype modifications of T-cells and their shift towards a Th2 response in patients with systemic lupus erythematos supplemented with monthly different regimens of vitamin D. Lupus 24:490–498
60. Sahebari M, Nabavi N, Salehi M (2014) Correlation between serum 25(OH)D values and lupus disease activity: an original article and a systematic review with meta-analysis focusing on serum VitD confounders. Lupus 23:1164–1177
61. Stagi S, Cavalli L, Bertini F et al (2014) Vitamin D levels in children, adolescents, and young adults with juvenile-onset systemic lupus erythematosus: a cross-sectional study. Lupus 23(10):1059–1065
62. Cutolo M (2013) Further emergent evidence for the vitamin D endocrine system involvement in autoimmune rheumatic disease risk and prognosis. Ann Rheum Dis 72:473–475
63. Reynolds J, Ray D, Alexander MY et al (2015) Role of vitamin D in endothelial function and endothelial repair in clinically stable systemic lupus erythematosus. Lancet 385(Suppl 1):S83
64. Kokic V, Martinovic Kaliterna D et al (2015) Relationship between vitamin D, IFN-γ, and E2 levels in systemic lupus erythematosus. Lupus. pii: 0961203315605367. [Epub ahead of print]

The Impact of aPL Detection on Pregnancy

13

Maria Tiziana Bertero, Anna Kuzenko, and Mario Bazzan

The coexistence of antiphospholipid syndrome (APS) diagnosis represents a further risk factor for adverse outcome in patients with systemic lupus erythematosus (SLE) during pregnancy [1, 2]. A quarter to half of patients with SLE are antiphospholipid antibody (aPL)-positive [3]. aPL are autoantibodies directed toward plasma proteins with affinity for anionic phospholipids: β2-glycoprotein I and prothrombin [4]. The revised APS classification criteria [5] emphasize the diagnostic value of three of them, namely, lupus anticoagulant (LA), anticardiolipin IgG or IgM isotype (aCL), and anti-β2-glycoprotein I IgG or IgM antibodies (anti-β2GPI), even though there are many more antibodies belonging to this family. Patients with a history of pregnancy morbidity or thrombosis and persistent aPL positivity are classified as affected by APS [6].

13.1 Pathogenesis of aPL-Induced Obstetric Manifestation

aPLs are widely accepted as pathogenic on the basis of studies on animal models and in vitro experiments [7]. The pathogenetic mechanisms of aPL have been studied since the discovery of the syndrome in the early 1980s with important advances in recent years which are summarized in the review of Giannakopoulos [8]. The mechanisms are multiple and not yet fully understood but the crucial point is that the presence of the abovementioned antibodies is necessary but usually insufficient

M.T. Bertero (✉) • A. Kuzenko
Clinical Immunology, Mauriziano Hospital, Largo Turati 62, Turin 10128, Italy
e-mail: tbertero@mauriziano.it; annakuzenko@gmail.com

M. Bazzan
Haematology and Thrombosis Unit, Giovanni Bosco Hospital,
Piazza del donatore di Sangue 3, Turin 10126, Italy
e-mail: bazzmar@yahoo.com

D. Roccatello, L. Emmi (eds.), *Connective Tissue Disease: A Comprehensive Guide-Volume 1*, Rare Diseases of the Immune System 5,
DOI 10.1007/978-3-319-24535-5_13

and requires other prothrombotic changes for the development of clinical manifestations of the syndrome. The so-called two hits theory has been proposed [9]: the first hit, represented by aPL, predisposes to thrombosis which occurs in the presence of another prothrombotic condition, the abovementioned "second hit." The antiphospholipid immune complexes do not recognize integrum endothelium, but do bind the injured vessel wall. The priming injuring factors can be recent infections, surgery, smoking, etc. The concomitance of the abovementioned exogenous prothrombotic factors multiplies significantly the odds ratio of thrombotic events [10]. Different pathogenetic mechanisms have been suggested to explain the nature of thrombotic and obstetric complications which only partially overlap. More details about aPL involvement in thrombosis will be found in another chapter. In obstetric APS, pregnancy itself probably accounts for the second hit, and experiments in naive mice demonstrated that passive transfer of IgG aPL is sufficient to induce fetal loss. Placental thrombosis with reduced blood flow has been thought for a long time to be the main cause of fetal growth restriction, late fetal loss, or premature delivery; for this reason initially treatment for obstetric APS (OAPS) consisted of low-dose aspirin (LDA) and heparin [11]. However, this mechanism did not explain early abortions, and moreover most placentas from APS patients did not show thrombosis evidence [9, 12]. aPLs are probably directly pathogenic: being anti-β2-glycoprotein I molecules strongly expressed on trophoblast, they represent a target for deposition of aPL, particularly anti-β2GPI. Non-thrombotic mechanisms have been identified on both the maternal (a reduction of endometrial angiogenesis) and the fetal side (a defective trophoblast invasiveness) [13]. Localized inflammatory responses inducing cell injury and apoptosis, decreased production of human chorionic gonadotropin, and growth factors are involved in aPL-mediated placental damage. Experimental observations suggest that complement activation plays an essential role in pregnancy loss, growth restriction, and preeclampsia. According to this acknowledged theory, C5a anaphylatoxin induces placental inflammation with expression of tissue factor (TF) by placental neutrophils and dysregulation of monocytes, endothelial cells, decidual cells, and trophoblast [8]. This evidence is still doubtful as complement deposition is found also in placentas without pregnancy morbidity. In animal models inhibition of complement in placenta rescues pregnancy, restores angiogenic balance, and prevents preeclampsia in mice, proving an important role for the complement system, both classical and alternative pathways [14]. The demonstration of a protective role of heparin through an anticomplement mechanism more than through the anticoagulant activity further supports the hypothesis of a role of complement in fetal loss. The use of complement inhibitor therapies to prevent or treat preeclampsia in these patients has been suggested, also on the basis of the effective use of eculizumab (humanized monoclonal IgG2/4 k antibody of that binds to C5) in catastrophic antiphospholipid syndrome (CAPS) cases [15]. The Task Force on Obstetric APS at the 14th International Congress on Antiphospholipid Antibodies proposed to consider new therapeutic agents such as complement inhibitors for refractory obstetric APS. An international trial with the participation of multiple centers should be planned [16]. Toll-like receptor 4 (TLR4) is another molecule which plays a role in aPL-mediated trophoblastic cell fusion and differentiation. Recent studies on experimental models on trophoblast fusion and differentiation using BeWo cells postulated hydroxychloroquine (HCQ) might inhibit TLR4 and consequently reduce the effect of aPL [17]. HCQ has already been used for the prevention of fetal losses by restoring the annexin V shield, an anticoagulant protection, disrupted by aPL at the trophoblastic cell surface [18]. For these reasons HCQ represents another candidate for cases who have failed with current treatments for OAPS [19].

13.2 Obstetric APS

As known [5], pregnancy complications included in APS criteria are the following (see Table 13.1):

(a) One or more unexplained deaths of a morphologically normal fetus at or beyond the 10th week of gestation, with normal fetal morphology documented by ultrasound or by direct examination of the fetus
(b) One or more premature births of a morphologically normal neonate before the 34th week of gestation because of: (i) eclampsia or severe preeclampsia defined according to standard definitions or (ii) recognized features of placental insufficiency
(c) Three or more unexplained consecutive spontaneous abortions before the 10th week of gestation, with maternal anatomic or hormonal abnormalities and paternal and maternal chromosomal causes excluded.

Table 13.1 APS classification criteria adapted from Miyakis (2006)

Clinical criteria		Laboratory criteria (all confirmed after at least 12 weeks apart)
Vascular thrombosis	Obstetric morbidity	
Venous, arterial, or microvessel thrombosis in any tissue or organ, confirmed by imaging studies	One or more unexplained deaths of a morphologically normal fetus at or beyond the 10th week of gestation	Lupus anticoagulant (LA) present in plasma, detected according to ISTH SSC guidelines
	One or more premature births of a morphologically normal neonate before the 34th week of gestation because of eclampsia, severe preeclampsia, or placental insufficiency	Anticardiolipin (aCL) antibodies of IgG or IgM isotype: present in serum or plasma at medium or high titer (>40 GPL or MPL or >99th percentile) measured by a standardized ELISA
	Three or more unexplained consecutive spontaneous abortions before the 10th week of gestation with exclusion of anatomic, hormonal, and chromosomal causes	Anti-beta2-glycoprotein I antibodies of IgG or IgM isotype, present in serum or plasma at titer >99th percentile, measured by a standardized ELISA

It can be noticed that, whereas other autoimmune diseases may affect the course of pregnancy, in this case pregnancy morbidity is a manifestation and a defining feature of OAPS [20]. As known, classification criteria in rheumatic diseases are continuously undergone to search to improve sensitivity and specificity. Current APS criteria are indeed under discussion: some debated aspects are the low specificity of early recurrent abortions, the weight of the single aPL positivity, and a more than 5 years interval between aPL test and clinical manifestations [21]. The Task Force on Obstetric APS, cited above, was created to carry out a critical appraisal – literature based – of the obstetric manifestations present in current classification criteria and the weight of the evidence of benefit provided by treatments in terms of avoiding recurrences [16]. But the laboratory classification criteria remain controversial, too. The Laboratory Diagnostics and Trends Task Force, who met at the abovementioned 14th International Congress on aPL, examined other antibodies shown to be directed to other proteins or their complex with antiphospholipids [22]. The report conclusions include the following:

- The necessity to develop international reference materials for anti-β2-glycoprotein I testing to reduce interlaboratory discrepancies
- The importance of further investigating the utility of anti-domain I assay (a targeted subpopulation of anti-β2-glycoprotein I considered particularly pathogenic)
- The contribution of antiprothrombin/antiphosphatidylserine antibodies (aPT/PS), appraised as more specific tests, to assess the risk of thrombosis in APS
- The restricted use of IgA isotype for aCL and anti-β2GPI in suspected cases of APS with negative aPL tests.

Gardiner et al. suggested including low-titer antibodies in the diagnosis of obstetric APS, to avoid missing APS cases [23]. The European Registry on Obstetric Antiphospholipid Syndrome described, in a preliminary first year report in 2012, a subgroup of patients, named OMAPS, who presented obstetric morbidity related to aPL, but not fulfilling APS criteria: these include two unexplained miscarriages, three nonconsecutive miscarriages, late preeclampsia, placental abruption, late premature birth, and two or more unexplained in vitro fertilization failures. Information about clinical, laboratory, and therapeutic characteristics was collected: the authors stated a better outcome even for these patients, if treated as classical APS [24]. Arachchillage et al. recently reported studies regarding non-criteria clinical and laboratory manifestations and addressed the question on whether they should be included within the spectrum of OAPS: non-criteria manifestations merit further observations and therapeutic approaches should be investigated [25].

13.3 Other Complications in Pregnancy with aPL Positivity

It should also be remembered that pregnant women with aPL have an increased risk of other (non-obstetric) problems [26]: thrombosis, bleeding risk due to ongoing therapy, thrombocytopenia, and catastrophic antiphospholipid syndrome (CAPS).

The latter is a severe complication characterized by multiorgan failure caused by microangiopathy, developing in a very short time in patients with antiphospholipid antibodies [27]. It is a very rare presentation of APS (1 %); the mortality rate, although reduced, is still 30 %. Data collected from the CAPS Registry showed that 4 % of 409 cases of CAPS were related to pregnancy or puerperium. In these cases differential diagnosis with HELLP (hemolysis, elevated liver enzymes, low platelet count), thrombotic thrombocytopenic purpura (TTP), hemolytic uremic syndrome (HUS), and acute fatty liver of pregnancy may be difficult. Early diagnosis and aggressive therapy allowed in the last 10 years an amelioration of prognosis; according to "CAPS Registry" the combination of anticoagulation plus corticosteroids plus plasma exchange is the most successful therapy [28]. When occurring during pregnancy, as soon as fetal maturity makes it possible, a prompt cesarean intervention is mandatory [29].

Positivity for aPL may be isolated or associated with other autoimmune diseases, mainly SLE. Obviously the presence of SLE with the risk of cardiac heart block due to SSA-Ro positivity, problems of disease activity, immunodepression and related infections, and other adverse effects of drugs may strongly affect maternal and fetal outcomes of the gestation [30]. This topic will be developed by other authors.

13.4 Risk Stratification

At present aPL, more than criteria, are considered risk factors for vascular thrombosis and/or for pregnancy complications. An innovative point of view advises a risk stratification in each aPL carrier. This evaluation could allow an individualized approach to prophylaxis and therapy. The global antiphospholipid syndrome score (GAPPS) has been recently proposed as a quantitative prediction scale of thrombosis or pregnancy loss risk in SLE. It is derived from the combination of aPL profile, cardiovascular risk factors, and autoimmune antibody profile [31]. Concerning pregnancy outcome, data from other authors outlined a correlation between prognosis and particular variables: some examples are previous thrombotic events [32], a diagnosis of SLE [33], and triple aPL positivity [19]. All these elements must be considered during preconceptional counseling in patients with aPL [13].

13.5 Prevention of Obstetric Adverse Events

Pregnancy in women with aPL should be considered at high risk, and the essential conditions to ameliorate prognosis are planning gestation, coordinated medical-obstetrical care, an agreed and well-defined management protocol, and a good neonatal unit [34]. If these provisions are met, the likelihood of a good pregnancy outcome is about 75–80 % (see Fig. 13.1). The pharmacological management includes LDA and heparin. In a recent meta-analysis Wu and colleagues compare 16 randomized controlled trials (RCTs) investigating effects on pregnancy in APS patients [35]: the combination of aspirin and unfractionated heparin (UFH) results

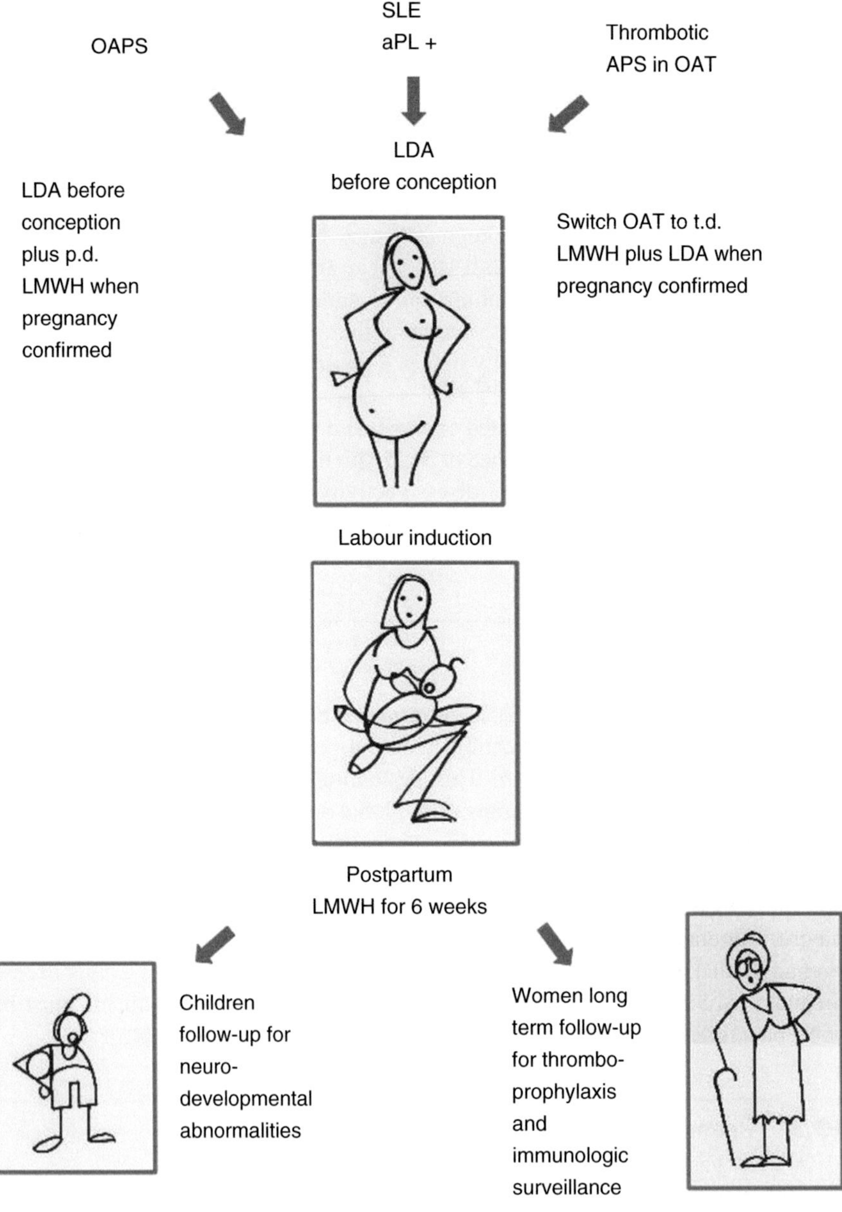

Fig. 13.1 Management protocol of pregnancy in aPL-positive patients. *OAPS* obstetric antiphospholipid syndrome, *aPL* antiphospholipid antibodies, *SLE* systemic lupus erythematosus, *OAT* oral anticoagulant therapy, *LDA* low-dose aspirin, *LMWH* low-molecular-weight heparin, *p.d.* prophylactic doses, *t.d.* therapeutic doses

in a higher birth rate than LDA alone, whereas aspirin plus LMWH seems to be superior to intravenous immunoglobulin (IVIg). LMWH is generally preferred to UFH because it has fewer adverse events and is easier to monitor [3].

The protocol of administration of LDA and LMWH differs depending on the situation of the patient (see Table 13.2) [36]. The recommendations for each different scenario include the following:

- LDA and prophylactic doses of LMWH for women with obstetric APS
- LDA and therapeutic doses of LMWH for women with thrombotic APS, switching from oral anticoagulant therapy (OAT) to heparin when pregnancy test becomes positive
- LDA to aPL carriers with SLE (also to reduce the risk of preeclampsia)
- An individualized approach based on the patient's history and on aPL profile for cases which do not fulfill APS criteria
- Postpartum thromboprophylaxis with LMWH in all patients with aPL.

No clear consensus about the timing of LDA prophylaxis starting exists. For some authors it would be preferable to start before conception [34]. It should be noted that current recommendations to treat patients aPL positive with fetal death are based on data from early recurrent abortions. Being difficult to plan a controlled trial on late fetal loss due to the rarity of complication but also for ethical reasons (nobody would be available for placebo arm), some authors propose to realize an international multicenter prospective registry instead of an RCT [16].

Even though treated with appropriate therapy, 20 % of APS patients have an unsuccessful pregnancy [33]: history of thrombosis, diagnosis of systemic lupus erythematosus, and triple antiphospholipid antibody positivity have been identified as risk factors.

In a European multicenter retrospective study, 10 % out of 196 pregnancies in APS patients with thrombosis and triple antiphospholipid positivity were prescribed other treatments, i.e., low-dose prednisone, hydroxychloroquine, IVIg, and plasma exchange (PE) in addition to conventional therapy. The authors concluded that APS pregnant patients with previous thrombosis and triple aPL positivity treated with additional therapy had a more favorable pregnancy outcome [37]. To the present the

Table 13.2 Prophylaxis of pregnancy complications in patients with aPL

Clinical situations	Management
Obstetric APS	LDA plus prophylactic doses of LMWH
APS with previous thrombosis	LDA plus therapeutic doses of LMWH
aPL-positive SLE	LDA
Isolated aPL positivity	No treatment or LDA
Puerperium in all patients aPL positive	Thromboprophylaxis with LMWH for 6 weeks

APS antiphospholipid syndrome, *aPL* antiphospholipid antibodies, *LDA* low-dose aspirin, *LMWH* low-molecular-weight heparin

advisable additional therapy is not known: for each of the mentioned management data are available on literature but we do not have at the moment a comparative trial [38, 39]. The following question was posed by Mekinian in a recently published paper: "Is there a place for hydroxychloroquine to improve pregnancy outcome in obstetrical APS?" [40].

Another observation is that prophylaxis with LDA and LMWH, although having increased fetal survival, does not allow a complete elimination of some neonatal complications such as intrauterine growth restriction (IUGR), premature birth, and newborn small for gestational age (SGA) [41].

13.6 Delivery

Perioperative management of patients on anticoagulant therapy involves assessing risks of both bleeding and thromboembolism [42]. In APS patient, moreover, an invasive procedure like the delivery is an established trigger factor for CAPS, too.

While LDA is normally stopped at 34° weeks of gestation, pregnant women with aPL often undergo labor and delivery under LMWH treatment. Even if this treatment does not increase blood loss at delivery, it may represent a risk with the use of spinal/epidural anesthesia. The unpredictable timing of labor and delivery in these patients may be an additional problem among anesthesiologists, particularly if a neuraxial technique is required. On the other hand, APS is an important risk factor for adverse pregnancy and maternal outcomes, in particular for women with previous thrombosis. Therefore withdrawal of LMWH for a long time further increases the already high risk of vascular events. Inducing labour could avoid further risks associated with unpredictable and uncontrollable situations: it allows planning the time of delivery (trying to avoid a cesarean section), optimal assistance of a multidisciplinary and expert medical team, and interruption of anticoagulant prophylaxis for as short a time as possible [43].

13.7 Preconceptional Counseling

All women with aPL should be informed of the importance of planning pregnancy.

The collection of complete anamnestic information associated with the evaluation of laboratory test, to estimate maternal and fetal risks, should ideally be done before conception and possibly with both members of the couple. In this setting obstetric history, any associated autoimmune systemic diseases, and current treatment should be investigated. An agreed and well-defined management protocol should be proposed, and time for answering questions and doubts should be provided to the couple (see Table 13.3).

Before the pregnancy starts, some more exams should be prescribed such as thyroid function and echocardiography. Revision of therapy to remove teratogenic drugs is mandatory.

Table 13.3 Preconceptional counseling

Anamnestic information
Age
Previous pregnancies
Family history of thrombosis, bleeding, preeclampsia
Associated SLE
Recent flares
Current therapy
Organ damage
Renal involvement
Heart valve lesions
Laboratory
Presence of SSA/SSB
Forbidden drugs
OAT
Antiepileptic drugs
ACE inhibitor
Comorbidities (thyroid dysfunction, hypertension, diabetes, etc.)

In rare circumstances pregnancy is contraindicated or postponed, according to tailored evaluation involving different specialists and the couple. These are pulmonary hypertension, heart failure, chronic renal failure, recent lupus flare, and stroke within the previous 6 months [34]. During gestation regular placental Doppler studies are helpful to estimate the risk of preeclampsia and placental insufficiency.

13.7.1 Long-Term Follow-Up of OAPS Patients

In the cohort of OAPS of the Piedmont Consortium, 16 out of 49 patients had a positive history for both vascular and obstetric APS. It should be noted that 8/16 patients developed a thrombosis after the pregnancy complication: that means that if these women had been followed up, the vascular event could have been avoided (data not published). An increased risk of subsequent thrombosis in OAPS has been proved by Martinez-Zamora: 12-year thrombotic cumulative incidence was higher in APS-recurrent spontaneous abortion (RSA) patients compared with aPL carriers, RSA of unknown etiology, and RSA in thrombophilic genetic defects (19, 3 % vs. 0 %, 0 %, 4,8 %, respectively) [44].

Since 2001 primary thromboprophylaxis for OAPS has been proposed, after evaluation of thrombotic event rate during long-term follow-up [45].

Another aspect deserving of long-term surveillance is the possible – albeit rare – appearance of immunological manifestations suggestive of systemic autoimmune disease, namely, SLE [46].

13.7.2 Long-Term Outcome of Children Born from OAPS Patients

Even if children born to mothers with APS do not seem to be at increased risk of developing the same autoimmune disease as their mothers, recently their long-term follow-up has become a subject of study. Possible correlation has been hypothesized between neurodevelopment abnormalities and mother disease or the presence of aPL or prematurity or drugs [36].

13.8 Assisted Reproductive Technology

It is not rare that a patient with APS chooses to undergo assisted reproduction technology [13]. The most serious adverse event of in vitro fertilization is thrombosis. The noticeable and rapid increase in levels of endogenous estrogens may cause an ovarian hyperstimulation syndrome (OHSS) that can ultimately result in pulmonary embolism or venous thromboembolism [47]. Friendly ovarian stimulation, single embryo transfer, avoidance of OHSS, stopping heparin before ovum retrieval and starting again after the maneuver, and use of natural estrogens avoiding oral route all may represent the safest approach [48].

13.9 Contraception

As pregnancy outcome in APS patients is strongly improved when pregnancy is planned, the importance of a good contraception is obvious. The choice of an effective and safe method permits avoiding pregnancy during immunological activity and/or forbidden drugs. Doctors should give information about thrombotic risk related to combined hormonal contraception that is contraindicated in APS patients. Progesterone-only contraceptives, levonorgestrel intrauterine device (IUD), and progesterone implant represent effective alternatives. Immunorheumatologists should broach this topic with patients and further suggest a more detailed counseling with gynecologists [49].

Conclusions

Numerous studies nowadays show a success rate of 70–80 % in pregnancies of women with APS. The live birth rate has significantly improved in the last 10–15 years; this is consistent with the prophylaxis strategies based on low-dose aspirin and heparin. However the role of pregnancy planning and of a multidisciplinary care in changing pregnancy outcome for these patients should also be mentioned [20].

References

1. Clowse ME, Magder LS, Witter F, Petri M (2006) Early risk factors for pregnancy loss in lupus. Obstet Gynecol 107(2 Pt 1):293–299
2. Canti V, Castiglioni MT, Rosa S, Franchini S, Sabbadini MG, Manfredi AA et al (2012) Pregnancy outcomes in patients with systemic autoimmunity. Autoimmunity 45(2):169–175

3. Lateef A, Petri M (2012) Management of pregnancy in systemic lupus erythematosus. Nat Rev Rheumatol 8(12):710–718
4. de Groot PG (2014) Platelets as pivot in the antiphospholipid syndrome. Blood 124(4):475–476
5. Miyakis S, Lockshin MD, Atsumi T, Branch DW, Brey RL, Cervera R et al (2006) International consensus statement on an update of the classification criteria for definite antiphospholipid syndrome (APS). J Thromb Haemost JTH 4(2):295–306
6. Taraborelli M, Andreoli L, Tincani A (2012) Much more than thrombosis and pregnancy loss: the antiphospholipid syndrome as a 'systemic disease'. Best Pract Res Clin Rheumatol 26(1):79–90
7. Pierangeli SS, Chen PP, Raschi E, Scurati S, Grossi C, Borghi MO et al (2008) Antiphospholipid antibodies and the antiphospholipid syndrome: pathogenic mechanisms. Semin Thromb Hemost 34(3):236–250
8. Giannakopoulos B, Krilis SA (2013) The pathogenesis of the antiphospholipid syndrome. N Engl J Med 368(11):1033–1044
9. Meroni PL, Borghi MO, Raschi E, Tedesco F (2011) Pathogenesis of antiphospholipid syndrome: understanding the antibodies. Nat Rev Rheumatol 7(6):330–339
10. Urbanus RT, Siegerink B, Roest M, Rosendaal FR, de Groot PG, Algra A (2009) Antiphospholipid antibodies and risk of myocardial infarction and ischaemic stroke in young women in the RATIO study: a case-control study. Lancet Neurol 8(11):998–1005
11. Ziakas PD, Pavlou M, Voulgarelis M (2010) Heparin treatment in antiphospholipid syndrome with recurrent pregnancy loss: a systematic review and meta-analysis. Obstet Gynecol 115(6):1256–1262
12. Oku K, Amengual O, Atsumi T (2012) Pathophysiology of thrombosis and pregnancy morbidity in the antiphospholipid syndrome. Eur J Clin Invest 42(10):1126–1135
13. Ostensen M, Andreoli L, Brucato A, Cetin I, Chambers C, Clowse ME et al (2015) State of the art: reproduction and pregnancy in rheumatic diseases. Autoimmun Rev 14(5):376–386
14. Salmon JE, de Groot PG (2008) Pathogenic role of antiphospholipid antibodies. Lupus 17(5):405–411
15. Espinosa G, Berman H, Cervera R (2011) Management of refractory cases of catastrophic antiphospholipid syndrome. Autoimmun Rev 10(11):664–668
16. de Jesus GR, Agmon-Levin N, Andrade CA, Andreoli L, Chighizola CB, Porter TF et al (2014) 14th International Congress on Antiphospholipid Antibodies Task Force report on obstetric antiphospholipid syndrome. Autoimmun Rev 13(8):795–813
17. Marchetti T, Ruffatti A, Wuillemin C, de Moerloose P, Cohen M (2014) Hydroxychloroquine restores trophoblast fusion affected by antiphospholipid antibodies. J Thromb Haemost JTH 12(6):910–920
18. Rand JH, Wu XX, Quinn AS, Ashton AW, Chen PP, Hathcock JJ et al (2010) Hydroxychloroquine protects the annexin A5 anticoagulant shield from disruption by antiphospholipid antibodies: evidence for a novel effect for an old antimalarial drug. Blood 115(11):2292–2299
19. Ruffatti A, Tonello M, Cavazzana A, Bagatella P, Pengo V (2009) Laboratory classification categories and pregnancy outcome in patients with primary antiphospholipid syndrome prescribed antithrombotic therapy. Thromb Res 123(3):482–487
20. Borchers AT, Naguwa SM, Keen CL, Gershwin ME (2010) The implications of autoimmunity and pregnancy. J Autoimmun 34(3):J287–J299
21. Bertero M, Kuzenko A (2013) Risk assessment in patients with antiphospholipid antibodies. Minerva Med 104(6):639–648
22. Bertolaccini ML, Amengual O, Andreoli L, Atsumi T, Chighizola CB, Forastiero R et al (2014) 14th International Congress on Antiphospholipid Antibodies Task Force. Report on antiphospholipid syndrome laboratory diagnostics and trends. Autoimmun Rev 13(9):917–930
23. Gardiner C, Hills J, Machin SJ, Cohen H (2013) Diagnosis of antiphospholipid syndrome in routine clinical practice. Lupus 22(1):18–25
24. Alijotas-Reig J, Ferrer-Oliveras R, Group ES (2012) The European Registry on Obstetric Antiphospholipid Syndrome (EUROAPS): a preliminary first year report. Lupus 21(7):766–768

25. Arachchillage DR, Machin SJ, Mackie IJ, Cohen H (2015) Diagnosis and management of non-criteria obstetric antiphospholipid syndrome. Thromb Haemost 113(1):13–19
26. Andreoli L, Fredi M, Nalli C, Reggia R, Lojacono A, Motta M et al (2012) Pregnancy implications for systemic lupus erythematosus and the antiphospholipid syndrome. J Autoimmun 38(2–3):J197–J208
27. Sciascia S, Lopez-Pedrera C, Roccatello D, Cuadrado MJ (2012) Catastrophic antiphospholipid syndrome (CAPS). Best Pract Res Clin Rheumatol 26(4):535–541
28. Cervera R (2012) CAPS registry. Lupus 21(7):755–757
29. Gomez-Puerta JA, Espinosa G, Cervera R (2013) Catastrophic antiphospholipid syndrome: diagnosis and management in pregnancy. Clin Lab Med 33(2):391–400
30. Ateka-Barrutia O, Khamashta MA (2013) The challenge of pregnancy for patients with SLE. Lupus 22(12):1295–1308
31. Sciascia S, Sanna G, Murru V, Roccatello D, Khamashta MA, Bertolaccini ML (2013) GAPSS: the global anti-phospholipid syndrome score. Rheumatology 52(8):1397–1403
32. Bramham K, Hunt BJ, Germain S, Calatayud I, Khamashta M, Bewley S et al (2010) Pregnancy outcome in different clinical phenotypes of antiphospholipid syndrome. Lupus 19(1):58–64
33. Ruffatti A, Tonello M, Visentin MS, Bontadi A, Hoxha A, De Carolis S et al (2011) Risk factors for pregnancy failure in patients with anti-phospholipid syndrome treated with conventional therapies: a multicentre, case-control study. Rheumatology 50(9):1684–1689
34. Danza A, Ruiz-Irastorza G, Khamashta M (2012) Antiphospohlipid syndrome in obstetrics. Best Pract Res Clin Obstet Gynaecol 26(1):65–76
35. Wu CQ, Kustec V, Brown RN, Martin MC, Filion KB (2014) The medical management of antiphospholipid syndrome in pregnancy: a meta-analysis. Obstet Gynecol 123(Suppl 1):178S–179S
36. Nalli C, Iodice A, Andreoli L, Lojacono A, Motta M, Fazzi E et al (2014) The effects of lupus and antiphospholipid antibody syndrome on foetal outcomes. Lupus 23(6):507–517
37. Ruffatti A, Salvan E, Del Ross T, Gerosa M, Andreoli L, Maina A et al (2014) Treatment strategies and pregnancy outcomes in antiphospholipid syndrome patients with thrombosis and triple antiphospholipid positivity. A European multicentre retrospective study. Thromb Haemost 112(4):727–735
38. Bramham K, Thomas M, Nelson-Piercy C, Khamashta M, Hunt BJ (2011) First-trimester low-dose prednisolone in refractory antiphospholipid antibody-related pregnancy loss. Blood 117(25):6948–6951
39. Bontadi A, Ruffatti A, Marson P, Tison T, Tonello M, Hoxha A et al (2012) Plasma exchange and immunoadsorption effectively remove antiphospholipid antibodies in pregnant patients with antiphospholipid syndrome. J Clin Apher 27(4):200–204
40. Mekinian A, Lazzaroni MG, Kuzenko A, Alijotas-Reig J, Ruffatti A, Levy P et al (2015) The efficacy of hydroxychloroquine for obstetrical outcome in anti-phospholipid syndrome: data from a European multicenter retrospective study. Autoimmun Rev 14(6):498–502
41. A K (2014) Obstetric antiphospholipid syndrome: analysis of 30 patients. Presented at the 8th international conference on reproduction, pregnancy and rheumatic diseases, Trondheim, pp 25–27
42. Raso S, Sciascia S, Kuzenko A, Castagno I, Marozio L, Bertero MT (2015) Bridging therapy in antiphospholipid syndrome and antiphospholipid antibodies carriers: case series and review of the literature. Autoimmun Rev 14(1):36–42
43. Butwick AJ, Carvalho B (2011) Anticoagulant and antithrombotic drugs in pregnancy: what are the anesthetic implications for labor and cesarean delivery? J Perinatol Off J Calif Perinat Assoc 31(2):73–84
44. Martinez-Zamora MA, Peralta S, Creus M, Tassies D, Reverter JC, Espinosa G et al (2012) Risk of thromboembolic events after recurrent spontaneous abortion in antiphospholipid syndrome: a case-control study. Ann Rheum Dis 71(1):61–66
45. Erkan D, Merrill JT, Yazici Y, Sammaritano L, Buyon JP, Lockshin MD (2001) High thrombosis rate after fetal loss in antiphospholipid syndrome: effective prophylaxis with aspirin. Arthritis Rheum 44(6):1466–1467

46. Gomez-Puerta JA, Martin H, Amigo MC, Aguirre MA, Camps MT, Cuadrado MJ et al (2005) Long-term follow-up in 128 patients with primary antiphospholipid syndrome: do they develop lupus? Medicine 84(4):225–230
47. Henriksson P, Westerlund E, Wallen H, Brandt L, Hovatta O, Ekbom A (2013) Incidence of pulmonary and venous thromboembolism in pregnancies after in vitro fertilisation: cross sectional study. BMJ 346:e8632
48. Bellver J, Pellicer A (2009) Ovarian stimulation for ovulation induction and in vitro fertilization in patients with systemic lupus erythematosus and antiphospholipid syndrome. Fertil Steril 92(6):1803–1810
49. Sammaritano LR (2014) Contraception in patients with systemic lupus erythematosus and antiphospholipid syndrome. Lupus 23(12):1242–1245

Systemic Lupus Erythematosus and Antiphospholipid Syndrome

14

Jose A. Gómez-Puerta and Ricard Cervera

14.1 Introduction

The antiphospholipid syndrome (APS) is defined by the occurrence of venous and arterial thromboses, often multiple, and recurrent fetal losses, frequently accompanied by a moderate thrombocytopenia, in the presence of antiphospholipid antibodies (aPL), namely, lupus anticoagulant (LA), anticardiolipin antibodies (aCL), or anti-β_2-glycoprotein I (β_2GPI) antibodies [1]. The APS can be found in patients having neither clinical nor laboratory evidence of another definable condition (primary APS), or it may be associated with other diseases, mainly systemic lupus erythematosus (SLE), but occasionally with other autoimmune conditions [1], infections [2], drugs [1], and malignancies [3] (Table 14.1).

Primary APS patients rarely progress to SLE. Only 8 % of 128 patients, who were followed up for about 9 years, developed lupus, and a positive Coombs' test was a clinically significant predictor of progression [4].

The aPL can appear in different scenarios, such as asymptomatic "carrier" patients for aPL, "classical" APS with recurrent venous and/or arterial thrombosis, APS affecting otherwise healthy women with recurrent pregnancy loss, patients with aPL positivity with non-thrombotic aPL manifestations (i.e., thrombocytopenia, hemolytic anemia, or *livedo reticularis*) [5], or, in a small subset of patients, as a life-threatening form characterized by a rapid development of microthrombosis that led to rapid multiorgan failure, which is termed catastrophic APS [6].

J.A. Gómez-Puerta (✉)
Grupo de Inmunología Celular e Inmunogenética (GICIG), and Sección de Reumatología, Facultad de Medicina, Universidad de Antioquia, Medellín, Colombia
e-mail: jgomezpuerta@mail.harvard.edu

R. Cervera
Department of Autoimmune Diseases, Hospital Clinic, Villarroel, 170, Barcelona, Catalonia, 08036, Spain
e-mail: rcervera@clinic.cat

D. Roccatello, L. Emmi (eds.), *Connective Tissue Disease: A Comprehensive Guide-Volume 1*, Rare Diseases of the Immune System 5,
DOI 10.1007/978-3-319-24535-5_14

Table 14.1 Diseases where aPL have been described

Systemic autoimmune diseases: systemic lupus erythematosus, rheumatoid arthritis, systemic sclerosis, primary Sjogren's syndrome, dermato- and polymyositis, vasculitis (polyarteritis nodosa, microscopic polyarteritis, giant cell arteritis, Behçet's disease, relapsing polychondritis, leukocytoclastic vasculitis)
Infections: viral (HIV infection; mononucleosis; rubella; parvovirus; hepatitis A, B, C; mumps), bacterial (syphilis, Lyme disease, tuberculosis, leprosy, infective endocarditis, rheumatic fever, *Klebsiella*), protozoal (malaria, toxoplasmosis)
Malignancies: solid tumors (lung, colon, cervix, prostate, liver, kidney, thymus, esophagus, maxilla, ovary, breast), hematologic (myeloid and lymphatic leukemias, polycythemia vera, myelofibrosis), lymphoproliferative diseases (Hodgkin's disease, non-Hodgkin's lymphoma, lymphosarcoma, cutaneous T-cell lymphoma/Sezary syndrome), paraproteinemias (monoclonal gammapathies, Waldenström macroglobulinemia, myeloma)
Nonmalignant hematologic conditions: idiopathic thrombocytopenic purpura, sickle-cell disease, pernicious anemia
Drugs: procainamide, phenothiazines, ethosuximide, chlorothiazide, quinine, oral contraceptives, anti-TNFα therapies
Other conditions: diabetes mellitus, autoimmune thyroid disease, inflammatory bowel diseases, dialysis, Klinefelter's syndrome, Ehlers-Danlos syndrome

14.2 Epidemiology of aPL

Prevalence of the aPL in the general population ranges between 1 and 5 %. However, only a minority of these individuals develop the APS. Some estimates indicate that the incidence of the APS is around 5 new cases per 100,000 persons per year and the prevalence around 40–50 cases per 100,000 persons [7]. Cross-sectional studies of aPL in SLE underestimate the true prevalence, because many SLE patients make these antibodies intermittently. In fact, aPL can disappear after thrombotic events in some SLE patients, demonstrating the importance of prospective studies in SLE. Previous estimates have suggested that 30 % of SLE patients will develop APS. In the Hopkins Lupus Cohort, after 20 years of follow-up, there was a 50 % chance of having an arterial or venous thrombosis event if the SLE patient had aPL.

Recently, the APS ACTION (AntiPhospholipid Syndrome Alliance For Clinical Trials and InternatiOnal Networking) group published a literature review focused in the prevalence of aPL in the general population with pregnancy morbidity, stroke, myocardial infarction (MI), and deep vein thrombosis (DVT). The authors estimated that aPL are positive in approximately 13 % of patients with stroke, 11 % with MI, 9.5 % of patients with DVT, and 6 % of patients with pregnancy morbidity [8].

The prevalence of the catastrophic APS is scarce (less than 1 % of all cases of APS) [6], but its potentially lethal outcome emphasizes its importance in clinical medicine today [9, 10]. In order to put together all the published case reports as well as the new diagnosed cases from all over the world, an international registry of patients with catastrophic APS ("CAPS Registry") was created in 2000 by the *European Forum on Antiphospholipid Antibodies*. Currently, it documents the entire clinical, laboratory, and therapeutic data of more than 500 patients whose data has been fully registered. This registry can be freely consulted on the Internet (http://ontocrf.costaisa.com/es/web/caps).

14.3 Pathogenesis of aPL-Mediated Events

Several mechanisms have been proposed for the development of thrombosis in relation with the presence of aPL. Available data indicate that many of the autoantibodies associated with APS are directed against a number of plasma proteins and proteins expressed on, or bound to, the surface of vascular endothelial cells or platelets. The involvement of aPL in clinically important normal procoagulant and anticoagulant reactions and on certain cells altering the expression and secretion of various molecules may offer a basis for definitive investigations of possible mechanisms by which aPL may develop thrombotic events in patients with APS [11].

A major advance came in the early 1990s with the simultaneous recognition by different groups that aPL required a plasma protein "cofactor" to bind cardiolipin on ELISA plates. β_2-glycoprotein I (β_2GPI) was identified as this cofactor. β2GPI-dependent autoantibodies seem to be the main pathogenic subpopulation of aPL.

Some evidence shows that a second hit (i.e., infections, trauma, drugs, among others) is required for thrombus formation in APS. This requirement is less clear for fetal loss. The theory of a second hit is especially important in the case of catastrophic APS.

In addition to placental thrombosis, other mechanisms for direct effects of aPL on placental tissues have been proposed. aPL decrease the levels of annexin V, a potent natural anticoagulant present in placenta and vascular endothelium. Another postulated mechanism is that aPL displace annexin V from trophoblast with resulting increased exposure of anionic phospholipids and acceleration of thrombin generation. Annexin V appears to play a thrombomodulatory role in the placental circulation where it is necessary for maintenance of placental integrity (Table 14.2) [12, 13].

14.4 Clinical Manifestations

APS is characterized by either venous or arterial thrombosis affecting any kind of blood vessels. Single-vessel involvement or multiple vascular occlusions may give rise to a wide variety of presentations. The baseline characteristics and new APS features during the follow-up of a cohort of 1,000 patients with APS ("Euro-Phospholipid Project") are collected in Table 14.3 [14].

14.4.1 Venous and Arterial Involvement

Any combination of vascular occlusive events may occur in the same individual and the time interval between them also varies considerably from weeks to months or even years.

Table 14.2 Possible pathogenic mechanisms of the aPL [11–13]

Inhibition of anticoagulant reactions:
Inhibition of β_2GPI anticoagulant activity
Inhibition of the protein C pathway
Inhibition of protein C activation
Inhibition of activated protein C
Inhibition of antithrombin activity
Displacement of annexin A5
Cell-mediated events:
On endothelial cells:
Enhanced endothelial cell procoagulant activity
Increased expression and activation of tissue factor
Expression of adhesion molecules
Impaired fibrinolysis
Dysregulation of eicosanoids
Decreased endothelial cell prostacyclin production
Increased platelet thromboxane A_2 production
Impaired function of endothelial nitric oxide synthase
On monocytes:
Expression of tissue factor
Increase oxidative stress
On platelets:
Enhanced platelet activation/aggregation
On plasmacytoid dendritic cells:
Increased expression of toll-like receptor 7 and toll-like receptor 8

Venous occlusions in form of DVT, particularly affecting the veins of the lower limbs, are the most common clinical manifestation of the APS [15].

Other less common manifestations include superficial thrombophlebitis, chronic venous stasis, secondary malleolar ulceration, and venous occlusions occurring at sites of venous access.

The thoracic branches of the aorta may be affected, and an "aortic arch syndrome" with absent brachial pulse has been documented. Patients with APS commonly present with thrombotic problems, but there is a subgroup of patients who develop aneurysms with no evidence of vasculitis. Arterial stenosis can also play a role in APS. It may affect arteries of varying sizes and sites. So far, arterial stenosis affecting the renal, celiac, and intracranial arteries has been observed. The underlying pathology and mechanism for these stenotic lesions are unknown but may

Table 14.3 Most common manifestations in the APS, according to the "Euro-Phospholipid Project" at baseline and during the 10-year follow-up

	Baseline	0–5 year	5–10 year
	(*n* = 1,000)	(*n* = 1,000)	(*n* = 796)[a]
Manifestations	%	%	%
Deep vein thrombosis	38.9	2.1	2.7
Superficial thrombophlebitis in legs	11.7	0.9	1.0
Stroke	19.8	2.4	3.6
Transient ischemic attack	11.1	2.3	3.0
Epilepsy	7.0	1.7	1.9
Pulmonary embolism	14.1	2.1	1.7
Cardiac manifestations			
Valve thickening/dysfunction	11.6	1.7	3.6
Myocardial infarction	5.5	0.9	1.2
Vegetations	2.7	1.4	0.9
Livedo reticularis	24.1	2.6	6.9
Thrombocytopenia (<100,000/μl)	29.6	3.7	6.3
Autoimmune hemolytic anemia	9.7	0.9	3.9
Obstetric manifestations	**(*n* = 1580)**	**(*n* = 105)**	**(*n* = 83)**
Preeclampsia	5.2	7.6	4.8
Early fetal losses (<10 weeks)	35.4	17.1	15.7
Late fetal losses (≥10 weeks)	16.9	6.7	2.4
Live births	47.7	76.2	68.7

Modified from Cervera et al. [22]

[a]Number of patients that continued in the study in 2004

[b]Obstetric manifestations related to number of pregnancies (*n*). Some women had more than one pregnancy

involve thrombosis, accelerated atherosclerosis, and/or proliferation of smooth muscle [16].

14.4.2 Neurologic Involvement

Involvement of cerebral large vessels is frequent in APS, and patients usually present clinically with transient ischemic attacks (TIA) and strokes. Additionally, a wide spectrum of other neurologic features has been described, including chorea, epilepsy, multiple sclerosis-like lesions, psychiatric features, migraine, and also dementia, among others.

The association of aPL with recurrent stroke has been demonstrated in prospective studies. Patients with cerebral ischemia and APS are younger than the general stroke population. In particular, the strongest association of aPL with stroke is seen in patients under 50 years of age, with a prevalence of aPL reported to be from 4 to 46 % in this population.

In a large prospective study [17], aCL were an independent risk factor for ischemic stroke and TIA in women after multivariate adjustment for other cardiovascular risk factors, including age, systolic blood pressure, diabetes, cigarette smoking, and plasma C-reactive protein and cholesterol levels.

Cognitive dysfunction varies from global dysfunction in the context of multi-infarct dementia to subtle cognitive deficits in otherwise asymptomatic patients with aPL.

14.4.3 Cardiac Involvement

A variety of cardiac valve lesions have been associated with aPL in primary APS and SLE. Echocardiographic studies have shown that SLE patients with aPL have a higher prevalence of valvular lesions (mainly mitral and aortic lesions) than those without aPL. The valvular lesions consist mainly of superficial or intravascular fibrin deposits and their subsequent organization: vascular proliferation, fibroblast influx, and rigidity, leading to functional abnormalities. These may represent a potential cardiac source of stroke. It has been shown that the prevalence of valvular abnormalities, particularly left-sided valve lesions, is higher in SLE patients with aPL than in those without. Our group [18] showed that patients with SLE and aPL have an increased frequency of mitral valve vegetations and mitral regurgitation than aPL-negative patients (16 % vs 1.2 % and 38 % vs 12 %, respectively). In this study, 9 of 50 patients with mitral valve disease had cerebrovascular occlusions during follow-up, showing that valvular lesions can be a source for emboli and a possible cause of ischemic stroke in aPL patients, as reported by other authors. In patients with SLE, particularly women between 35 and 44 years of age, the risk of cardiovascular events is over ten times higher than in healthy women of similar age.

14.4.4 Pulmonary Involvement

Pulmonary manifestations – including pulmonary embolism and infarction; pulmonary hypertension; adult respiratory distress syndrome (ARDS); intra-alveolar hemorrhage; primary thrombosis of lung vessels, both large and small; and pulmonary capillaritis – may be associated with this syndrome. Less commonly, a postpartum syndrome and fibrosing alveolitis associated with APS have been described.

The prevalence of pulmonary hypertension in APS associated with SLE and primary APS has been estimated to be between 1.8 % and 3.5 %, respectively. In a prospective analysis of 500 patients with SLE, a statistically significant association between pulmonary hypertension and the presence of IgA aCL above 2 SD has been described.

14.4.5 Renal Involvement

Renal involvement can be present in patients with either primary or SLE-associated APS. Clinical and laboratory features of renal involvement in APS include hypertension, hematuria, acute renal failure, and progressive chronic renal insufficiency with mild levels of proteinuria that can progress to nephrotic-range proteinuria. The main lesions are renal artery stenosis, venous renal thrombosis, and glomerular lesions (APS nephropathy) that may be acute (thrombotic microangiopathy) and/or chronic (arteriosclerosis, arterial fibrous intimal hyperplasia, tubular thyroidization, arteriolar occlusions, and focal cortical atrophy). APS can also cause end-stage renal disease and allograft vascular thrombosis [19].

14.4.6 Osteoarticular Involvement

Osteonecrosis (ON) or avascular necrosis of bone is a well-recognized complication in patients with SLE and APS. The pathogenesis of ON is probably multifactorial, of which abnormal hemostatic state such as the presence of aPL may play an important role. In patients with aPL, bilateral involvement of the femoral head is often found, but some patients follow an asymptomatic course. Atypical site ON (talus, vertebral, carpal lunate) and/or multiple ON (more than three bones affected) are not uncommon in patients with APS.

By definition, frank and sustained arthritis are not usually seen in patients with primary APS. However, arthralgias are not uncommon. Other anecdotal features, such as stress fractures, have been occasionally reported in association with aPL. The management of patients with aPL and ON without venous or arterial thrombosis is still controversial. A high diagnostic suspicion is crucial in order to prevent the onset of ON in new territories and to avoid the need of joint replacement [20].

14.4.7 Obstetric APS

A large proportion of pregnancy losses related to aPL occurs in the fetal period (greater than 10 weeks of gestation). However, fetal deaths at these gestational ages normally account for only a small proportion of all pregnancy losses in the general population, which occur more frequently before 10 weeks of gestation.

The most characteristic feature of obstetrical APS is miscarriage. Currently, recurrent miscarriage is a potentially treatable condition when it is associated with aPL. Additionally, several other serious obstetric complications have been associated with APS, including preeclampsia, fetal growth restriction, uteroplacental insufficiency, fetal distress, and medically induced preterm delivery. Preeclampsia is also associated with APS. Although 11–17 % of women with preeclampsia will test positive for aPL, the association is strongest in women with severe preterm preeclampsia (less than 34 weeks of gestation). Other infrequent reported maternal APS complications include postpartum cardiopulmonary syndrome, chorea gravidarum, and postpartum cerebral infarct among others [21].

In the "Euro-Phospholipid Project," baseline obstetric manifestations included early fetal losses (<10 weeks) in 35 % of patients, late fetal losses (>10 weeks) in 17 %, and prematurity in 10 % of cases [14].

14.5 Follow-Up, Outcome, and Organ Damage in APS

Under an appropriate treatment (usually, anticoagulation), most patients with diagnosis of APS have a satisfactory outcome. However, some patients can develop new manifestations. The 10-year follow-up report from the "Euro-Phospholipid Project" was recently published [22]. During the 10-year period, the most frequent manifestation was thrombosis. The most common thrombotic events were strokes (5.3 %), TIA (4.7 %), DVT (4.3 %), and pulmonary embolism (3.5 %). Other APS-related manifestations were also commonly observed, including thrombocytopenia (8.7 %), *livedo reticularis* (8.1 %), autoimmune hemolytic anemia (4 %), valve thickening/dysfunction (4.6 %), epilepsy (3.2 %), and skin ulcers (3.1 %).

Given that APS affect predominantly young patients, assessment of organ damage is crucial, but publications in that field are limited. A retrospective analysis was recently published that focused in morbidity, mortality, and organ damage in 135 APS patients. Patients were clustered according to the initial event: arterial thrombosis, DVT, or pregnancy morbidity. One-fourth of the patients progressed to organ damage in a mean time of 10 years from disease onset. The highest morbidity was attributed to neurologic damage, which was more common among patients with arterial thrombosis as an initial manifestation.

In the "Euro-Phospholipid Project," a 5-year survival rate of 94 % was reported. During this follow-up period, 53 (5.3 %) patients died. The main causes of death included bacterial infection (21 %), MI (19 %), stroke (13 %), hemorrhage (11 %), malignancy (11 %), catastrophic APS (9 %), and pulmonary embolism (9 %), among others.

During the 10-year period, 93 (9.3 %) patients (72 female and 21 male) died, leading to a survival rate of 91 % at 10-year follow-up. There were no differences in survival probabilities between patients with primary APS and those associated with SLE. The most common causes of death were severe thrombotic events, including MI, strokes and pulmonary embolism (36 % of total deaths), infections (27 %: bacterial 21 %, other 6 %), and hemorrhages (11 %). Five out of the nine (56 %) patients who developed catastrophic APS died [22].

14.6 Laboratory Abnormalities in APS

A wide variety of laboratory abnormalities can be found in patients with APS, depending on the organ involvement. The most common immunological features are depicted in Table 14.4. Detection of the LA must be performed according to the guidelines of the International Society on Thrombosis and Hemostasis (Scientific Subcommittee on Lupus Anticoagulants/Phospholipid-Dependent Antibodies) [23].

Table 14.4 Most common immunological findings in the APS, according to the "Euro-Phospholipid Project"

Parameter	%
aCL	87.9
IgG and IgM aCL	32.1
IgG aCL alone	43.6
IgM aCL alone	12.2
LA	53.6
LA alone	12.1
LA and aCL	41.5
ANA	59.7
Anti-dsDNA	29.2
Anti-Ro/SS-A	14
Anti-La/SS-B	5.7
Anti-RNP	5.9
Anti-Sm	5.5
Rheumatoid factor	7.8
Cryoglobulins	3.6

14.7 APS Classification Criteria

In 1999, a preliminary set of classification criteria was established after an expert workshop held in Sapporo, Japan [24]. Later, another workshop was held in Sydney, Australia, in which the experts proposed some modifications to the previous criteria, such as the inclusion of anti-β2GPI antibodies. Although no new clinical criteria were added, some particular features were remarked on, such as associated APS features, including cardiac valve involvement, *livedo reticularis*, thrombocytopenia, APS nephropathy, and non-thrombotic central nervous system manifestations (i.e., cognitive dysfunction) [25] (Table 14.5).

The preliminary classification criteria for catastrophic APS were formulated at a workshop in Taormina, Italy, in 2002, during the 10th International Congress on aPL, and published as a consensus statement in 2003 (Table 14.6) [26].

14.7.1 Assessment of the Classification Criteria

The revised APS classification criteria [25] provide a more uniform basis for selecting patients for APS research by emphasizing risk stratification. They strongly recommend investigating coexisting inherited and acquired thrombosis risk factors in patients with APS, especially in those who are included in clinical trials. A recent assessment of the 2006 revised APS classification criteria has shown that only 59 % of the patients meeting the 1999 APS Sapporo classification criteria met the revised criteria [27]. Therefore, it is expected that these revised criteria will have positive implications in APS research by means of limiting the inclusion of a heterogeneous group of patients and also by providing a risk-stratified approach. Furthermore,

Table 14.5 Revised classification criteria for the APS [25]

Clinical criteria
1. Vascular thrombosis[a]
One or more clinical episodes of arterial, venous, or small vessel thrombosis, in any tissue or organ. Thrombosis must be confirmed by imaging or Doppler studies or histopathology, with the exception of superficial venous thrombosis. For histopathologic confirmation, thrombosis should be present without significant evidence of inflammation in the vessel wall
2. Pregnancy morbidity
(a) One or more unexplained deaths of a morphologically normal fetus at or beyond the 10th week of gestation, with normal fetal morphology documented by ultrasound or by direct examination of the fetus
(b) One or more premature births of a morphologically normal neonate before the 34th week of gestation because of (a) eclampsia or severe preeclampsia defined according to standard definitions or (b) recognized features of placental insufficiency[b]
(c) Three or more unexplained consecutive spontaneous abortions before the 10th week of gestation, with maternal anatomic or hormonal abnormalities and paternal and maternal chromosomal causes excluded
In studies of populations of patients who have more than one type of pregnancy morbidity, investigators are strongly encouraged to stratify groups of subjects according to a, b, or c above
Laboratory criteria[c]
1. Anticardiolipin antibody of IgG and/or IgM isotype in serum or plasma, present in medium or high titer (i.e., >40 GPL or MPL or > the 99th percentile or > mean + 3SD of 40 healthy controls), on 2 or more occasions, at least 12 weeks apart, measured by a standardized enzyme-linked immunosorbent assay
2. Lupus anticoagulant present in plasma, on 2 or more occasions at least 12 weeks apart, detected according to the guidelines of the International Society on Thrombosis and Hemostasis (Scientific Subcommittee on Lupus Anticoagulants/Phospholipid-Dependent Antibodies)
3. Anti-β_2-glycoprotein I antibody of IgG and/or IgM isotype in serum or plasma, present on 2 or more occasions, at least 12 weeks apart, measured by a standardized enzyme-linked immunosorbent assay, according to recommended procedures
Definite APS is present if at least one of the clinical criteria and one[c] of the laboratory criteria are met, with the first measurement of the laboratory test performed at least 12 weeks from the clinical manifestation[d]

[a]Coexisting inherited or acquired factors for thrombosis are *not* a reason for excluding patients from APS trials. However, two subgroups of APS patients should be recognized, according to (a) the *presence* and (b) the *absence* of additional risk factors for thrombosis. Indicative (but not exhaustive) cases include age (>55 in men and >65 in women) and the presence of any of the established risk factors for cardiovascular disease (hypertension, diabetes mellitus, elevated LDL or low HDL cholesterol, cigarette smoking, family history of premature cardiovascular disease, body mass index $\geq$30 kg/m^2, microalbuminuria, estimated GFR <60 mL/min), inherited thrombophilias, oral contraceptives, nephrotic syndrome, malignancy, immobilization, surgery. Thus, patients who fulfill criteria should be stratified according to contributing causes of thrombosis

[b]Generally accepted features of placental insufficiency include: (1) abnormal or non-reassuring fetal surveillance test(s), e.g., a nonreactive non-stress test, suggestive of fetal hypoxemia; (2) abnormal Doppler flow velocimetry waveform analysis suggestive of fetal hypoxemia, e.g., absent end-diastolic flow in the umbilical artery; (3) oligohydramnios, e.g., an amniotic fluid index of 5 cm or less; or (4) a postnatal birth weight less than the 10th percentile for the gestational age

Table 14.5 (continued)

[c]Investigators are strongly advised to classify APS patients in studies into one of the following categories:

I: More than one laboratory criteria present (any combination)

IIa: Anticardiolipin antibody present alone

IIb: Lupus anticoagulant present alone

IIc: Anti-β_2-glycoprotein I antibody present alone

[d]Classification of APS should be avoided if less than 12 weeks or more than 5 years separate the positive aPL test and the clinical manifestation

Table 14.6 Preliminary criteria for the classification of catastrophic APS [26]

1. Evidence of involvement of three or more organs, systems, and/or tissues[a]
2. Development of manifestations simultaneously or in less than a week
3. Confirmation by histopathology of small vessel occlusion in at least one organ or tissue[b]
4. Laboratory confirmation of the presence of antiphospholipid antibodies (lupus anticoagulant and/or anticardiolipin antibodies)[c]

Definite catastrophic APS: All four criteria

Probable catastrophic APS:

All four criteria, except for only two organs, systems, and/or tissues involvement

All four criteria, except for the absence of laboratory confirmation at least 6 weeks apart due to the early death of a patient never tested for aPL before the catastrophic APS

1, 2, and 4

1, 3, and 4 and the development of a third event in more than a week but less than a month, despite anticoagulation

[a]Usually, clinical evidence of vessel occlusions, confirmed by imaging techniques when appropriate. Renal involvement is defined by a 50 % rise in serum creatinine, severe systemic hypertension (>180/100 mmHg), and/or proteinuria (>500 mg/24 h)

[b]For histopathologic confirmation, significant evidence of thrombosis must be present, although vasculitis may coexist occasionally

[c]If the patient had not been previously diagnosed as having an APS, the laboratory confirmation requires that presence of antiphospholipid antibodies must be detected on two or more occasions at least 6 weeks apart (not necessarily at the time of the event), according to the proposed preliminary criteria for the classification of definite APS (9)

although the APS classification criteria are not meant for clinical purposes, they are the best available tool to avoid overdiagnosis of APS in clinical practice.

Regarding the classification criteria for the catastrophic APS, a validation study showed that they have a sensitivity of 90.3 %, a specificity of 99.4 %, a positive predictive value of 99.4 %, and a negative predictive value of 91.1 % [28].

14.8 Assessment of Thrombosis Risk in APS Patients

Several attempts have been made in order to identify the individual risk of thrombosis in patients positive for aPL [29–31]. A study of pregnant women with APS reported that patients with triple aPL positivity (i.e., positivity for LA, aCL, and anti-β_2GPI) and/or previous thromboembolism had an increased likelihood of poor neonatal outcomes than patients with double or single aPL positivity and no thrombosis history. More recently, a global APS score (GAPSS) was developed in a cohort of 211 SLE from a single center [31]. GAPSS is derived from the combination of independent risk for both thrombosis and loss of pregnancy, taking into account a panel of seven different aPL, conventional cardiovascular risk factors, the autoimmune antibody profile (i.e., antinuclear, anti-dsDNA, or anti-ENA antibodies), and the use of thromboprophylactic drugs. The authors assigned the risk factors identified by multivariate analysis-weighted points proportional to the ß-regression coefficient values. Finally, six factors were included in the model, and they included IgG/IgM aCL (5 points), IgG/IgM anti-β_2GPI antibodies (4 points), LA (4 points), IgG/IgM anti-phosphatidylserine-prothrombin complex antibodies (3 points), hyperlipidemia (3 points), and arterial hypertension (1 point). A GAPSS cutoff value of ≥10 points appears to have the best diagnostic yield.

14.9 Therapy

Treatment decisions in APS fall into four main areas: prophylaxis, prevention of further thromboses of large vessels, management of pregnancy in association with aPL, and treatment of acute thrombotic microangiopathy, mainly catastrophic APS.

Elimination of aPL may be accomplished by several therapeutic regimens, including high-dose steroid administration, immunosuppression (e.g., cyclophosphamide), or plasma exchange. The decrease or elimination is, however, temporary, and antibodies rapidly return (within 1–3 weeks) on cessation of therapy. Therefore, therapy should not primarily be directed at effectively reducing the aPL levels, and the use of immunotherapy is generally not indicated, unless required for the treatment of the underlying condition, e.g., SLE, or in acute life-threatening situations, such as the catastrophic APS. The risk of recurrence of thrombosis is markedly increased in the first 6 months after discontinuation therapy, suggesting a "rebound" phenomenon. Therefore, for patients who have already experienced thrombotic events, lifelong treatment with anticoagulants is essential [32].

In cases of first venous event, low-risk aPL profile or a known transient precipitating factor (e.g., oral contraceptives), anticoagulation could be limited to 3–6 months and antiaggregants, as well as avoidance of the triggering factors, may indeed be sufficiently effective for future thromboprophylaxis [33].

Patients with definite APS with a first venous thrombosis event should receive oral anticoagulant therapy to a target INR 2.0–3.0. Patients with definite APS and arterial thrombosis should receive oral anticoagulant therapy to a target around 3.0 or receive a combined therapy with antiaggregant plus anticoagulation with a INR target between 2.0 and 3.0 [34].

Long-term anticoagulation with oral vitamin K antagonists such as warfarin is the cornerstone treatment in APS. However, novel oral anticoagulation therapies have been developed during the last years; these therapies are direct anti-Xa inhibitors and included rivaroxaban, apixaban, and edoxaban as well as a direct thrombin inhibitor named dabigatran etexilate. Although these are promising therapies for patients with arterial or venous thrombosis, data in APS is scare but prospective clinical trials are ongoing. However, a recent report described three cases who developed new APS features (i.e., cerebral emboli, stroke, and porto-mesenteric venous thrombosis) in patients who were switched from oral warfarin to new anticoagulants (one case dabigatran and two cases rivaroxaban) [35].

The thrombocytopenia occurring during the course of the APS is usually mild and does not require any active intervention. However, in a minority of cases, it can be severe and refractory to prednisone therapy. In these cases, immunosuppressive therapy (e.g., azathioprine), intravenous immunoglobulins, or rituximab may be effective.

A recently published non-randomized prospective pilot study has shown the efficacy and safety *of* rituximab for the treatment of non-criteria aPL manifestations in patients with classic APS [36]. According to the results, rituximab may be effective in controlling some non-criteria aPL manifestations, such as thrombocytopenia and skin ulcers.

It is important to consider that the presence of moderate to severe thrombocytopenia in patients with ongoing thromboses is not a contraindication for anticoagulation.

Management of the catastrophic APS includes an aggressive approach with a combined treatment that includes anticoagulation with heparin, high-dose steroids, plasma exchange, and/or intravenous immunoglobulins [26]. For patients with refractory catastrophic APS, rituximab and eculizumab are good alternatives. A recent publication [37] demonstrated that 75 % of patients with refractory catastrophic APS treated with rituximab recovered from the acute catastrophic APS episode; however, 20 % of them died at the time of the event. Eculizumab, a humanized monoclonal antibody against complement protein C5, is currently approved for the treatment of paroxysmal nocturnal hemoglobinuria and is a promising therapy in catastrophic APS [38]. Eculizumab treatment benefits patients with microangiopathies, reducing intravascular hemolysis and blocking complement-mediated pathogenic effects. Recently, a few case reports have described the benefits of eculizumab therapy in catastrophic APS patients who were refractory to conventional therapy or for the prevention of recurrent catastrophic APS after renal transplantation [39].

14.10 Prevention

In patients with aPL who have never suffered from a thrombotic event (primary thromboprophylaxis), energetic attempts must be made to avoid or to treat any associated risk factors – e.g., antihypertensives, cholesterol-lowering agents, treatment of active nephritis, avoidance of smoking, or sedentarism.

Individual decisions should be made based on several aspects, including the aPL profile (type of antibodies, level, and persistence), the coexistence of other prothrombotic factors, the presence of an underlying autoimmune disease (specially SLE) [34], and, potentially, the GAPSS score.

Care should be also taken with the administration of oral contraceptives. There may be a case for the prophylactic treatment of individuals with high levels of IgG aCL or persistent LA activity with antiaggregants (aspirin, 75–150 mg daily), specially in those with added risk factors [40], although a recently published trial has not confirmed the benefits of aspirin in the APS primary thromboprophylaxis [41]. For higher-risk patients (patients with SLE and persistently positive LA), primary thromboprophylaxis with hydroxychloroquine and low-dose aspirin is recommended [34].

On the other hand, prophylaxis of venous thrombosis is required for patients undergoing surgical procedures (particularly, hip surgery), those requiring long stays in bed, or during the puerperium. The use of low-molecular-weight subcutaneous heparin is recommended in those circumstances.

Low-dose aspirin (50–100 mg daily) administered from the beginning of pregnancy until just prior to delivery is the accepted standard therapy for the prevention of fetal loss today. This may be combined with daily subcutaneous heparin in the face of previous fetal losses using aspirin [42, 43]. In cases of ongoing anticoagulation, warfarin administration should be discontinued as soon as pregnancy is diagnosed, since it is teratogenic, and switched to heparin plus low-dose aspirin. In addition, close monitoring of pregnancy with Doppler techniques, in order to detect early placental vascular insufficiency, and delivery with the first signs of fetal distress are mandatory [44].

Some potential alternatives for the treatment of refractory obstetric APS include double antiaggregant therapy, intravenous immunoglobulins, and biologic therapies, especially antitumor necrosis factor alpha agents and plasma exchange sessions [45].

References

1. Gómez-Puerta JA, Cervera R (2014) Diagnosis and classification of the antiphospholipid syndrome. J Autoimmun 48–49:20–25
2. Cervera R, Asherson RA, Acevedo ML et al (2004) Antiphospholipid syndrome associated with infections: clinical and microbiological characteristics of 100 patients. Ann Rheum Dis 63:1312–1317
3. Gómez-Puerta JA, Cervera R, Espinosa G et al (2006) Antiphospholipid antibodies associated with malignancies: clinical and pathological characteristics of 120 patients. Semin Arthritis Rheum 35:322–332
4. Gómez-Puerta JA, Martin H, Amigo MC et al (2005) Long-term follow-up in 128 patients with primary antiphospholipid syndrome: do they develop lupus? Medicine 84:225–230
5. Asherson RA, Bucciarelli S, Gomez-Puerta JA, Cervera R (2009) History, classification, and subsets of the antiphospholipid syndrome. In: Cervera R, Reverter JC, Khamashta MA (eds) Antiphospholipid syndrome in systemic autoimmune diseases. Elsevier, Amsterdam, pp 1–12
6. Cervera R, Rodríguez-Pintó I, Espinosa G, on behalf of the Task Force on Catastrophic Antiphospholipid Syndrome (2014) Catastrophic antiphospholipid syndrome: task force report summary. Lupus 23:1283–1285
7. Mehrania T, Petri M (2009) Epidemiology of the antiphospholipid syndrome. In: Cervera R, Reverter JC, Khamashta MA (eds) Antiphospholipid syndrome in systemic autoimmune diseases. Elsevier, Amsterdam, pp 13–34
8. Andreoli L, Chighizola CB, Banzato A, Pons-Estel GJ, de Jesus GR, Erkan D (2013) The estimated frequency of antiphospholipid antibodies in patients with pregnancy morbidity, stroke, myocardial infarction, and deep vein thrombosis. Arthritis Care Res 65:1869–1873

9. Cervera R, Espinosa G, Bucciarelli S, Gomez-Puerta JA, Font J (2006) Lessons from the catastrophic antiphospholipid syndrome (CAPS) registry. Autoimmun Rev 6:81–84
10. Cervera R, Bucciarelli S, Plasin MA et al (2009) Catastrophic antiphospholipid syndrome (CAPS): descriptive analysis of a series of 280 patients from the "CAPS Registry". J Autoimmun 32:240–245
11. Meroni PL, Borghi MO, Raschi E, Tedesco F (2011) Pathogenesis of antiphospholipid syndrome: understanding the antibodies. Nat Rev Rheumatol 7:330–339
12. Espinosa G, Cervera R, Font J, Shoenfeld Y (2003) Antiphospholipid syndrome: pathogenic mechanisms. Autoimmun Rev 2:86–93
13. Giannakopoulos B, Krilis SA (2013) The pathogenesis of the antiphospholipid syndrome. N Engl J Med 368:1033–1044
14. Cervera R, Piette JC, Font J et al (2002) Antiphospholipid syndrome: clinical and immunologic manifestations and patterns of disease expression in a cohort of 1,000 patients. Arthritis Rheum 46:1019–1027
15. Cervera R, Espinosa G, Reverter JC (2009) Systemic manifestations of the antiphospholipid syndrome. In: Cervera R, Reverter JC, Khamashta MA (eds) Antiphospholipid syndrome in systemic autoimmune diseases. Elsevier, Amsterdam, pp 105–116
16. Sangle SR, D'Cruz DP, Jan W et al (2003) Renal artery stenosis in the antiphospholipid (Hughes) syndrome and hypertension. Ann Rheum Dis 62:999–1002
17. Janardhan V, Wolf PA, Kase CS et al (2004) Anticardiolipin antibodies and risk of ischemic stroke and transient ischemic attack: the Framingham cohort and offspring study. Stroke 35:736–741
18. Khamashta MA, Cervera R, Asherson RA et al (1990) Association of antibodies against phospholipids with heart valve disease in systemic lupus erythematosus. Lancet 335:1541–1544
19. Pons-Estel GJ, Cervera R (2014) Renal involvement in antiphospholipid syndrome. Curr Rheumatol Rep 16:397
20. Gómez-Puerta JA, Pons-Estel GJ (2010) Skeletal involvement in antiphospholipid syndrome. Curr Rheumatol Rev 6:25–31
21. Gómez-Puerta JA, Sanin-Blair J, Galarza-Maldonado C (2009) Pregnancy and catastrophic antiphospholipid syndrome. Clin Rev Allergy Immmunol 36:85–90
22. Cervera R, Serrano R, Pons-Estel GJ et al (2015). Morbidity and mortality in the antiphospholipid syndrome during a 10-year period: a multicentre prospective study of 1000 patients. Ann Rheum Dis 74:1011-1018
23. Brandt JT, Triplett DA, Alving B, Scharrer I (1995) Criteria for the diagnosis of lupus anticoagulants: an update. On behalf of the Subcommittee on Lupus Anticoagulant/Antiphospholipid Antibody of the Scientific and Standardisation Committee of the ISTH. Thromb Haemost 74:1185–1190
24. Wilson WA, Gharavi AE, Koike T et al (1999) International consensus statement on preliminary classification criteria for definite antiphospholipid syndrome: report of an international workshop. Arthritis Rheum 42:1309–1311
25. Miyakis S, Lockshin MD, Atsumi T et al (2006) International consensus statement on an update of the classification criteria for definite antiphospholipid syndrome (APS). J Thromb Haemos 4:295–306
26. Asherson RA, Cervera R, de Groot PG et al (2003) Catastrophic antiphospholipid syndrome: international consensus statement on classification criteria and treatment guidelines. Lupus 12:530–534
27. Kaul M, Erkan D, Sammaritano L, Lockshin MD (2007) Assessment of the 2006 revised antiphospholipid syndrome classification criteria. Ann Rheum Dis 66:927–930
28. Cervera R, Font J, Gomez-Puerta JA et al (2005) Validation of the preliminary criteria for the classification of catastrophic antiphospholipid syndrome. Ann Rheum Dis 64:1205–1209
29. Ruffatti A, Calligaro A, Hoxha A et al (2010) Laboratory and clinical features of pregnant women with antiphospholipid syndrome and neonatal outcome. Arthritis Care Res 62:302–307
30. Otomo K, Atsumi T, Amengual O et al (2012) Efficacy of the antiphospholipid score for the diagnosis of antiphospholipid syndrome and its predictive value for thrombotic events. Arthritis Rheum 64:504–512

31. Sciascia S, Sanna G, Murru V, Roccatello D, Khamashta MA, Bertolaccini ML (2013) GAPSS: the global anti-phospholipid syndrome score. Rheumatol (Oxford) 52:1397–1403
32. Lim W, Crowther MA, Eikelboom JW (2006) Management of antiphospholipid antibody syndrome: a systematic review. JAMA 295:1050–1057
33. Coloma Bazan E, Donate Lopez C, Moreno Lozano P, Cervera R, Espinosa G (2013) Discontinuation of anticoagulation or antiaggregation treatment may be safe in patients with primary antiphospholipid syndrome when antiphospholipid antibodies became persistently negative. Immunol Res 56:358–361
34. Ruiz-Irastorza G, Cuadrado MJ, Ruiz-Arruza I et al (2011) Evidence-based recommendations for the prevention and long-term management of thrombosis in antiphospholipid antibody-positive patients: report of a task force at the 13th International Congress on antiphospholipid antibodies. Lupus 20:206–218
35. Schaefer JK, McBane RD, Black DF, Williams LN, Moder KG, Wysokinski WE (2014) Failure of dabigatran and rivaroxaban to prevent thromboembolism in antiphospholipid syndrome: a case series of three patients. Thromb Haemost 112:947–950
36. Erkan D, Vega J, Ramon G, Kozora E, Lockshin MD (2013) A pilot open-label phase II trial of rituximab for non-criteria manifestations of antiphospholipid syndrome. Arthritis Rheum 65:464–471
37. Berman H, Rodriguez-Pinto I, Cervera R et al (2013) Rituximab use in the catastrophic antiphospholipid syndrome: descriptive analysis of the CAPS registry patients receiving rituximab. Autoimmun Rev 12:1085–1090
38. Shapira I, Andrade D, Allen SL, Salmon JE (2012) Brief report: induction of sustained remission in recurrent catastrophic antiphospholipid syndrome via inhibition of terminal complement with eculizumab. Arthritis Rheum 64:2719–2723
39. Canaud G, Kamar N, Anglicheau D et al (2013) Eculizumab improves posttransplant thrombotic microangiopathy due to antiphospholipid syndrome recurrence but fails to prevent chronic vascular changes. Am J Transplant 13:2179–2185
40. Alarcon-Segovia D, Boffa MC, Branch W et al (2003) Prophylaxis of the antiphospholipid syndrome: a consensus report. Lupus 12:499–503
41. Erkan D, Harrison MJ, Levy R et al (2007) Aspirin for primary thrombosis prevention in the antiphospholipid syndrome: a randomized, double-blind, placebo-controlled trial in asymptomatic antiphospholipid antibody-positive individuals. Arthritis Rheum 56:2382–2391
42. Tincani A, Branch W, Levy RA et al (2003) Treatment of pregnant patients with antiphospholipid syndrome. Lupus 12:524–529
43. Carmona F, Font J, Azulay M et al (2001) Risk factors associated with fetal losses in treated antiphospholipid syndrome pregnancies: a multivariate analysis. Am J Reprod Immunol 46:274–279
44. Cervera R, Balasch J (2004) The management of pregnant patients with antiphospholipid syndrome. Lupus 13:683–687
45. Gomez-Puerta JA, Cervera R (2013) Are there additional options for the treatment of refractory obstetric antiphospholipid syndrome? Lupus 22:754–755

Disease Activity Indices and Prognosis of Systemic Lupus Erythematosus

15

Luca Iaccarino, Maddalena Larosa, and Andrea Doria

15.1 Introduction

Systemic lupus erythematosus (SLE) is an autoimmune rheumatic disease characterized by a heterogeneous group of clinical features and laboratory abnormalities. Disease presentation appears highly changeable [1], and quantification of disease activity is still variably applied in clinical trials and clinical practice since no gold standard clinimetric measurement of lupus activity has been identified to date.

Prognosis of SLE has dramatically improved since the 1950s; however, SLE patients still display a 4.6-fold higher standardized mortality rate and a poorer quality of life compared to their counterparts in the general population [2]. Persistent disease activity and drug side effects are associated with damage accrual, which in turn is predictive of more damage and poor prognosis.

In this chapter, we review the various instruments that are used to assess disease activity, as well as SLE prognosis, including survival, causes of death, and prognostic predictors.

15.2 Disease Activity Indices

Lupus activity can be defined as the sum of all clinical manifestations and serological abnormalities related to ongoing immune inflammatory pathways involved in SLE. From the clinical point of view, lupus activity encompasses inflammatory and noninflammatory manifestations and persistent serologic abnormalities including

L. Iaccarino • M. Larosa • A. Doria (✉)
Rheumatology Unit, Department of Medicine, University of Padua,
Via Giustiniani 2, Padua 35128, Italy
e-mail: adoria@unipd.it

D. Roccatello, L. Emmi (eds.), *Connective Tissue Disease: A Comprehensive Guide-Volume 1*, Rare Diseases of the Immune System 5,
DOI 10.1007/978-3-319-24535-5_15

Table 15.1 Major disease activity scores of SLE

Global indices	Organ-specific indices
PGA	BILAG
SLEDAI	CLASI
SLEPDAI	DAS28
SLAM	
ECLAM	

PGA physician global assessment, *SLEDAI* systemic lupus erythematosus activity index, *SLEPDAI* systemic lupus erythematosus pregnancy activity index, *SLAM* systemic lupus activity measure, *ECLAM* European Consensus Lupus activity measurement, *BILAG* British Isles Lupus Assessment Group, *CLASI* Cutaneous Lupus Erythematosus Disease Area and Severity Index, *DAS28* Disease Activity Score-28

the presence of autoantibodies, especially anti-double-stranded (ds) DNA antibody and low C3 and/or C4.

The physician's opinion is often considered the "gold standard" for the evaluation of disease activity; however, it is not reliable due to important limitations including the physician's personal experience and the weight which has to be assigned to the involvement of various organs [3].

Since the 1980s, nearly 60 different indices for assessing SLE activity have been elaborated [3]. Among them, two types of disease activity measurements can be identified: global activity scores, which provide an overall measurement of disease activity, and specific organ/system activity scores which assess disease activity in a single organ or system. Table 15.1 reports the most commonly used SLE disease activity indices.

Global score indices are very useful for comparing cohorts of SLE patients, as well as subjects with different disease manifestations. In addition, they are easy to assess and can be used retrospectively. However, the final score of a global activity tool might be the result of low activity in several organs or high activity in one single organ. In addition, they may underscore the severity of the disease [3].

On the other hand, specific organ/system scales are able to identify the extreme variability of SLE manifestations and allow for the assessment of disease activity and clinical response in specific organs. Therefore, they may be used as a cutoff for defining entry criteria into clinical trials. However, they are not very sensitive, and training is required to improve the performance of assessors.

15.3 Global Score Activity Indices

The *Physician Global Assessment (PGA)* is an important and useful outcome evaluation of lupus disease activity that is based on the physicians' overall judgment. It provides a score based on clinical evaluation ranging between 0 and 3, where 0 means absence of disease activity and 3 is the highest disease activity which the examiner can expect considering all patients with lupus, in other words the most active patient in the "universe of lupus" and not in that particular patient.

The *systemic lupus erythematosus disease activity index (SLEDAI)* was developed at the University of Toronto in 1992 and it is composed of 24 items [4]. The score of severe clinical manifestations of SLE, such as vasculitis and renal and neurological involvement, is higher compared to other less severe disease manifestations, e.g., joint and skin manifestations. Serology, including anti-dsDNA, C3, and C4, is also taken into consideration. Only descriptors that are present in the 10 days prior to evaluation should be scored. The total SLEDAI score can vary from 0 to 105.

SLEDAI provides an overall evaluation of disease activity and is especially useful for comparing cohorts of SLE patients. Notably, it allows comparisons of patients with different disease manifestations. It is easy to assess, straightforward, and can also be retrospectively evaluated. Nonetheless, the SLEDAI score has some drawbacks: first, the final score might be due to low activity in different organs or high activity in one single organ; second, the same score may be due to the involvement of different organs; third, it may underscore the severity of the disease; and, lastly, the decrease in score due to the improvement in a specific organ system may be masked by the worsening in another organ system.

Since the first publication of the SLEDAI index, several modifications have been made including the Safety of Estrogens in Lupus Erythematosus National Assessment (SELENA) – SLEDAI and the SLEDAI-2000 (SLEDAI-2K). There are also simplified English and Spanish versions of the SLEDAI without immunological tests, which make the index easier to assess: the MEX-SLEDAI [3].

SELENA-SLEDAI [5] emphasizes new or recurrent disease activity in some descriptors (seizure, cranial nerve disorders, cerebrovascular accidents, skin rash, alopecia, mucosal ulcers, proteinuria) in order to identify disease flares rather than persistent disease activity.

In 2002, Gladman et al. published an updated version of the original SLEDAI, called SLEDAI-2K [6]. The modification was made in order to identify persistent active disease manifestations and not only new onset or flares. In the SLEDAI-2K, ongoing rashes, proteinuria, alopecia, and mucosal lesions have to be scored (Table 15.2). The SLEDAI-2K is widely used in clinical practice.

On the basis of the SLEDAI score, we can subdivide disease activity into five levels: 0 = inactive disease, from 1 to 5 = mild SLE activity, from 6 to 10 = moderately active lupus, from 11 to 19 = active SLE, and ≥20 = very active lupus.

In order to better standardize the assessment of SLE activity during pregnancy, SLEDAI was modified into the SLE-Pregnancy Disease Activity Index (SLEPDAI) [7]. This includes the 24 SLEDAI descriptors, 15 of which were modified in order to differentiate signs or symptoms caused by lupus activity from those related to pregnancy. Notably, preeclampsia-eclampsia is considered an exclusion criterion for some CNS descriptors including seizure, headache and cerebral infarctions, and HELLP (hemolysis, elevated liver enzymes, and low platelets) syndrome for thrombocytopenia. SLEPDAI has not been formally validated; nevertheless, it has been used in some studies.

Table 15.2 The systemic lupus erythematosus disease activity index 2000 (SLEDAI-2K)

Weight	Score	Descriptor	Definition
8		Seizure	Recent onset, exclude metabolic, infectious, or drug causes
8		Psychosis	Altered ability to function in normal activity due to severe disturbance in the perception of reality. Includes hallucinations, incoherence, marked loose associations, impoverished thought content, marked illogical thinking, bizarre, disorganized, or catatonic behavior. Exclude uremia and drug causes
8		Organic brain syndrome	Altered mental function with impaired orientation, memory, or other intellectual function, with rapid-onset and fluctuating clinical features, inability to sustain attention to environment, plus at least 2 of the following: perceptual disturbance, incoherent speech, insomnia or daytime drowsiness, or increased or decreased psychomotor activity. Exclude metabolic, infectious, or drug causes
8		Visual disturbance	Retinal changes of SLE. Include cytoid bodies, retinal hemorrhages, serous exudate, or hemorrhages in the choroid, or optic neuritis. Exclude hypertension, infection, or drug causes
8		Cranial nerve disorder	New onset of sensory or motor neuropathy involving cranial nerves
8		Lupus headache	Severe, persistent headache; may be migraine, but must be nonresponsive to narcotic analgesia
8		Cerebrovascular accident	New onset of cerebrovascular accident(s). Exclude arteriosclerosis
8		Vasculitis	Ulceration, gangrene, tender finger nodules, periungual infarction, splinter hemorrhages, or biopsy or angiogram proof of vasculitis
4		Arthritis	≥2 joints with pain and signs of inflammation (i.e., tenderness, swelling, or effusion)
4		Myositis	Proximal muscle aching/weakness, associated with elevated creatine phosphokinase/aldolase or electromyogram changes or a biopsy showing myositis
4		Urinary casts	Heme-granular or red blood cell casts
4		Hematuria	>5 red blood cells/high power field. Exclude stone, infection, or other cause
4		Proteinuria	>0.5 g/24 h
4		Pyuria	>5 white blood cells/high power field. Exclude infection
2		Rash	Inflammatory-type rash
2		Alopecia	Abnormal, patchy, or diffuse loss of hair
2		Mucosal ulcers	Oral or nasal ulcerations

Table 15.2 (continued)

Weight	Score	Descriptor	Definition
2		Pleurisy	Pleuritic chest pain with pleural rub or effusion, or pleural thickening
2		Pericarditis	Pericardial pain with at least 1 of the following: rub, effusion, or electrocardiogram or echocardiogram confirmation
2		Low complement	Decrease in CH50, C3, or C4 below the lower limit of normal for testing laboratory
2		Increased DNA binding	Increased DNA binding by Farr assay above normal range for testing laboratory
1		Fever	>38 °C. Exclude infectious cause
1		Thrombocytopenia	<100,000 platelets/$\times 10^9$/L, exclude drug causes
1		Leukopenia	<3,000 white blood cells/$\times 10^9$/L, exclude drug causes

Weighted score of SLEDAI-2K has to be scored in the score column if the descriptor is present at the time of the visit or in the preceding 10 days

The European Consensus Lupus Activity Measurement (ECLAM) was developed in 1992 through the analysis of symptoms and laboratory abnormalities reported in a cohort of 704 European patients affected with SLE. It comprises 15 weighted clinical and serological descriptors. The laboratory variables are hemoglobin, white blood cells, lymphocytes, platelets, proteinuria, urinary sediment, and complement levels, which are used in routine clinical practice. ECLAM has a high inter-rater concordance and can be retrospectively calculated [8].

The Systemic Lupus Erythematosus Activity Measure (SLAM), modified later into SLAM-R [8], is composed of 31 clinical manifestations or laboratory abnormalities that are usually found in SLE. Similarly to other global scores, a numerical value is attributed to each item based on different degrees of severity, with a total sum indicative of overall disease activity.

15.4 Organ-Specific Activity Indices

The British Isles Lupus Assessment Group (BILAG) index was first proposed in 1988 and later revised in 2004. It includes 97 items, most of which can be assessed by physical exams; in fact, only serum creatinine, urine dipstick, and total blood cell count are scored, while no serologic tests are included [7]. Each item is evaluated qualitatively by clinical assessment or quantitatively by considering laboratory values as well. BILAG includes nine organs/systems, i.e., general, mucocutaneous, neurological, musculoskeletal, cardiovascular, respiratory, renal, hematological, and gastrointestinal.

Only features that are related to active lupus and that were present in the 4 weeks prior to evaluation should be taken into consideration. Actually, BILAG was developed on the basis of the intention-to-treat principle. Hence, each of the nine systems is scored by an alphabetic character: BILAG A stands for "Action," BILAG B for "Beware," BILAG C for "Containment," BILAG D for "Discount," and BILAG E for "no Evidence" [8]. Although it has recently been proposed, a total score obtained by attributing a numeric value to the alphabetic character has rarely been used.

It should be noted that BILAG is the only transitional index where each item has to be recorded as new, same, worse, or improving rather than simply present or absent. These features are relevant when assessing the effect of a therapeutic intervention in a clinical trial.

BILAG is able to identify the extreme variability of SLE by assessing disease activity and clinical response in specific organs. It is reliable, sensitive to change, and widely used as a cutoff for entry criteria in clinical trials. Although it would appear to be the most complete SLE activity index, it is time consuming and quite complex to perform; thus, training is needed to improve the performance of the assessors. A software program (British Lupus Integrated Prospective System (BLIPS)) was created to help physicians calculate BILAG.

The Cutaneous Lupus Erythematosus Disease Area and Severity Index (CLASI) was developed in 2005 to evaluate the activity and damage of lupus skin manifestations. It consists of two scores: the first summarizes the activity of skin manifestations, while the second measures disease-related skin damage. Activity is scored taking into account the following lesions: erythema, scales/hyperkeratosis, mucous membrane involvement, acute hair loss, and non-scarring alopecia. Damage is scored in terms of dyspigmentation and scarring, including scarring alopecia. The scores are calculated by a simple addition based on the extent of the lesions. The degree of involvement of each skin lesion is calculated according to the involvement of specific anatomic areas (i.e., malar area, neck, arms, etc.), scored on the basis of the worst skin lesion present within that area [9].

The Disease Activity Score (DAS)-28 is a validated and widely used clinimetric measurement in clinical trials and in routine clinical practice for patients with rheumatoid arthritis (RA). This is a standardized disease activity index that is highly correlated with the physician's and patient's overall assessment. By using DAS28, we can both classify patients with RA as having low, moderate, or high disease activity and define disease remission. Although it was only validated for patients with RA, DAS28 has been used for monitoring patients affected with other rheumatic conditions including SLE [10]. It assesses 28 joints (for swelling and tenderness), erythrocyte sedimentation rate (ESR) or C-reactive protein (CRP) levels, and the patient's overall health.

15.5 Evaluation of Disease Activity Over Time

Variations in disease activity over time are commonly recognized in SLE patients regardless of therapy. Unfortunately, disease activity indices measure disease activity at a single time point; thus by looking at only one measurement, we cannot have a comprehensive view of the variation of disease activity over time.

The *Adjusted Mean SLEDAI-2K (AMS)* was recently proposed to better summarize SLE activity over multiple visits. AMS is equivalent to the area under the curve of the SLEDAI-2K over time divided by time interval [11]. AMS is determined as follows: "(a) calculate the area under the curve between two visits: the length of time between two visits multiplied by the average of the two SLEDAI-2K values; (b) add up all the calculated areas; and (c) divide the result by the total length of the time period. AMS shares the same units as SLEDAI-2K and it is interpreted in the same way."

By performing a longitudinal series of disease activity measurements, three different patterns of SLE activity were identified: relapsing remitting (RRD), clinical quiescent (CQD), and chronic active disease (CAD). CQD means no disease activity over time, CAD means persistent disease activity, and RRD indicates periods of disease activity interspersed with periods of inactive disease [12]. However, the frequency of disease activity patterns differs among studies as a consequence of the different definitions that are used. In our SLE cohort, we observed that every year 50 % of patients have CQD, while the remaining 50 % retained some kind of disease activity, being either CAD (in most cases) or RRD. After 7 years of follow-up, only one-third of patients could be considered in CQD, while 65 % displayed either relapsing or persistent disease activity [12].

15.6 Prognosis of Systemic Lupus Erythematosus

Survival of patients with SLE has improved over the past few decades [13]. Before 1955, the 5-year survival rate in SLE was less than 50 %; nowadays, the average 10-year survival rate exceeds 90 %, and the 15-year survival rate is approximately 80 % [14].

The main contributing factors toward improved survival were initially the availability of corticosteroids, dialysis, antibiotics, and antihypertensive agents. Afterward, the use of immunosuppressants and an improvement in disease classification leading to early diagnosis and treatment, and more recently the more appropriate use of conventional therapies as well as the tendency to follow patients with SLE in specialized clinics, the so-called lupus clinics, have all resulted in increased survival [4, 14–16].

Causes of death can be subdivided into those related to SLE itself and those related to disease complications. Causes related to SLE itself include active disease, i.e., active nephritis, CNS involvement, visceral vasculitis, and end-organ failure. Causes related to complications include infections, neoplasm, and atherosclerosis.

In 1976, Urowitz first reported a bimodal mortality pattern: deaths in the first few years of illness are typically caused by severe disease or infections due to immunosuppressive therapy, whereas late deaths are generally related to myocardial infarction or strokes, both attributed to accelerated atherosclerosis [17, 18]. Nowadays, deaths due to SLE have been further reduced, thanks to a more appropriate use of traditional treatments and to the introduction of new drugs such as mycophenolate mofetil, belimumab, and rituximab. However, intervening infections or cardiovascular events remain the major causes of deaths in the long term, followed by an increased incidence of malignancies [19, 20].

15.6.1 Prognostic Factors in SLE

It has been hypothesized that several specific factors may influence the prognosis of patients with SLE. They can be subdivided into two groups: unrelated or related to SLE.

15.6.2 Factors Unrelated to SLE

Prognostic factors unrelated to SLE include race, gender, age at SLE onset, socioeconomic status, and environment. In general, whites tend to have a better outcome than nonwhites, with mortality rates being higher in nonwhites. Low socioeconomic status and poor compliance seem to negatively influence the survival and morbidity of SLE patients with lupus. The effect of gender, age at disease onset, or environment on SLE prognosis remains elusive [16].

15.6.3 Factors Related to SLE

SLE-related factors include year of diagnosis, time from disease onset to diagnosis, disease activity and remission, SLE manifestations, disease treatment, and damage accrual.

15.6.3.1 Age at Diagnosis

Year of diagnosis is a critical aspect in the prognosis of SLE patients since the treatment has changed over the decades. For example, patients diagnosed with SLE in the 1950s, 1960s, and 1970s were treated more aggressively and for a longer period of time with corticosteroids and cyclophosphamide than patients diagnosed more recently.

15.6.3.2 Lag Time Between Symptoms and Diagnosis

In our cohort of 487 SLE patients recruited between 1970 and 2008, the mean lag time between onset and diagnosis was 59 months in patients diagnosed before 1980, a figure that is similar to what was reported by Wallace in 1981 [21], 28 months in those diagnosed between 1980 and 1989, 15 months in those diagnosed between 1990 and 1999, and 9 months after 2000. It is noteworthy that the difference was significant between the first and the second group, probably as a consequence of the introduction of antinuclear antibody (ANA) testing, and between the second and the third group, probably due to better knowledge of autoimmunity and autoimmune diseases. By contrast, the difference was not significant between the third and fourth group, supporting the concept that from 1990 until now nothing relevant has been introduced which could have improved the SLE diagnostic process. Disease progression in the time that elapses between disease onset and diagnosis is one of the major contributors to the improvement of survival and quality of life in SLE patients since early diagnosis and treatment increase SLE remission rate and improve patient prognosis [1, 14, 22].

15.6.3.3 Overall Disease Activity

Overall disease activity at first visit, at time of renal biopsy, or over time (AMS) proved to be an important predictor of mortality in a number of cohorts [23–26]. Moreover, Cook et al. [27] found an increase in the relative risk (RR) of mortality depending on the progressive increase in SLEDAI score: RR 1.28 for SLEDAI 1-5, RR 2.34 for SLEDAI 6-10, RR 4.74 for SLEDAI 11-19, and RR 14.11 for SLEDAI >20 (compared with SLEDAI = 0).

15.6.3.4 Disease Manifestations

In Cook's cohort [27], some SLEDAI descriptors were found to be risk factors for death, including organic brain syndrome, retinal changes, cranial nerve disorders, proteinuria, pleurisy, fever, thrombocytopenia, and leukopenia. Moreover, Doria et al. [14] pointed out that the survival curves of patients affected with mild SLE (i.e., skin and musculoskeletal involvement) are similar to those of patients with severe lupus (i.e., renal involvement and CNS lupus) but only for up to 15 years after diagnosis; thereafter, the survival curves of patients with severe SLE rapidly worsen. By contrast, patients with mild disease have a survival rate similar to their counterparts in the general population [14].

15.6.3.5 Disease Remission

As shown by a large multicenter inception SLE cohort, disease remission and particularly early remission are predictive of better outcome in SLE patients [28]. As an example, renal survival is higher in patients who achieve either complete or partial disease remission as compared to severely affected patients, and overall survival at 20 years is significantly increased only in SLE patients who have complete disease remission [25, 29].

Indeed, remission within 1 year from disease onset is associated with a significant reduction in disease flares, organ damage, and overall cumulative dosage of corticosteroids [28], meaning a greater chance for lasting disease quiescence.

Unfortunately, remission in SLE is not clearly defined by any of the available disease activity scores. According to SLEDAI, remission may be defined as SLEDAI = 0, whereas SLEDAI ≥3 is considered persistent disease activity. Many authors have raised the question regarding what significance should be given to serological abnormalities such as anti-dsDNA antibodies or complement levels in patients without clinical manifestations of lupus, the so-called serologically active clinical quiescent disease. Based on clinical practice, three levels of remission in SLE can be identified: (a) complete remission may be defined as no clinical or serological signs of disease activity in patients who are treatment-free; (b) clinical remission off corticosteroids can be defined as the absence of signs and symptoms of urinary and hematological abnormalities in patients with or without serological abnormalities who are corticosteroid-free; and (c) clinical remission on corticosteroids can be defined as the absence of signs and symptoms of urinary and hematological abnormalities in patients with or without serological abnormalities who are taking low-dose corticosteroids (≤5 mg/day prednisone or equivalent) [30].

15.6.3.6 Disease Treatment

Improved therapeutic approaches for SLE have led to better disease control, thereby reducing mortality related to active disease. However, they can be responsible for drug-related adverse events which may affect long-term prognosis. The drugs which mostly seem to affect long-term prognosis are corticosteroids and immunosuppressants which are able to decrease disease activity, but their prolonged use has been associated with increased cholesterol levels and a high frequency of cardiovascular events and infections [16]. On the other hand, hydroxychloroquine seems to be associated with lower cholesterol levels, suggesting a protective role of this drug against coronary artery disease [17].

15.6.3.7 Damage Accrual

Damage is defined as irreversible tissue injury occurring after SLE diagnosis and lasting at least 6 months. Damage is evaluated by the SLICC (Systemic Lupus International Collaborating Clinics) damage index (SDI), which encompasses 12 organ systems [31]. While disease activity tends to decline over time in patients with SLE, damage tends to increase. Since lupus patients nowadays live longer than they did a few decades ago, they tend to accumulate more damage, which is secondary to both active disease and long-standing treatment, especially corticosteroid chronic exposure [32, 33]. Notably, SLE patients with active disease (CAD or RRD) accumulate more organ damage compared to patients in remission. It has been shown that long-standing active SLE may drive an 8 % increased risk of organ damage [30]. High AMS scores were also found to be associated with damage and cardiovascular disease in SLE [34].

Damage is one of the main determinants of poor long-term prognosis in SLE patients. Indeed, damage accrual can lead to more damage, which, in turn, leads to disability, productivity loss, and, in the most severe cases, death [30].

A prospective study showed that 25 % of lupus patients with a SLICC-DI >0 at baseline had died at 10 years vs. only 7.3 % of patients with no damage at study entry; notably, renal damage and cardiovascular disease were associated with a higher risk of death during the follow-up [35]. In another prospective follow-up study, an increase in SLICC-DI ≥2 up to the third year of disease was found to increase the RR of mortality to 7.7 [36]; renal failure and cardiovascular disease were again the major predictors of death.

15.7 Quality of Life and Loss of Productivity

Health-related quality of life (HRQL) in SLE patients is usually evaluated by the SF-36 (Medical Outcomes Study Short Form) which consists of 36 items among 8 domains measuring diverse components of psychophysical health, i.e., physical function, role limitations due to emotional or physical problems, social function, mental health, general health perception, vitality, and pain [37]. HRQL has been shown to be lower in SLE patients as compared to their counterparts in the general population. Organ damage was associated with an overall decrease in physical, social, and mental performance, and poor coping strategies [38, 39] and new organ damage were a predictor of a further decline in HRQL [38].

Everyday activities and the ability to work are also affected in SLE patients [22, 40, 41]. It has been shown that two-third of SLE patients have a decreased ability to perform routine activities, both at home and in the workplace, thus worsening their psychological and financial well-being [42]. One-third of patients with SLE had an occupational disability with a decrease in the number of working hours per week and 50 % of patients left their jobs within 15 years of SLE diagnosis [43]. A number of studies showed SLE-related damage to be associated with work disability and loss of productivity [44–46], which was particularly significant in case of neuropsychiatric SLE or deforming arthritis [46]. Longer disease duration, fatigue, comorbidities, and poor mental status also negatively influence the patients' productivity [46].

Conclusions

Despite their limitations, disease activity and damage indices have helped physicians to better standardize the assessment and management of SLE, which has certainly contributed to the improvement in survival of SLE patients in the last decades. Unfortunately, disease mortality is still high and is mostly due to disease complications, especially in patients with active and severe disease and damage accrual. Moreover, the HRQL of SLE patients is still poorer than that of their healthy counterparts. On the other hand, some indicators of a favorable outcome have emerged in the last few years. Early diagnosis and treatment, close control of disease activity, follow-up of patients in specialized lupus clinics, and prolonged remission all seem to be associated with better outcome.

References

1. Doria A, Zen M, Canova M, Bettio S, Bassi N, Nalotto L, Rampudda M, Ghirardello A, Iaccarino L (2010) SLE diagnosis and treatment: when early is early. Autoimmun Rev 10:55–60
2. Lopez R, Davidson JE, Beeby MD et al (2012) Lupus disease activity and the risk of subsequent organ damage and mortality in a large lupus cohort. Rheumatology 51:491–498
3. Griffiths B, Mosca M, Gordon C (2005) Assessment of patients with systemic lupus erythematosus and the use of lupus disease activity indices. Best Pract Res Clin Rheumatol 19:685–708
4. Urowitz MB, Gladman DD (1998) Measures of disease activity and damage in SLE. Clin Rheumatol 12:405–413
5. Buyon JP, Petri MA, Kim MY et al (2005) The effect of combined estrogen and progesterone hormone replacement therapy on disease activity in systemic lupus erythematosus: a randomized trial. Ann Intern Med 142:953–962
6. Gladman DD, Ibañez D, Urowitz MB (2002) Systemic lupus erythematosus disease activity index 2000. J Rheumatol 29:288–291
7. Buyon GP, Kalunian CK, Ramsey-Goldman R et al (1999) Assessing disease activity in SLE patients during pregnancy. Lupus 8:677–684
8. Romero-Diaz J, Isenberg D, Ramsey-Goldman R (2011) Measures of adult systemic lupus erythematosus: updated version of British Isles Lupus Assessment Group (BILAG 2004),

European Consensus Lupus Activity Measurements (ECLAM), Systemic Lupus Activity Measure, Revised (SLAM-R), Systemic Lupus Activity Questionnaire for Population Studies (SLAQ), Systemic Lupus Erythematosus Disease Activity Index 2000 (SLEDAI-2 K), and Systemic Lupus International Collaborating Clinics/American College of Rheumatology Damage Index (SDI). Arthritis Care Res (Hoboken) 63(Suppl 11):S37–S46

9. Albrecht JL, Taylor L, Berlin JA et al (2005) The CLASI (Cutaneous Lupus Erythematosus Disease Area and Severity Index): an outcome instrument for cutaneous lupus erythematosus. Invest Dermatol 125:889–894
10. Ceccarelli F, Perricone C, Massaro L et al (2014) The role of disease activity score 28 in the evaluation of articular involvement in systemic lupus erythematosus. ScientificWorldJournal 2014:236842
11. Ibañez D, Urowitz MB, Gladman DD (2003) Summarizing disease features over time: I. Adjusted mean SLEDAI derivation and application to an index of disease activity in lupus. J Rheumatol 30:1977–1982
12. Zen M, Bassi N, Nalotto L et al (2012) Disease activity patterns in a monocentric cohort of SLE patients: a seven-year follow-up study. Clin Exp Rheumatol 30:856–3
13. Ruiz-Irastorza G, Khamashta MA, Castellino G, Hughes GR (2001) Systemic lupus erythematosus. Lancet 357:1027–1032
14. Doria A, Iaccarino L, Ghirardello A et al (2006) Long-term prognosis and causes of death in systemic lupus erythematosus. Am J Med 119:700–706
15. Doria A, Canova M, Tonon M et al (2008) Infections as triggers and complications of systemic lupus erythematosus. Autoimmun Rev 8:24–28
16. Wallace DJ, Hahn BH (2007) Dubois' lupus erythematosus, 7th edn. Lippincott Williams & Wilkins, Philadelphia, Chapter 69
17. Urowitz MB, Bookman AA, Koehler BE, Gordon DA, Smythe HA, Ogryzlo MA (1976) The bimodal mortality pattern of systemic lupus erythematosus. Am J Med 60:221–225
18. Doria A, Shoenfeld Y, Wu R et al (2003) Risk factors for subclinical atherosclerosis in a prospective cohort of patients with systemic lupus erythematosus. Ann Rheum Dis 62:1071–1077
19. Iaccarino L, Bettio S, Zen M, Nalotto L, Gatto M, Ramonda R et al (2013) Premature coronary heart disease in SLE: can we prevent progression? Lupus 22:1232–1242
20. Fei Y, Shi X, Gan F, Li X, Zhang W, Li M et al (2014) Death causes and pathogens analysis of systemic lupus erythematosus during the past 26 years. Clin Rheumatol 33:57–63
21. Pistiner M, Wallace DJ, Nessim S, Metzger AL, Klinenberg JR (1991) Lupus erythematosus in the 1980s: a survey of 570 patients. Semin Arthritis Rheum 21:55–64
22. Doria A, Rinaldi S, Ermani M, Salaffi F, Iaccarino L, Ghirardello A et al (2005) Health related quality of life in Italian patients with systemic lupus erythematosus. II. Role of clinical, immunological and psychological determinants. Rheumatology 43:1580–1586
23. Abu-Shakra M, Urowitz MB, Gladman DD et al (1995) Mortality studies in systemic lupus erythematosus. Results from a single center. II Predictors variables for mortality. J Rheumatol 2:1265–1270
24. Golet JR, Mackenzie T, Levinton C et al (1993) The long term prognosis of lupus nephritis; the impact of disease activity. J Rheumatol 20:59–65
25. Moroni G, Quaglini S, Gallelli B et al (2007) The long-term outcome of 93 patients with proliferative lupus nephritis. Nephrol Dial Transplant 22:2531–2539
26. Ibanez D, Urowitz MB, Gladman DD et al (2003) Summarizing disease features over time: I. adjusted mean SLEDAI derivation and application to an index of disease activity in lupus. J Rheumatol 30:1977–1982
27. CooK RJ, Gladman DD, Pericak D et al (2000) Prediction of short term mortality in SLE with time dependent measures of disease activity. J Rheumatol 27:1892–1895
28. Nossent J, Kiss E, Rozman B et al (2010) Disease activity and damage accrual during the early disease course in a multinational inception cohort of patients with systemic lupus erythematosus. Lupus 19:949–956
29. Chen YE, Korbet SM, Katz RS et al (2008) Value of a complete or partial remission in severe lupus nephritis. Clin J Am Soc Nephrol 3:46–53

30. Doria A, Gatto M, Zen M, Iaccarino L, Punzi L (2014) Optimizing outcome in SLE: treating-to-target and definition of treatment goals. Autoimmun Rev 13:770–777
31. Gladman DD, Urowitz MB, Goldsmith CH, Fortin P, Ginzler E, Gordon C et al (1997) The reliability of the Systemic Lupus International Collaborating Clinics/American College of Rheumatology Damage Index in patients with systemic lupus erythematosus. Arthritis Rheum 40:809–813
32. Thamer M, Hernán MA, Zhang Y et al (2009) Prednisone, lupus activity, and permanent organ damage. J Rheumatol 36:560–564
33. Stoll T, Sutcliffe N, Mach J et al (2004) Analysis of the relationship between disease activity and damage in patients with systemic lupus erythematosus – a 5-yr prospective study. Rheumatology 43:1039–4
34. Ibañez D, Gladman DD, Urowitz MB (2005) Adjusted mean Systemic Lupus Erythematosus Disease Activity Index-2K is a predictor of outcome in SLE. J Rheumatol 32:824–827
35. Rahman P, Gladman DD, Urowitz MB et al (2001) Early damage as measured by the SLICC/ACR damage index is a predictor of mortality in systemic lupus erythematosus. Lupus 10:93–96
36. Manger K, Manger B, Repp R et al (2002) Definition of risk factors for death, end stage renal disease, and thromboembolic events in a monocentric cohort of 338 patients with systemic lupus erythematosus. Ann Rheum Dis 61:1065–1070
37. Ware JE Jr, Sherbourne CD (1992) The MOS 36-item short-form health survey (SF-36). I. Conceptual framework and item selection. Med Care 30:473–483
38. Mok CC, Ho LY, Cheung MY, Yu KL, To CH (2009) Effect of disease activity and damage on quality of life in patients with systemic lupus erythematosus: a 2-year prospective study. Scand J Rheumatol 38:121–127
39. Rinaldi S, Ghisi M, Iaccarino L et al (2006) Influence of coping skills on health-related quality of life in patients with systemic lupus erythematosus. Arthritis Rheum 55:427–433
40. Rinaldi S, Doria A, Salaffi F, Ermani M, Iaccarino L, Ghirardello A et al (2004) Health related quality of life in Italian patients with systemic lupus erythematosus. I. Relationship between physical and metal dimension and impact of age. Rheumatology 43:1574–1579
41. Khanna S, Pal H, Pandey RM, Handa R (2004) The relationship between disease activity and quality of life in systemic lupus erythematosus. Rheumatology 43:1536–1540
42. Bertsias G, Ioannidis JP, Boletis J et al (2008) EULAR recommendations for the management of systemic lupus erythematosus. Report of a Task Force of the EULAR Standing Committee for International Clinical Studies Including Therapeutics. Ann Rheum Dis 67:195–205
43. Yelin E, Trupin L, Katz P, Criswell L, Yazdany J, Gillis J et al (2007) Work dynamics among persons with systemic lupus erythematosus. Arthritis Rheum 57:56–63
44. Bertoli AM, Fernández M, Alarcón GS, Vilá LM, Reveille JD (2007) Systemic lupus erythematosus in a multiethnic US cohort LUMINA (XLI): factors predictive of self reported work disability. Ann Rheum Dis 66:12–17
45. Mok CC, Cheung MY, Ho LY, Yu KL, To CH (2008) Risk and predictors of work disability in Chinese patients with systemic lupus erythematosus. Lupus 17:1103–1107
46. Al Dhanhani AM, Gignac MA, Su J, Fortin PR (2009) Work disability in systemic lupus erythematosus. Arthritis Rheum 61:378–385

Conventional Treatment of Systemic Lupus Erythematosus

16

Giacomo Quattrocchio, Fernando Fervenza, and Dario Roccatello

Systemic lupus erythematosus (SLE) is a chronic, multisystem disease which may have a variable course and multifaceted organ involvement [1]. Each patient may manifest different symptoms and variable disease activity and severity, with periods of quiescence alternating with flares of activity, as well as therapy-related adverse effects. Moreover, SLE patients frequently have numerous comorbidities, such as hyperlipidemia and hypertension, which represent risk factors for accelerated atherosclerosis and cardiovascular disease [2] and depression, which can seriously compromise health-related quality of life [3].

According to an international task force of specialists and a patients' representatives [4], four overarching principles should always be considered in the decision-making process in SLE: (I) management of SLE should be based on shared decisions between informed patients and their physicians; (II) treatment should be aimed at ensuring

G. Quattrocchio
SCDU Nephrology and Dialysis, Giovanni Bosco Hospital,
Piazza del donatore di Sangue 3, Turin 10154, Italy
e-mail: g.quattrocchio@libero.it

F. Fervenza
Division of Nephrology and Hypertension, Department of Internal Medicine, Mayo Clinic College of Medicine, 200 First Street SW, Rochester, MN 55905, USA
e-mail: fervenza.fernando@mayo.edu

D. Roccatello (✉)
SCDU Nephrology and Dialysis, Giovanni Bosco Hospital,
Piazza del donatore di Sangue 3, Turin 10154, Italy

Center of Research of Immunopathology and Rare Diseases- Coordinating Center of Piemonte and Valle d'Aosta Network for Rare Diseases, Department of Rare, Immunologic, Hematologic and Immunohematologic Diseases, S. Giovanni Bosco Hospital Turin,
Piazza del donatore di Sangue 3, Torino 10154, Italy
e-mail: dario.roccatello@unito.it

D. Roccatello, L. Emmi (eds.), *Connective Tissue Disease: A Comprehensive Guide-Volume 1*, Rare Diseases of the Immune System 5,
DOI 10.1007/978-3-319-24535-5_16

long-term survival, preventing organ damage, and optimizing health-related quality of life by controlling disease activity and minimizing comorbidities and drug toxicity; (III) management of the disease requires an understanding of its many aspects and manifestations, which may have to be targeted in a multidisciplinary manner; and (IV) patients need regular, long-term monitoring and review/adjustment of therapy [5].

The treatment target of SLE should be remission of systemic symptoms and organ manifestations or attainment of the lowest possible disease activity, measured by at least one validated disease activity index and/or by organ-specific markers [4, 6–10].

Conventional management of SLE patients includes nonpharmacologic measures and pharmacological therapies and can be categorized according to organ involvement.

16.1 Nonpharmacologic Measures

Sun protection. Ultraviolet light is a known risk factor for inducing or exacerbating cutaneous and systemic manifestations of SLE, and photosensitivity is highly prevalent in SLE patients [11]. Therefore, patients should avoid intense exposure to sunlight and other sources of ultraviolet light and should be instructed to always use sunscreen with a sun protection factor (SPF) of at least 30. They should avoid medications that can cause photosensitivity and should wear sun-protective clothing.

Smoking cessation. Complete cessation of smoking is a very important issue because smoking is associated with worse skin disease, more active systemic disease [12, 13], and is an additional risk factor for an already increased prevalence of cardiovascular disease [2].

Exercise. SLE patients often complain of fatigue, with consequent inactivity and loss of muscle mass. Furthermore, steroid therapy can cause muscle weakness and bone demineralization. Thus, regular aerobic exercise should be encouraged [14].

Diet. A diet including moderate protein and energy content, but rich in vitamins, minerals, and mono/polyunsaturated fatty acids, can promote a beneficial protective effect against tissue damage and suppression of inflammatory activity, in addition to helping the treatment of dyslipidemia, obesity, systemic arterial hypertension, and metabolic syndrome [15].

Furthermore, as a consequence of reduced sun exposure, SLE patients often have low serum levels of 25-hydroxy vitamin D [16] that may require supplementation.

Immunization. Influenza and pneumococcal vaccines can be administered to SLE patients, even if their efficacy may be decreased [17]. Likewise, human papillomavirus vaccine [18] and hepatitis B vaccine [19] appear to be safe in patients with inactive disease.

16.2 Conventional Pharmacologic Therapies

Therapy for SLE must be tailored to the individual patients as multispecialty experts have indicated in treat-to-target in SLE recommendations [4].

The therapeutic approach is multifaceted and is usually based on the predominant disease manifestations. However, some general principles may apply to all patients.

In general, regardless of the use of other treatments, some experts believe that antimalarials, like chloroquine and the preferred hydroxychloroquine, should be considered in all SLE patients unless contraindicated [4]. Nonrandomized studies have suggested favorable effects on various SLE outcomes [20], such as reduction of flares, improvement of skin manifestations, prevention of damage accrual, and possible reduction in mortality risk [21–28]. Furthermore, antimalarial drugs have antiplatelet and antithrombotic effects; they improve lipid profile and may have an osteoprotective effect.

Specific therapy is based upon clinical manifestations, organ involvement, and disease severity [4].

16.3 Constitutional Symptoms

Fatigue and fever are common symptoms in patients with SLE and may be the result of multifactorial etiologies.

Fatigue may depend on anemia, diabetes, depression, hypothyroidism, or fibromyalgia. These conditions should be investigated and treated if they are present. Low-dose glucocorticoids and antimalarials could be of some benefit [29].

Fever may be secondary to an underlying infection in patients treated with immunosuppressive therapy. If it is associated with disease activity, it usually responds to NSAIDs, acetaminophen, and low-moderate doses of steroids.

16.4 Management of Cutaneous Manifestations

The skin is frequently involved in clinical manifestations of SLE, and up to 80 % of patients have some type of cutaneous involvement in the course of their disease.

Cutaneous lupus erythematosus (CLE) may present in a variety of clinical forms. The three recognized subtypes of cutaneous LE are acute cutaneous LE (ACLE), subacute cutaneous LE (SCLE), and chronic cutaneous LE (CCLE) [30]:

ACLE may be either localized (most often as a malar or "butterfly" rash) or generalized. Multisystem involvement as a component of SLE is common, with prominent musculoskeletal symptoms.

SCLE is highly photosensitive, with predominant distribution on the upper back, shoulders, neck, and anterior chest. SCLE is frequently associated with positive anti-Ro antibodies and may be triggered by a variety of medications.

Classic discoid LE is the most common form of CCLE, with indurated scaly plaques on the scalp, face, and ears and characteristic scarring and pigmentary change. Less common forms of CCLE include hyperkeratotic LE, lupus tumidus, lupus profundus, and chilblain lupus. Common cutaneous diseases associated with, but not specific for LE, include vasculitis, livedo reticularis, alopecia, digital manifestations such as periungual telangiectasia and Raynaud phenomenon, photosensitivity, and bullous lesions.

The goal of treatment of the various forms of cutaneous lupus is to prevent long-term skin sequelae, such as telangiectasia, hyperpigmentation or hypopigmentation, alopecia, and scarring [31].

Treatment initially includes preventive (e.g., photoprotective) strategies and topical therapies (corticosteroids and calcineurin inhibitors). For skin disease that cannot be controlled by these interventions, oral antimalarial agents (most commonly hydroxychloroquine) are often beneficial. Additional systemic conventional therapies include corticosteroids, immunosuppressive, immunomodulatory, and various other drugs [30].

Prevention. Preventive measures are able to prevent skin lesions in most patients who must thus avoid sun exposure during peak daylight hours as well as medications that may cause photosensitivity [32]. Sunscreens that block both ultraviolet-A and ultraviolet-B radiation, with an SPF of at least 30 (according to some authors >55), should be used regularly, applying them 30–60 min prior to exposure and then every 4–6 h. Furthermore, patients should be instructed to wear sun-protective clothing and to quit smoking since it is associated with active cutaneous manifestations of SLE and decreased effectiveness of antimalarial agents [33].

Topical therapy. The initial treatment of cutaneous lupus is based on topical glucocorticoids, starting with a low potency agent such as hydrocortisone for early superficial involvement and escalating to more potent, fluorinated corticosteroids for thicker lesions. Ointments are generally considered more effective than creams, and lotions are frequently used for scalp lesions [34].

In case of facial lesions, fluorinated topical corticosteroids should be used for no more than 2 weeks in order to avoid skin atrophy or other side effects.

Tacrolimus ointment and pimecrolimus cream may be used in resistant lesions [35–37], but recently, an increased risk of skin cancer has been reported. Some authors recommend topical retinoids [31, 38], but their efficacy and safety have not been verified.

Pulse dye laser has demonstrated effectiveness in treating acute flares of lupus tumidus [39].

Antimalarial drugs. Patients who are unresponsive to topical or intralesional therapy should be treated with an antimalarial. These agents are effective due to a number of mechanisms including photoprotection, lysosomal stabilization, influence on apoptosis, inhibitory effect on Toll-like receptor-mediated activation of the innate immune response and inhibition of antigen presentation, prostaglandin synthesis, lipid peroxidation, and proinflammatory cytokine synthesis [40].

The agent of choice is hydroxychloroquine [41, 42], given at 200–400 mg per day, without exceeding 6.5 mg/kg per day. Hydroxychloroquine may be more effective at higher blood concentrations, so some authors suggest monitoring blood drug concentration [43]. Potential side effects include severe retinopathy (preliminary and then regular ophthalmologic examination are necessary), gastrointestinal upset, headache, and rashes.

Chloroquine (250–500 mg/day) or quinacrine (50–100 mg/day) are more potent agents that can be used in patients who are unresponsive to hydroxychloroquine. Quinacrine has a much lower risk of retinal toxicity and can be effectively associated with both chloroquine and hydroxychloroquine [23, 42]. Improvement with antimalarials may require 6–12 weeks to be seen. They have been associated with flares of psoriasis and should not be given to individuals with G6PD deficiency.

Long-term use of antimalarials may result in yellow skin and nails (quinacrine) which fluoresce under Wood's light, or hyperpigmentation.

Immunosuppressive and other agents. Patients with refractory, severe cutaneous SLE may be treated with a variety of other drugs, such as systemic glucocorticoids, methotrexate, azathioprine (AZA), cyclosporine, cyclophosphamide (CYC), chlorambucil, and mycophenolate mofetil (MMF) [44].

Some results have been obtained with dapsone, thalidomide, lenalidomide, gold, retinoids, intravenous immunoglobulin, diphenylhydantoin, clofazimine, sulfasalazine, interferon alpha, cefuroxime, danazol, and extracorporeal photophoresis [30, 44–48].

16.5 Management of Musculoskeletal Manifestations

Articular involvement is extremely common in patients with SLE. Initial therapy is based on nonsteroidal anti-inflammatory drugs (NSAIDs), acetaminophen, or both, which are generally effective for relieving minor symptoms. The most severe adverse effects associated with NSAIDs include renal and hepatic impairment, gastrointestinal discomfort, bleeding, cardiovascular risk, and aseptic meningitis. Naproxen might have greater relative cardiovascular safety than other NSAIDs. NSAIDs with high selectivity for cyclooxygenase-2 (COX-2), such as celecoxib, are recommended by experts to reduce adverse effects, whereas those with less selectivity, such as piroxicam and ketorolac, should be avoided [47].

In non-responders, antimalarials like hydroxychloroquine 200–400 mg per day are usually added to NSAIDs [20, 47, 49]. In acute phases of disease, low doses of glucocorticoids, such as prednisone 5–10 mg/day, may sometimes be necessary for a short period of time.

Methotrexate, an antifolate agent with anti-inflammatory effects, leads to significant reductions in SLEDAI scores and allows reduction of steroid doses [47, 50].

Azathioprine, a purine analog that inhibits nucleic acid synthesis with activity on both cellular and humoral immunity, or mycophenolate mofetil, a reversible inhibitor of the enzyme inosine monophosphate dehydrogenase with antiproliferative effects toward activated B and T cells, are effective options in cases of methotrexate intolerance or refractory disease [47, 51].

16.6 Management of Neuropsychiatric Manifestations

Nervous system involvement can manifest in 20–70 % of patients prior to the diagnosis of SLE or during the course of the disease [52]. Patients may present a wide range of neurological and psychiatric features, which are classified using the ACR case definitions for 19 neuropsychiatric syndromes, of which cognitive dysfunction, mood disorder, headache, and peripheral neuropathy are the most common [53, 54]. Nervous system involvement is common in both children and adults with SLE and is associated with worse prognosis and more cumulative damage. Neuropsychiatric lupus (NPSLE) can occur in the absence of either serologic activity or other systemic disease manifestations [54]. The pathogenic etiologies of NPSLE manifestations are likely to be multifactorial and may involve autoantibody production, microangiopathy, intrathecal production of proinflammatory cytokines, and premature atherosclerosis [55]. Approximately one-third of all neuropsychiatric syndromes in patients with SLE are primary manifestations of SLE-related autoimmunity. Anticardiolipin autoantibodies are the most common autoantibodies in NSPLE patients and correlate with cognitive impairment, depression, psychosis, chorea, and migraine [56, 57].

Diagnosis of NPSLE requires the exclusion of secondary causes, such as infections, metabolic derangements, hypertension, and drug toxicity [58]. Clinical assessment steers the selection of appropriate investigations, which include measurement of autoantibodies, analysis of cerebrospinal fluid, electrophysiological studies, neuropsychological assessment, and neuroimaging to evaluate brain structure and functional syndromes [54, 59].

The general management of patients with NPSLE includes symptomatic and immunosuppressive therapies, but evidence of the efficacy of the most commonly used treatment modalities is largely limited to uncontrolled clinical trials and anecdotal experience [60]. Antimalarial agents, such as hydroxychloroquine 200–400 mg daily, can be used as maintenance therapy to prevent disease flares. Furthermore, they may improve fatigue and possibly cognitive dysfunction and could lead to a reduction in prednisone dose [47, 49]. Treatments usually focus on the specific neuropsychiatric symptoms rather than on treating the underlying SLE [47]. The key to treatment is to first establish the correct diagnosis on the basis of ACR case definitions [61]. Moreover, for many NPSLE syndromes, symptomatic treatment, such as anticonvulsants, antidepressants, and antipsychotics, may be needed in addition to immunomodulatory therapy [47, 62].

Although the prognosis is variable, studies suggest a more favorable outcome for primary NPSLE manifestations compared to neuropsychiatric events attributable to non-SLE causes [54, 59].

Specific therapy depends upon the nature of the underlying process (inflammatory or thrombotic). In some cases, differentiation between these processes may not be feasible and in some patients both mechanisms may be operant. When NPSLE is believed to reflect an inflammatory/neurotoxic process (especially aseptic meningitis, optic neuritis, transverse myelitis, peripheral neuropathy, refractory seizures, psychosis, acute confusional state), and in the presence of generalized lupus activity, management includes glucocorticoids alone. If no improvement is observed, immunosuppressants, such as azathioprine or cyclophosphamide, or rituximab (anti-CD20 monoclonal antibody) should be added [62–65].

In severe, life-threatening NPSLE, high-dose glucocorticoids, mycophenolate mofetil, plasmapheresis, and intravenous immunoglobulins can be used [66–68].

Antiplatelet and/or anticoagulation therapy is recommended for NPSLE related to antiphospholipid antibodies, especially for thrombotic cerebrovascular disease [4]. Anticoagulation may be superior to antiplatelet therapy for the secondary prevention of arterial events in antiphospholipid antibody syndrome (APS) [69–72]. Antiplatelet/anticoagulation therapy has also been used in antiphospholipid-associated ischemic optic neuropathy and chorea, as well as in myelopathy refractory to immunosuppressive therapy [73–75]. In severe cases, rituximab has showed beneficial effects [57]. Data from cohort studies [76–78], but not from a randomized controlled trial [79], support the potential benefit of antiplatelet agents in the primary prevention of cerebrovascular disease (and other thrombotic events) in SLE patients with persistently positive, moderate-to-high titers of antiphospholipid antibodies.

Patients with peripheral neuropathies (10–15 %) should be treated with glucocorticoids alone (prednisone 1–2 mg/kg/day) or – in severe cases – associated with immunosuppressive therapy such as cyclophosphamide 1.5–2 mg/kg/day orally, or intermittent monthly intravenous doses of 600–750 mg/m^2 [64]. Immunoglobulins and plasma exchange have been used in refractory cases [47, 80–82]. Administering gabapentin (initial dose of 100 mg three times daily), pregabalin (initial dose of 75 mg twice a day), a low-dose of tricyclic antidepressant such as amitriptyline (initial dose of 25 mg/day), or carbamazepine has resulted in long-term benefits in patients with pain or intolerable paresthesia and an abnormal nerve conduction test [83].

16.7 Management of Renal Manifestations

Kidney involvement is a common complication of SLE and increases both morbidity and mortality in SLE patients, mainly in African-Americans [84–86]. Up to 70 % of patients with SLE develop lupus nephritis during the first 10 years of disease, and its prevalence is substantially higher in African-American and Hispanic individuals than in Caucasians [47, 87–89]. Lupus nephritis (LN) is defined according to the ACR classification criteria by two characteristics: urinary protein >0.5 g per day or >3+ by dipstick analysis, or a urinary protein-to-creatinine ratio of >0.5, and active urinary sediment (>5 red blood cells per high-power field, >5 white blood cells per high-power field in the absence of infection, or the presence of red or white blood cell casts) [90].

Early recognition and treatment of renal involvement are strongly recommended, and, as is the case for other organ manifestations, each patient should be evaluated for antimalarial administration [4]. Renal biopsy plays a critical role in the diagnosis, treatment, management, and follow-up of LN; thus, routine biopsy has been advocated by some nephrologists in SLE patients with any signs of kidney disease [91]. However, some authors feel that the role of renal biopsy in predicting outcome, treatment, and prognosis is controversial [92].

The original World Health Organization (WHO) classification of LN that was introduced in 1974 has more recently evolved into the 2003 International Society of Nephrology (ISN)/Renal Pathology Society (RPS) classification [93], which recognizes six classes of lupus nephritis. The histological findings provide the basis for the treatment recommendations for LN. Kidney Disease: Improving Global Outcomes (KDIGO), American College of Rheumatology (ACR), and European League Against Rheumatism and European Renal Association-European Dialysis and Transplant Association (EULAR/ERA-EDTA) have developed specific treatment guidelines, which can sometimes present little differences [90, 94, 95]. Generally speaking:

- Class I LN patients, as well as class II LN patients with proteinuria <1 g/day, only require treatment as dictated by the extrarenal clinical manifestations of lupus.
- Class II LN patients with proteinuria >3 g/day require a RAS-blocking agent and an antimalarial agent. Glucocorticoids (prednisone 1 mg/kg/day) or a calcineurin inhibitor should be considered.
- Class III (focal) LN, class IV (diffuse) LN patients as well as class V (membranous) LN patients with severe nephrotic syndrome, elevated serum creatinine levels, and/or associated proliferative disease should receive initial combined steroid and immunosuppressive (induction) treatment, aimed at inducing remission by controlling immunologic activity, and a subsequent longer period of less intensive (maintenance) treatment to consolidate remission and prevent relapses [4, 47, 90, 94, 95].
- Class V (membranous) LN with normal kidney function and non-nephrotic-range proteinuria should be treated with antiproteinuric and antihypertensive medications. These subjects should receive corticosteroids and immunosuppressives if dictated by the extrarenal manifestations of systemic lupus [94].
- Class VI (advanced sclerosis) LN should be treated with corticosteroids and immunosuppressives only as dictated by the extrarenal manifestations of systemic lupus [94].

Induction therapy. Glucocorticoids rapidly reduce inflammation and modulate the innate and adaptive immune systems, resulting in an amelioration of SLE-related manifestations of LN [96]. The dose of glucocorticoid treatment depends on the severity of the disease. High doses of oral prednisone (1.0–1.5 mg/kg) and/or intravenous methylprednisolone (1 g or 15 mg/kg) for three consecutive days (pulse therapy) are used to treat severe disease.

Immunosuppressive induction treatment could consist of either intravenous/oral cyclophosphamide or mycophenolate mofetil [94]. The choice between intravenous cyclophosphamide and oral MMF depends upon the clinical features (MMF may be preferable in African-Americans and Hispanics) and upon patient preference (e.g., a young woman may want to avoid the potential ovarian toxicity of cyclophosphamide).

Cyclophosphamide is an alkylating and cytotoxic agent that cross-links DNA and DNA-associated proteins and thereby inhibits DNA replication, leading to cell death. It exerts its cytotoxic effect on both resting and dividing lymphocytes; however, the precise mechanisms through which it provides therapeutic benefits in autoimmune diseases are not well established. The first dosing regimen was the NIH protocol, which involves intravenous infusion of cyclophosphamide (0.5–1.0 g/m^2 body surface area) once a month for 6 months and then once every 3 months for an additional 2 years [97, 98]. In another protocol, known as the Euro-Lupus regimen, cyclophosphamide is given intravenously at a dose of 500 mg every 2 weeks for

3 months, followed by azathioprine 2 mg/kg/day for at least 2 years [99]. A comparison between "mini-pulse" cyclophosphamide (the Euro-Lupus regimen) and the conventional NIH regimen showed no difference in efficacy in terms of mortality, renal function, or overall SLE damage score after 10 years of follow-up [100]. Oral cyclophosphamide 1.0–1.5 mg/kg/day (maximum dose of 150 mg/day) for 2–4 months has been used as an alternative to i.v. cyclophosphamide with equivalent efficacy in prospective observational studies [101, 102].

The main adverse effects of cyclophosphamide treatment include severe infections, alopecia, malignancies (lymphomas and bladder carcinoma), and infertility [103]. Intravenous infusions of 2-mercaptoethanesulphonate sodium (mesna) can be given to decrease the risk of bladder damage that occurs with i.v. cyclophosphamide treatment [104]. In addition, treatment with gonadotropin-releasing hormone might protect against premature ovarian failure during cyclophosphamide treatment [105]. Finally, prophylactic treatment to prevent Pneumocystis pneumonia should be considered.

MMF, a reversible inhibitor of the inosine monophosphate dehydrogenase enzyme with antiproliferative effects toward activated B and T cells, is an alternative to cyclophosphamide as the initial therapy for proliferative LN. The Aspreva Lupus Management Study (ALMS) compared 24-weeks induction therapy with daily glucocorticoids associated with either oral MMF (target dosage 3 g/day) or monthly intravenous cyclophosphamide (0.75 g/m^2 first dose, followed by five infusions of 0.5–1 g/m^2) in 370 patients with class III, IV, and V LN [106]. No differences were found in either primary (a prespecified decrease in urine protein/creatinine ratio and stabilization or improvement in serum creatinine) or secondary end points (complete renal remission, systemic disease activity and damage, and safety). In a post hoc analysis, however, MMF therapy was associated with a significantly higher response rate in African-American and Hispanic patients (60 versus 39 %, odds ratio 2.4, 95 % CI 1.1–5.4) [107]. In a meta-analysis and a Cochrane review, which included 45 trials involving 2,559 patients, there were no significant differences between cyclophosphamide- and MMF-based induction therapy with respect to mortality, incidence of ESRD, and relapse during induction [108, 109].

Azathioprine is an alternative therapeutic option [94]: an RCT involving European subjects compared initial therapy with azathioprine (2 mg/kg/day for 2 years) combined with i.v. methylprednisolone (1×3 pulses of 1,000 mg repeated after 2 and 6 weeks) followed by oral prednisone, to i.v. cyclophosphamide (750 mg/m^2, 13 pulses over 2 years) with oral prednisone [110]. After 2 years, there was no difference in response rate, though there were fewer adverse effects in subjects receiving azathioprine. However, supplementary studies on these cohorts showed a higher late-relapse rate and higher risk of doubling of SCr after azathioprine. Furthermore, there was more chronicity on later biopsies after azathioprine [111].

Cyclosporine has been used in a small ($n=40$), open-label RCT, in comparison to cyclophosphamide as initial therapy combined with corticosteroids for proliferative LN [94, 112]. Cyclosporine (4–5 mg/kg/day) was used for 9 months and then tapered over the next 9 months. Cyclophosphamide was used in a different regimen than in most published trials: eight i.v. pulses (10 mg/kg) were given in the first 9 months, followed by four to five oral pulses (10 mg/kg) over the next 9 months. There were no differences in response or remission at 9 or 18 months, or in relapse rate after 40 months of follow-up. Infections and leukopenia did not differ between the groups.

Tacrolimus and steroids with or without MMF have been reported as a possible alternative to i.v. cyclophosphamide and steroids as induction therapy for active LN in studies on Chinese patients [113–115]. These regimens could be used in patients who cannot tolerate either cyclophosphamide or MMF, or in those with associated proliferative and membranous LN.

Plasmapheresis has not shown efficacy in patients with LN [116], although some benefit has been suggested in observational studies in selected patients [117].

Intravenous immunoglobulin (most commonly 400 mg/kg/day for four to five daily doses) administration has immunomodulatory properties and could be a reasonable option in patients who are refractory to initial induction therapy or have a concomitant infection [118, 119].

Maintenance therapy. Up to 50 % of patients have proliferative LN relapse following reduction in or cessation of immunosuppressive therapy [120]. Relapse rates range from 5 to 15 per 100 patient-years, with an average of about 8 per 100 patient-years for the first 5 years of follow-up [121]. Relapse is more common when partial rather than complete remission is obtained with induction treatment. After induction therapy, at least 3 years of immunosuppressive maintenance treatment is recommended to consolidate remission and prevent relapses [4, 122, 123]. Treatment options include glucocorticoids and the following immunosuppressive agents: cyclophosphamide, azathioprine, and mycophenolate mofetil. However, these drugs show considerable toxicity and are not effective in all patients [124].

KDIGO and ACR guidelines recommend MMF or azathioprine maintenance for LN patients who respond to standard induction therapy [90, 94].

Two recent randomized trials of maintenance therapy in lupus nephritis compared AZA (2 mg/kg/day) with MMF (2 g/day) for 3 years [125, 126]. In the ALMS maintenance trial, after induction therapy with 24 months of either high-dose "NIH protocol" intravenous cyclophosphamide or MMF, immunosuppressors were associated with up to 10 mg/day of prednisone at the discretion of the investigator, and only patients who had undergone successful induction therapy were enrolled [125]. In the MAINTAIN trial, after receiving the Euro-Lupus induction regimen (500 mg of intravenous cyclophosphamide every 2 weeks for 3 months), and regardless of response, patients with at least 0.5 g/day of proteinuria were included and were administered corticosteroids on a defined taper [126]. Despite the differences, both trials demonstrate that maintenance therapy with either MMF or AZA is overall well tolerated and leads to excellent results at 3–4 years of follow-up in the majority of patients. Both agents yielded extremely low rates of creatinine doubling, end-stage renal disease, and death. The ALMS trial suggests that MMF may be more effective and better tolerated than AZA, especially in higher-risk minority patients. So, for now, clinicians should feel confident when using either of these agents for the maintenance treatment of lupus nephritis [127].

In patients who are MMF or AZA intolerant, calcineurin inhibitors with low-dose corticosteroids [128, 129] or cyclophosphamide [130] can be used.

Relapsing and resistant lupus nephritis. LN is a relapsing condition, and relapses are associated with the development of chronic kidney disease [131]. Furthermore, pathologic findings in LN may change with a relapse, and such changes cannot be clinically predicted with certainty.

A relapse of LN after complete or partial remission should be treated with the same initial therapy followed by the maintenance therapy that was effective in inducing the original remission [94].

A repeat kidney biopsy during relapse should be considered if there is a suspicion that the histological class of LN has changed, or if there is uncertainty about whether increasing creatinine and/or worsening proteinuria represents disease activity or chronicity [94].

Patients who have failed more than one of the recommended initial regimens may be considered for treatment with rituximab [94, 132–134], intravenous immunoglobulins [94, 118, 119, 135], or calcineurin inhibitors [94, 136–138].

As regard to rituximab, an original regimen, initially employed as a rescue therapy in refractory LN, has been recently proposed in order to minimize the long-term effects of both corticosteroids and the immunosuppressive agents used for remission maintenance. It was based on an intensified B-lymphocyte depletion consisting of four weekly doses of rituximab (375 mg/m^2) followed by two more doses after 1 and 2 months, associated with two IV administrations of 10 mg/kg of cyclophosphamide and three pulses of methylprednisolone (15 mg/kg) followed by oral prednisone (0.8 mg/die, rapidly tapered to 5 mg/day in 10 weeks) without further immunosuppressive maintenance therapy [132].

16.8 Management of Cardiac Manifestations

Cardiac involvement is common among SLE patients and can frequently be recognized by echocardiography and other noninvasive tests. It is usually mild and may manifest as pericardial disease, myocardial dysfunction, valvular lesions, and coronary artery disease [139–141].

Pericarditis is the most common cardiac abnormality and can be life threatening. Pericardial effusion occurs in about 50 % of patients during the course of the disease and is frequently observed when SLE is clinically active [142]. NSAIDs and moderate to high doses of corticosteroids (0.5–1 mg/kg/day of prednisone in divided doses) with/without hydroxychloroquine are often effective, but more aggressive immunosuppressive therapy (azathioprine, mycophenolate, or methotrexate) is required for severe or refractory cases [47, 49, 57]. Colchicine may be considered for patients who do not respond to NSAIDs or glucocorticoids or who have a relapsing course. Pericardial tamponade is rare and is most often associated with low C4 levels at presentation; it should be treated with high-dose corticosteroids. The prognosis of lupus pericarditis is generally good and relapse or progression to fibrotic disease is uncommon, but some patients may require a pericardial window [143].

Myocarditis is uncommon and often asymptomatic with a prevalence of about 10 % in SLE patients. It is more frequently observed in African-Americans and in patients with active disease [144]. It may manifest as resting tachycardia, ST- and T-wave abnormalities, or ventricular hypokinesis. Alternative causes of myocarditis, such as uremia and drug toxicity (cyclophosphamide, antimalarials, phenothiazines), should be ruled out, if necessary by myocardial biopsy [145]. Patients with severe myocarditis may respond to high-dose intravenous glucocorticoids (methylprednisolone 1000 mg for 3 days), followed by subsequent oral prednisone, sometimes combined with immunosuppressors [49, 146]. The efficacy of intravenous immunoglobulins has been reported [147].

Valvular lesions, often involving the mitral valve, may range from small nodules to verrucous Libman-Sacks endocarditis [148]. The prevalence is about 10 % of SLE patients. Heart valve disease is better detected by transesophageal echocardiography and is often associated with antiphospholipid antibodies [148–150]. Infective endocarditis must always be ruled out in patients who often undergo immunosuppressive therapy. Glucocorticoids and cytotoxic treatment appear to be of no use. Anticoagulants or antiplatelet agents can be considered for patients with significant vegetations or associated antiphospholipid syndrome and must be prescribed in case of thromboembolic events.

Coronary artery disease has an increased prevalence and an accelerated course in SLE patients compared to the general population [151]. The pathogenesis is likely multifactorial and is related to traditional risk factors (hypertension, hyperlipidemia, diabetes), systemic inflammation, and steroid therapy [152]. A healthy lifestyle (not smoking, regular physical activity) and adequate blood pressure and glycemic control should be pursued, like in the general population. The lowest possible glucocorticoid dosage needed to control the disease should be administered in an effort to possibly discontinue use altogether [4]. Antimalarials should be considered for their multifaceted, favorable effects on coagulation and lipid profile [4, 20, 26, 40]. Statins may be beneficial due to their pleiotropic action [153, 154].

16.9 Management of Pulmonary Manifestations

Pulmonary involvement is observed in up to 50 % of SLE patients during their disease course [155]. Clinical manifestations include pleuritis, inflammatory and fibrotic forms of interstitial lung disease, alveolar hemorrhage, shrinking lung syndrome (SLS), pulmonary hypertension (PH), airway disease, and thromboembolic disease.

Inflammation of the pleura may manifest with or without effusion and it usually responds to NSAIDS. In resistant serositis, moderate- to high-dose glucocorticoids (prednisone 0.5–1 mg/kg/day) and/or hydroxychloroquine is usually effective [47, 57, 155, 156]. Immunosuppressive treatment, like oral cyclophosphamide, is rarely necessary.

Interstitial lung disease has been described in about 9 % of SLE patients. It may manifest with cough, dyspnea, and decreased exercise tolerance, and it is recognized by pulmonary function tests and high-resolution CT scanning [155, 156]. Treatment of severe inflammatory forms includes high-dose glucocorticosteroids associated with intravenous cyclophosphamide, followed by either azathioprine or mycophenolate mofetil; alternative therapies are calcineurin inhibitors, intravenous immunoglobulins, or rituximab [49, 157].

Pulmonary hemorrhage is a rare, life-threatening complication in SLE [158, 159] that needs to be distinguished from infection, pulmonary embolism, and vasculitis, in some cases by lung biopsy when necessary. It has a very high mortality rate and should be treated with high-dose intravenous glucocorticoids combined with cyclophosphamide [155, 160]. In some cases, efficacy of plasmapheresis has been reported [161].

Shrinking lung syndrome is a rare respiratory complication associated with SLE, whose pathogenesis remain controversial. Patients present dyspnea alone or associated with chest pain and orthopnea, lung volume reduction with no parenchymal abnormalities, and a restrictive ventilatory defect on pulmonary function tests [162]. Treatment of SLS includes theophylline, an increase in corticosteroid dosage, and intensification of immunosuppressive medication with either methotrexate or cyclophosphamide [163].

Pulmonary hypertension is a rare manifestation in SLE that can occur at any time during the course of the disease. It has a multifactorial pathogenesis (thromboembolism, pulmonary vasculitis, hypoxia, and fibrosis from interstitial lung disease) and can be independent of lupus disease activity in other systems. Echocardiograms are a screening tool but may yield false positives, and right heart catheterization must be performed to confirm the diagnosis. Early identification is important and can alter the natural history of this dangerous complication of lupus [164, 165]. PH may benefit from systemic glucocorticoids associated with intravenous cyclophosphamide [166], as well as endothelin receptor antagonists, phosphodiesterase type 5 inhibitors, and prostanoids [167].

Upper airways and bronchial involvement in SLE may be treated with glucocorticoids and immunosuppressors as with other respiratory lesions [168].

Finally, pulmonary thromboembolic disease is a manifestation of antiphosholipid syndrome (APS), which is discussed in detail separately.

16.10 Management of Gastrointestinal Manifestations

Gastrointestinal symptoms in SLE patients occur in about 50 % of patients and are usually mild. More than half of the symptoms are caused by adverse reactions to medications and viral or bacterial infections. SLE can involve the entire GI tract and the liver. The most common SLE-related gastroenteropathies are lupus enteritis, protein-losing enteropathy (PLE), intestinal pseudo-obstruction, pancreatitis, peritonitis, and liver dysfunction [169, 170].

Lupus enteritis due to mesenteric vasculitis is a life-threatening disorder that may be complicated by infarction and bowel perforation. It may respond to high-dose intravenous pulse steroids associated with immunosuppressive agents [171].

Lupus protein-losing enteropathy is characterized by diarrhea, edema, and hypoalbuminemia. A diagnosis can be made using 99m Tc-labeled albumin scintigraphy. Glucocorticoids are the mainstay of treatment, but immunosuppressive therapy may be required [172].

Intestinal pseudo-obstruction is a rare syndrome described in recent decades that is characterized by ineffective propulsion of the intestine without an apparent mechanical cause. It preferentially involves the small rather than the large bowel, and it is usually observed with active lupus serology. Management of this disorder should include immunomodulators, mainly corticosteroids and cyclophosphamide, prokinetics, and parenteral nutrition when required. Intravenous immunoglobulins may be a good alternative [173].

Pancreatitis occurs in about 5 % of patients and may result from vasculitis or thrombosis, as well as from some drugs (including steroids and immunosuppressors). It generally responds to intravenous fluids, restriction of oral intake, and cessation of the implicated drugs. Therapy with glucocorticoids and azathioprine may be associated with reduced mortality [174]. In severe cases, plasmapheresis and intravenous immunoglobulins may be helpful [170].

Acute and chronic ascites due to lupus peritonitis is extremely rare and may be treated with prednisone and antimalarials [175].

Liver test abnormalities have been described in up to 60 % of patients at some point during the course of their disease. Prior treatment with potentially hepatotoxic drugs, or viral hepatitis, may be the cause of liver disease in SLE patients. However, in rare cases, elevated liver enzymes may be due to concurrent autoimmune hepatitis (AIH). Remission of acute hepatitis was achieved in all cases after starting immunosuppressive therapy [176].

16.11 Management of Hematologic Manifestations

Hematologic abnormalities are common findings in patients with SLE and can be a sign of disease activity as well as an effect of immunosuppressive treatment or infections [177].

The main hematological manifestations of SLE are leukopenia, thrombocytopenia, anemia, and the antiphospholipid syndrome. The first three items are included in the Systemic Lupus International Collaborating Clinics (SLICC) classification Criteria [178].

Leukopenia is common in SLE and usually reflects disease activity.

Neutropenia may be due to increased peripheral destruction of granulocytes, changes in marginal and splenic pool, or increased margination and decreased marrow production. Mild neutropenia requires no specific therapy. Patients with severe neutropenia with opportunistic infections or at the risk of such infection can be successfully treated with G-CSF [179].

Lymphopenia is observed in about 50 % of patients. Specific therapy is not indicated, but the presence and degree of lymphopenia may be related to disease activity. Severely low lymphocyte count may predispose patients to opportunistic infections such that prophylactic therapy should be considered, especially in patients on immunosuppressive therapy [177].

Thrombocytopenia is usually due to increased peripheral destruction commonly mediated by antiplatelet antibodies. Many patients can be watched without specific therapy. Glucocorticoids are the mainstay of therapy for treating acute conditions. Either danazol or hydroxychloroquine can be added to glucocorticoid therapy, followed by slow tapering of the glucocorticoids [180]. If these therapies are not effective, an attempt with additional immunosuppressive therapy may be warranted in the form of cyclophosphamide [181]. Very low-dose cyclosporin or vincristine can also be considered [177]. For emergent treatment of thrombocytopenia, both high-dose glucocorticoid and IVIG have proven to be effective and can be used together [182]. Apheresis should be considered in patients with thrombocytopenia and life-threatening bleeding that does not respond to other therapies [183]. Recent data show that rituximab is an effective therapy in patients with refractory thrombocytopenia [184]. Splenectomy should be kept as a last resort in patients with SLE [185]. Finally, there are newer treatments for immune thrombocytopenia (ITP) such as eltrombopag that perhaps may be used in SLE [186].

Patients with SLE may also develop an autoimmune hemolytic anemia. Its clinical presentation varies from mild to severe anemia and may be associated with other autoimmune manifestations. Glucocorticoids (prednisone 1 mg/kg/day) are used as first-line therapy. Patients who are refractory to conventional therapy should be treated with immunosuppressive drugs, danazol or rituximab [187–190]. Plasmapheresis and intravenous immunoglobulins may be effective in some cases [191, 192].

Antiphospholipid syndrome complicates 10–15 % of cases of SLE and is characterized by recurrent venous or arterial thrombosis or pregnancy morbidity and persistent antiphospholipid antibodies. Therapeutic approach is based on the use of antiplatelet and anticoagulant agents, and in some cases, good results are reported with rituximab. APS is discussed in detail separately.

16.12 Pediatric SLE

SLE onset occurs during childhood in approximately 15 % of patients with SLE. The treatment of pediatric SLE follows the same guidelines as the treatment of adult patients. The aim of effective disease management with early immunosuppression is to achieve symptomatic resolution and improvement of the quality of life by maintaining sustained remission and thereby preventing tissue damage in young as well as in adult patients. However, in the management of children and adolescents, clinicians must consider problems related to physical growth, bone health, psychological development, appearance, and fertility. A multidisciplinary approach including instructing the family is therefore warranted [193].

Key Points and Practical Recommendations

- SLE is a multifaceted disease that can affect several organs.
- SLE manifestations should be managed in a multidisciplinary manner.
- Treatment must be tailored according to the clinical presentation, and a shared decision must be made with the informed patient.
- The goals of treatment are remission of systemic symptoms and organ manifestations and prevention of flares and of damage accrual.
- Antimalarials should be considered in virtually all patients.
- If glucocorticoid administration cannot be discontinued, the dosage should be the lowest possible while still allowing disease control.
- Table 16.1 shows the main drugs that are used for SLE treatment and their main indications, dosage, and warning.

Table 16.1 Drugs for SLE treatment

Drug	Indications	Dosage	Warning
Hydroxychloroquine	Virtually all SLE patients, unless contraindicated	400 mg/day initially, then 200 mg/day	Baseline eye examination and then every 6–12 months thereafter
NSAIDs	Fever, musculoskeletal manifestations, headache, serositis	It depends on drug and individual response	Renal, gastrointestinal, and cardiovascular adverse effects
Glucocorticoids	Any organ manifestations, refractory to other treatment	i.v. methylprednisolone (15 mg/kg) for 3 consecutive days, followed by prednisone 1–1.5 mg/kg/day in severe disease	Glycemic control, blood pressure monitoring, bone protection, gastrointestinal and muscular toxicity, glaucoma, and cataracts
		Prednisone 0.5 mg/kg/day for moderate activity	Use the lowest dosage needed to control disease
		Prednisone 0.1–0.2 mg/kg/day for mild activity	
Cyclophosphamide (CYC)	Severe organ-threatening SLE, in particular renal and neuropsychiatric involvement	NIH protocol: i.v. CYC 0.5–1.0 g/m^2 body surface area once a month for 6 months, followed by the same dose once every 3 months for 24 months	Infections, alopecia, malignancies, infertility
		Euro-Lupus regimen: i.v. CYC 500 mg every 2 weeks for 3 months	i.v. MESNA (2-mercaptoethanesulphonate sodium) to prevent bladder toxicity
		Oral CYC 2–3 mg/kg/day for 2–4 months	Gonadotropin-releasing hormone for ovarian protection

Azathioprine (AZA)	Musculoskeletal, neuropsychiatric, and cutaneous manifestations	Oral AZA 2–3 mg/kg/day	Bone marrow suppression, hepatotoxicity, gastrointestinal intolerance
	Serositis		Monitor blood counts and liver function tests
	Induction and maintenance therapy in nephritis		
Mycophenolate mofetil (MMF)	Induction and maintenance therapy of renal manifestations	Oral MMF 3 g/day for 6 months, then 2 g/day for at least 3 years	Gastrointestinal intolerance, bone marrow suppression, infections
Methotrexate	Cutaneous and musculoskeletal manifestations	10–15 mg/week	Bone marrow suppression, hepatitis, stomatitis

References

1. Von Feldt JM (1995) Systemic lupus erythematosus. Recognizing its various presentations. Postgrad Med 97:79–83, 86 passim
2. Gustafsson JT, Svenungsson E (2014) Definitions of and contributions to cardiovascular disease in systemic lupus erythematosus. Autoimmunity 47:67–76
3. Dua AB, Touma Z, Toloza S et al (2013) Top 10 recent developments in health-related quality of life in patients with systemic lupus erythematosus. Curr Rheumatol Rep 15:380–389
4. van Vollenhoven RF, Mosca M, Bertsias G et al (2014) Treat-to-target in systemic lupus erythematosus: recommendations from an international task force. Ann Rheum Dis 73:958–967
5. Mosca M, Tani C, Aringer M et al (2010) European League Against Rheumatism recommendations for monitoring patients with systemic lupus erythematosus in clinical practice and in observational studies. Ann Rheum Dis 69:1269–1274
6. Gladman D, Ginzler E, Goldsmith C et al (1996) The development and initial validation of the Systemic Lupus International Collaborating Clinics/American College of Rheumatology damage index for systemic lupus erythematosus. Arthritis Rheum 39:363–369
7. Petri M, Purvey S, Fang H et al (2012) Predictors of organ damage in systemic lupus erythematosus: the Hopkins Lupus Cohort. Arthritis Rheum 64:4021–4028
8. Ibanez D, Urowitz MB, Gladman DD (2003) Summarizing disease features over time: I. Adjusted mean SLEDAI derivation and application to an index of disease activity in lupus. J Rheumatol 30:1977–1982
9. Andrade RM, Alarcon GS, Fernandez M et al (2007) Accelerated damage accrual among men with systemic lupus erythematosus: XLIV. Results from a multiethnic US cohort. Arthritis Rheum 56:622–630
10. Lopez R, Davidson JE, Beeby MD et al (2012) Lupus disease activity and the risk of subsequent organ damage and mortality in a large lupus cohort. Rheumatology (Oxford) 51:491–498
11. Lehmann P, Homey B (2009) Clinic and pathophysiology of photosensitivity in lupus erythematosus. Autoimmun Rev 8:456–461
12. Takvorian SU, Merola JF, Costenbader KH (2014) Cigarette smoking, alcohol consumption and risk of systemic lupus erythematosus. Lupus 23:537–544
13. Ghaussy NO, Sibbitt W Jr, Bankhurst AD, Qualls CR (2003) Cigarette smoking and disease activity in systemic lupus erythematosus. J Rheumatol 30:1215–1221
14. Yuen HK, Cunnigham MA (2014) Optimal management of fatigue in patients with systemic lupus erythematosus: a systematic review. Ther Clin Risk Manag 10:775–786
15. Klack K, Bonfa E, Borba Neto EF (2012) Diet and nutritional aspects in systemic lupus erythematosus. Rev Bras Reumatol 52:384–408
16. Toloza SM, Cole DE, Gladman DD et al (2010) Vitamin D insufficiency in a large female SLE cohort. Lupus 19:13–19
17. Murdaca G, Orsi A, Spanò F et al (2014) Influenza and pneumococcal vaccinations of patients with systemic lupus erythematosus: current views upon safety and immunogenicity. Autoimmun Rev 13:75–84
18. Mok CC, Ho LY, Fong LS, To CH (2013) Immunogenicity and safety of a quadrivalent human papillomavirus vaccine in patients with systemic lupus erythematosus: a case-control study. Ann Rheum Dis 72:659–664
19. Kuruma KA, Borba EF, Lopes MH et al (2007) Safety and efficacy of hepatitis B vaccine in systemic lupus erythematosus. Lupus 16:350–354
20. Ruiz-Irastorza G, Ramos-Casals M, Brito-Zeron P, Khamashta MA (2010) Clinical efficacy and side effects of antimalarials in systemic lupus erythematosus: a systematic review. Ann Rheum Dis 69:20–28
21. Tsakonas E, Joseph L, Esdaile JM et al (1998) A long-term study of hydroxychloroquine withdrawal on exacerbations in systemic lupus erythematosus. The Canadian Hydroxychloroquine Study Group. Lupus 7:80–85

22. Bezerra EL, Vilar MJ, da Trindade Neto PB et al (2005) Double-blind, randomized, controlled clinical trial of clofazimine compared with chloroquine in patients with systemic lupus erythematosus. Arthritis Rheum 52:3073–3078
23. Cavazzana I, Sala R, Bazzani C et al (2009) Treatment of lupus skin involvement with quinacrine and hydroxychloroquine. Lupus 18:735–739
24. Fessler BJ, Alarcon GS, McGwin G Jr et al (2005) Systemic lupus erythematosus in three ethnic groups: XVI. Association of hydroxychloroquine use with reduced risk of damage accrual. Arthritis Rheum 52:1473–1480
25. Ibanez D, Gladman DD, Urowitz MB (2005) Adjusted mean systemic lupus erythematosus disease activity index-2K is a predictor of outcome in SLE. J Rheumatol 32:824–827
26. Ruiz-Irastorza G, Egurbide MV, Pijoan JI et al (2006) Effect of antimalarials on thrombosis and survival in patients with systemic lupus erythematosus. Lupus 15:577–583
27. Urowitz MB, Gladman DD, Tom BD et al (2008) Changing patterns in mortality and disease outcomes for patients with systemic lupus erythematosus. J Rheumatol 35:2152–2158
28. Zheng ZH, Zhang LJ, Liu WX et al (2012) Predictors of survival in Chinese patients with lupus nephritis. Lupus 21:1049–1056
29. Jones DW, Wright D, Jankowski TA (2014) Clinical inquiry. What treatments relieve arthritis and fatigue associated with systemic lupus erythematosus? J Fam Pract 63:607–617
30. Walling HW, Sontheimer RD (2009) Cutaneous lupus erythematosus: issues in diagnosis and treatment. Am J Clin Dermatol 10:365–381
31. Callen JP (2006) Cutaneous lupus erythematosus: a personal approach to management. Australas J Dermatol 47:13–27
32. Millard TP, Hawk JL, McGregor JM (2000) Photosensitivity in lupus. Lupus 9:3–10
33. Bourré-Tessier J, Peschken CA, Bernatsky S et al (2013) Association of smoking with cutaneous manifestations in systemic lupus erythematosus. Arthritis Care Res (Hoboken) 65:1275–1280
34. Sigges J, Biazar C, Landmann A, the EUSCLE Co-Authors et al (2013) Therapeutic strategies evaluated by the European Society of Cutaneous Lupus Erythematosus (EUSCLE) Core Set Questionnaire in more than 1000 patients with cutaneous lupus erythematosus. Autoimmun Rev 12:694–702
35. Avgerinou G, Papafragkaki DK, Nasiopoulou A et al (2012) Effectiveness of topical calcineurin inhibitors as monotherapy or in combination with hydroxychloroquine in cutaneous lupus erythematosus. J Eur Acad Dermatol Venereol 26:762–767
36. Pothinamthong P, Janjumratsang P (2012) A comparative study in efficacy and safety of 0.1% tacrolimus and 0.05% clobetasol propionate ointment in discoid lupus erythematosus by modified cutaneous lupus erythematosus disease area and severity index. J Med Assoc Thai 95:933–940
37. Khondker L, Wahab MA, Khan SI (2012) Efficacy of topical application of pimecrolimus cream in the treatment of discoid lupus erythematosus. Mymensingh Med J 21:259–264
38. Kuhn A, Ruland V, Bonsmann G (2011) Cutaneous lupus erythematosus: update of therapeutic options part II. J Am Acad Dermatol 65:195–213
39. Truchuelo MT, Boixeda P, Alcántara J et al (2012) Pulsed dye laser as an excellent choice of treatment for lupus tumidus: a prospective study. J Eur Acad Dermatol Venereol 26:1272–1279
40. Wallace DJ, Gudsoorkar VS, Weisman MH, Venuturupalli SR (2012) New insights into mechanisms of therapeutic effects of antimalarial agents in SLE. Nat Rev Rheumatol 8:522–533
41. Kuhn A, Ruland V, Bonsmann G (2011) Cutaneous lupus erythematosus: update of therapeutic options part I. J Am Acad Dermatol 65:179–193
42. Chang AY, Piette EW, Foering KP et al (2011) Response to antimalarial agents in cutaneous lupus erythematosus: a prospective analysis. Arch Dermatol 147:1261–1267
43. Francès C, Cosnes A, Duhaut P et al (2012) Low blood concentration of hydroxychloroquine in patients with refractory cutaneous lupus erythematosus: a French multicenter prospective study. Arch Dermatol 148:479–484
44. Hansen CB, Dahle KW (2012) Cutaneous lupus erythematosus. Dermatol Ther 25:99–111

45. Cuadrado MJ, Karim Y, Sanna G et al (2005) Thalidomide for the treatment of resistant cutaneous lupus: efficacy and safety of different therapeutic regimens. Am J Med 118:246–250
46. Cortés-Hernández J, Ávila G, Vilardell-Tarrés M, Ordi-Ros J (2012) Efficacy and safety of lenalidomide for refractory cutaneous lupus erythematosus. Arthritis Res Ther 14:R265
47. Xiong W, Lahita RG (2014) Pragmatic approaches to therapy for systemic lupus erythematosus. Nat Rev Rheumatol 10:97–107
48. Privette ED, Werth VP (2013) Update on pathogenesis and treatment of CLE. Curr Opin Rheumatol 25:584–590
49. Muangchan C, van Vollenhoven RF, Bernatsky SR et al (2015) Treatment algorithms in systemic lupus erythematosus. Arthritis Care Res (Hoboken). doi:10.1002/acr.22589, Epub ahead of print
50. Sakthiswary R, Suresh E (2014) Methotrexate in systemic lupus erythematosus: a systematic review of its efficacy. Lupus 23:225–235
51. Artifoni M, Puéchal X (2012) How to treat refractory arthritis in lupus? Joint Bone Spine 79:347–350
52. Jennekens FG, Kater L (2002) The central nervous system in systemic lupus erythematosus. Part 1. Clinical syndromes: a literature investigation. Rheumatology (Oxford) 41:605–618
53. Hanly JG (2004) ACR classification criteria for systemic lupus erythematosus: limitations and revisions to neuropsychiatric variables. Lupus 13:861–864
54. Muscal E, Brey RL (2010) Neurologic manifestations of systemic lupus erythematosus in children and adults. Neurol Clin 28:61–73
55. Hanly JG (2001) Neuropsychiatric lupus. Curr Rheumatol Rep 3:205–212
56. McLaurin EY, Holliday SL, Williams P et al (2005) Predictors of cognitive dysfunction in patients with systemic lupus erythematosus. Neurology 64:297–303
57. Lisnevskaia L, Murphy G, Isenberg D (2014) Systemic lupus erythematosus. Lancet 384:1878–1888
58. Hanly JG, Su L, Farewell V et al (2009) Prospective study of neuropsychiatric events in systemic lupus erythematosus. J Rheumatol 36:1449–1459
59. Hanly JG (2014) Diagnosis and management of neuropsychiatric SLE. Nat Rev Rheumatol 10:338–347
60. O'Neill SG, Schrieber L (2005) Immunotherapy of systemic lupus erythematosus. Autoimmmunity Rev 4:395–402
61. The American College of Rheumatology nomenclature and case definitions for neuropsychiatric lupus syndromes (1999). Arthritis Rheum 42:599–608
62. Bertsias GK, Ioannidis JP, Aringer M et al (2010) EULAR recommendations for the management of systemic lupus erythematosus with neuropsychiatric manifestations: report of a task force of the EULAR standing committee for clinical affairs. Ann Rheum Dis 69:2074–2082
63. Mok CC, Lau CS, Wong RW (2003) Treatment of lupus psychosis with oral cyclophosphamide followed by azathioprine maintenance: an open-label study. Am J Med 115:59–62
64. Barile-Fabris L, Ariza-Andraca R, Olguín-Ortega L et al (2005) Controlled clinical trial of IV cyclophosphamide versus IV methylprednisolone in severe neurological manifestations in systemic lupus erythematosus. Ann Rheum Dis 64:620–625
65. Fernandes Moça Trevisani V, Castro AA, Ferreira Neves Neto J, Atallah AN (2013) Cyclophosphamide versus methylprednisolone for treating neuropsychiatric involvement in systemic lupus erythematosus. Cochrane Database Syst Rev 2:CD002265
66. Tomietto P, D'Agostini S, Annese V et al (2007) Mycophenolate mofetil and intravenous dexamethasone in the treatment of persistent lupus myelitis. J Rheumatol 34:588–591
67. Neuwelt CM (2003) The role of plasmapheresis in the treatment of severe central nervous system neuropsychiatric systemic lupus erythematosus. Ther Apher Dial 7:173–182
68. Milstone AM, Meyers K, Elia J (2005) Treatment of acute neuropsychiatric lupus with intravenous immunoglobulin (IVIG): a case report and review of the literature. Clin Rheumatol 24:394–397
69. Khamashta MA, Cuadrado MJ, Mujic F et al (1995) The management of thrombosis in the antiphospholipid-antibody syndrome. N Engl J Med 332:993–997
70. Muñoz-Rodriguez FJ, Font J, Cervera R et al (1999) Clinical study and follow-up of 100 patients with the antiphospholipid syndrome. Semin Arthritis Rheum 29:182–190

71. Tektonidou MG, Ioannidis JP, Boki KA et al (2000) Prognostic factors and clustering of serious clinical outcomes in antiphospholipid syndrome. Q J Med 93:523–530
72. Ruiz-Irastorza G, Hunt BJ, Khamashta MA (2007) A systematic review of secondary thromboprophylaxis in patients with antiphospholipid antibodies. Arthritis Rheum 57:1487–1495
73. Cervera R, Asherson RA, Font J et al (1997) Chorea in the antiphospholipid syndrome. Clinical, radiologic, and immunologic characteristics of 50 patients from our clinics and the recent literature. Med (Baltimore) 76:203–212
74. D'Cruz DP, Mellor-Pita S, Joven B et al (2004) Transverse myelitis as the first manifestation of systemic lupus erythematosus or lupus-like disease: good functional outcome and relevance of antiphospholipid antibodies. J Rheumatol 31:280–285
75. Heinlein AC, Gertner E (2007) Marked inflammation in catastrophic longitudinal myelitis associated with systemic lupus erythematosus. Lupus 16:823–826
76. Tarr T, Lakos G, Bhattoa HP et al (2007) Analysis of risk factors for the development of thrombotic complications in antiphospholipid antibody positive lupus patients. Lupus 16:39–45
77. Hereng T, Lambert M, Hachulla E et al (2008) Influence of aspirin on the clinical outcomes of 103 anti-phospholipid antibodies-positive patients. Lupus 17:11–15
78. Tektonidou MG, Laskari K, Panagiotakos DB et al (2009) Risk factors for thrombosis and primary thrombosis prevention in patients with systemic lupus erythematosus with or without antiphospholipid antibodies. Arthritis Rheum 61:29–36
79. Erkan D, Harrison MJ, Levy R et al (2007) Aspirin for primary thrombosis prevention in the antiphospholipid syndrome: a randomized, double-blind, placebo-controlled trial in asymptomatic antiphospholipid antibody-positive individuals. Arthritis Rheum 56: 2382–2391
80. Popescu A, Kao AH (2011) Neuropsychiatric systemic lupus erythematosus. Curr Neuropharmacol 9:449–457
81. Zandman-Goddard G, Blank M, Shoenfeld Y (2009) Intravenous immunoglobulins in systemic lupus erythematosus: from the bench to the bedside. Lupus 18:884–888
82. Navarrete MG, Brey RL (2000) Neuropsychiatric systemic lupus erythematosus. Curr Treat Options Neurol 2:473–485
83. Attal N, Bouhassira D (2015) Pharmacotherapy of neuropathic pain: which drugs, which treatment algorithms? Pain 156(Suppl 1):S104–S114
84. Bernatsky S, Boivin JF, Joseph L et al (2006) Mortality in systemic lupus erythematosus. Arthritis Rheum 54:2550–2557
85. Cervera R, Khamashta MA, Font J et al (2003) Morbidity and mortality in systemic lupus erythematosus during a 10-year period: a comparison of early and late manifestations in a cohort of 1,000 patients. Med (Baltimore) 82:299–308
86. Schwartz N, Goilav B, Putterman C (2014) The pathogenesis, diagnosis and treatment of lupus nephritis. Curr Opin Rheumatol 26:502–509
87. Dooley MA, Aranow C, Ginzler EM (2004) Review of ACR renal criteria in systemic lupus erythematosus. Lupus 13:857–860
88. Kasitanon N, Magder LS, Petri M (2006) Predictors of survival in systemic lupus erythematosus. Med (Baltimore) 85:147–156
89. Alarcon GS, McGwin GJ, Petri M et al (2002) Baseline characteristics of a multiethnic lupus cohort: PROFILE. Lupus 11:95–101
90. Hahn BH, McMahon MA, Wilkinson A et al (2012) American College of Rheumatology guidelines for screening, treatment, and management of lupus nephritis. Arthritis Care Res (Hoboken) 64:797–808
91. Bihl GR, Petri M, Fine DM (2006) Kidney biopsy in lupus nephritis: look before you leap. Nephrol Dial Transplant 21:1749–1752
92. Giannico G, Fogo AB (2013) Lupus nephritis: is the kidney biopsy currently necessary in the management of lupus nephritis? Clin J Am Soc Nephrol 8:138–145
93. Weening JJ, D'Agati VD, Schwartz MM et al (2004) International Society of Nephrology Working Group on the Classification of Lupus Nephritis; Renal Pathology Society Working Group on the Classification of Lupus Nephritis: the classification of glomerulonephritis in systemic lupus erythematosus revisited. Kidney Int 65:521–530

94. KDIGO (2012) KDIGO clinical practice guideline for glomerulonephritis. Kidney Int Suppl 2:221–232
95. Bertsias GK, Tektonidou M, Amoura Z et al (2012) Joint European League Against Rheumatism and European Renal Association-European Dialysis and Transplant Association (EULAR/ERA-EDTA) recommendations for the management of adult and paediatric lupus nephritis. Ann Rheum Dis 71:1771–1782
96. Tseng CE, Buyon JP, Kim M et al (2006) The effect of moderate-dose corticosteroids in preventing severe flares in patients with serologically active, but clinically stable, systemic lupus erythematosus: findings of a prospective, randomized, double-blind, placebo-controlled trial. Arthritis Rheum 54:3623–3632
97. Steinberg AD (1986) The treatment of lupus nephritis. Kidney Int 30:769–787
98. Gourley MF, Austin HA 3rd, Scott D et al (1996) Methylprednisolone and cyclophosphamide, alone or in combination, in patients with lupus nephritis. A randomized, controlled trial. Ann Intern Med 125:549–557
99. Houssiau FA, Vasconcelos C, D'Cruz D et al (2002) Immunosuppressive therapy in lupus nephritis: the Euro-Lupus Nephritis Trial, a randomized trial of low-dose versus high-dose intravenous cyclophosphamide. Arthritis Rheum 46:2121–2131
100. Houssiau FA, Vasconcelos C, D'Cruz D et al (2010) The 10-year follow-up data of the Euro-Lupus Nephritis Trial comparing low-dose and high-dose intravenous cyclophosphamide. Ann Rheum Dis 6:61–64
101. McKinley A, Park E, Spetie D et al (2009) Oral cyclophosphamide for lupus glomerulonephritis: an underused therapeutic option. Clin J Am Soc Nephrol 4:1754–1760
102. Chan TM, Tse KC, Tang CS et al (2005) Long-term outcome of patients with diffuse proliferative lupus nephritis treated with prednisolone and oral cyclophosphamide followed by azathioprine. Lupus 14:265–272
103. Petri M, Jones RJ, Brodsky RA (2003) High-dose cyclophosphamide without stem cell transplantation in systemic lupus erythematosus. Arthritis Rheum 48:166–173
104. Monach PA, Arnold LM, Merkel PA (2010) Incidence and prevention of bladder toxicity from cyclophosphamide in the treatment of rheumatic diseases: a data-driven review. Arthritis Rheum 62:9–21
105. Somers EC, Marder W, Christman GM et al (2005) Use of a gonadotropin-releasing hormone analog for protection against premature ovarian failure during cyclophosphamide therapy in women with severe lupus. Arthritis Rheum 5:2761–2767
106. Appel GB, Contreras G, Dooley MA et al (2009) Mycophenolate mofetil versus cyclophosphamide for induction treatment of lupus nephritis. J Am Soc Nephrol 20:1103–1112
107. Isenberg D, Appel GB, Contreras G et al (2010) Influence of race/ethnicity on response to lupus nephritis treatment: the ALMS study. Rheumatology (Oxford) 49:128–140
108. Henderson LK, Masson P, Craig JC et al (2013) Induction and maintenance treatment of proliferative lupus nephritis: a meta-analysis of randomized controlled trials. Am J Kidney Dis 61:74–87
109. Henderson L, Masson P, Craig JC et al (2012) Treatment for lupus nephritis. Cochrane Database Syst Rev 12:CD002922
110. Grootscholten C, Ligtenberg G, Hagen EC et al (2006) Azathioprine/methylprednisolone versus cyclophosphamide in proliferative lupus nephritis. A randomized controlled trial. Kidney Int 70:732–742
111. Grootscholten C, Bajema IM, Florquin S et al (2007) Treatment with cyclophosphamide delays the progression of chronic lesions more effectively than does treatment with azathioprine plus methylprednisolone in patients with proliferative lupus nephritis. Arthritis Rheum 56:924–937
112. Zavada J, Pesickova S, Rysava R et al (2010) Cyclosporine A or intravenous cyclophosphamide for lupus nephritis: the Cyclofa-Lune study. Lupus 19:1281–1289
113. Liu Z, Zhang H, Liu Z et al (2015) Multitarget therapy for induction treatment of lupus nephritis: a randomized trial. Ann Intern Med 162:18–26
114. Chen W, Tang X, Liu Q et al (2011) Short-term outcomes of induction therapy with tacrolimus versus cyclophosphamide for active lupus nephritis: a multicenter randomized clinical trial. Am J Kidney Dis 57:235–244

115. Li X, Ren H, Zhang Q et al (2012) Mycophenolate mofetil or tacrolimus compared with intravenous cyclophosphamide in the induction treatment for active lupus nephritis. Nephrol Dial Transplant 27:1467–1472
116. Lewis EJ, Hunsicker LG, Lan SP et al (1992) A controlled trial of plasmapheresis therapy in severe lupus nephritis. The Lupus Nephritis Collaborative Study Group. N Engl J Med 326:1373–1379
117. Euler HH, Schroeder JO, Harten P et al (1994) Treatment-free remission in severe systemic lupus erythematosus following synchronization of plasmapheresis with subsequent pulse cyclophosphamide. Arthritis Rheum 37:1784–1794
118. Levy Y, Sherer Y, George J et al (2000) Intravenous immunoglobulin treatment of lupus nephritis. Semin Arthritis Rheum 29:321–327
119. Wenderfer SE, Thacker T (2012) Intravenous immunoglobulin in the management of lupus nephritis. Autoimmune Dis 2012:589359. doi:10.1155/2012/589359, Epub 2012 Sep 27
120. Ioannidis JP, Boki KA, Katsorida ME et al (2000) Remission, relapse, and re-remission of proliferative lupus nephritis treated with cyclophosphamide. Kidney Int 57:258–264
121. Grootscholten C, Berden JH (2006) Discontinuation of immunosuppression in proliferative lupus nephritis: is it possible? Nephrol Dial Transplant 21:1465–1469
122. Laskari K, Tzioufas AG, Antoniou A et al (2011) Longterm followup after tapering mycophenolate mofetil during maintenance treatment for proliferative lupus nephritis. J Rheumatol 38:1304–1308
123. Yap DY, Ma MK, Mok MM et al (2013) Long-term data on corticosteroids and mycophenolate mofetil treatment in lupus nephritis. Rheumatology (Oxford) 52:480–486
124. Bomback AS, Appel GB (2010) Updates on the treatment of lupus nephritis. J Am Soc Nephrol 21:2028–2035
125. Dooley MA, Jayne D, Ginzler EM et al (2011) Mycophenolate versus azathioprine as maintenance therapy for lupus nephritis. N Engl J Med 365:1886–1895
126. Houssiau FA, D'Cruz D, Sangle S et al (2010) Azathioprine versus mycophenolate mofetil for long-term immunosuppression in lupus nephritis: results from the MAINTAIN nephritis trial. Ann Rheum Dis 69:2083–2089
127. Morris HK, Canetta PA, Appel GB (2013) Impact of the ALMS and Maintain trials on the management of lupus nephritis. Nephrol Dial Transplant 28:1371–1376
128. Moroni G, Doria A, Mosca M et al (2006) A randomized pilot trial comparing cyclosporine and azathioprine for maintenance therapy in diffuse lupus nephritis over four years. Clin J Am Soc Nephrol 1:925–932
129. Griffiths B, Emery P, Ryan V et al (2010) The BILAG multi-centre open randomized controlled trial comparing ciclosporin vs azathioprine in patients with severe SLE. Rheumatology (Oxford) 49:723–732
130. Contreras G, Pardo V, Leclercq B et al (2004) Sequential therapies for proliferative lupus nephritis. N Engl J Med 350:971–980
131. Gibson KL, Gipson DS, Massengill SA et al (2009) Predictors of relapse and end stage kidney disease in proliferative lupus nephritis: focus on children, adolescents, and young adults. Clin J Am Soc Nephrol 4:1962–1967
132. Roccatello D, Sciascia S, Rossi D et al (2011) Intensive short-term treatment with rituximab, cyclophosphamide and methylprednisolone pulses induces remission in severe cases of SLE with nephritis and avoids further immunosuppressive maintenance therapy. Nephrol Dial Transplant 26:3987–3992
133. Davies RJ, Sangle SR, Jordan NP et al (2013) Rituximab in the treatment of resistant lupus nephritis: therapy failure in rapidly progressive crescentic lupus nephritis. Lupus 22:574–582
134. Gunnarsson I, Jonsdottir T (2013) Rituximab treatment in lupus nephritis – where do we stand? Lupus 22:381–389
135. Rauova L, Lukac J, Levy Y et al (2001) High-dose intravenous immunoglobulins for lupus nephritis – a salvage immunomodulation. Lupus 10:209–213
136. Ogawa H, Kameda H, Amano K et al (2010) Efficacy and safety of cyclosporine A in patients with refractory systemic lupus erythematosus in a daily clinical practice. Lupus 19:162–169

137. Miyasaka N, Kawai S, Hashimoto H (2009) Efficacy and safety of tacrolimus for lupus nephritis: a placebo-controlled double-blind multicenter study. Mod Rheumatol 19: 606–615
138. Gordon S, Denunzio T, Uy A (2013) Success using tacrolimus in patients with proliferative and membranous lupus nephritis and refractory proteinuria. Hawaii J Med Public Health 72(9 Suppl 4):18–23
139. Mandell BF (1987) Cardiovascular involvement in systemic lupus erythematosus. Semin Arthritis Rheum 17:126–141
140. Doria A, Iaccarino L, Sarzi-Puttini P et al (2005) Cardiac involvement in systemic lupus erythematosus. Lupus 14:683–686
141. Miner JJ, Kim AH (2014) Cardiac manifestations of systemic lupus erythematosus. Rheum Dis Clin North Am 40:51–60
142. Man BL, Mok CC (2005) Serositis related to systemic lupus erythematosus: prevalence and outcome. Lupus 14:822–826
143. Rosenbaum E, Krebs E, Cohen M et al (2009) The spectrum of clinical manifestations, outcome and treatment of pericardial tamponade in patients with systemic lupus erythematosus: a retrospective study and literature review. Lupus 18:608–612
144. Apte M, McGwin G Jr, Vilá LM et al (2008) Associated factors and impact of myocarditis in patients with SLE from LUMINA, a multiethnic US cohort (LV). [corrected]. Rheumatology (Oxford) 47:362–367
145. Schattner A, Liang MH (2003) The cardiovascular burden of lupus: a complex challenge. Arch Intern Med 163:1507–1510
146. Zawadowski GM, Klarich KW, Moder KG et al (2012) A contemporary case series of lupus myocarditis. Lupus 21:1378–1384
147. Micheloud D, Calderón M, Caparrros M, D'Cruz DP (2007) Intravenous immunoglobulin therapy in severe lupus myocarditis: good outcome in three patients. Ann Rheum Dis 66:986–987
148. Moyssakis I, Tektonidou MG, Vasilliou VA et al (2007) Libman-Sacks endocarditis in systemic lupus erythematosus: prevalence, associations, and evolution. Am J Med 120:636–642
149. Roldan CA, Qualls CR, Sopko KS, Sibbitt WL Jr (2008) Transthoracic versus transesophageal echocardiography for detection of Libman-Sacks endocarditis: a randomized controlled study. J Rheumatol 35:224–229
150. Zuily S, Regnault V, Selton-Suty C et al (2011) Increased risk for heart valve disease associated with antiphospholipid antibodies in patients with systemic lupus erythematosus: meta-analysis of echocardiographic studies. Circulation 124:215–224
151. Bartels CM, Buhr KA, Goldberg JW et al (2014) Mortality and cardiovascular burden of systemic lupus erythematosus in a US population-based cohort. J Rheumatol 41:680–787
152. Schoenfeld SR, Kasturi S, Costenbader KH (2013) The epidemiology of atherosclerotic cardiovascular disease among patients with SLE: a systematic review. Semin Arthritis Rheum 43:77–95
153. Riboldi P, Gerosa M, Meroni PL (2005) Statins and autoimmune diseases. Lupus 14:765–768
154. Tu H, Li Q, Xiang S et al (2012) Dual effects of statins therapy in systemic lupus erythematosus and SLE-related atherosclerosis: the potential role for regulatory T cells. Atherosclerosis 222:29–33
155. Mittoo S, Fell CD (2014) Pulmonary manifestations of systemic lupus erythematosus. Semin Respir Crit Care Med 35:249–254
156. Keane MP, Lynch JP 3rd (2000) Pleuropulmonary manifestations of systemic lupus erythematosus. Thorax 55:159–166
157. Kobayashi A, Okamoto H (2012) Treatment of interstitial lung diseases associated with connective tissue diseases. Expert Rev Clin Pharmacol 5:219–227
158. Badsha H, Teh CL, Kong KO et al (2004) Pulmonary hemorrhage in systemic lupus erythematosus. Semin Arthritis Rheum 33:414–421

159. Virdi RP, Bashir A, Shahzad G et al (2012) Diffuse alveolar hemorrhage: a rare life-threatening condition in systemic lupus erythematosus. Case Rep Pulmonol 2012:836017. doi:10.1155/2012/836017, Epub 2012 May 27
160. Schwab EP, Schumacher HR Jr, Freundlich B, Callegari PE (1993) Pulmonary alveolar hemorrhage in systemic lupus erythematosus. Semin Arthritis Rheum 23:8–15
161. Erickson RW, Franklin WA, Emlen W (1994) Treatment of hemorrhagic lupus pneumonitis with plasmapheresis. Semin Arthritis Rheum 24:114–123
162. Calderaro DC, Ferreira GA (2012) Presentation and prognosis of shrinking lung syndrome in systemic lupus erythematosus: report of four cases. Rheumatol Int 32:1391–1396
163. Karim MY, Miranda LC, Tench CM et al (2002) Presentation and prognosis of the shrinking lung syndrome in systemic lupus erythematosus. Semin Arthritis Rheum 31:289–298
164. Pope J (2008) An update in pulmonary hypertension in systemic lupus erythematosus – do we need to know about it? Lupus 17:274–277
165. Prabu A, Gordon C (2013) Pulmonary arterial hypertension in SLE: what do we know? Lupus 22:1274–1285
166. Jais X, Launay D, Yaici A et al (2008) Immunosuppressive therapy in lupus- and mixed connective tissue disease-associated pulmonary arterial hypertension: a retrospective analysis of twenty-three cases. Arthritis Rheum 58:521–531
167. Provencher S, Granton JT (2015) Current treatment approaches to pulmonary arterial hypertension. Can J Cardiol 31:460–477
168. Carmier D, Marchand-Adam S, Diot P, Diot E (2010) Respiratory involvement in systemic lupus erythematosus. Rev Mal Respir 27:e66–e78
169. Ebert EC, Hagspiel KD (2011) Gastrointestinal and hepatic manifestations of systemic lupus erythematosus. J Clin Gastroenterol 45:436–441
170. Tian XP, Zhang X (2010) Gastrointestinal involvement in systemic lupus erythematosus: insight into pathogenesis, diagnosis and treatment. World J Gastroenterol 16:2971–2977
171. Janssens P, Arnaud L, Galicier L et al (2013) Lupus enteritis: from clinical findings to therapeutic management. Orphanet J Rare Dis 8:67. doi:10.1186/1750-1172-8-67
172. Law ST, Ma KM, Li KK (2012) The clinical characteristics of lupus related protein-losing enteropathy in Hong Kong Chinese population: 10 years of experience from a regional hospital. Lupus 21:840–847
173. García López CA, Laredo-Sánchez F, Malagón-Rangel J et al (2014) Intestinal pseudo-obstruction in patients with systemic lupus erythematosus: a real diagnostic challenge. World J Gastroenterol 20:11443–11450
174. Nesher G, Breuer GS, Temprano K et al (2006) Lupus-associated pancreatitis. Semin Arthritis Rheum 35:260–267
175. Liu R, Zhang L, Gao S et al (2014) Gastrointestinal symptom due to lupus peritonitis: a rare form of onset of SLE. Int J Clin Exp Med 7:5917–5920
176. Beisel C, Weiler-Normann C, Teufel A, Lohse AW (2014) Association of autoimmune hepatitis and systemic lupus erythematodes: a case series and review of the literature. World J Gastroenterol 20:12662–12667
177. Fayyaz A, Igoe A, Kurien BT et al (2015) Haematological manifestations of lupus. Lupus Sci Med 2(1):e000078
178. Petri M, Orbai AM, Alarcón GS et al (2012) Derivation and validation of the Systemic Lupus International Collaborating Clinics classification criteria for systemic lupus erythematosus. Arthritis Rheum 64:2677–2686
179. Euler HH, Harten P, Zeuner RA et al (1997) Recombinant human granulocyte colony stimulating factor in patients with systemic lupus erythematosus associated neutropenia and refractory infections. J Rheumatol 24:2153–2157
180. Arnal C, Piette JC, Leone J et al (2002) Treatment of severe immune thrombocytopenia associated with systemic lupus erythematosus: 59 cases. J Rheumatol 29:75–83
181. Roach BA, Hutchinson GJ (1993) Treatment of refractory, systemic lupus erythematosus-associated thrombocytopenia with intermittent low-dose intravenous cyclophosphamide. Arthritis Rheum 36:682–684

182. Roldan R, Roman J, Lopez D et al (1994) Treatment of hemolytic anemia and severe thrombocytopenia with high-dose methylprednisolone and intravenous immunoglobulins in SLE. Scand J Rheumatol 23:218–219
183. Sakamoto H, Takaoka T, Usami M et al (1985) Apheresis: clinical response to patients unresponsive to conventional therapy. Trans Am Soc Artif Intern Organs 31:704–770
184. Lateef A, Lahiri M, Teng GG et al (2010) Use of rituximab in the treatment of refractory systemic lupus erythematosus: Singapore experience. Lupus 19:765–770
185. Hakim AJ, Machin SJ, Isenberg DA (1998) Autoimmune thrombocytopenia in primary antiphospholipid syndrome and systemic lupus erythematosus: the response to splenectomy. Semin Arthritis Rheum 28:20–25
186. Saleh MN, Bussel JB, Cheng G, Meyer O, Bailey CK, Arning M et al (2013) Safety and efficacy of eltrombopag for treatment of chronic immune thrombocytopenia: results of the long-term, open-label EXTEND study. Blood 121:537–545
187. Gomard-Mennesson E, Ruivard M, Koenig M et al (2006) Treatment of isolated severe immune hemolytic anaemia associated with systemic lupus erythematosus: 26 cases. Lupus 15:223–231
188. Alba P, Karim MY, Hunt BJ (2003) Mycophenolate mofetil as a treatment for autoimmune haemolytic anaemia in patients with systemic lupus erythematosus and antiphospholipid syndrome. Lupus 12:633–635
189. Letchumanan P, Thumboo J (2011) Danazol in the treatment of systemic lupus erythematosus: a qualitative systematic review. Semin Arthritis Rheum 40:298–306
190. Abdwani R, Mani R (2009) Anti-CD20 monoclonal antibody in acute life threatening haemolytic anaemia complicating childhood onset SLE. Lupus 18:460–464
191. Nesher G, Hanna VE, Moore TL et al (1994) Thrombotic microangiographic hemolytic anemia in systemic lupus erythematosus. Semin Arthritis Rheum 24:165–172
192. Zandman-Goddard G, Levy Y, Shoenfeld Y (2005) Intravenous immunoglobulin therapy and systemic lupus erythematosus. Clin Rev Allergy Immunol 29:219–228
193. Arıcı ZS, Batu ED, Ozen S (2015) Reviewing the recommendations for lupus in children. Curr Rheumatol Rep 17:17

Innovative Therapies in Systemic Lupus Erythematosus

17

Roberta Fenoglio, Fernando Fervenza, and Dario Roccatello

Systemic lupus erythematosus (SLE) is a particularly challenging disease to study due to the broad spectrum of clinical manifestations and varying patterns of disease activity. The existing standard of care for SLE depends primarily on disease severity and has been in place for over 60 years. NSAIDS (aspirin, ibuprofen, and diclofenac) and antimalarials (hydroxychloroquine) are used in mild forms of the disease. Corticosteroids are vital in moderate to severe disease with additional immunosuppressives, such as mycophenolate mofetil (MMF), azathioprine (AZT), cyclophosphamide (CYC), and cyclosporine, being effective in severe cases of SLE. The efficacy of current SLE medications has been questioned by treatment-related adverse side effects secondary to corticosteroid use and untargeted immunosuppression and by the increasing number of patients (pts) with refractory disease. Over the last decades, there have been significant advances in the understanding of the immunopathology of SLE. A variety of novel therapeutic targets have been identified and there have been many studies in patients with SLE in an attempt to translate these new treatments into clinical practice [1] (Table 17.1).

R. Fenoglio
SCDU Nephrology and Dialysis, Giovanni Bosco Hospital,
Piazza del donatore di Sangue 3, Turin 10154, Italy
e-mail: robyfenoglio@hotmail.com

F. Fervenza (✉)
Division of Nephrology and Hypertension, Department of Internal Medicine, Mayo Clinic College of Medicine, 200 First Street SW, Rochester, MN 55905, USA
e-mail: fervenza.fernando@mayo.edu

D. Roccatello
SCDU Nephrology and Dialysis, Giovanni Bosco Hospital,
Piazza del donatore di Sangue 3, Turin 10154, Italy

Department of Rare, Immunologic, Hematologic and Immunohematologic Diseases, Center of Research of Immunopathology and Rare Diseases – Coordinating Center of Piemonte and Valle d'Aosta Network for Rare Diseases, Giovanni Bosco Hospital, University of Turin, Piazza del donatore di Sangue 3, Turin 10154, Italy
e-mail: dario.roccatello@unito.it

D. Roccatello, L. Emmi (eds.), *Connective Tissue Disease: A Comprehensive Guide-Volume 1*, Rare Diseases of the Immune System 5,
DOI 10.1007/978-3-319-24535-5_17

Table 17.1 Summary of trials in SLE immunotherapies

Molecular target	Drug name	Mechanism of action	Trials
Targeting cell surface receptors: B-cell inhibition or depletion			
Anti-CD20	Rituximab	B-cell lysis or apoptosis	Phase II/III EXPLORER and LUNAR trials
	Ocrelizumab	B-cell lysis	Phase III BELONG and BEGIN trials
Anti-CD22	Epratuzumab	B-cell apoptosis	Phase IIb EMBLEM trial
Targeting soluble mediators to inhibit B-cell growth and function			
Anti-Blys, BCMA, TACI	Belimumab	Blys inhibition blocks soluble Blys	Phase III BLISS 52 and BLISS 76
	Blisibimod	Blys inhibition blocks soluble Blys	Phase II PEARL
	Tabalumab	Blys inhibition blocks membrane-bound and soluble Blys	Phase III NCT01196091 trial
	Atacicept	Inhibition of B-cell activation	Phase II/III APRIL-SLE[a]
Co-stimulatory modulation			
CD28/CTLA4 co-ligands	Abatacept	Blockade of the co-stimulatory interaction between T and B cells	Phase III trial
CD40-CD40L	Anti-CD40L Ab	Blockade of B-cell maturation and function	IDEC-131 trial
			BG9588 trial
Anti-cytokine therapy			
Anti-IL-6 R	Tocilizumab	Inhibition of IL-6 receptor	Phase I trial
Anti-IL6	Sirukumab	Attenuation of the biological activity of IL-6	Phase I trial
			Phase II NCT01273389 trial in LN[a]
Anti-IL-10	Anti-IL-10 (B-N10)	Attenuation of the biological activity of IL-10	Pilot trial
Anti-IFN-α	Sifalimumab	Inhibition of type I IFN-induced mRNAs	Phase I trial
			NCT01283139 trial[a]
	Rontalizumab	Inhibition of type I IFN-induced mRNAs	Phase II ROSE study, randomized trial
Targeting Fcγ receptor IIB			
FcγRIIB	Anti-FcγRIIB (SM101)	Interaction with the response to immune complexes	Phase II trial[a]

Table 17.1 (continued)

Molecular target	Drug name	Mechanism of action	Trials
Anti-TWEAK			
Anti-TWEAK	BIIB023	Inhibition of renal cell proliferation and apoptosis, vascular changes, and fibrosis	Phase I trial NCT0149935[a]

[a]Trial ongoing

Biological therapy has proven to be effective in inflammatory diseases such as rheumatoid arthritis, multiple sclerosis, and inflammatory bowel disease but its efficacy in SLE is still controversial [2]. Conventional therapies including corticosteroids, azathioprine, hydroxychloroquine, cyclophosphamide, and MMF have been utilized for the treatment of SLE. However, it has been estimated that more than 50 % of pts affected by SLE have suboptimal disease control: while 40 % of them have chronic active disease, the remaining 10 % suffer from relapsing-remitting disease with frequent exacerbations [3]. This situation requires frequent changes of therapy and, in particular, increased steroid dosage [4]. High-dose corticosteroids have significantly deleterious effects that may contribute to the development of damage and, hence, long-term morbidity and premature mortality [5]. Consequently, there is a need for developing new and innovative treatment options to help improve prognosis and reduce the burden of iatrogenic morbidity.

17.1 Targets of Therapy

Disturbances of T- and B-cell functions are involved in autoimmune diseases. In particular, B lymphocytes play a pivotal role in the pathogenesis of autoimmune diseases. The main alteration of the immune system in SLE is the production of a large number of autoantibodies directed against antigens that are present in all cells. B cells also contribute to immune dysregulation by presenting antigens, regulating T-cell functions, and producing cytokines (IL-4, IL-6, IL-10) and chemokines that affect other cells of the immune system [6].

T cells have important regulatory and effector functions, both of which are abnormal in pts with SLE. Elevated levels of some cytokines, chemokines, and/or growth factors made by monocytes, macrophages, and endothelial cells also drive lupus disease activity and organ damage [2]. These include interleukin (IL)-10, IL-12, IL-6, and MCP-1, tumor necrosis factor (TNF) alpha, INF-α, INF-γ, and B-cell-activating factor (BAFF)/B-lymphocyte stimulator (BLyS) [7]. Appropriate targets for therapeutic modulation include T/B-lymphocyte signaling, inhibition of T-cell activation and B-cell activation and/or maturation, TNF-alpha inhibition, and antibodies to IFN, ILs, and anti-CD40L and CTLA4Ig (Fig. 17.1).

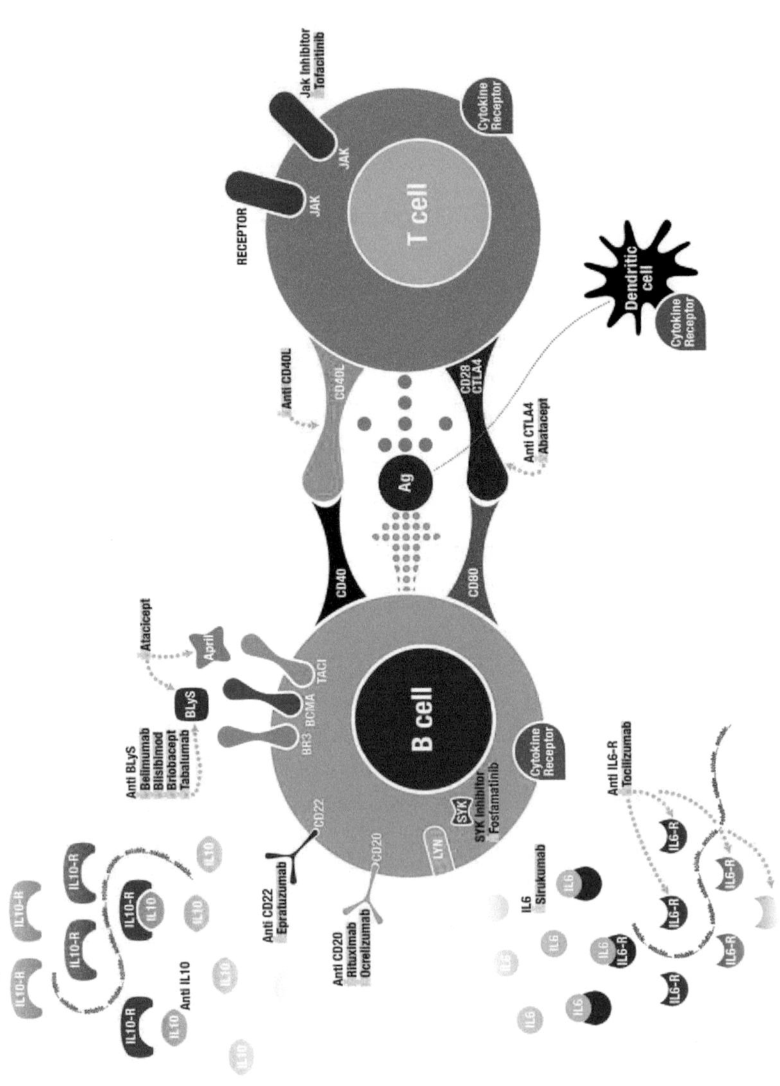

Fig. 17.1 Target of biological drugs in SLE

17.2 Targeting Cell Surface Receptors: B-Cell Inhibition or Depletion

B cells are involved in the pathogenesis of SLE and are therefore a potential therapeutic target. Current biological drugs are directed toward three main targets that are present on B lymphocytes [8]: (1) CD20, an activated-glycosylated phosphoprotein expressed on the surface of all B cells starting from the pro-B phase (CD45R+, CD117+) and progressively increasing in concentration until maturity. In humans, CD20 is encoded by the MS4A1 gene. This gene encodes a member of the membrane-spanning 4A gene family. Members of this nascent protein family are characterized by common structural features and similar intron/exon splice boundaries and display unique expression patterns within hematopoietic cells and non-lymphoid tissues. This gene encodes a B-lymphocyte surface molecule that plays a role in the development and differentiation of B cells into plasma cells. Alternative splicing of this gene results in two transcript variants that encode the same protein. The protein has no known natural ligand and its function is to enable optimal B-cell immune response, specifically against T-independent antigens. It acts as a calcium channel in the cell membrane. The drugs targeting CD20 are: rituximab, ocrelizumab, atumumab [9]. (2) CD22, a molecule belonging to the SIGLEC family of lectins. It is found on the surface of mature B cells and to a lesser extent on some immature B cells. CD22 is a sugar binding transmembrane protein which specifically binds sialic acid with an immunoglobulin (Ig) domain located at its N-terminus. The presence of Ig domains makes CD22 a member of the immunoglobulin superfamily. CD22 works as an inhibitory receptor for B-cell receptor (BCR) signaling. The drug targeting CD22 currently under evaluation is epratuzumab [10]. (3) BR3 (BlyS-receptor), B-cell maturation antigen (BCMA) and transmembrane activator and calcium modulator and cyclophilin ligand interactor (TACI). B-cell activating factor, also known as tumor necrosis factor ligand superfamily member 13B, is a protein that in humans is encoded by the TNFSF13B gene. BAFF, also known as BlyS, is expressed in B-cell lineage cells and acts as a potent B-cell activator. It has also been shown to play an important role in the proliferation and differentiation of B cells. BAFF is expressed as a membrane-bound type II transmembrane protein on various cell types including monocytes and bone marrow stromal cells. The transmembrane form can be cleaved from the membrane, thus generating a soluble protein fragment. BAFF steady-state concentrations depend on B cells and also on the expression of BAFF-binding receptors. BAFF is the natural ligand of three unusual tumor necrosis factor receptors named BAFF-R (BR3), TACI, and BCMA, all of which have differing binding affinities for it. These receptors are expressed mainly on mature B lymphocytes and their expression varies depending on B-cell maturation. TACI binds less effective than BR3 since its affinity is higher for a protein similar to BAFF, called a proliferation-inducing ligand (APRIL). BCMA displays an intermediate binding phenotype and will work with either BAFF or APRIL to varying degrees. Signaling through BAFF-R and BCMA stimulates B lymphocytes to undergo proliferation and to counter apoptosis. The drugs targeting BR3, BMCA and TACI currently available or under investigation are belimumab, atacicept [11].

17.2.1 Rituximab (Anti-CD20)

Rituximab (RTX) is a chimeric monoclonal antibody against CD20, an antigen expressed on B cells; it was used for the first time in 1997 to treat non-Hodgkin lymphomas [12]. In 2006, it was approved for the treatment of rheumatoid arthritis (RA), in combination with methotrexate for pts who were non-responsive to treatment with anti-TNF agents. The first report of the use of RTX in SLE was in 2002; since then it has been effectively used off-label in a number of pts with autoimmune diseases. RTX acts via antibody-dependent, cell-mediated cytotoxicity and complement-dependent cytotoxicity and apoptosis to effectively deplete B cells for 6–9 months in over 80 % of pts [13]. Re-population of B cells, which typically occurs 6–9 months after RTX administration, predominantly involves a subset of naïve or antigenically inexperienced transitional B cells similar to what occurs after bone marrow transplantation [14]. The removal of memory B cells by RTX and the reconstitution of a population of naïve transitional cells assign a strong role to this biological agent in the treatment of SLE [15]. Early case reports followed by case series suggested some benefit in the treatment of SLE [16]. Two randomized double-blind, placebo-controlled trials (EXPLORER and LUNAR) were designed to objectively assess the efficacy and safety of RTX. However, despite expectations, neither trial achieved the primary goal [17]. The EXPLORER trial recruited 257 pts with moderate to severe SLE who met four of the American College of Rheumatology (ACR) criteria for SLE including testing positive for antinuclear antibodies, active disease at screening, and stable use of one immunosuppressive drug at entry which was continued during the study (methotrexate, azathioprine, or MMF). Pts received intravenous placebo or RTX 1 gr on days 1,15,168, and 182. Major clinical response was 15.9 versus 12.4 % and partial clinical response was 12.5 versus 17.2 % for the placebo and RTX groups, respectively. The RTX group showed a significant improvement in anti-dsDNA and complement levels. The main flaws in this trial were study design and pt background. For instance, concomitant use of corticosteroids and immunosuppressants may have masked the benefits of RTX. The total follow-up duration was only 52 weeks. Furthermore, most of the open-label trial studies were conducted in pts with very active disease who failed conventional therapy, whereas pts in the EXPLORER trial may have had less active disease. A post hoc analysis of this trial suggested that RTX reduced the risk of severe flares and lowered mean severe flare rates [18].

The LUNAR trial was performed in pts with active proliferative lupus nephritis (LN) (class III or IV and urine protein to creatinine ratio >1). The trial compared RTX therapy (1 gr on days 1, 15, 168, and 182 days) versus placebo when added to a background of steroids and MMF. A total of 144 pts were randomized to receive treatment or placebo. At week 52 there were no differences in the RTX arm versus the standard of therapy, although there were more responders in the RTX group (57 % vs 46 % in the placebo group). Improvement in anti-dsDNA and complement levels was more marked in RTX-treated pts. Like the EXPLORER trial, African Americans showed a trend of better response compared to Caucasians [19]. However, when the data was evaluated at 78-weeks follow-up, there were significant differences in favor of RTX regarding the proportion of pts who achieved proteinuric remission or required additional immunosuppression [20].

Despite the failure of the randomized controlled trials to achieve their primary endpoint, many clinicians continue to use rituximab in daily practice, based on their personal experience, the long-term outcome data in the LUNAR trial, and large case series showing success in patients with refractory disease. A review [12] published in 2009 evaluated the clinical efficacy of RTX in 188 pts with refractory SLE included in 35 studies. Clinical response was reported in 91 % of the RTX-treated pts. The most common indication was LN, followed by articular, mucocutaneous, and hematological disease. RTX was used in conjunction with glucocorticoids in all pts, and 22 % of them were treated with intravenous pulse methylprednisolone and cyclophosphamide. Another systematic review summarized 26 published reports (300 pts) regarding the efficacy of RTX in refractory LN [21]. A European registry study [22] evaluated 164 pts with LN treated with RTX, glucocorticoids, and cyclophosphamide or MMF. At 1 year, complete and partial clinical response was observed in 30 % and 37 % of the pts, respectively. A higher response rate was found in pts with class III or mixed types of LN compared to class IV or pure class V lupus nephritis. Similarly, Hickman et al. documented the clinical and immunological responses of 15 heterogeneous pts who received RTX for drug refractory SLE. This study showed that repeated courses of RTX appear safe and effective in inducing prolonged remission in pts with severe, refractory lupus disease allowing a significant reduction of corticosteroids [23]. In another study, 54 patients with active LN received three methylprednisolone pulses followed by oral prednisone and RTX 1 g at days 3 and 18 (17 patients) or MMF 2–2.5 g/day (17 patients) or six CYC pulses (0.5 g every fortnight) (20 patients). At 4 months MMF, AZA or cyclosporine was associated to prednisone as a consolidation/maintenance therapy in all groups. At 12 months, complete remission was present in 70.6 % of patients on RTX, in 52.9 % on MMF, and in 65 % on CYC. Partial remission was reached in 29.4 % on RTX, 41.2 % on MMF, and 25 % on CYC [24].

The RING study (RTX for Lupus Nephritis with Remission as a Goal, NCT01673295), an ongoing trial led by Houssiau and colleagues, is aiming to evaluate the addition of rituximab in patients who have had 6 months of standard of care but failed to achieve a complete remission. This trial will formally assess whether rituximab is effective in refractory LN.

An alternative way of using rituximab, that has been defined "instead of" drug rather than an "add-on," opted to omit oral steroids. A single-center observational cohort study was performed on 50 consecutive patients with biopsy-proven LN, not on oral steroids and who were treated with methylprednisolone (500 mg) and rituximab (1 g) on days 1 and 15 and followed by MMF as maintenance and no oral steroids [25]. Fifty-two percent of patients achieved complete renal remission at 1 year; there were few extrarenal flares; and of the 45 patients who stayed on the regimen, only 2 required longer than 2 weeks of oral steroids over a median follow-up of 163 weeks. This work is now being taken forward in a large, open-labeled, randomized, controlled, multicenter trial (the RITUXILUP trial, NCT01773636 at www.clinicaltrials.gov). It is designed as a non-inferiority trial to demonstrate that the RITUXILUP regimen is not inferior in inducing CR at 1 year compared to standard of care with methylprednisolone, MMF, and tapering oral steroids. The estimated completion date is 2018.

A different approach to minimize the long-term effects not only of corticosteroids but also of the immunosuppressive drugs used for remission maintenance was based on the use of a regimen of intensified B-lymphocyte depletion (IBLD). It consisted of rituximab 375 mg/sm on days 1, 8, 15, and 22 and 2 more doses after 1 and 2 months, associated with 2 IV administrations of 10 mg/kg of cyclophosphamide and three infusions of methylprednisolone (15 mg/kg) followed by oral prednisone (0.8 mg/die, rapidly tapered to 5 mg/day in 10 weeks). No further immunosuppressive maintenance therapy has been given. This regimen has been initially employed as a rescue therapy in refractory LN [26].

Presently, in a 4-year observation period, 12 SLE pts with multiorgan involvement including class IV or III/V (ISN/RPS) glomerulonephritis have been treated. IBLD obtained a complete depletion of CD20+ BL for 12–18 months. Patients had been followed up for 49 months. Significant decreases were found in the levels of ESR, anti-dsDNA antibodies, and proteinuria. C4 values significantly increased. Three patients relapsed after 36, 41, and 72 months, respectively, and all achieved complete remission after retreatment. These data suggest a promising role of RTX protocols of "intensified induction therapy" in selected patients for whom avoiding immunosuppressive maintenance therapy is particularly appealing [27].

17.2.2 Adverse Effects of RTX Therapy

In the EXPLORER study [18], the rates of adverse effects (AEs) or severe adverse effects (SAEs) were similar between the RTX and placebo groups of pts. Infusion reactions (starting from the third infusion) and neutropenia were more common in RTX users. The rates of severe infections were not significantly higher in RTX-treated pts. Although the LUNAR study [19] reported similar SAE and AE rates in the rituximab and placebo groups, neutropenia, leukopenia, hypotension, infusion-related reactions, herpes zoster, and opportunistic infections occurred more frequently in RTX-treated pts. Data from the French registry [28] revealed that 13 % of SLE pts developed infusion-related reactions to the drug that were severe in 12 % and with delayed onset in 29 %. Serum sickness-like reactions occurred in 4 % of pts and severe infections were observed in 9 % of pts. Data from rheumatoid arthritis registries reported an association between repeated infusion of RTX and hypogammaglobulinemia [29]. Since pts with SLE are usually more immunocompromised than RA pts, RTX-induced hypogammaglobulinemia may be a serious concern [23] Progressive multifocal leukoencephalopathy (PML) is a rare, progressive and typically fatal demyelinating disease of the central nervous system caused by the JC virus. The literature reports 50 cases of PML in rheumatic diseases. Because of the high frequency in SLE, PML should be suspected in any patient who presents with new-onset neurological symptoms [30].

17.2.3 Ocrelizumab (Anti-CD20)

Another anti-CD20 monoclonal antibody, ocrelizumab, was studied in LN, with a background of MMF or EUROLUPUS regimen, but the trial (BELONG study) was discontinued early due to an imbalance in the rate of SAEs in pts treated with ocrelizumab and MMF [2]. In a subgroup analysis, there was a greater treatment effect of ocrelizumab when combined with the EUROLUPUS regimen [31]. It has not been studied further.

17.2.4 Epratuzumab (Anti-CD22)

Epratuzumab is a humanized monoclonal antibody targeting CD22, a transmembrane protein expressed on mature B cells that influences their migration and activation [32]. Epratuzumab is able to reduce CD22 while minimizes B-cell destruction and impact on the immune system. Indeed, epratuzumab eliminates up to 45 % of circulating B cells while rituximab eliminates >90 % of B cells. Epratuzumab has shown therapeutic potential in SLE presumably by modulating the proliferation and trafficking of activated B cells [33]. Rossi et al. showed that the mechanism of action of epratuzumab on B cells is twofold: one via binding to CD22, which also occurs with F(ab)2, and the other via engagement of FcγR-bearing effector cells. It also induces a marked decrease of CD22 (>80 %), CD19 (>50 %), CD21 (>50 %), and CD79b (>30 %), on the B-cell surface in peripheral blood mononuclear cells obtained from normal controls or SLE patients. The other mechanism of action of epratuzumab is trogocytosis which is Fc dependent and causes the transfer of epratuzumab opsonized B cells to FcγR-expressing monocytes, natural killer cells, and granulocytes. Epratuzumab also induces moderate antibody-dependent cellular cytotoxicity without complement-dependent cytotoxicity and this may explain the absence of infusion-related reactions in humans. The pronounced and persistent loss of CD22 on B cells by epratuzumab-mediated internalization and trogocytosis is expected to make B cells less active and less viable, and the accompanying decrease of CD19 could further enhance this effect [34]. Nearly all of the published studies on epratuzumab as an additive to the traditional treatment in moderate to severe SLE patients reported an improvement in disease activity after the first cycle of therapy. The benefits were persistent in pts who were maintained on regular epratuzumab administration every 12 weeks, as in the SL0006 trial [35]. The first trial involving SLE patients was carried out by Dorner et al. in 2006 [32]. It was a phase II, open-label, single-center study. All pts received 360 mg/m^2 epratuzumab intravenously every 2 weeks for a total of four doses in the absence of additional corticosteroid or immunosuppressive therapies. Both outcome and safety profile were good. A total of 14 pts with moderate disease activity were enrolled in this study. Results were sufficiently promising to support further drug development. ALLEVIATE 1 and ALLEVIATE 2 were two randomized, double-blind, controlled trials assessing the efficacy of epratuzumab (360 mg/m^2 or 720 mg/m^2 or placebo) in addition to standard of care therapies in severe SLE pts assessed by BILAG scores [36]. Total BILAG scores were lower in both epratuzumab arms versus placebo at week 48. The treatment also allowed for a reduction in steroid use, suggesting a significant clinical benefit. A follow-up study noted that pts in the treatment arm maintained both amelioration of the disease and improved health-related quality of life scores over approximately 4 years [37]. Thus, these encouraging results led to the development of the EMBODY 1 trial, a large ongoing-phase III, double-blind randomized placebo-controlled trial to further evaluate the long-term efficacy of epratuzumab [38].

17.3 Targeting Soluble Mediators to Inhibit B-Cell Growth and Function

The BAFF axis comprises two ligands (BAFF and APRIL) and three receptors (BCMA, TACI, BR3) [39]. BAFF is a vital B-cell survival factor and overexpression of BAFF in both mice and humans is associated with SLE. The anti-BAFF monoclonal antibody (mAb), belimumab, was recently approved for the treatment of adult SLE pts, and additional BAFF antagonists (blisibimod, tabalumab, atacicept, bribacept) are presently being evaluated in SLE pts in phase III trials [40].

17.3.1 Belimumab

Belimumab is a human immunoglobulin (Ig)-G1λ monoclonal antibody which blocks the binding of the soluble form of the cytokine BLyS, also known as B-cell activating factor, to the TACI receptor, BCMA receptor, and BAFF receptor 3 (BR3) on B cells and thus interrupts the B-cell survival role of BLyS [41]. As a result, it has been deduced that the inhibition of BAFF/BLyS by belimumab has therapeutic implications in SLE. In 2011, belimumab was licensed as an add-on biological agent to standard therapy for pts with SLE, excluding those with active LN and CNS involvement. Belimumab is administered on a weight-based dosing schedule, i.e., 10 mg/kg, as an hour-long intravenous infusion fortnightly for three infusions and then monthly thereafter. Two phase III trials – BLISS-52 and BLISS-76 – demonstrated that a significantly greater proportion of pts responded to belimumab plus standard SLE therapy than to placebo plus standard therapy [42, 43]. The studies included 865 and 826 pts, respectively. In each of these trials, pts were randomized to receive 10 mg/kg belimumab, 1 mg/kg belimumab, or placebo. Pts were given the drug intravenously on days 0, 14, and 28 and then every 28 days thereafter for the duration of the study. The primary efficacy endpoint was the composite responder index (SRI) at week 52: belimumab achieved significantly better results than placebo in both studies. In addition, the drug significantly delayed time to disease flare and led to a significant reduction in steroid dosage.

The BLISS trials were not designed to specifically assess the effects of belimumab on renal parameters. Pts with severe active lupus nephritis were excluded from these studies, including those with proteinuria (Pto) >6 g/24 h or serum creatinine (Crs) >2.5 mg/dl and those who required dialysis or high doses of prednisone within 90 days of study initiation. A post hoc pooled analysis was conducted to derive information about the potential effect of belimumab on renal parameters and in pts who were receiving MMF therapy at baseline. More pts receiving belimumab with renal involvement at baseline showed renal improvement at week 52 than controls [44]. Data from this pooled analysis suggest that belimumab may provide additional benefits to pts receiving MMF therapy with baseline SELENA-SLEDAI renal involvement, including an improvement of renal biomarkers, and that it may be useful in pts who have shown improvement with standard therapy, including MMF, but continue to have some degree of renal abnormality. The limitations of this analysis include the small number of pts and the post hoc nature of this analysis.

Pts treated with belimumab have increased susceptibility to infection, the most common being pharyngitis, bronchitis, cystitis, and viral gastroenteritis. In clinical trials, severe infections have been reported in 6 % of belimumab-treated pts as compared to 5.2 % in placebo controls [41]. The susceptibility to infection after belimumab treatment may be a consequence of alterations in the signaling pathways involving BAFF/BLys and the TACI receptor. TACI plays a complex role in host immunity involving the activation of B cells and T-cell-independent immune regulation [45]. It has been postulated that the post-belimumab low BAFF/BLys levels result in a reduction in TACI signaling, lowering host immunity against pathogens such as polysaccharide-encapsulated bacteria.

A recent Italian study [4] evaluated the efficacy and safety in the real-life experience of a single center after the first year of licensed use in Italy. The study group was made up of 18 SLE pts with active disease despite standard therapy; they received belimumab (10 mg/kg) in addition to their current treatment. The authors noticed a significant reduction in SLEDAI scores after 3 months of treatment, followed by a significant decrease in steroid intake after 9 months of treatment, thus suggesting that the effects of belimumab can be seen over time for disease activity control and steroid sparing at different time points. Changes in serology were not found possibly due to the fact that nearly half the pts had low titers of anti-dsDNA and/or slightly reduced complement at the start of the treatment. Long-term follow-up is needed to evaluate the true effects of the drug in terms of clinical stabilization, improvement of laboratory parameters, lack of chronic damage accrual, and stable reduction of steroid intake.

Taken together, these results highlight the efficacy and tolerability of belimumab as a novel biologic for the treatment of SLE. It would be useful to investigate the efficacy of this drug in specific subpopulations in future trials. Additionally, comparing belimumab to current therapies would also be useful to determine how best to prescribe the treatment (induction and maintenance [46]), in order to determine which pts are most likely to benefit from this therapy.

17.3.2 Blisibimod

Blisibimod is a fusion protein consisting of four BAFF-binding domains fused to the N-terminus of the fragment crystallizable region (Fc) of a human antibody. A recent phase II clinical trial (PEARL-SC) [47] showed that high-dose blisibimod (200 mg once weekly) produced significantly higher responder rates compared to placebo in patients with a ≥8 point reduction in SLEDAI. Similarly, patients with severe SLE at baseline (SLEDAI ≥10 and on corticosteroid treatment) showed even greater benefits, with 41.7 % of responders achieving a ≥8 SLEDAI point decrease in the high-dose blisibimod group compared to placebo. These results were associated with a significant decrease in anti-ds DNA and an increase in C3/C4 in the blisibimod arm compared to placebo – which was still sustained after 6 months. On the basis of this trial, the efficacy and tolerability of blisibimod administration (one subcutaneous injection weekly for 1 year) together with standard of care therapies as compared to placebo are being assessed in patients with highly active and refractory SLE [48].

17.3.3 Tabalumab

Tabalumab is a human IgG4 monoclonal antibody targeting membrane-bound and soluble BAFF. A phase III, multicenter, randomized, double-blind, placebo-controlled study to evaluate the efficacy and safety of subcutaneous tabalumab in SLE pts was expected to be completed in May 2015. In addition to standard of care therapy pts with active SLE are randomized to receive high dose (120 mg subcutaneous injection every fortnight for 1 year), low dose (alternating placebo and tabalumab 120 mg subcutaneous injection every fortnight for 1 year), or placebo [1].

17.3.4 Atacicept (TACI-Ig Fusion Protein)

Atacicept is a recombinant fusion protein containing both human IgG and the extracellular section of the B-cell surface receptor TACI. Thus, it is able to inhibit activation of the TACI receptor by both APRIL and BLyS. A landmark study [49] in a murine lupus model established that low (20 μg) and high (100 μg) TACI-Ig infusions in SLE mice resulted in a significant attenuation of proteinuria in a dose-dependent manner. Similarly, atacicept resulted in significantly lower mortality rates with 100 % survival among mice in the high-dose treatment arm compared to only 47 % survival in the control arm. A previous phase I, randomized, placebo-controlled double-blind trial showed that atacicept resulted in a 45–60 % attenuation in mature B cells as well as significant dose-dependent decreases in autoantibody levels compared to placebo [50]. There were no significant differences in the number and severity of adverse events between intervention and placebo arms of the trial. The results from murine studies and this phase I trial are now been followed by a phase II/III study (APRIL-SLE) testing the efficacy of TACI-Ig compared to placebo in ameliorating disease severity in SLE [48].

17.3.5 Briobacept (BR3-Fc)

Briobacept is a protein containing both IgG and the ligand-binding section of the BAFF-R that inhibits BLyS and thus induces B-cell apoptosis. In a SLE mice model,

Kayagaki et al. demonstrated that three weekly infusion of 100 μg briobacept for 5 weeks was effective at inhibiting dsDNA autoantibody formation [51]. Mice treated with briobacept had 100 % survival at about 6 months posttreatment compared to 40 % survival among the control mice. Furthermore, briobacept significantly ameliorated nephritis, and at 40 weeks none of the mice had significant proteinuria. These promising results warrant further investigation in randomized human SLE studies [52].

17.4 Blockade of T-Cell Co-stimulation

17.4.1 Abatacept (CTLA-4Ig Fusion Protein)

Blockade of the co-stimulatory interactions between T and B cells can induce immunological tolerance. The most well-characterized T-lymphocyte co-stimulatory ligand is CD28, a glycoprotein which interacts with the co-stimulatory receptors B7-1 (CD80) and B7-2 (CD86). CTLA4 (cytotoxic T-lymphocyte antigen) is expressed on activated T cells and interacts with B7 with higher affinity than CD28 resulting in a negative feedback mechanism that inhibits T-cell activation [1]. Abatacept is a fusion protein composed of the Fc region of the immunoglobulin IgG1 fused to the extracellular domain of CTLA-4. It binds to the CD80 and CD86 molecule preventing T-cell activation. Abatacept has demonstrated efficacy in both rheumatoid arthritis and psoriatic arthritis, and earlier studies have presented evidence of efficacy in SLE. Combination therapy with CTLA4Ig and cyclophosphamide significantly reduces proteinuria and autoantibody titers and improves mortality in murine LN [53]. However, a recent randomized double-blind trial failed to show a reduction in the proportion of pts with a new SLE flare [54]. There were, however, some improvements in quality of life. A phase II/III trial in proliferative LN failed to meet the primary endpoint of time to complete renal response, defined as a glomerular filtration rate within 10 % of the pre-flare/screening value, urinary protein/creatinine ratio <0.26 mg/mg, and inactive urinary sediment at 12 months [55]. However, when the same data were analyzed using different outcome measures, the study showed positive data in favor of abatacept pointing to the need to find appropriate definitions of response and trial design when evaluating novel therapies in LN [56]. Currently, abatacept remains an off-label therapeutic option.

17.4.2 Anti-CD40 Ligand

CD40L, also called CD154, is a protein that is primarily expressed on activated T cells and is a member of the TNF superfamily of molecules. It binds to CD40 on antigen-presenting cells (APC), which leads to several effects depending on the target cell type. Altogether, CD40L has three binding partners: CD40, $\alpha 5\beta 1$integrin, and $\alpha IIb\beta 3$. CD154 acts as a co-stimulatory molecule and is particularly important on a subset of T cells called T follicular helper cells (TFH cells). CD154 promotes B-cell maturation by engaging CD40 on the B-cell surface facilitating cell-cell communication. CD40L is over-expressed in murine lupus models, and monoclonal antibodies against CD40L are effective in treating murine LN. There have been two clinical trials of humanized anti-CD40L monoclonal antibodies (IDEC-131 and BG9588) in SLE pts. The first study failed to demonstrate clinical improvement as compared to placebo at 20 weeks [57]. The second trial showed initial promise with reduced anti-dsDNA titers and increasing complement levels, but was discontinued prematurely due to unexpected thromboembolic side effects [58]. Given the lack of efficacy and the toxicity demonstrated in these studies, it is unlikely that anti-CD40L will progress to larger clinical trials in SLE pts [1].

17.5 Cytokine Therapies

17.5.1 Tocilizumab (Interleukin-6 Receptor Inhibitor)

IL-6 is a pleiotropic cytokine with both proinflammatory and anti-inflammatory properties and it has been implicated in LN pathogenesis. In lupus mouse models, exogenous IL-6 increases autoantibody production and accelerates nephritis progression. In SLE pts, IL-6 levels have been shown to correlate with clinical activity and anti-dsDNA antibody levels. Urinary IL-6 excretion is increased in pts with active SLE nephritis and decreases after treatment [59]. Tocilizumab is a fully humanized monoclonal antibody against the IL-6 receptors that prevents binding of IL-6 to both membrane-bound and soluble IL-6 receptors [1]. A phase I dose finding study [60] evaluated 16 pts with moderately active disease who received tocilizumab (2–4–8 mg/kg) twice weekly for 3 months. The drug led to a reduction in inflammatory markers of disease activity and autoantibody levels, while proteinuria remained unchanged. The majority of pts developed dose-related neutropenia, and high rates of infections were recorded. Results of randomized trials of tocilizumab in SLE are upcoming.

17.5.2 Sirukumab

Sirukumab is a human, anti-IL-6 monoclonal antibody that binds to IL-6 with affinity and specificity. It inhibits IL-6-mediated STAT-3 phosphorylation and thus attenuates the biological activity of IL-6. Sirukumab has been tested in a phase I, double-blind, placebo-controlled study to evaluate the safety and pharmacokinetics of multiple intravenous infusions in 31 pts with cutaneous lupus erythematosus (CLE) and 15 pts with systemic lupus erythematosus (SLE) [61]. The drug was generally well tolerated in both CLE and SLE pts with mild, stable, or active disease. No clinically relevant changes from baseline were observed in the overall scores; the treatment group showed a tendency to improve in the BILAG musculoskeletal domain. However, due to the limited sample size, duration of therapy, exploratory nature, and the fact that the study was not designed to evaluate efficacy, the results should be interpreted cautiously. A phase II study testing the efficacy of sirukumab in LN is currently being conducted (NCT01273389).

17.5.3 Anti-IL-10 Antibody

Several studies have confirmed the presence of increased levels of IL-10 in SLE pts. While IL-10 promotes the proliferation of B cells, it is also capable of reducing proinflammatory responses [62]. Despite the uncertainty of the effects of antagonizing IL-10 in human SLE, a small study was performed with a follow-up period of 6 months [63]. Joint symptoms and cutaneous lesions improved in all pts and that persisted for 6 months. The need for prednisone was significantly reduced by month 6. To date, there have been no further clinical trials to evaluate the potential efficacy of this therapy in SLE.

17.6 Targeting Interferon (IFN)-α

Microarray gene expression analysis has shown widespread activation of IFN-inducible genes in SLE pts that correlates with disease activity [64]. In addition, IFN pathway activation has been associated with LN activity.

17.6.1 Sifalimumab

Sifalimumab, a fully human anti-IFN-α monoclonal antibody, induced a dose-dependent inhibition of type I IFN-induced mRNAs in whole blood in a phase I study. No increase in viral infections was observed, and a general trend toward improvement in disease activity was seen [65]. Further studies examining the efficacy of sifalimumab in SLE are currently ongoing (NCT01283139).

17.6.2 Rontalizumab

Rontalizumab is a recombinant humanized monoclonal antibody to IFN-α. The efficacy and safety of rontalizumab were assessed in a phase II trial in adults with moderate to severe, nonrenal SLE [66]. Overall, response rates at 24 weeks were similar for rontalizumab and placebo. However, rontalizumab was more effective at reducing lupus disease activity in pts taking >10 mg/kg of steroids daily. A further analysis showed a greater benefit in pts who had a low IFN-α signature (type I IFN-induced mRNAs) suggesting that higher antibody doses may be required to attenuate IFN-α activity in pts with high gene signature [67].

17.7 Complement Therapies: Eculizumab

The complement system plays a significant role in SLE [68]. Early components of the complement cascade are critical in the clearance of immune complexes and apoptotic material. Activation of terminal complement components is associated with exacerbations of disease [69]. Eculizumab is a recombinant humanized monoclonal IgG2/4 antibody that specifically binds to the terminal complement component 5, or C5, and inhibits the cleavage of C5 to C5a (a potent anaphylatoxin with prothrombotic and proinflammatory properties) and C5b by the C5 convertase, thus preventing the generation of the terminal complement complex C5b-9 [70]. It is conceivable that in LN, eculizumab might prevent direct complement-mediated injury to intrinsic glomerular cells and attenuate kidney inflammation by reducing renal leukocyte recruitment. Wang at al. studied [71] the contribution of activated terminal complement components to the inflammatory processes in the pathogenesis of glomerulonephritis in C5 sufficient NZB/W F1 mice using a mAb specific for murine C5. Treatment with an antimurine C5 mAb results in marked amelioration of the course of renal disease and in dramatic prolongation of survival. These data point toward an important role for the complement system in LN models. Disappointedly, a phase I trial of eculizumab in SLE showed safety and tolerability, but no clinical benefit [72]. To date, there have been no further clinical trials studying the potential role of eculizumab in SLE.

17.8 Targeting Fcγ Receptor IIB

Receptors for the Fc domains of IgG (Fcγ R) play a critical role in linking humoral and cellular immune responses [73]. The various Fcγ R genes may contribute to differences in infectious and immune-related diseases in various ethnic populations. Polymorphisms of Fcγ R have been identified as genetic factors influencing susceptibility to disease or disease course in autoimmune diseases. In SLE, activated and inhibitory Fcγ Rs play a role in the pathogenesis of SLE, the initiation of autoimmunity, development of inflammatory lesions, and immune clearance mechanisms [74]. Modulating Fcγ receptor signaling is a potential candidate for immunotherapy. In murine lupus model, treatment with recombinant soluble FcγRIIB significantly delayed the onset of proteinuria, reduced histopathological findings, and improved survival. Presently, a soluble FcγRIIB (SM101) is being tested in a phase II trial in SLE [1].

17.9 Anti-TWEAK

The cytokine tumor necrosis factor (TNF)-like weak inducer of apoptosis (TWEAK, TNFSF12) is a member of the TNF superfamily that is prominently featured in normal and pathological remodeling of tissues. TWEAK, which is expressed primarily as a soluble cytokine by infiltrating leukocytes, mediates multiple activities through its receptor FGF-inducible molecule 14 (Fn14, TNFRSF12) which is upregulated locally on epithelial and mesenchymal cell types in injured and diseased target tissues including the kidney [75]. The role of TWEAK in promoting inflammatory response, renal cell proliferation and apoptosis, vascular changes, and fibrosis, together with an increasing appreciation for the locally elevated levels of TWEAK in LN patients, suggests that TWEAK may play an active role in the kidney in the context of LN. BIIB023 is a monoclonal antibody against TWEAK that is currently undergoing clinical development for the treatment of LN. To date, BIIB023 has completed a phase I double-blind, placebo-controlled, single-dose study in subjects with rheumatoid arthritis [76]. BIIB023 treatment was well tolerated across all dose groups in this study. No dose-dependent safety findings were observed in any of the dose groups. In addition, there was no increase in infection rate associated with the use of BIIB023 in this study. BIIB023 is currently being tested for the treatment of LN in the ATLAS Study. The primary aim of this study is to evaluate the efficacy of BIIB023 in patients with active LN as an add-on after initial therapy with standard of care in order to induce a complete or partial renal response as assessed by proteinuria and renal function in subjects with ISN/RPS class III or IV LN. Secondary objectives include assessment of the effect of BIIB023 on renal histopathology, the effect of BIIB023 on extrarenal SLE disease activity/manifestations, and the PK and immunogenicity of BIIB023 (clinical trial NCT01499355).

17.10 Janus Kinase (JAK) and Spleen Tyrosine Kinase (Syk) Inhibitors

17.10.1 Tofacitinib (JAK Inhibitor)

Cytokines are key mediators of the development and homeostasis of hematopoietic cells that are critical for host defense but also for the development of autoimmune and inflammatory diseases. In a subgroup of cytokines, signaling requires association with a family of cytoplasmic protein tyrosine kinases known as JAK. JAKs have recently attracted significant attention as therapeutic targets in inflammation and autoimmunity, and a selective Jak inhibitor, tofacitinib, has been developed [77]. Targeting JAKs in pts with SLE awaits future studies.

17.10.2 Fostamatinib (SyK Inhibitor)

The non-receptor tyrosine kinase, spleen tyrosine kinase (Syk), is primarily expressed in hematopoietic cells and appears to be particularly important in B cells. Syk is involved in signal transduction processes and appears to regulate allergic, inflammatory, and autoimmune responses. Inhibitors of Syk are potentially useful in treating rheumatoid arthritis, lupus, and hematological disorders [78]. SyK inhibitors have been shown to prevent the development of renal disease and to treat established murine LN. These data suggest that Syk inhibitors may be of therapeutic benefit in human lupus and related disorders [79]. Fosfamatinib is a Syk inhibitor being evaluated for the management of autoimmune rheumatic diseases [80].

17.11 Anti-inflammatory Therapies

Anti-inflammatory drugs with the potential to be more effective than current therapies, e.g., corticosteroids, are also available [81].

17.11.1 Laquinimod

Laquinimod is a small-molecule derivative of quinolone-3-carboxamide. It has been studied extensively as therapy for multiple sclerosis and a phase II trial in LN and lupus arthritis has just been completed (www.clinicaltrials.gov). In experimental autoimmune encephalitis, laquinimod behaves like an anti-inflammatory agent, decreasing infiltration of the central nervous system by monocytes and reducing proinflammatory cytokine and transcription factor expression, such as MCP-1 (monocyte protein 1) and NF-κB (nuclear factor-κB), respectively [82]. Laquinimod also appears to modulate the inflammatory environment by polarizing T cells toward Tregs and away from TH1 and TH17 phenotypes [83]. Laquinimod may also have a role in modulating autoimmunity as it suppresses major histocompatibility class II antigen presentation and downregulates epitope spreading as well.

17.11.2 Synthetic Retinoids

Small-molecule synthetic retinoids that are ligands for α/β-retinoic acid receptors alone have been used to treat experimental autoimmune uvo-retinitis and experimental autoimmune encephalitis [84, 85]. A trial of one such agent, tamibarotene, is planned in SLE (clinical trial NCT01226147). In experimental inflammatory diseases, retinoid AM80 increased gene expression of an NF-κB repression factor. It may also increase Tregs and decrease T_H17 cells.

17.12 Proteasome Inhibitor: Bortezomib

Proteasomes are large protein complexes located in the nucleus and cytoplasm that degrade abnormal and misfolded proteins – a function that is crucial for the control of the cell cycle, the regulation of gene expression, and overall cell homeostasis. The catalytic subunits that can be found in the immunoproteasome differ from those in the proteasome. The immunoproteasome is constitutively expressed in immune cells, but its expression in other tissues can be induced by inflammatory cytokines such as IFN-γ. Its specific role is to generate peptides that can be presented by major histocompatibility complex class I (MHC-I) molecules [86]. Proteasome inhibitor is a promising therapeutic approach for targeting long-lived plasma cells (PCs) [87]. In SLE, autoantibodies produced by long-lived plasma cells are major players in disease pathogenesis. Bortezomib administration in a lupus mouse model resulted in a significant reduction of both short- and long-lived plasma cells in the spleen and bone marrow (BM), and it was much more efficient in depleting BM total and long-lived plasma cells compared to cyclophosphamide or dexamethasone. Of note, the anti-dsDNA antibody titers were significantly decreased [88]. These observations were supported by other reports [89]. The treatment with bortezomib was not associated with overt toxicity or severe immunosuppression. Interestingly, evaluation of renal biopsies of mice treated with bortezomib showed that besides eliminating anti-dsDNA antibody-secreting plasma cells, bortezomib also exerted a protective effect on podocyte ultrastructure [90]. Alexander et al. reported the clinical features and the serological response of 13 pts treated with bortezomib [91]. Treatment was generally well tolerated. Disease activity and anti-dsDNA antibody titers decreased in all 13 patients. Patients with active LN experienced a decrease in proteinuria within 6 weeks of treatment and an increase in complement levels. Thus, preliminary data shows promise for the use of proteasome inhibitors in pts resistant to conventional therapies but further studies are needed.

References

1. Jordan N, Lutalo PMK, D'Cruz D (2013) Novel therapeutic agents in clinical development for systemic lupus erythematosus. BMC J 11:120–130
2. Gottenberg J-E, Lorenzo N, Sordet C, Theulin A, Chatelus E, Sibilia J (2014) When biologics should be used in systemic lupus erythematosus? Presse Med 43:e181–e185
3. Ginzler EM, Moldovan I (2004) Systemic lupus erythematosus trials: successes and issues. Curr Opin Rheumatol 16:499–504
4. Andreoli L, Reggia R, Pea L, Frassi M, Zanola A, Cartella S, Franceschini F, Tincani A (2014) Belimumab for the treatment of refractory systemic lupus erythematosus: real-life experience in the first year of use in 18 Italian patients. IMAJ 16:651–653
5. Zonana-Nacach A, Barr SG, Magder LS, Petri M (2000) Damage in systemic lupus erythematosus and its association with corticosteroids. Arthritis Rheum 43:1801–1808
6. Dorner T, Radbruch A, Gerd R, Burmester GR (2009) B-cell-direct therapies for autoimmune disease. Nat Rev Rheumatol 5:433–441
7. Schiffer L, Bethunaickan R, Ramanujam M et al (2008) Activated renal macrophages are markers of disease onset and disease remission in lupus nephritis. J Immunol 180:1938–1947
8. Doria A, Iaccarino L (2013) Terapia del LES. Ital J Public Health 2(1):37–53
9. Cragg MS, Walshe CA, Ivanov AO, Glennie MJ (2005) The biology of CD20 and its potential as a target for mAb therapy. Curr Dir Autoimmune 8:140–174
10. Harvey PR, Gordon C (2013) B-cell targeted therapies in systemic lupus erythematosus: successes and challenges. BioDrugs 27(2):85–95
11. Zhou T, Zhang J, Carter R, Kimberly R (2003) BLyS and B cell autoimmunity. Curr Dir Autoimmun 6:21–37
12. Ramos-Casals M, Soto MJ, Cuadrado MJ, Khamashta MA (2009) Rituximab in systemic lupus erythematosus: a systematic review of off-label use in 188 cases. Lupus 18(9):767–776
13. Anolik JH et al (2003) The relationship of FcgammaRIIIa genotype to degree of B cell depletion by rituximab in the treatment of systemic lupus erythematosus. Arthritis Rheum 48:455–459
14. Leandro MJ, Cooper N, Cambridge G et al (2007) Bone marrow B lineage cells in patients with rheumatoid arthritis following rituximab therapy. Rheumatology 46:29–36
15. Beckwith H, Lightstone L (2014) Rituximab in systemic lupus erythematosus and lupus nephritis. Nephron Clin Pract 128:250–254

16. Favas C, Isenberg DA (2009) B-cell-depletion therapy in SLE – what are the current prospects for its acceptance? Nat Rev Rheumatol 5:711–716
17. Merrill JT, Neuwelt CM, Wallace DJ et al (2010) Efficacy and safety of rituximab in moderately-to-severely active systemic lupus erythematosus: the randomized, double-blind, phase II/III systemic lupus erythematosus evaluation of rituximab trial. Arthritis Rheum 62:222–233
18. Merrill J et al (2011) Assessment of flares in lupus patients enrolled in a phase II/III study of rituximab (EXPLORER). Lupus 20:709–716
19. Rovin BH, Furie R, Latinis K et al (2012) Efficacy and safety of rituximab in patients with active proliferative lupus nephritis: the Lupus Nephritis Assessment with Rituximab study. Arthritis Rheum 64:1215–1226
20. Lightstone L (2012) The landscape after LUNAR: rituximab's crater-filled path. Arthritis Rheum 64:962–965
21. Weidenbusch M, Rommele C, Schrottle A, Anders HJ (2013) Beyond the LUNAR trial. Efficacy of rituximab in refractory lupus nephritis. Nephrol Dial Transplant 28:106–111
22. Diaz-Lagares C, Croca S, Sangle S et al (2012) Efficacy of rituximab in 164 pts with biopsy-proven lupus nephritis: pooled data from European cohorts. Autoimmun Rev 11:357–364
23. Hickman RA, Hira-Kazal R, Yee C-S, Toescu V (2015) The efficacy and safety of rituximab in a chart review study of 15 pts with systemic lupus erythematosus. Clin Rheumatol 34:263–271
24. Moroni G, Raffiotta F, Trezzi B, Giglio E, Mezzina N, Del Papa N, Meroni P, Messa P, Sinico AR (2014) Rituximab vs mycophenolate and vs cyclophosphamide pulses for induction therapy of active lupus nephritis: a clinical observational study. Rheumatology (Oxford) 53(9):1570–1577
25. Condon MB, Ashby D, Pepper RJ, Cook HT, Levy JB, Griffith M, Cairns TD, Lightstone L (2013) Prospective observational single-centre cohort study to evaluate the effectiveness of treating lupus nephritis with rituximab and mycophenolate mofetil but no oral steroids. Ann Rheum Dis 72:1280–1286
26. Roccatello D, Sciascia S, Rossi D, Alpa M, Naretto C, Baldovino S, Menegatti E, La Grotta R, Modena V (2011) Intensive short-term treatment with rituximab, cyclophosphamide and methylprednisolone pulses induces remission in severe cases of SLE with nephritis and avoids further immunosuppressive maintenance therapy. Nephrol Dial Transplant 26(12):3987–3992
27. Roccatello D, Sciascia S, Baldovino S, Rossi D, Alpa M, Naretto C, Di Simone D, Simoncini M, Menegatti E. A 4-year observation in lupus nephritis patients treated with an intensified B-lymphocyte depletion without immunosuppressive maintenance treatment-Clinical response compared to literature and immunological re-assessment. Autoimmun Rev. 2015;14(12):1123–1130
28. Terrier B, Amoura Z, Ravaud P et al (2010) Safety and efficacy of rituximab in systemic lupus erythematosus: results from 136 pts from the French Autoimmunity and Rituximab registry. Arthritis Rheum 62:2458–2466
29. van Vollenhoven RF, Emery P, Bingham CO et al (2013) Long-term safety of rituximab in rheumatoid arthritis: 9.5-year follow up of the global clinical trial programme focus on adverse events of interest in RA pts. Ann Rheum Dis 72:1496–1502
30. Molloi ES (2011) PML and rheumatology: the contribution of disease and drugs. Cleve Clin J Med 78:S28–S32
31. Mysler EF, Spindler AJ, Guzman R, Bijl M, Jayne D, Furie RA et al (2013) Efficacy and safety of ocrelizumab in active proliferative lupus nephritis: results from a randomized, double-bind, phase III study. Arthritis Rheum 65:2368–2379
32. Dorner T, Kaufmann J, Wegener WA et al (2006) Initial clinical trial of epratuzumab (humanized anti-CD22 antibody) for immunotherapy of systemic lupus erythematosus. Arthritis Res Ther 8:R74
33. Jacobi AM, Goldenberg DM, Hiepe F et al (2006) Differential effects of epratuzumab on peripheral blood B cells of patients with systemic lupus erythematosus versus normal control. Ann Rheum Dis 67:450–457

34. Al Rayes H, Touma Z (2014) Profile of epratuzumab and its potential in the treatment of systemic lupus erythematosus. Drug Des Devel Ther 8:2303–2310
35. Wallace DJ, Goldenberg DM (2013) Epratuzumab for systemic lupus erythematosus. Lupus 22(4):400–405
36. Traczewski P, Rudnicka L (2011) Treatment of systemic lupus erythematosus with epratuzumab. Br J Clin Pharmacol 71:175–182
37. Strand V, Petri M, Kalunian K, Gordon C, Wallace DJ, Hobbs K et al (2014) Epratuzumab for patients with moderate to severe flaring SLE: health-related quality of life outcomes and corticosteroid use in the randomized controlled ALLEVIATE trials and extension study SL0006. Rheumatology (Oxford) 53(3):502–511
38. ClinicalTrials.gov. Identifier NCT01262365, a phase 3, randomized, double-blind, placebo-controlled, multicenter study of the efficacy and safety of four 12-week treatment cycles (48 weeks total) of epratuzumab in systemic lupus erythematosus subjects with moderate to severe disease (EMBODY 1); 14th Dec 2010 – [cited 30th Mar 2014])
39. Stohl W (2013) Future prospects in biologic therapy for systemic lupus erythematosus. Nat Rev Rheumatol 9:705–720
40. Stohl W (2014) Therapeutic targeting of the BAFF/APRIL axis in systemic lupus erythematosus. Expert Opin Ther Targets 18(4):473–489
41. Pisetsky DS, Grammer AC, Ning TC, Lipsky PE (2011) Are autoantibodies the target of B cell-direct therapy? Nat Rev Rheumatol 7:551–556
42. Navarra SV, Guzman RM, Gallacher AE et al (2011) Efficacy and safety of belimumab in patients with active systemic lupus erythematosus: a randomized, placebo-controlled, phase 3 trial. Lancet 377:721–731
43. Furie R, Petri M, Zamani O et al (2011) A phase III, randomized, placebo-controlled study of belimumab, a monoclonal antibody that inhibits B lymphocyte stimulator, in patients with systemic lupus erythematosus. Arthritis Rheum 63:3918–3930
44. Dooley MA, Houssiau F, Aranow C, D'Cruz DP, Askanase A, Roth DA, Zhong ZJ, Cooper S, Freimuth WW, Ginzler EM (2013) Effects of belimumab treatment on renal outcomes: results from the phase 3 belimumab clinical trials in patients with SLE. Lupus 22:63
45. Fried AJ, Bonilla FA (2009) Pathogenesis, diagnosis, and management of primary antibody deficiencies and infections. Clin Microbiol Rev 22:396–414
46. Kraaij T, Huizinga TW, Rabelink TJ, Teng YK (2014) Belimumab after rituximab as maintenance therapy in lupus nephritis. Rheumatology 53(11):2122–2124
47. Furie RA, Leon G, Thomas M, Petri MA, Chu AD, Hislop C et al (2014) A phase 2, randomised, placebo-controlled clinical trial of blisibimod, an inhibitor of B cell activating factor, in patients with moderate-to-severe systemic lupus erythematosus, the PEARL-SC study. Ann Rheum Dis. http://dx.doi.org/10.1136/annrheumdis-2013-205144
48. Kamala A, Khamashta M (2014) The efficacy of novel B cell biologics as the future of SLE treatment: a review. Autoimmun Rev 13(11):1094–1101
49. Gross JA, Johnston J, Mudri S, Enselman R, Dillon SR, Madden K et al (2000) TACI and BCMA are receptors for a TNF homologue implicated in B-cell autoimmune disease. Nature 404:995–999
50. Dall'Era M, Chakravarty E, Wallace D, Genovese M, Weisman M, Kavanaugh A et al (2007) Reduced B lymphocyte and immunoglobulin levels after atacicept treatment in patients with systemic lupus erythematosus: results of a multicenter, phase Ib, double-blind, placebo-controlled, dose-escalating trial. Arthritis Rheum 56(12):4142–4150
51. Kayagaki N, Yan M, Seshasayee D, Wang H, Lee W, French DM et al (2002) BAFF/BLyS receptor 3 binds the B cell survival factor BAFF ligand through a discrete surface loop and promotes processing of NF-kappaB2. Immunity 17(4):515–524
52. Mok MY (2010) The immunological basis of B-cell therapy in systemic lupus erythematosus. Int J Rheum Dis 13(1):3–11
53. Cunane G, Chan OT, Cassafer G, Brindis S, Kaufman E, Yen TS, Daikh DI (2004) Prevention in renal damage in murine lupus nephritis by CTLA-4Ig and cyclophosphamide. Arthritis Rheum 50:1539–1548

54. Merrill JT, Burgos-Vargas R, Westhovens R, Chalmers A, D'Cruz D, Wallace DJ, Bae SC, Sigal L, Becker JC, Kelly S, Raghupathi K, Li T, Peng Y, Kinaszczuk M, Nash P (2010) The efficacy and safety of abatacept in patients with non-life-threatening manifestations of systemic lupus erythematosus: results of a twelve month, multicenter, exploratory, phase IIb, randomized, double-blind, placebo-controlled trial. Arthritis Rheum 62:3077–3087
55. Furie R, Nicholis K, Cheng TT, Houssiau F, Burgos-Vargas R, Chen SL et al (2011) Efficacy and safety of abatecept over 12 months in patients with lupus nephritis: results from a multicenter, randomized, double blind, placebo-controlled phase II/III study. Arthritis Rheum 63:S 962–S 963
56. Wofsy D, Hillson JL, Diamond B (2013) Comparison of alternative primary outcome measures for use in a lupus nephritis trial. Arthritis Rheum 65(6):1586–1591
57. Kalumian KC, Davis JC Jr, Merrill JT, Totoritis MC, Wofsy D (2002) Treatment of systemic lupus erythematosus by inhibition of T cell costimulation with anti-CD154: a randomized, double blind, placebo-controlled trial. Arthritis Rheum 46:3251–3258
58. Boumpas DT, Furie R, Manzi S, Illei GG, Wallace DJ, Balow JE, Vaishnaw A (2003) A short course of BG9588 (anti-CD40 ligand antibody) improves serologic activity and decreases hematuria in patients with proliferative lupus glomerulonephritis. Arthritis Rheum 48:719–727
59. Liang B, Gardner DB, Griswold DE et al (2006) Antiinterleukin-6 monoclonal antibody inhibits its autoimmune responses in a murine model of systemic lupus erythematosus. Immunology 119:296–305
60. Illei GG, Shirota Y, Yarboro C et al (2010) Tocilizumab in systemic lupus erythematosus: data on safety, preliminarily efficacy, and impact on circulating plasma cells from an open label phase I dosage-escalation study. Arthritis Rheum 62:542–552
61. Szepietowski JC, Nilganuwong S, Wozniacka A, Kuhn A et al (2013) Phase I randomized, double-blind, placebo-controlled, multiple intravenous, dose-ascending study of Sirukumab in cutaneous or systemic lupus erythematosus. Arthritis Rheum 65:2661–2671
62. Rajadhyaksha AG, Mehra S, Nadkar MY (2013) Biologics in SLE: current status. JAPI 61:262–267
63. Llorente L, Richaud-Patin Y, Garcia-Padilla C et al (2000) Clinical and biologic effects of anti-interleukin-10 monoclonal antibody administration in systemic lupus erythematosus. Arthritis Rheum 43:1790–1800
64. Crow MK, Wohlgemuth J (2003) Microarray analysis of gene expression in lupus. Arthritis Rheum Ther 5:279–287
65. Merrill JT, Wallace DJ, Petri M et al (2011) Safety profile and clinical activity of sifalimumab, a fully human anti-interferon alpha monoclonal antibody, in systemic lupus erythematosus: a phase I, multicentre, double-blind randomised study. Ann Rheum Dis 70(11):1905–1913
66. McBride JM, Jiang J, Abbas AR et al (2012) Safety and pharmacodynamics of rontalizumab in patients with systemic lupus erythematosus: results of a phase I, placebo-controlled, double-blind, dose-escalation study. Arthritis Rheum 64(11):3666–36769
67. Kirou KA, Gkrouzman E (2013) Anti-interferon alpha treatment in SLE. Clin Immunol 148(3):303–312
68. Hein E, Nielsen LA, Nielsen CT, Munthe-Fog L, Skjoedt MO, Jacobsen S, Garred P (2015) Ficolins and the lectin pathway of complement in patients with systemic lupus erythematosus. Mol Immunol 63(2):209–214
69. Cordeiro AC, Isenberg DA (2008) Novel therapies in lupus – focus on nephritis. Acta Reumatol Port 33:157–169
70. Hillmen P, Young NS, Schubert J, Brodsky RA, Socié G, Muus P et al (2006) The complement inhibitor eculizumab in paroxysmal nocturnal hemoglobinuria. N Engl J Med 355:1233–1243
71. Wang Y, Hu Q, Madri J, Rollins SA, Chodera A, Matis LA (1996) Amelioration of lupus-like autoimmune disease in NZB/WF1 mice after treatment with a blocking monoclonal antibody specific for complement component C5. Proc Natl Acad Sci 93(16):8563–8568

72. Barilla-Labarca ML, Toder K, Furie R (2013) Targeting the complement system in systemic lupus erythematosus and other diseases. Clin Immunol 148(3):313–321
73. Baumann U, Schimidt RE, Gessner JE (2003) New insights into the pathophysiology and *in vivo* Function of IgG Fc receptors through gene deletion studies. Arch Immunol Ther Exp 51:399–406
74. Pradhan V, Patwardhan M, Ghosh K (2008) Fc gamma receptor polymorphisms in systemic lupus erythematosus and their correlation with the clinical severity of the disease. Indian J Hum Genet 14(3):77–78
75. Michaelson JS, Wisniacki N, Burkly LC, Putterman C (2012) Role of TWEAK in lupus nephritis: a bench-to-bedside review. J Autoimmun 39(3):130–142
76. Wisniacki NC, Codding CE (2011) Phase I, randomized, double-blind, placebo-controlled, single dose, dose escalation study to evaluate the safety, tolerability and pharmacokinetics of BIIB023 (Anti-TWEAK) in subjects with rheumatoid arthritis. Arthritis Rheum 63:S858
77. Ghoreschi K, Gadina M (2014) Jakpot! New small molecules in autoimmune and inflammatory diseases. Exp Dermatol 23(1):7–11
78. Norman P (2014) Spleen tyrosine kinase inhibitors: a review of the patent literature 2010–2013. Expert Opin Ther Pat 24(5):573–595
79. Bahjat FR, Pine PR, Reitsma A, Cassafer G, Baluom M, Grillo S, Chang B, Zhao FF, Payan DG, Grossbard EB, Daikh DI (2008) An orally bioavailable spleen tyrosine kinase inhibitor delays disease progression and prolongs survival in murine. Lupus 58(5):1433–1444
80. Morales-Torres J (2012) The status of fostamatinib in the treatment of rheumatoid arthritis. Expert Rev Clin Immunol 8(7):609–615
81. Rovin BH, Parikh SV (2014) Lupus nephritis: the evolving role of novel therapeutics. Am J Kidney Dis 63(4):677–690
82. Mishra MK, Wang J, Silva C, Mack M, Yong VW (2012) Kinetics of proinflammatory monocytes in a model of multiple sclerosis and its perturbation by laquinimod. Am J Pathol 181(2):642–651
83. Jolivel V, Luessi F, Masri J et al (2013) Modulation of dendritic cell properties by laquinimod as a mechanism for modulating multiple sclerosis. Brain 136:1048–1066
84. Keino H, Watanabe T, Sato Y, Okada AA (2011) Oral administration of retinoic acid receptor-alpha/beta-specific ligand Am80 suppresses experimental autoimmune uveoretinitis. Invest Ophthalmol Vis Sci 52(3):1548–1556
85. Klemann C, Raveney BJ, Klemann AK et al (2009) Synthetic retinoid AM80 inhibits Th17 cells and ameliorates experimental autoimmune encephalomyelitis. Am J Pathol 174(6):2234–2245
86. Markopoulou A, Kyttaris VC (2013) Small molecules in the treatment of systemic lupus erythematosus. Clin Immunol 148(3):359–368
87. Hiepe F, Dorner T (2011) Long-lived autoreactive plasma cells drive persistent autoimmune inflammation. Nat Rev Rheumatol 7:170–178
88. Neubert K et al (2008) The proteasome inhibitor bortezomib depletes plasma cells and protects mice with lupus-like disease from nephritis. Nat Med 14:748–755
89. Starke C, Frey S, Ubronaviciute V, Schett G, Winkler T, Voll R (2011) Depletion of autoreactive short- and long-lived plasma cells within nephritic kidneys of lupus mice by bortezomib. Ann Rheum Dis 2011;70:S91
90. Hainz N et al (2012) The proteasome inhibitor bortezomib prevents lupus nephritis in the NZB/W F1 mouse model by preservation of glomerular and tubulo-interstitial architecture. Nephron Exp Nephrol 120:e47–e58
91. Alexander T, Sarfert R, Klotsche J, Kuhl A et al (2015) The proteasome inhibitor bortezomib depletes plasma cells and ameliorates clinical manifestations of refractory systemic lupus erythematosus. Ann Rheum Dis 0:1–5

SLE in 21st Century

18

Graham Hughes

Clinical and translational research in systemic lupus erythematosus (SLE) has advanced the available diagnostic and therapeutic options, translating into better patient outcomes.

Five-year survival in patients with SLE has improved from 50 % in the 1950s to over 90 % currently.

There has been major progress in the understanding of the intricate pathogenesis underlying SLE, most notably the critical role of auto B cells in autoantibody formation, antigen presentation, and T-cell activation.

After the heterogeneous results with the use of rituximab in SLE (good in real life, bad in controlled trials), the approval of belimumab by the FDA in 2011 was a significant milestone for the treatment of SLE. Furthermore murine models and early phase studies of epratuzumab and sifalimumab have shown promising results, and multicenter randomized controlled trials with long-term follow-ups are ongoing.

18.1 Which Are the Challenges for the Twenty-First Century?

Future research will focus on the goals of increasing survival, limiting organ damage, and improving quality of life for patients with SLE.

Early diagnosis is still an unmet need in SLE, as the diverse and nonspecific presentations can still lead to delay in diagnosis. Disease monitoring remains difficult due to the low sensitivity of current disease activity markers. Management of refractory disease, especially nephritis and cutaneous and neuropsychiatric

G. Hughes
The London Lupus Centre, 1st Floor, St Olaf House, London Bridge Hospital, London SE1 2PR, UK
e-mail: londonlupuscentre@hcahealthcare.co.uk

D. Roccatello, L. Emmi (eds.), *Connective Tissue Disease: A Comprehensive Guide-Volume 1*, Rare Diseases of the Immune System 5,
DOI 10.1007/978-3-319-24535-5_18

manifestations, remains unsatisfactory. End-stage renal failure, scarring cutaneous lesions, and neurological damage especially that resulting from antiphospholipid syndrome remain major complications of the disease. Cardiovascular disease secondary to accelerated atherosclerosis has emerged as an important contributor to the higher morbidity and mortality in long-standing disease. Damage due to both disease and treatment, especially corticosteroid-associated damage, tends to accumulate over time.

Large international collaborations have resulted in development of new composite outcome indices and insights into disease pathogenesis. Multiple newer biologic agents targeting specific immune system pathways and effectors are undergoing evaluation.

Hopefully, these efforts will lead to development of newer therapeutic agents in SLE, a dire need.

Part II

Sjögren Syndrome

Classification Criteria of Sjögren's Syndrome

19

Chiara Baldini and Stefano Bombardieri

19.1 Introduction

Primary Sjögren's syndrome (pSS) is a complex autoimmune disease characterized by a progressive dysfunction of the salivary glands associated to a variety of systemic manifestations, including lymphoproliferative disorders [1–3]. Thus, pSS can be considered as a heterogeneous autoimmune entity possessing both organ-specific and systemic features and encompassing a wide spectrum of clinical manifestations, serological abnormalities, and scattered complications [4–9]. The complexity of SS clinical presentation is moreover increased by the fact that SS may occur alone, as a primary condition, or in association with other connective tissue diseases, including rheumatoid arthritis (RA), systemic lupus erythematosus (SLE), and systemic sclerosis (SSc), as secondary SS (sSS) variants [10–13]. This complexity makes it difficult to classify the disease and to identify a homogeneous group of patients with a common etiopathogenesis or prognosis. This is probably the most important reason for explaining why it remains an unresolved issue to reach a scientific consensus on universally accepted classification criteria for pSS [14, 15]. The American-European Consensus Group (AECG) criteria are the currently used classification criteria for Sjögren's syndrome (SS) and were derived after proper modifications and revisions from the preliminary European criteria [16, 17]; nonetheless, the recent American College of Rheumatology/Sjögren's International Collaborative Clinical Alliance (ACR/SICCA) criteria [18] that are based exclusively on objective tests clearly set the need for the scientific community to discuss extensively the concept of a new classification system for patients with SS [19–21].

Herewith a critical historical overview of the different criteria sets for SS will be provided from the beginning up to the more recent proposals.

C. Baldini • S. Bombardieri (✉)
Rheumatology Unit, University of Pisa, via Roma 67, Pisa, Italy
e-mail: s.bombardieri@int.med.unipi.it

D. Roccatello, L. Emmi (eds.), *Connective Tissue Disease: A Comprehensive Guide-Volume 1*, Rare Diseases of the Immune System 5,
DOI 10.1007/978-3-319-24535-5_19

19.2 Sets of Classification Criteria Proposed for pSS over the Time: The Long Journey to the Preliminary European Criteria 1993

During the First International Seminar on pSS, held in Copenhagen in May 1986, the four – at that time – most widely used criteria for definition of pSS were presented. Namely, the four different sets of criteria were the Copenhagen (1976) [22], the Japanese (1977) [23], the Greek (1979) [24], and the San Diego criteria (1986) [25]. In 1975, the San Francisco criteria for SS had been previously proposed in the USA [26]. Table 19.1 summarizes their similarities and dissimilarities. All these criteria sets were mainly focused on assessing the glandular signs and symptoms of the disease utilizing different procedures with different (and in many cases still not assessed) levels of sensitivity, specificity, and reliability. The attitude of the criteria sets versus the histology and the serological patients' profiles differed significantly from one set to another. In particular, the Copenhagen and the Japanese criteria were focused mainly on the objective assessment of functional impairment of the salivary and lachrymal glands, while histology and serology were not considered obligatory for diagnosis. The Greek proposal emphasized the role of focal sialadenitis and the subjective complaints of the disease, while the California criteria introduced the presence of autoantibodies and histopathology as distinct items.

Overall, in spite of their differences, these proposed classification criteria might hypothetically select and correctly classify patients affected by pSS, when used by single groups of investigators, but they were not free from disadvantages. The San Francisco criteria, for example, emphasizing the specificity of focal sialadenitis on minor salivary gland biopsies and the role of the objective tests in the diagnosis of pSS, appeared to be quite stringent and not completely able to properly diagnosed patients with a milder sicca syndrome, especially at the onset of the disease. The Copenhagen criteria on the other hand required the presence of two abnormal test assessing the dryness of the eyes and two abnormal tests assessing the dryness of the mouth, but they did not require as a mandatory item the salivary gland biopsy. Another drawback of the Copenhagen criteria was moreover that they pointed out that it was up to the local pSS center to decide which objective tests to select, and therefore, the tests used may vary slightly from center to center. Finally, another potential drawback was represented by the fact that some of the criteria sets did not consider the presence of autoantibodies.

During the First International Seminar on pSS, the comparison of all these criteria sets made it possible to focus on the lack of homogeneity in the diagnostic tools for pSS and therefore on the potential discrepancies observed in clinical studies and/or in the epidemiological surveys [27].

In 1988, 2 years after the First International Seminar on pSS held in Copenhagen in 1986, a workshop was held in Pisa sponsored by the Epidemiology Committee of the Commission of the European Communities (EEC-COMAC) involving 29 experts, representing 11 European countries and Israel. The aim of this collaboration was to define and validate simple standardized diagnostic tools for pSS and to design a multicenter study to define classification criteria for SS [17, 28]. The

Table 19.1 Similarities and dissimilarities of the historical criteria sets for SS: Copenhagen, Japanese, Greek, San Diego, and San Francisco criteria

	Copenhagen (1976)	Japanese (1977)	Greek (1979)	San Diego (1986)	San Francisco (1975, 1984)
Definition of probable/definite SS	–	+	+	+	+
Definition of pSS/sSS	+	–	+	–	+
Subjective xeroftalmia	–	+	+	–	–
Subjective xerostomia	–	+	+	+	–
Objective tests exclusively (no subjective symptoms)	+	–	–	–	+
Parotid gland swelling (history)	–	+	+	–	–
Ocular tests:					
Schirmer-I test	+ (≤10 mm/5′)	+ (≤10 mm/5′)	+ (≤10 mm/5′)	+ (<9 mm/5′)	+ (≤10 mm/5′)
Breakup time	+ (≤10 s)	–	–	–	+
Rose bengal (van Bijsterveld score)	+ (≥4)	+(≥2)	+ (≥4)	+(≥4)	+(≥4)
Fluorescein test	–	+	–	+	–
At least two abnormal tests as evidence of KCS	+	+	–	+	+
Oral tests:					
Unstimulated whole saliva	+	–	–	+	
Stimulated parotid flow rate	–	–	+	+	–
Scintigraphy	+	–	–	–	–
Sialography	–	+	–	–	–
Minor salivary obligatory criterion	No	No	Yes	Yes	Yes
Focus score (minor salivary glands biopsy)	>1	>1	≥2	≥2	>1
Serological findings					

(continued)

Table 19.1 (continued)

	Copenhagen (1976)	Japanese (1977)	Greek (1979)	San Diego (1986)	San Francisco (1975, 1984)
Antinuclear antibodies	–	–	–	+	–
Anti-SS-A/Ro	–	–	–	+	–
Anti-SS-B/La	–	–	–	+	–
IgM-rheumatoid factor	–	–	–	+	–

novelty was represented by the fact that previously proposed classification criteria had generally been formulated by experts on the basis of clinical experience or derived from data coming from a single center. The preliminary European classification criteria, on the contrary, represented the first attempt to create the criteria for pSS through a multicenter study aimed at deriving and validating standardized methodologies directly from real patients. A simple questionnaire (20 questions: 13 regarding the ocular involvement and 7 regarding the oral involvement) for dry eyes and dry mouth was validated. Data from 480 patients (240p SS and 240 controls) were gathered. Univariate and multivariate analysis and stepwise multiple regression were used to select those questions and combinations of questions that showed the best performance in correctly classifying patients and controls. Thus, a simplified questionnaire consisting of three questions for dry eyes and three for dry mouth emerged from this section of the study. For part II, each center recruited 40 patients – 10 with pSS, 10 with sSS, 10 with other connective tissue disorders (CTDs) without SS, and 10 controls. The CTD diagnoses were made on the basis of the standard criteria for the various diseases, while the diagnosis of pSS was based at the best of the clinical skills of the expert observer clinician as gold standard. In these patients a limited set of proposed diagnostic tests were validated (including Schirmer-I test, rose bengal test, tear breakup time, tear fluid lactoferrin level, stimulated and unstimulated saliva flow, biopsy of the minor salivary glands, parotid sialography, and salivary gland scintigraphy). The exact procedure to be followed for each test was described in the protocol. The data in part II were subjected to the same analysis of part I, with the addition of a classification tree in order to determine the optimal classification strategy. From the analysis the consensus group established a set of four objective criteria for the diagnosis of SS. These four criteria and the two subjective criteria are presented in Table 19.2. The preliminary European criteria were based on any four out of six items including ocular and oral symptoms (such as oral and ocular dryness), ocular and oral signs (such as positive Schirmer-I test, rose bengal score, parotid sialography, scintigraphy, and unstimulated salivary flow), immunological parameters, and focal sialadenitis. For primary pSS, the presence of four out of six items had good sensitivity (93.5 %) and specificity (94 %). Some exclusion criteria were also added to this classification set for pSS and, namely, preexisting lymphoma, acquired immunodeficiency syndrome, sarcoidosis, and graft-versus-host disease [17].

Table 19.2 European preliminary criteria for Sjögren's syndrome

I. Ocular symptoms: a positive response to at least one of the following questions:
1. Have you had daily, persistent, troublesome dry eyes for more than 3 months?
2. Do you have a recurrent sensation of sand or gravel in the eyes?
3. Do you use tear substitutes more than 3 times a day?
II. Oral symptoms: a positive response to at least one of the following questions:
1. Have you had a daily feeling of dry mouth for more than 3 months?
2. Have you had recurrently or persistently swollen salivary glands as an adult?
3. Do you frequently drink liquids to aid in swallowing dry food?
III. Ocular signs – that is, objective evidence of ocular involvement defined as a positive result for at least one of the following two tests:
1. Schirmer-I test (≤5 mm in 5 min)
2. Rose bengal score or other ocular dye score (≥4 according to van Bijsterveld's scoring system)
IV. Histopathology: focus score ≥1 on minor salivary gland biopsy (focus defined as an aggregation of at least 50 mononuclear cells; focus score defined as the number of foci per 4 mm^2 of glandular tissue)
V. Salivary gland involvement: objective evidence of salivary gland involvement defined by a positive result for at least one of the following diagnostic tests:
1. Unstimulated whole salivary flow (<1.5 ml in 15 min)
2. Parotid sialography showing the presence of diffuse sialectasias (punctate, cavitary, or destructive pattern), without evidence of obstruction in the major ducts
3. Salivary scintigraphy showing delayed uptake, reduced concentration, and/or delayed excretion of tracer
VI. Autoantibodies: presence in the serum of the following autoantibodies:
1. Antibodies to Ro(SSA) or La(SSB) antigens or both
2. Antinuclear antibodies
3. Rheumatoid factor
Exclusion criteria
Preexisting lymphoma
Acquired immunodeficiency syndrome (AIDS)
Sarcoidosis
Graft-versus-host disease

Furthermore, for the diagnosis of sSS, all the serological tests were excluded, and the consensus group established that it was sufficient, the presence of at least three out five items.

In 1996, the criteria set was validated on a total of 278 cases (157 SS patients and 121 non-SS controls) collected from 16 centers in 10 countries, and the criteria confirmed to have a sensitivity of 97.5 % and a specificity of 94.2 % [29].

After their validation the European classification criteria received a large acceptance by the scientific community because of their good combination of sensitivity and specificity. In fact, when previously proposed, the criteria had been used to classify patients with pSS, and controls enrolled in the European study all showed a very high specificity (range 97.9–100 %) but a low sensitivity (range 22.9–72.2 %)

which make them less useful for epidemiological surveys. Other potential advantageous characteristics of the European criteria were that they distinguished between pSS and sSS but avoid the concept of definite/possible SS. Furthermore, they – as do the Copenhagen criteria – rely on unstimulated or basal tests and did not require as mandatory for the diagnosis invasive tests such as the minor salivary gland biopsy.

Nonetheless, during the subsequent International Symposia on SS, the European criteria for the classification of SS generated an extensive discussion. The key point of debate was that these criteria could be fulfilled in the absence of either autoantibodies or positive findings on labial salivary gland biopsy and, then, can also be met by patients with sicca symptoms, but not strictly primary SS. Furthermore, a criteria set in which two out of the six items were devoted to subjective complaints cannot allow to correctly classify patients with SS but without symptoms [30].

19.3 From the European Classification Criteria to the American-European Classification Criteria

The preliminary European criteria raised objections concerning the misclassification of patients who could fulfill the items for ocular and oral symptoms and signs but not the histological or the autoimmunity criterion. As a consequence of the abovementioned criticisms which were raised against them, the SS Foundation proposed that a joint effort be undertaken by the Europe Study Group on classification criteria for SS and a group of American experts. A detailed analysis of the European database of the patients and controls collected during the validation phase of the European Criteria was undertaken. A receiver-operating characteristic (ROC) curve of the revised criteria was constructed based on the analysis of 180 cases provided by 16 centers from 10 European countries. In more details, patient and control populations included 76 patients affected by pSS, 41 patients with a diagnosis of CTD without SS, and 63 control (no SS) subjects. Based on this, the ROC curve analyzes the condition "positivity of any four out of the six items" and the condition "positivity of four out of six items with the exclusion of the cases in which both serology and histopathology were negative"; the second condition had a lower sensitivity (89.5 % vs 97.4 %) but a higher specificity (95.2 % vs 89.4 %). The presence of any three of the four objective criteria items showed a slightly lower accuracy (90.5 %) but a specificity of 95.2 % and a sensitivity of 84.2 %. This combination was, therefore, judged reliable as well. The American-European Consensus Group, then, even maintaining the previous European scheme of six items, introduced the obligatory rule that for a definite diagnosis of pSS, either the minor salivary gland biopsy or serology had to be positive (see Table 19.3) [16]. Other modifications were proposed and included in the European criteria set to make the item definitions more precise. In particular, it was specified that Schirmer-I test should be performed with standardized paper strips in unanesthetized and closed eyes following the European and the Japanese tradition. Moreover, as rose bengal is not available in many countries, other ocular dye scores (i.e., fluorescein stain and lissamine green) were

Table 19.3 American-European Consensus Group Criteria. Revised international classification criteria for Sjögren's syndrome

I. Ocular symptoms: a positive response to at least one of the following questions:
1. Have you had daily, persistent, troublesome dry eyes for more than 3 months?
2. Do you have a recurrent sensation of sand or gravel in the eyes?
3. Do you use tear substitutes more than 3 times a day?
II. Oral symptoms: a positive response to at least one of the following questions:
1. Have you had a daily feeling of dry mouth for more than 3 months?
2. Have you had recurrently or persistently swollen salivary glands as an adult?
3. Do you frequently drink liquids to aid in swallowing dry food?
III. Ocular signs – that is, objective evidence of ocular involvement defined as a positive result for at least one of the following two tests:
1. Schirmer-I test, performed without anesthesia (<5 mm in 5 min)
2. Rose bengal score or other ocular dye score (>4 according to van Bijsterveld's scoring system)
IV. Histopathology: in minor salivary glands (obtained through normal-appearing mucosa) focal lymphocytic sialadenitis, evaluated by an expert histopathologist, with a focus score >1, defined as a number of lymphocytic foci (which are adjacent to normal-appearing mucous acini and contain more than 50 lymphocytes) per 4 mm^2 of glandular tissue
V. Salivary gland involvement: objective evidence of salivary gland involvement defined by a positive result for at least one of the following diagnostic tests:
1. Unstimulated whole salivary flow (<1.5 ml in 15 min)
2. Parotid sialography showing the presence of diffuse sialectasias (punctate, cavitary, or destructive pattern), without evidence of obstruction in the major ducts
3. Salivary scintigraphy showing delayed uptake, reduced concentration, and/or delayed excretion of tracer
VI. Autoantibodies: presence in the serum of the following autoantibodies:
1. Antibodies to Ro(SSA) or La(SSB) antigens or both
Revised rules for classification
For primary SS
In patients without any potentially associated disease, primary SS may be defined as follows:
(a) The presence of any 4 of the 6 items is indicative of primary SS, as long as either item IV (histopathology) or VI (serology) is positive
(b) The presence of any 3 of the 4 objective criteria items (i.e., items III, IV, V, VI)
(c) The classification tree procedure represents a valid alternative method for classification, although it should be more properly used in clinical-epidemiological survey
For secondary SS
In patients with a potentially associated disease (for instance, another well-defined connective tissue disease), the presence of item I or item II plus any 2 from among items III, IV, and V may be considered as indicative of secondary SS
Exclusion criteria
Past head and neck radiation treatment
Hepatitis C infection
Acquired immunodeficiency syndrome (AIDS)
Preexisting lymphoma

(continued)

Table 19.3 (continued)

Sarcoidosis
Graft-versus-host disease
Use of anticholinergic drugs (since a time shorter than fourfold the half-life of the drug)

suggested to replace it. They also defined a positive minor salivary glands biopsy as one focus of lymphocytes or more specifying that it/they had to be adjacent to normal-appearing mucous acini per 4 mm^2 glandular tissue. Finally, a consensus on the list of exclusion criteria was also reached. In comparison to the exclusion criteria adopted by the European preliminary criteria, the category "anticholinergic" drugs was introduced instead of "antidepressant, antihypertensive, parasympatholytic drugs, and neuroleptic agents," the term sialadenosis was deleted, and the definition past head and neck radiation treatment added. Finally, it was decided to add the hepatitis C virus (HCV) infection as an exclusion criterion considering the sicca symptoms observed in some patients with HCV as one of the extrahepatic manifestations of the virus which has to be differentiated from SS.

For sSS it was established that in patients with a potentially associated disease, it has to be considered as indicative of the disorder and the presence of the item I or II plus any two from among items III, IV, and V [31].

Overall, the American-European Revised Classification Criteria, even preserving many aspects of the European preliminary criteria, appear to be more stringent [32, 33]. In particular in 2006, the comparability of the Copenhagen, San Diego, European, and AECG criteria sets was assessed prospectively, examining 222 consecutive patients referred to the Department of Rheumatology of Ljubljana. The authors found that 90 out of 222 patients (41 %) fulfilled at least one classification criteria set. The highest number of patients fulfilled the European criteria (36 %), followed by the Copenhagen criteria (28 %), the AECG criteria (26 %), and the San Diego criteria (9 %) sets. The AECG criteria resulted therefore to be highly specific and quite restrictive [32].

19.4 Classification Criteria for pSS: Present and Future

The AECG criteria represent the most commonly employed tool to classify patients with primary and secondary SS in clinical trials, in epidemiological studies, and in clinical practice, given their high sensibility and specificity [34–36]. However, according to results derived from clinical settings, the higher specificity of the AECG criteria in comparison with preliminary criteria might lead to the exclusion of a considerable proportion of patients with classical features and long-term outcome complications of SS [37, 38]. Recently, the American College of Rheumatology (ACR)/Sjögren's International Collaborative Clinical Alliance (SICCA) endorsed new classification criteria for pSS [18, 39, 40]. These criteria were derived from 1107 participants. According to the ACR/SICCA criteria, for SS diagnosis, two out of the following three are required: (a) positive anti-Ro/SSA and anti-La/SSB or positive rheumatoid factor and ANA ≥1:320, (b) ocular staining score ≥3 (sum total score 0–12; 0–6 score for staining of the cornea with fluorescein, 0–3 score for staining of both the nasal and temporal conjunctivae with lissamine green), and (c) focal lymphocytic sialadenitis with focus score ≥1 in labial gland biopsy. The ACR/SICCA criteria do not target the general population but individuals suspected to be affected by SS and were aimed at selecting homogenous patients to be enrolled in clinical trials.

Interestingly, Rasmussen et al.[41] recently compared the performance of the new ACR and the AECG classification criteria for SS and found concordant results when applied to a homogeneous cohort of patients with sicca symptoms, providing no clear evidence for increased value of the new ACR criteria over the old AECG criteria from the clinical and biological perspective 11. In this scenario, the entire scientific community is making an international effort to create novel criteria able to overcome the limitations of both the existing criteria set. In fact, a major limitation of the ACR classification criteria is represented by the fact that they require an evaluation by a practitioner specialized in eyes and lip biopsy and may oversee patient's subjective symptoms; on the other hand, AECG criteria rely on the employment of obsolete objective tests like sialography and scintigraphy. From this perspective, the addition of salivary gland ultrasonography (SGUS) has been proposed in order to replace more painful or invasive tests [42–46]. Despite the encouraging results obtained, however, the employment of SGUS as an adjunctive item in classification criteria needs further validation and standardization. In parallel a number of studies have been designed searching for novel and specific biomarkers for pSS, but their results are still in progress [47–49].

In 2013, an ACR-European classification criteria working group has been found in order to elaborate novel classification criteria derived from the existing ones. In fact, the burden of creating a completely novel set of classification criteria has not appeared justified, considering the lack of novel specific biomarkers for the disease. Hopefully, the novel criteria will be able to select homogenous patients opening new avenues for clinical trials and epidemiological studies.

References

1. Mavragani CP, Moutsopoulos HM (2010) The geoepidemiology of Sjogren's syndrome. Autoimmun Rev 9(5):A305–A310
2. Moutsopoulos HM (2014) Sjogren's syndrome: a forty-year scientific journey. J Autoimmun 51:1–9
3. Epstein JB, Villines DC, Sroussi HY (2015) Oral symptoms and oral function in people with Sjogren's syndrome. Clin Exp Rheumatol 33(1):132–133
4. Baldini C, Pepe P, Quartuccio L, Priori R, Bartoloni E, Alunno A, Gattamelata A, Maset M, Modesti M, Tavoni A, De Vita S, Gerli R, Valesini G, Bombardieri S (2014) Primary Sjogren's syndrome as a multi-organ disease: impact of the serological profile on the clinical presentation of the disease in a large cohort of Italian patients. Rheumatology (Oxford). 53(5): 839–844
5. Ramos-Casals M, Brito-Zeron P, Solans R, Camps MT, Casanovas A, Sopena B et al (2014) Systemic involvement in primary Sjogren's syndrome evaluated by the EULAR-SS disease

activity index: analysis of 921 Spanish patients (GEAS-SS Registry). Rheumatology (Oxford) 53(2):321–331

6. Voulgarelis M, Dafni UG, Isenberg DA, Moutsopoulos HM (1999) Malignant lymphoma in primary Sjogren's syndrome: a multicenter, retrospective, clinical study by the European Concerted Action on Sjogren's Syndrome. Arthritis Rheum 42(8):1765–1772
7. Malladi AS, Sack KE, Shiboski SC, Shiboski CH, Baer AN, Banushree R et al (2012) Primary Sjogren's syndrome as a systemic disease: a study of participants enrolled in an international Sjogren's syndrome registry. Arthritis Care Res (Hoboken) 64(6):911–918
8. Quartuccio L, Isola M, Baldini C, Priori R, Bartoloni Bocci E, Carubbi F, Maset M, Gregoraci G, Della Mea V, Salvin S, De Marchi G, Luciano N, Colafrancesco S, Alunno A, Giacomelli R, Gerli R, Valesini G, Bombardieri S, De Vita S (2014) Biomarkers of lymphoma in Sjögren's syndrome and evaluation of the lymphoma risk in prelymphomatous conditions: results of a multicenter study. J Autoimmun 51:75–80
9. ter Borg EJ, Kelder JC (2014) Lower prevalence of extra-glandular manifestations and anti-SSB antibodies in patients with primary Sjogren's syndrome and widespread pain: evidence for a relatively benign subset. Clin Exp Rheumatol 32(3):349–353
10. Theander E, Jacobsson LT (2008) Relationship of Sjogren's syndrome to other connective tissue and autoimmune disorders. Rheum Dis Clin North Am 34(4):935–947, viii-ix
11. Ramos-Casals M, Brito-Zeron P, Font J (2007) The overlap of Sjogren's syndrome with other systemic autoimmune diseases. Semin Arthritis Rheum 36(4):246–255
12. Baldini C, Mosca M, Della Rossa A, Pepe P, Notarstefano C, Ferro F et al (2013) Overlap of ACA-positive systemic sclerosis and Sjogren's syndrome: a distinct clinical entity with mild organ involvement but at high risk of lymphoma. Clin Exp Rheumatol 31(2):272–280
13. Shavit L, Grenader T (2014) Clinical manifestations and outcome of ANCA-related pauci-immune glomerulonephritis in patients with Sjogren's syndrome. Clin Exp Rheumatol 32(2 Suppl 82):S19–S25
14. Baldini C, Talarico R, Tzioufas AG, Bombardieri S (2012) Classification criteria for Sjogren's syndrome: a critical review. J Autoimmun 39(1–2):9–14
15. Goules AV, Tzioufas AG, Moutsopoulos HM (2014) Classification criteria of Sjogren's syndrome. J Autoimmun 48–49:42–45
16. Vitali C, Bombardieri S, Jonsson R, Moutsopoulos HM, Alexander EL, Carsons SE et al (2002) Classification criteria for Sjogren's syndrome: a revised version of the European criteria proposed by the American-European Consensus Group. Ann Rheum Dis 61(6):554–558
17. Vitali C, Bombardieri S, Moutsopoulos HM, Balestrieri G, Bencivelli W, Bernstein RM et al (1993) Preliminary criteria for the classification of Sjogren's syndrome. Results of a prospective concerted action supported by the European Community. Arthritis Rheum 36(3):340–347
18. Shiboski SC, Shiboski CH, Criswell L, Baer A, Challacombe S, Lanfranchi H et al (2012) American College of Rheumatology classification criteria for Sjogren's syndrome: a data-driven, expert consensus approach in the Sjogren's International Collaborative Clinical Alliance cohort. Arthritis Care Res (Hoboken) 64(4):475–487
19. Vitali C, Bootsma H, Bowman SJ, Dorner T, Gottenberg JE, Mariette X et al (2013) Classification criteria for Sjogren's syndrome: we actually need to definitively resolve the long debate on the issue. Ann Rheum Dis 72(4):476–478
20. Quartuccio L, Baldini C, Priori R, Bartoloni E, Carubbi F, Giacomelli R et al (2014) The classification criteria for Sjogren syndrome: issues for their improvement from the study of a large Italian cohort of patients. Ann Rheum Dis 73(7):e35
21. Bowman SJ, Fox RI (2014) Classification criteria for Sjogren's syndrome: nothing ever stands still! Ann Rheum Dis 73(1):1–2
22. Manthorpe R, Oxholm P, Prause JU, Schiodt M (1986) The Copenhagen criteria for Sjogren's syndrome. Scand J Rheumatol Suppl 61:19–21
23. Homma M, Tojo T, Akizuki M, Yamagata H (1986) Criteria for Sjogren's syndrome in Japan. Scand J Rheumatol Suppl 61:26–27
24. Skopouli FN, Drosos AA, Papaioannou T, Moutsopoulos HM (1986) Preliminary diagnostic criteria for Sjogren's syndrome. Scand J Rheumatol Suppl 61:22–25

25. Fox RI, Robinson CA, Curd JG, Kozin F, Howell FV (1986) Sjogren's syndrome. Proposed criteria for classification. Arthritis Rheum 29(5):577–585
26. Daniels TE, Silverman S Jr, Michalski JP, Greenspan JS, Sylvester RA, Talal N (1975) The oral component of Sjogren's syndrome. Oral Surg Oral Med Oral Pathol 39(6):875–885
27. Prause JU, Manthorpe R, Oxholm P, Schiodt M (1986) Definition and criteria for Sjogren's syndrome used by the contributors to the First International Seminar on Sjogren's syndrome – 1986. Scand J Rheumatol Suppl 61:17–18
28. (1989) Workshop on diagnostic criteria for Sjogren's syndrome. Pisa, September 30–October 1, 1988. Clin Exp Rheumatol 7(2):111–219
29. Vitali C, Bombardieri S, Moutsopoulos HM, Coll J, Gerli R, Hatron PY et al (1996) Assessment of the European classification criteria for Sjogren's syndrome in a series of clinically defined cases: results of a prospective multicentre study. The European Study Group on Diagnostic Criteria for Sjogren's Syndrome. Ann Rheum Dis 55(2):116–121
30. Fox RI (1996) Fifth international symposium on Sjogren's syndrome. Arthritis Rheum 39(2):195–196
31. Devauchelle-Pensec V, Morvan J, Rat AC, Jousse-Joulin S, Pennec Y, Pers JO et al (2011) Effects of rituximab therapy on quality of life in patients with primary Sjogren's syndrome. Clin Exp Rheumatol 29(1):6–12
32. Novljan MP, Rozman B, Jerse M, Rotar Z, Vidmar G, Kveder T et al (2006) Comparison of the different classification criteria sets for primary Sjogren's syndrome. Scand J Rheumatol 35(6):463–467
33. Langegger C, Wenger M, Duftner C, Dejaco C, Baldissera I, Moncayo R et al (2007) Use of the European preliminary criteria, the Breiman-classification tree and the American-European criteria for diagnosis of primary Sjogren's Syndrome in daily practice: a retrospective analysis. Rheumatol Int 27(8):699–702
34. Binard A, Devauchelle-Pensec V, Fautrel B, Jousse S, Youinou P, Saraux A (2007) Epidemiology of Sjogren's syndrome: where are we now? Clin Exp Rheumatol 25(1):1–4
35. Trontzas PI, Andrianakos AA (2005) Sjogren's syndrome: a population based study of prevalence in Greece. The ESORDIG study. Ann Rheum Dis 64(8):1240–1241
36. Hernandez-Molina G, Avila-Casado C, Nunez-Alvarez C, Cardenas-Velazquez F, Hernandez-Hernandez C, Luisa Calderillo M et al (2015) Utility of the American-European Consensus Group and American College of Rheumatology Classification Criteria for Sjogren's syndrome in patients with systemic autoimmune diseases in the clinical setting. Rheumatology (Oxford) 54(3):441–448
37. Brun JG, Madland TM, Gjesdal CB, Bertelsen LT (2002) Sjogren's syndrome in an out-patient clinic: classification of patients according to the preliminary European criteria and the proposed modified European criteria. Rheumatology (Oxford) 41(3):301–304
38. Sanchez-Guerrero J, Perez-Dosal MR, Cardenas-Velazquez F, Perez-Reguera A, Celis-Aguilar E, Soto-Rojas AE et al (2005) Prevalence of Sjogren's syndrome in ambulatory patients according to the American-European Consensus Group criteria. Rheumatology (Oxford) 44(2):235–240
39. Whitcher JP, Shiboski CH, Shiboski SC, Heidenreich AM, Kitagawa K, Zhang S et al (2010) A simplified quantitative method for assessing keratoconjunctivitis sicca from the Sjogren's Syndrome International Registry. Am J Ophthalmol 149(3):405–415
40. Daniels TE, Criswell LA, Shiboski C, Shiboski S, Lanfranchi H, Dong Y et al (2009) An early view of the international Sjogren's syndrome registry. Arthritis Rheum 61(5):711–714
41. Rasmussen A, Ice JA, Li H, Grundahl K, Kelly JA, Radfar L et al (2014) Comparison of the American-European Consensus Group Sjogren's syndrome classification criteria to newly proposed American College of Rheumatology criteria in a large, carefully characterised sicca cohort. Ann Rheum Dis 73(1):31–38
42. Cornec D, Jousse-Joulin S, Marhadour T, Pers JO, Boisramé-Gastrin S, Renaudineau Y, Saraux A, Devauchelle-Pensec V (2014) Salivary gland ultrasonography improves the diagnostic performance of the 2012 American College of Rheumatology classification criteria for Sjögren's syndrome. Rheumatology (Oxford) 53(9):1604–1607

43. Carotti M, Ciapetti A, Jousse-Joulin S, Salaffi F (2014) Ultrasonography of the salivary glands: the role of grey-scale and colour/power Doppler. Clin Exp Rheumatol 32(1 Suppl 80):S61–S70
44. Hammenfors DS, Brun JG, Jonsson R, Jonsson MV (2015) Diagnostic utility of major salivary gland ultrasonography in primary Sjogren's syndrome. Clin Exp Rheumatol 33(1):56–62
45. Song GG, Lee YH (2014) Diagnostic accuracies of sialography and salivary ultrasonography in Sjogren's syndrome patients: a meta-analysis. Clin Exp Rheumatol 32(4):516–522
46. Nieto-Gonzalez JC, Monteagudo I, Bello N, Martinez-Estupinan L, Naredo E, Carreno L (2014) Salivary gland ultrasound in children: a useful tool in the diagnosis of juvenile Sjogren's syndrome. Clin Exp Rheumatol 32(4):578–580
47. Baldini C, Gallo A, Perez P, Mosca M, Alevizos I, Bombardieri S (2012) Saliva as an ideal milieu for emerging diagnostic approaches in primary Sjogren's syndrome. Clin Exp Rheumatol 30(5):785–790
48. Alevizos I, Illei GG (2010) MicroRNAs in Sjogren's syndrome as a prototypic autoimmune disease. Autoimmun Rev 9(9):618–621
49. Asashima H, Inokuma S, Onoda M, Oritsu M (2013) Cut-off levels of salivary beta2-microglobulin and sodium differentiating patients with Sjogren's syndrome from those without it and healthy controls. Clin Exp Rheumatol 31(5):699–703

Etiopathogenesis of Sjogren's Syndrome 20

Adrianos Nezos and Clio P. Mavragani

20.1 Introduction

Sjogren's syndrome (SS) is a chronic, relatively common autoimmune disease primarily affecting middle-aged women. Its prevalence has been reported up to 0.5–1.0 % of the general population. The major SS characteristic is the accumulation of periepithelial lymphocytic cell infiltrates in the exocrine glands, mainly labial and lachrymal glands, resulting in oral and ocular dryness. Approximately half of the patients with SS experiences systemic disease manifestations with periepithelial mononuclear infiltrates in parenchymal organs such as kidneys, lung, and liver. Immunocomplex deposition resulting in palpable purpura, glomerulonephritis, and vasculitis can also occur [1, 2]. The latter set of manifestations have been designated as adverse predictors for non-Hodgkin lymphoma (NHL) development [1, 3]. The disease typically occurs in two forms: primary and SS associated with other autoimmune disorders, such as lupus, rheumatoid arthritis, and systemic sclerosis [2]. Although the upstream events leading to the development of SS have not been fully understood, the interactions between genetic, epigenetic, and environmental contributors seem to underlie its pathogenesis.

20.2 Etiological Factors

20.2.1 Genetics

The contribution of heritable components in disease pathogenesis is supported by the heightened prevalence of SS in monozygotic twins, in conjunction with the

A. Nezos • C.P. Mavragani (✉)
Department of Physiology, University of Athens, Athens, Greece
e-mail: kmauragan@med.uoa.gr

D. Roccatello, L. Emmi (eds.), *Connective Tissue Disease: A Comprehensive Guide-Volume 1*, Rare Diseases of the Immune System 5,
DOI 10.1007/978-3-319-24535-5_20

familial aggregation of the disease. Major histocompatibility complex (MHC) alleles together with single nucleotide polymorphisms (SNPs) outside the human leukocyte antigen (HLA) locus have been proposed to have a role in SS pathogenesis. The latter includes several genes involved in the immune innate and adaptive response, mainly related to interferon (IFN), nuclear factor kappa-light-chain-enhancer of activated B cells (NF-κB), as well as B-cell activation and differentiation pathways. In detail, variants in the IFN regulating factor 5 transportin 3 (IRF5-TNPO3) locus and signal transducer and activator of transcription 4 (STAT4) have been consistently shown to confer increased SS susceptibility [4–9]. IRF5 encodes a transcription factor central to the innate and adaptive immune response, while TNPO3 encodes a nuclear import receptor that mediates nuclear entry of splicing factors. These findings along with the MHC associations were recently confirmed in two SS large-scale association studies both in Caucasian and in Han Chinese populations [10, 11].

Genetic variants involve genes implicated either in the suppression or in the activation of the NF-κB pathway. Tumor necrosis factor alpha-induced protein 3 (TNFAIP3), a gene encoding the A20 protein, [10–12], and TNFAIP3-interacting protein 1 (TNIP1) [10, 13] have been shown to have a role in inhibiting NF-κB. Conversely, NF-κB pathway seems to be activated by the mutation His159Tyr of the B-cell activating factor (BAFF) receptor. These genetic variants may be involved in the development of NHL in the contest of SS [10, 12, 14].

Moreover, the presence of SNPs of genes implicated in B-cell maturation and activation such as early B-cell factor 1 [4, 10, 15] or germinal center formation such as the lymphotoxin-α LTA/LTB/tumor necrosis factor (TNF) gene have been also found to increase the risk for SS development [16, 17].

Besides, SNPs in the chemokine gene CCL11 were associated with the formation of germinal center (GC)-like structures in salivary gland tissues, possibly leading to enhanced migration of immune cells in the inflamed salivary glands [18]. Finally, a functional deletion of 6.7 Kb of the leukocyte immunoglobulin-like receptor A3, a soluble receptor for class I MHC antigens implicated in modulation of immune function, has been detected in patients with SS of both Caucasian [19] and Chinese [20] origin [21–23]. In patients with SS, the presence of this functional deletion has been associated with leucopenia and the presence of autoantibodies against Ro/SSA and La/SSB antigens [20].

20.2.2 Epigenetics

Several studies have implicated epigenetic influences in the development of SS. Small noncoding RNAs, such as microRNAs mir146a and miR-155, which regulate the expression of genes linked to innate immune responses, were found differentially expressed in peripheral blood mononuclear cells from SS patients compared to healthy controls, in association with glandular manifestations [24, 25]. Defective resolution of inflammatory process has been proposed as a potential mechanism of mir146a contribution in disease process [25]. Deep sequencing of small RNAs from SS patients disclosed previously unidentified microRNAs with significant disease specificity [26–28].

Alteration of methylation patterns has been also evaluated in SS. A recent genome-wide methylation analysis in patients with SS identified distinct patterns in naive CD4+ T cells compared to healthy controls. Important genes in SS pathogenesis – including LTA and IFN signature pathway genes – were found to be hypomethylated in SS patients [29]. Forkhead box P3 (FOXP3), the major regulator of the T regulatory cell development, was found to be hypermethylated in CD4+ T cells from SS patients, leading to a suppression at mRNA and protein levels [30]. Global DNA methylation was shown to be reduced in SS-derived salivary gland epithelial cells (SGEC). Defective PKC-δ function of the infiltrating B cells and alterations of methylating mediators such as DNA methyltransferase 1 (DNMT1) have been reported in patients with SS [31]. On the other hand, a coordinated overexpression of methylating enzymes implicated in both de novo and maintenance methylation has been observed at the level of SS salivary gland possibly as a compensatory response aimed at controlling inappropriate overexpression of endogenous retroelements [32].

20.2.3 Role of Environment

20.2.3.1 Viruses

Given the previously reported activated status of SGECs along with the upregulation of IFN-related genes in the setting of SS, the implication of viruses in disease initiation has been long suspected. Cytomegalovirus, Epstein-Barr virus (EBV), human herpes virus type-6, human T-cell lymphotropic virus type 1 (HTLV-1), retroviruses, hepatitis C virus, and enteroviruses have been all proposed as potential triggers [33, 34]. EBV virus-encoded small RNA (EBER) from EBV-infected cells in association with the SS-related autoantigen La/SSB were previously shown to induce TLR3-mediated activation of the type I IFN pathway [35]. Of interest, in a recent study, evidence of latent and lytic EBV infection was demonstrated in salivary gland tissues demonstrating ectopic lymphoid structure formation in association with production of autoantibodies against Ro52 autoantigens by EBV-infected perifollicular plasma cells. These data strongly suggest chronic EBV infection as a potential contributor of survival and perpetuation of autoreactive B cells in the setting of SS [36]. Endogenous retroviral elements have been also proposed as potential primary triggers in generation of type I IFN responses among primary SS patients [32].

20.2.3.2 Stress

The occurrence of major stressful life events prior to disease onset in association with an inability to effectively cope against environmental challenges [37], in conjunction with an hypofunctional hypothalamic-pituitary-adrenal axis (HPA), have been previously proposed as potential SS triggers in genetically susceptible individuals [38]. On the other hand, antibodies against neuropeptides have been viewed as putative determinants in personality characteristics and psychopathology features of patients with primary SS [39], implying a key role of neuroendocrine interactions in disease pathogenesis [40].

20.2.3.3 Hormonal Factors

The active role of the endocrine system in SS pathogenesis is supported by the clear female preponderance and by the perimenopausal disease onset. Data from animal models also suggest the contribution of estrogen deficiency in SS development [34, 41]. In view of the immunomodulatory actions of estrogens in normal SGECs, the intrinsic epithelial activation observed in SS could be linked to alteration of these mechanisms [42, 43]. On the other hand, reduced androgen levels – especially the active testosterone form, previously shown to inhibit apoptosis in SGEC – could lead to enhanced apoptosis in menopausal SS patients, promoting further autoimmune-related tissue injury [44–46].

20.3 Histopathology

The main histopathological lesion in SS consists of periepithelial lymphocytic cell infiltrates in exocrine glands (mainly salivary and lachrymal glands) as well as in parenchymal organs (liver, lung, kidney). Biopsy of minor salivary gland (MSG) tissues obtained from the lower lip is considered the gold standard for SS histopathological diagnosis; an average focus score >1 according to Chisholm [47] is compatible with SS diagnosis according to the widely accepted American/European criteria [48] and the more recently proposed criteria by the American College of Rheumatology [49]. The Chisholm focus score [47] is calculated as the number of lymphocytic foci per 4 mm^2 surface in at least four informative lobules, with a focus being defined as a cluster of at least 50 lymphocytes. In the ocular surface, the activation of proinflammatory pathways with local production of cytokines and metalloproteinases results into damage of both corneal and bulbar conjunctival epithelia (keratoconjunctivitis sicca) [50]. Reduced transcript levels of the PAX6 gene – a regulator of corneal development – in impression cytology specimens derived from SS patients were recently shown to associate with ocular surface damage [51].

Parenchymal organs (lung, kidney liver) from SS patients can present histopathological features similar to those seen in exocrine tissues, such as peribronchial lymphocytic infiltrates in transbronchial specimens, focal lymphocytic infiltrates around renal tubular epithelium, or around the biliary duct epithelial cells. As a result, small airway obstructive disease, interstitial nephritis with associated renal tubular acidosis, and primary biliary cirrhosis-like manifestations may occur in these patients (as reviewed in [3]). Taken together, these findings confirm the crucial role of the epithelium in disease pathophysiology, and therefore, the term "autoimmune epithelitis" has been earlier proposed [52].

20.4 Cells and Cytokines in SS

It has long been established – in both SS human and mouse model studies – that the extent of cellular infiltrates in MSG tissues is highly variable and can be classified into mild, intermediate, and severe, according to the Tarpley biopsy score [53]. Furthermore, the degree of lesion severity in the affected tissues is associated with the composition of cellular infiltrates [54].

20.4.1 T Lymphocytes

CD4+ T cells have been originally viewed as the principal cell population in salivary gland infiltrates of SS patients; however, recent data revealed a different expression of cellular components in relation to the severity of the histopathological lesion, with B cells prevailing in advanced and CD4+ cells in mild lesions, respectively [54]. Th1 cytokine patterns (such as IFN-γ) were shown to predominate over Th2 patterns, in association with more severe glandular infiltrates. Th1 pattern seems to promote tissue injury through production and release of plasminogen activation system components [54–57]. Interleukin-33 (IL-33) – a recently identified cytokine of the IL-1 family with both extracellular and nuclear functions – has been also found to be increased in both serum and salivary gland tissues of SS patients (mainly in focus scores 2 and 3). IL-33 synergistically acts with IL-12 and IL-23 for the induction of IFN-γ secretion by natural killers (NK) and NKT cells [58].

Th17 cells (an IL-17-producing CD4+ subtype) have been also detected in the SS salivary gland tissue [59], especially in patients with advanced lesions. Their role in the immunopathogenesis of the disease has been also supported by recent observations in experimental models [60, 61]. A reduced function of the suppressor of cytokine signaling 3 (SOCS3) has been postulated as a possible mechanism involved in the deregulated expression of IL-17 in SS [62]. Another source of IL-17 in SS salivary gland tissues is the "double negative" (DN) T-cell subset (absence of both CD4 and CD8 molecules) [63]. IL-22, also produced by Th17 and a subset of NK cells [64] as well as IL-7 along with CD4+ T cells bearing the IL-7 receptor, has been also detected in salivary SS gland tissues [65].

The follicular cells – an IL-21 producer CD4+ subset – are actively involved in lymphoid follicle formation, and they were also found to be present in salivary gland tissues characterized by the presence of high focus scores and GC structures [66, 67]. Of interest, SS-derived SGECs were shown to directly induce T follicular cells differentiation in co-culture experiments [68]. Finally, the adhesion and chemotactic molecule CX3CL1 and its receptor CX3CR1 have been also proposed as potential participants in the ectopic GC formation in SS salivary glands [69].

Regulatory T lymphocytes – a Th population with a controlling role against undesired lymphocytic activation – have been also studied in the setting of SS with conflicting results [70, 71]. A newly identified regulatory cell subtype includes CD4+ cells expressing glucocorticoid-induced TNFR-related (GITR) (a key role protein in the maintenance of immunological self-tolerance) protein. GITR was found expanded in both SS salivary gland tissues and periphery, possibly in an attempt to control excessive autoimmune-driven inflammation [72]. Altered B-cell regulatory function mediated by the T-cell deficiency of the calcium sensors stromal interaction molecules 1 and 2 (STIM1 and STIM2) has been also proposed as a putative mechanism of disease development in both humans and animal models [73].

20.4.2 B Lymphocytes

B-cell hyperactivity has been long appreciated as a main disease feature, as indicated by the presence of hypergammaglobulinemia and both specific and nonspecific serum autoantibodies including antinuclear, anti-ribonucleoproteinic complexes Ro/SSA and La/SSB, rheumatoid factor (RF), and cryoglobulins. Autoantibodies against α-fodrin, carbonic anhydrase, and muscarinic antibodies have been also described, with the latter being involved in SS-related secretory dysfunction [74]. The underlying mechanisms for B-cell hyperresponsiveness in the setting of SS remain to be elucidated. However, the following mechanisms have been proposed: abnormal retention of pre-switch Ig transcripts in circulating memory B cells, prolonged translocation of BCR in lipid rafts of B cells resulting in increased signaling, and heightened BAFF levels in both serum and saliva [75]. BAFF is a member of the (TNF) family essential for the development and survival of B lymphocytes. The development of an SS phenotype reminiscent of human SS in the BAFF transgenic mice is indicative of its central role in disease pathogenesis [76].

In MSG tissues, B cells were found as a predominant cell type in advanced SS. MSG lesions with oligoclonal B-cell populations and germinal center formation have been proposed as predictors of lymphoma development [54, 77, 78]; interestingly, recent data suggested the presence of locally produced anti-Ro(SSA) and/or anti-La(SSB) at the level of salivary glands [79].

Naive peripheral B cells (CD19+, CD27+, IgD+) were found to be increased in SS patients compared to controls [80, 81]. Memory (CD19+, CD27+, IgD-) B cells are reduced in the periphery [80, 81], possibly because of their retention in inflamed salivary gland tissues [82]. Un-switched memory B cells (CD19+, CD27+, IgD+) have been recently shown to display an altered transcriptional profile in SS and in a subset of sicca patients compared to healthy individuals [83]. Accumulation of autoreactive clones in both naive and memory B-cell compartment and in another CD21-/low B-cell population suggests defective checkpoint immune tolerance mechanisms operating in SS similarly to other autoimmune diseases [81, 84] (Fig. 20.1).

20.4.3 Macrophages/Dendritic Cells

Increased numbers of macrophages have been reported in advanced SS MSG lesions, with the presence of IL-18 secreting macrophages being associated with clinical and serological risk factors for SS lymphomagenesis [85]. Additionally,

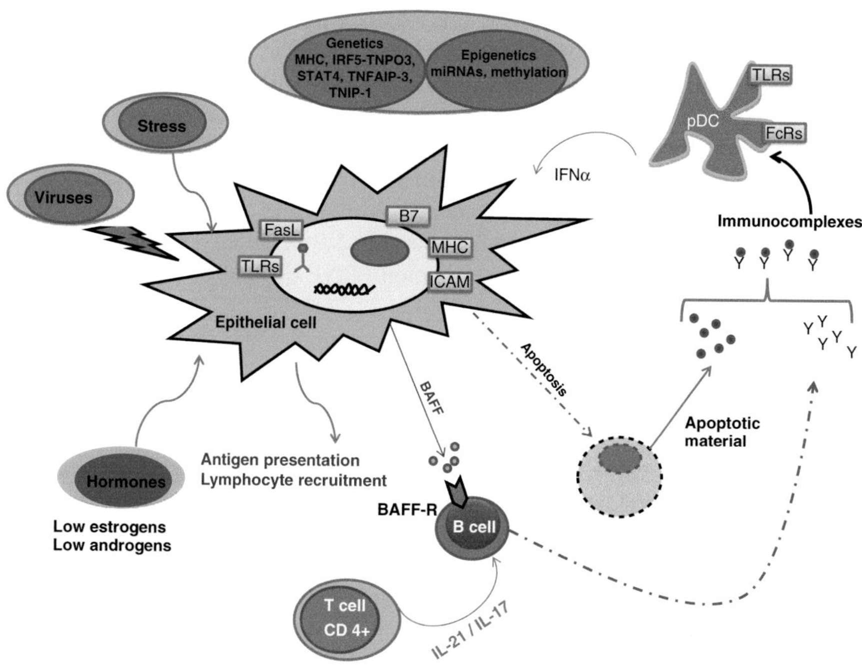

Fig. 20.1 Proposed model of Sjogren's Syndrome etiopathogenesis

IL-34 – a recently identified proinflammatory cytokine which promotes the growth and differentiation of CD14+ monocytes – was also found to be overexpressed in SS MSGs [86]. In a recent report, increased phagocytic uptake of necrotic material in the peripheral blood was described, possibly related to a defective DNAase activity [87].

Dendritic cells (DCs) – involved in both disease initiation and tolerance – have also been considered as main contributors in disease pathogenesis. So far, two major types of DCs are recognized, namely, myeloid DCs (mDCs) and plasmacytoid DCs (pDCs). The latter have been shown to produce type I IFN through TLR-7 and TLR-9 [88]. Type I IFN inducible genes have been found to be upregulated in SS peripheral blood and salivary gland tissues compared to controls; particularly, IFN-α itself strongly correlates with expression of LINE-1 retroviral elements at the level of salivary gland tissue. An overexpression of IFN inducible genes was also detected in peripheral blood cells in association with disease activity (as reviewed in [32]).

20.4.4 Epithelial Cells

Available evidence supports the intrinsic activating capacity of SGEC, as shown by the presence of numerous immune reactive molecules implicated in antigen presentation such as TLRs, CD91, and MHC I/II, costimulation (CD40, B.7/CD80, PD-L1), cell adhesion (ICAM.1/CD54), and apoptosis (Fas, FasL). Activated epithelial cells have been also shown to produce proinflammatory cytokines (IL-1, IL-6, IL-8, TNF-α, and adiponectin), chemokines, as well as BAFF [89, 90]. Some forms of the latter have been recently shown to promote survival of epithelial cells through an autocrine action [91]. Alterations in IkBa kinase – an essential negative regulator of NF-κB activation – and TNFAIP3 – a negative feedback regulator of TNF-α signaling through NF-κB – have been proposed as potential culprits for the sustained activation of NF-κB pathways in SS salivary epithelial cells [92].

20.5 Exocrine Gland Dysfunction

Growing evidence over the last years challenges the prevailing dogma according to which, loss of function in secretory epithelia is mainly attributed to destruction of the glandular tissue by lymphocytic infiltrates. The dissociation between the severity of sicca complaints and the extent of glandular autoimmune inflammation suggest alternative pathways as principal contributors to the defective glandular homeostasis. These include (a) increased apoptosis of salivary epithelial cells (caused by cytokines and hormonal changes); (b) inhibition of cholinergic neurotransmission induced by antimuscarinic M3 autoantibodies; (c) structural alterations arising either from abnormal tight junction protein levels, disorganization of the basal membrane in labial SGEC, overexpression of the bone morphogenetic protein-6 (BMP-6), or dysfunction of the Hippo signaling pathway; and (d) abnormal distribution and expression of the water channel aquaporin 5 in SS-derived SGEC, potentially related to the presence of antimuscarinic antibodies [34, 93–95].

Conclusion

SS epithelial cell plays a central role in disease pathogenesis serving as an antigen-presenting cell, recruiting B and T lymphocytes through lympho-attractant chemokines and ensuring B-cell lymphocyte survival and proliferation through BAFF production. The release of endogenous nucleic acids and autoantigens can occur as a result of increased apoptosis possibly caused by neuroendocrine, viral, or genetic/epigenetic insults. The consequent exposition of autoantigens can lead to the production of disease-specific autoantibodies against ribonucleoproteinic complexes. As a consequence, immunocomplexes are formed, leading to PDC activation and IFN-α production, which further causes B-cell activation through BAFF production as well as enhanced salivary epithelial cell apoptosis, closing this vicious inflammatory cycle.

Acknowledgments The authors are indebted to Professor Moutsopoulos for his continuous inspiration, guidance, and support.

References

1. Skopouli FN, Dafni U, Ioannidis JP, Moutsopoulos HM (2000) Clinical evolution, and morbidity and mortality of primary Sjogren's syndrome. Semin Arthritis Rheum 29(5):296–304
2. Mavragani CP, Moutsopoulos HM (2010) The geoepidemiology of Sjogren's syndrome. Autoimmun Rev 9(5):A305–A310
3. Mavragani CP, Moutsopoulos HM (2014) Sjogren syndrome. CMAJ 186(15):E579–E586
4. Nordmark G, Kristjansdottir G, Theander E, Appel S, Eriksson P, Vasaitis L et al (2011) Association of EBF1, FAM167A(C8orf13)-BLK and TNFSF4 gene variants with primary Sjogren's syndrome. Genes Immun 12(2):100–109
5. Gottenberg JE, Busson M, Loiseau P, Cohen-Solal J, Lepage V, Charron D et al (2003) In primary Sjogren's syndrome, HLA class II is associated exclusively with autoantibody production and spreading of the autoimmune response. Arthritis Rheum 48(8):2240–2245
6. Mann DL, Moutsopoulos HM (1983) HLA DR alloantigens in different subsets of patients with Sjogren's syndrome and in family members. Ann Rheum Dis 42(5):533–536
7. Cruz-Tapias P, Rojas-Villarraga A, Maier-Moore S, Anaya JM (2012) HLA and Sjogren's syndrome susceptibility. A meta-analysis of worldwide studies. Autoimmun Rev 11(4):281–287
8. Miceli-Richard C, Comets E, Loiseau P, Puechal X, Hachulla E, Mariette X (2007) Association of an IRF5 gene functional polymorphism with Sjogren's syndrome. Arthritis Rheum 56(12):3989–3994
9. Nordmark G, Kristjansdottir G, Theander E, Eriksson P, Brun JG, Wang C et al (2009) Additive effects of the major risk alleles of IRF5 and STAT4 in primary Sjogren's syndrome. Genes Immun 10(1):68–76
10. Lessard CJ, Li H, Adrianto I, Ice JA, Rasmussen A, Grundahl KM et al (2013) Variants at multiple loci implicated in both innate and adaptive immune responses are associated with Sjogren's syndrome. Nat Genet 45(11):1284–1292
11. Li Y, Zhang K, Chen H, Sun F, Xu J, Wu Z et al (2013) A genome-wide association study in Han Chinese identifies a susceptibility locus for primary Sjogren's syndrome at 7q11.23. Nat Genet 45(11):1361–1365
12. Nocturne G, Boudaoud S, Miceli-Richard C, Viengchareun S, Lazure T, Nititham J et al (2013) Germline and somatic genetic variations of TNFAIP3 in lymphoma complicating primary Sjogren's syndrome. Blood 122(25):4068–4076
13. Nordmark G, Wang C, Vasaitis L, Eriksson P, Theander E, Kvarnstrom M et al (2013) Association of genes in the NF-kappaB pathway with antibody-positive primary Sjogren's syndrome. Scand J Immunol 78(5):447–454
14. Sisto M, Lisi S, Lofrumento DD, Ingravallo G, De Lucro R, D'Amore M (2013) Salivary gland expression level of Ikappa Balpha regulatory protein in Sjogren's syndrome. J Mol Histol 44(4):447–454
15. Sun F, Li P, Chen H, Wu Z, Xu J, Shen M et al (2014) Association studies of TNFSF4, TNFAIP3 and FAM167A-BLK polymorphisms with primary Sjogren's syndrome in Han Chinese. J Hum Genet 58(7):475–479
16. Nezos A, Papageorgiou A, Fragoulis G, Ioakeimidis D, Koutsilieris M, Tzioufas AG et al (2014) B-cell activating factor genetic variants in lymphomagenesis associated with primary Sjogren's syndrome. J Autoimmun 51:89–98
17. Bolstad AI, Le Hellard S, Kristjansdottir G, Vasaitis L, Kvarnstrom M, Sjowall C et al (2012) Association between genetic variants in the tumour necrosis factor/lymphotoxin alpha/lymphotoxin beta locus and primary Sjogren's syndrome in Scandinavian samples. Ann Rheum Dis 71(6):981–988
18. Reksten TR, Johnsen SJ, Jonsson MV, Omdal R, Brun JG, Theander E et al (2014) Genetic associations to germinal centre formation in primary Sjogren's syndrome. Ann Rheum Dis 73(6):1253–1258
19. Kabalak G, Dobberstein SB, Matthias T, Reuter S, The YH, Dorner T et al (2009) Association of immunoglobulin-like transcript 6 deficiency with Sjogren's syndrome. Arthritis Rheum 60(10):2923–2925

20. Du Y, Su Y, He J, Yang Y, Shi Y, Cui Y et al (2014) Impact of the leucocyte immunoglobulin-like receptor A3 (LILRA3) on susceptibility and subphenotypes of systemic lupus erythematosus and Sjogren's syndrome. Ann Rheum Dis 74(11):2070–2075
21. Du Y, Cui Y, Liu X, Hu F, Yang Y, Wu X et al (2014) Contribution of functional LILRA3, but not nonfunctional LILRA3, to sex bias in susceptibility and severity of anti-citrullinated protein antibody-positive rheumatoid arthritis. Arthritis Rheumatol 66(4):822–830
22. Low HZ, Reuter S, Topperwien M, Dankenbrink N, Peest D, Kabalak G et al (2013) Association of the LILRA3 deletion with B-NHL and functional characterization of the immunostimulatory molecule. PLoS ONE 8(12):e81360
23. Ordonez D, Sanchez AJ, Martinez-Rodriguez JE, Cisneros E, Ramil E, Romo N et al (2009) Multiple sclerosis associates with LILRA3 deletion in Spanish patients. Genes Immun 10(6):579–585
24. Shi H, Zheng LY, Zhang P, Yu CQ (2014) miR-146a and miR-155 expression in PBMCs from patients with Sjogren's syndrome. J Oral Pathol Med 43(10):792–797
25. Pauley KM, Stewart CM, Gauna AE, Dupre LC, Kuklani R, Chan AL et al (2011) Altered miR-146a expression in Sjogren's syndrome and its functional role in innate immunity. Eur J Immunol 41(7):2029–2039
26. Tandon M, Gallo A, Jang SI, Illei GG, Alevizos I (2012) Deep sequencing of short RNAs reveals novel microRNAs in minor salivary glands of patients with Sjogren's syndrome. Oral Dis 18(2):127–131
27. Alevizos I, Alexander S, Turner RJ, Illei GG (2011) MicroRNA expression profiles as biomarkers of minor salivary gland inflammation and dysfunction in Sjogren's syndrome. Arthritis Rheum 63(2):535–544
28. Kapsogeorgou EK, Gourzi VC, Manoussakis MN, Moutsopoulos HM, Tzioufas AG (2011) Cellular microRNAs (miRNAs) and Sjogren's syndrome: candidate regulators of autoimmune response and autoantigen expression. J Autoimmun 37(2):129–135
29. Altorok N, Coit P, Hughes T, Koelsch KA, Stone DU, Rasmussen A et al (2014) Genome-wide DNA methylation patterns in naive CD4+ T cells from patients with primary Sjogren's syndrome. Arthritis Rheumatol 66(3):731–739
30. Yu X, Liang G, Yin H, Ngalamika O, Li F, Zhao M et al (2013) DNA hypermethylation leads to lower FOXP3 expression in CD4+ T cells of patients with primary Sjogren's syndrome. Clin Immunol 148(2):254–257
31. Thabet Y, Le Dantec C, Ghedira I, Devauchelle V, Cornec D, Pers JO et al (2013) Epigenetic dysregulation in salivary glands from patients with primary Sjogren's syndrome may be ascribed to infiltrating B cells. J Autoimmun 41:175–181
32. Mavragani CP, Crow MK (2010) Activation of the type I interferon pathway in primary Sjogren's syndrome. J Autoimmun 35(3):225–231
33. Nakamura H, Takahashi Y, Yamamoto-Fukuda T, Horai Y, Nakashima Y, Arima K et al (2015) Direct infection of primary salivary gland epithelial cells by HTLV-I that induces the niche of the salivary glands of Sjogren's syndrome patients. Arthritis Rheumatol 67(4):1096–1106
34. Mavragani CP, Moutsopoulos HM (2014) Sjogren's syndrome. Annu Rev Pathol 9:273–285
35. Iwakiri D, Zhou L, Samanta M, Matsumoto M, Ebihara T, Seya T et al (2009) Epstein-Barr virus (EBV)-encoded small RNA is released from EBV-infected cells and activates signaling from Toll-like receptor 3. J Exp Med 206(10):2091–2099
36. Croia C, Astorri E, Murray-Brown W, Willis A, Brokstad KA, Sutcliffe N et al (2014) Implication of Epstein-Barr virus infection in disease-specific autoreactive B cell activation in ectopic lymphoid structures of Sjogren's syndrome. Arthritis Rheumatol 66(9): 2545–2557
37. Karaiskos D, Mavragani CP, Makaroni S, Zinzaras E, Voulgarelis M, Rabavilas A et al (2009) Stress, coping strategies and social support in patients with primary Sjogren's syndrome prior to disease onset: a retrospective case-control study. Ann Rheum Dis 68(1):40–46
38. Johnson EO, Kostandi M, Moutsopoulos HM (2006) Hypothalamic-pituitary-adrenal axis function in Sjogren's syndrome: mechanisms of neuroendocrine and immune system homeostasis. Ann N Y Acad Sci 1088:41–51

39. Karaiskos D, Mavragani CP, Sinno MH, Dechelotte P, Zintzaras E, Skopouli FN et al (2010) Psychopathological and personality features in primary Sjogren's syndrome – associations with autoantibodies to neuropeptides. Rheumatology (Oxford) 49(9):1762–1769
40. Mavragani CP, Fragoulis GE, Moutsopoulos HM (2012) Endocrine alterations in primary Sjogren's syndrome: an overview. J Autoimmun 39(4):354–358
41. Ishimaru N, Arakaki R, Watanabe M, Kobayashi M, Miyazaki K, Hayashi Y (2003) Development of autoimmune exocrinopathy resembling Sjogren's syndrome in estrogen-deficient mice of healthy background. Am J Pathol 163(4):1481–1490
42. Tsinti M, Kassi E, Korkolopoulou P, Kapsogeorgou E, Moutsatsou P, Patsouris E et al (2009) Functional estrogen receptors alpha and beta are expressed in normal human salivary gland epithelium and apparently mediate immunomodulatory effects. Eur J Oral Sci 117(5): 498–505
43. Manoussakis MN, Tsinti M, Kapsogeorgou EK, Moutsopoulos HM (2012) The salivary gland epithelial cells of patients with primary Sjogren's syndrome manifest significantly reduced responsiveness to 17beta-estradiol. J Autoimmun 39(1–2):64–68
44. Konttinen YT, Fuellen G, Bing Y, Porola P, Stegaev V, Trokovic N et al (2012) Sex steroids in Sjogren's syndrome. J Autoimmun 39(1–2):49–56
45. Spaan M, Porola P, Laine M, Rozman B, Azuma M, Konttinen YT (2009) Healthy human salivary glands contain a DHEA-sulphate processing intracrine machinery, which is deranged in primary Sjogren's syndrome. J Cell Mol Med 13(7):1261–1270
46. Porola P, Virkki L, Przybyla BD, Laine M, Patterson TA, Pihakari A et al (2008) Androgen deficiency and defective intracrine processing of dehydroepiandrosterone in salivary glands in Sjogren's syndrome. J Rheumatol 35(11):2229–2235
47. Chisholm DM, Mason DK (1968) Labial salivary gland biopsy in Sjogren's disease. J Clin Pathol 21(5):656–660
48. Vitali C, Bombardieri S, Jonsson R, Moutsopoulos HM, Alexander EL, Carsons SE et al (2002) Classification criteria for Sjogren's syndrome: a revised version of the European criteria proposed by the American-European Consensus Group. Ann Rheum Dis 61(6):554–558
49. Shiboski SC, Shiboski CH, Criswell L, Baer A, Challacombe S, Lanfranchi H et al (2012) American College of Rheumatology classification criteria for Sjogren's syndrome: a data-driven, expert consensus approach in the Sjogren's International Collaborative Clinical Alliance cohort. Arthritis Care Res (Hoboken) 64(4):475–487
50. Stevenson W, Chauhan SK, Dana R (2012) Dry eye disease: an immune-mediated ocular surface disorder. Arch Ophthalmol 130(1):90–100
51. McNamara NA, Gallup M, Porco TC (2014) Establishing PAX6 as a biomarker to detect early loss of ocular phenotype in human patients with Sjogren's syndrome. Invest Ophthalmol Vis Sci 55(11):7079–7084
52. Moutsopoulos HM (1994) Sjogren's syndrome: autoimmune epithelitis. Clin Immunol Immunopathol 72(2):162–165
53. Tarpley TM Jr, Anderson LG, White CL (1974) Minor salivary gland involvement in Sjogren's syndrome. Oral Surg Oral Med Oral Pathol 37(1):64–74
54. Christodoulou MI, Kapsogeorgou EK, Moutsopoulos HM (2010) Characteristics of the minor salivary gland infiltrates in Sjogren's syndrome. J Autoimmun 34(4):400–407
55. Mitsias DI, Tzioufas AG, Veiopoulou C, Zintzaras E, Tassios IK, Kogopoulou O et al (2002) The Th1/Th2 cytokine balance changes with the progress of the immunopathological lesion of Sjogren's syndrome. Clin Exp Immunol 128(3):562–568
56. Oxholm P, Daniels TE, Bendtzen K (1992) Cytokine expression in labial salivary glands from patients with primary Sjogren's syndrome. Autoimmunity 12(3):185–191
57. Gliozzi M, Greenwell-Wild T, Jin W, Moutsopoulos NM, Kapsogeorgou E, Moutsopoulos HM et al (2013) A link between interferon and augmented plasmin generation in exocrine gland damage in Sjogren's syndrome. J Autoimmun 40:122–133
58. Awada A, Nicaise C, Ena S, Schandene L, Rasschaert J, Popescu I et al (2014) Potential involvement of the IL-33-ST2 axis in the pathogenesis of primary Sjogren's syndrome. Ann Rheum Dis 73(6):1259–1263

59. Katsifis GE, Rekka S, Moutsopoulos NM, Pillemer S, Wahl SM (2009) Systemic and local interleukin-17 and linked cytokines associated with Sjogren's syndrome immunopathogenesis. Am J Pathol 175(3):1167–1177
60. Lin X, Rui K, Deng J, Tian J, Wang X, Wang S et al (2014) Th17 cells play a critical role in the development of experimental Sjogren's syndrome. Ann Rheum Dis 74(6):1302–1310
61. Iizuka M, Tsuboi H, Matsuo N, Asashima H, Hirota T, Kondo Y et al (2015) A crucial role of RORgammat in the development of spontaneous Sialadenitis-like Sjogren's syndrome. J Immunol 194(1):56–67
62. Vartoukian SR, Tilakaratne WM, Seoudi N, Bombardieri M, Bergmeier L, Tappuni AR et al (2014) Dysregulation of the suppressor of cytokine signalling 3-signal transducer and activator of transcription-3 pathway in the aetiopathogenesis of Sjogren's syndrome. Clin Exp Immunol 177(3):618–629
63. Alunno A, Carubbi F, Bistoni O, Caterbi S, Bartoloni E, Bigerna B et al (2014) CD4(-)CD8(-) T-cells in primary Sjogren's syndrome: association with the extent of glandular involvement. J Autoimmun 51:38–43
64. Ciccia F, Guggino G, Rizzo A, Ferrante A, Raimondo S, Giardina A et al (2012) Potential involvement of IL-22 and IL-22-producing cells in the inflamed salivary glands of patients with Sjogren's syndrome. Ann Rheum Dis 71(2):295–301
65. Bikker A, Kruize AA, Wenting M, Versnel MA, Bijlsma JW, Lafeber FP et al (2012) Increased interleukin (IL)-7Ralpha expression in salivary glands of patients with primary Sjogren's syndrome is restricted to T cells and correlates with IL-7 expression, lymphocyte numbers and activity. Ann Rheum Dis 71(6):1027–1033
66. Kang KY, Kim HO, Kwok SK, Ju JH, Park KS, Sun DI et al (2011) Impact of interleukin-21 in the pathogenesis of primary Sjogren's syndrome: increased serum levels of interleukin-21 and its expression in the labial salivary glands. Arthritis Res Ther 13(5):R179
67. Szabo K, Papp G, Barath S, Gyimesi E, Szanto A, Zeher M (2013) Follicular helper T cells may play an important role in the severity of primary Sjogren's syndrome. Clin Immunol 147(2):95–104
68. Gong YZ, Nititham J, Taylor K, Miceli-Richard C, Sordet C, Wachsmann D et al (2014) Differentiation of follicular helper T cells by salivary gland epithelial cells in primary Sjogren's syndrome. J Autoimmun 51:57–66
69. Astorri E, Scrivo R, Bombardieri M, Picarelli G, Pecorella I, Porzia A et al (2014) CX3CL1 and CX3CR1 expression in tertiary lymphoid structures in salivary gland infiltrates: fractalkine contribution to lymphoid neogenesis in Sjogren's syndrome. Rheumatology (Oxford) 53(4):611–620
70. Furuzawa-Carballeda J, Sanchez-Guerrero J, Betanzos JL, Enriquez AB, Avila-Casado C, Llorente L et al (2014) Differential cytokine expression and regulatory cells in patients with primary and secondary Sjogren's syndrome. Scand J Immunol 80(6):432–440
71. Christodoulou MI, Kapsogeorgou EK, Moutsopoulos NM, Moutsopoulos HM (2008) Foxp3+ T-regulatory cells in Sjogren's syndrome: correlation with the grade of the autoimmune lesion and certain adverse prognostic factors. Am J Pathol 173(5):1389–1396
72. Alunno A, Petrillo MG, Nocentini G, Bistoni O, Bartoloni E, Caterbi S et al (2013) Characterization of a new regulatory CD4+ T cell subset in primary Sjogren's syndrome. Rheumatology (Oxford) 52(8):1387–1396
73. Cheng KT, Alevizos I, Liu X, Swaim WD, Yin H, Feske S et al (2012) STIM1 and STIM2 protein deficiency in T lymphocytes underlies development of the exocrine gland autoimmune disease, Sjogren's syndrome. Proc Natl Acad Sci U S A 109(36):14544–14549
74. Kyriakidis NC, Kapsogeorgou EK, Tzioufas AG (2014) A comprehensive review of autoantibodies in primary Sjogren's syndrome: clinical phenotypes and regulatory mechanisms. J Autoimmun 51:67–74
75. Youinou P, Devauchelle-Pensec V, Pers JO (2010) Significance of B cells and B cell clonality in Sjogren's syndrome. Arthritis Rheum 62(9):2605–2610

76. Mackay F, Woodcock SA, Lawton P, Ambrose C, Baetscher M, Schneider P et al (1999) Mice transgenic for BAFF develop lymphocytic disorders along with autoimmune manifestations. J Exp Med 190(11):1697–1710
77. Pablos JL, Carreira PE, Morillas L, Montalvo G, Ballestin C, Gomez-Reino JJ (1994) Clonally expanded lymphocytes in the minor salivary glands of Sjogren's syndrome patients without lymphoproliferative disease. Arthritis Rheum 37(10):1441–1444
78. Theander E, Vasaitis L, Baecklund E, Nordmark G, Warfvinge G, Liedholm R et al (2011) Lymphoid organisation in labial salivary gland biopsies is a possible predictor for the development of malignant lymphoma in primary Sjogren's syndrome. Ann Rheum Dis 70(8):1363–1368
79. Tengner P, Halse AK, Haga HJ, Jonsson R, Wahren-Herlenius M (1998) Detection of anti-Ro/SSA and anti-La/SSB autoantibody-producing cells in salivary glands from patients with Sjogren's syndrome. Arthritis Rheum 41(12):2238–2248
80. Karlsen M, Hansen T, Nordal HH, Brun JG, Jonsson R, Appel S (2015) Expression of toll-like receptor -7 and -9 in B cell subsets from patients with primary Sjogren's syndrome. PLoS ONE 10(3):e0120383
81. Corsiero E, Sutcliffe N, Pitzalis C, Bombardieri M (2014) Accumulation of self-reactive naive and memory B cell reveals sequential defects in B cell tolerance checkpoints in Sjogren's syndrome. PLoS ONE 9(12):e114575
82. Hansen A, Odendahl M, Reiter K, Jacobi AM, Feist E, Scholze J et al (2002) Diminished peripheral blood memory B cells and accumulation of memory B cells in the salivary glands of patients with Sjogren's syndrome. Arthritis Rheum 46(8):2160–2171
83. Roberts ME, Kaminski D, Jenks SA, Maguire C, Ching K, Burbelo PD et al (2014) Primary Sjogren's syndrome is characterized by distinct phenotypic and transcriptional profiles of IgD+ unswitched memory B cells. Arthritis Rheumatol 66(9):2558–2569
84. Saadoun D, Terrier B, Bannock J, Vazquez T, Massad C, Kang I et al (2013) Expansion of autoreactive unresponsive CD21(-/low) B cells in Sjogren's syndrome associated lymphoproliferation. Arthritis Rheum 65(4):1085–1096
85. Manoussakis MN, Boiu S, Korkolopoulou P, Kapsogeorgou EK, Kavantzas N, Ziakas P et al (2007) Rates of infiltration by macrophages and dendritic cells and expression of interleukin-18 and interleukin-12 in the chronic inflammatory lesions of Sjogren's syndrome: correlation with certain features of immune hyperactivity and factors associated with high risk of lymphoma development. Arthritis Rheum 56(12):3977–3988
86. Ciccia F, Alessandro R, Rodolico V, Guggino G, Raimondo S, Guarnotta C et al (2013) IL-34 is overexpressed in the inflamed salivary glands of patients with Sjogren's syndrome and is associated with the local expansion of pro-inflammatory CD14(bright)CD16+ monocytes. Rheumatology (Oxford) 52(6):1009–1017
87. Fragoulis GE, Vakrakou AG, Papadopoulou A, Germenis A, Kanavakis E, Moutsopoulos HM et al (2015) Impaired degradation and aberrant phagocytosis of necrotic cell debris in the peripheral blood of patients with primary Sjogren's syndrome. J Autoimmun 56:12–22
88. Ozaki Y, Ito T, Son Y, Amuro H, Shimamoto K, Sugimoto H et al (2010) Decrease of blood dendritic cells and increase of tissue-infiltrating dendritic cells are involved in the induction of Sjogren's syndrome but not in the maintenance. Clin Exp Immunol 159(3):315–326
89. Manoussakis MN, Kapsogeorgou EK (2010) The role of intrinsic epithelial activation in the pathogenesis of Sjogren's syndrome. J Autoimmun 35(3):219–224
90. Tzioufas AG, Kapsogeorgou EK, Moutsopoulos HM (2012) Pathogenesis of Sjogren's syndrome: what we know and what we should learn. J Autoimmun 39(1–2):4–8
91. Lahiri A, Varin MM, Le Pottier L, Pochard P, Bendaoud B, Youinou P et al (2014) Specific forms of BAFF favor BAFF receptor-mediated epithelial cell survival. J Autoimmun 51:30–37
92. Peng B, Ling J, Lee AJ, Wang Z, Chang Z, Jin W et al (2010) Defective feedback regulation of NF-kappaB underlies Sjogren's syndrome in mice with mutated kappaB enhancers of the IkappaBalpha promoter. Proc Natl Acad Sci U S A 107(34):15193–15198

93. Lee BH, Gauna AE, Perez G, Park YJ, Pauley KM, Kawai T et al (2013) Autoantibodies against muscarinic type 3 receptor in Sjogren's syndrome inhibit aquaporin 5 trafficking. PLoS ONE 8(1):e53113
94. Enger TB, Samad-Zadeh A, Bouchie MP, Skarstein K, Galtung HK, Mera T et al (2013) The Hippo signaling pathway is required for salivary gland development and its dysregulation is associated with Sjogren's syndrome. Lab Invest 93(11):1203–1218
95. Yin H, Cabrera-Perez J, Lai Z, Michael D, Weller M, Swaim WD et al (2013) Association of bone morphogenetic protein 6 with exocrine gland dysfunction in patients with Sjogren's syndrome and in mice. Arthritis Rheum 65(12):3228–3238

Autoantibodies in Sjögren's Syndrome and Laboratory Markers

21

Efstathia K. Kapsogeorgou and Athanasios G. Tzioufas

Abbreviations

ACA	Anti-centromere antibodies
AMA	Antimitochondrial antibodies
ANA	Antinuclear antibodies
Anti-CCP	Antibodies against cyclic citrullinated peptides
Anti-CAII	Anti-carbonic anhydrase II
ASMA	Anti-smooth muscle antibodies
MRs	Muscarinic receptors
NLS	Neonatal lupus syndrome
RF	Rheumatoid factor
SLE	Systemic lupus erythematosus
SS	Sjögren's syndrome
SSc	Systemic sclerosis

21.1 Introduction

Sjögren's syndrome (SS) is a heterogeneous autoimmune disease, mainly affecting middle-aged women (women:men, 9:1). Sicca syndrome-related symptoms, mainly of the eyes and mouth, are associated with the destruction and dysfunction of the exocrine glands. SS is characterized by various clinical spectra, ranging from local exocrinopathy to extraglandular, systemic manifestations that affect several organs.

E.K. Kapsogeorgou, PhD • A.G. Tzioufas, MD (✉)
Department of Pathophysiology, School of Medicine, National University of Athens, 75 MikrasAsias street, Athens 11527, Greece
e-mail: agtzi@med.uoa.gr

D. Roccatello, L. Emmi (eds.), *Connective Tissue Disease: A Comprehensive Guide-Volume 1*, Rare Diseases of the Immune System 5,
DOI 10.1007/978-3-319-24535-5_21

Extraglandular systemic manifestations are frequent in primary SS (pSS) and can be categorized as either related to periepithelial inflammation (involving the lung, the liver, or the kidneys) or to immune complex-mediated vasculitis (leading to peripheral neuropathy, glomerulonephritis, or purpura) [1]. The wide spectrum of disease features and outcomes implies the need for biomarkers permitting an early diagnosis of the disease and/or effective treatment, as well as the stratification of the patients according to distinct clinical phenotypes. Indeed, several clinical and laboratory parameters have been shown able to identify patients predisposed to develop lymphoma at the time of pSS diagnosis, supporting the notion that the identification of relevant disease biomarkers is a feasible goal.

The heterogeneity of clinical phenotypes and the diverse disease outcomes most probably reflect complex pathogenetic mechanisms operating in SS patients. The pathogenetic pathways underlying the disease are not fully delineated yet. Organ destruction is associated with periepithelial lymphocytic infiltrates of variable grade, whereas severe lesions have been linked to systemic disease [2, 3], suggesting that local and systemic autoimmune responses may be associated.

A plethora of autoreactive antibodies against intracellular autoantigens is produced in SS. Although the pathogenetic significance of these autoantibodies and the mechanisms governing their production are not fully elucidated, recent evidence confirms that the development of SS humoral autoimmune responses is an antigen-driven process. This is supported by the following: (a) certain autoantibodies are disease specific; (b) the majority of autoantibodies detected are of the IgG class, which is suggestive of an antigen-dependent T-cell help [4]; (c) autoimmune responses are mainly polyclonal and target multiple epitopes within the same or interacting autoantigens [4]; and (d) immunization of experimental animals with fragments of the autoantigens results in intra- and intermolecular spreading of the immune response, similar to that observed after immunization with foreign antigens [5, 6].

Epithelial cells, which are key regulators of local autoimmune responses in SS, may also be implicated in the development of humoral autoimmune responses by releasing autoantigens in apoptotic bodies or exosomes [1, 7, 8]. To date, several antibodies against autoantigens have been described in SS; some of them have been proved valuable for disease diagnosis, whereas others are the still under further investigation.

The main autoantibodies in SS and their clinical significance in disease diagnosis, prognosis, and patient classification, as well as laboratory markers with predictive value for disease outcome, are discussed in the following pages and summarized in Table 21.1.

21.2 Autoantibodies and Clinical Phenotypes

21.2.1 Anti-Ro/SSA and Anti-La/SSB Autoantibodies

The autoimmune response against the Ro/La heterogeneous ribonucleoprotein (RNP) complex characterizes SS and constitutes a diagnostic marker according to

Table 21.1 Prevalence of autoantibodies in SS patients and associations with disease features

Autoantibodies against	Prevalence (%)	Clinical associations
Ro/SSA	33–74	Younger age at diagnosis
		Exocrine gland hypofunction
		Severe infiltration of salivary glands
La/SSB	23–52	Parotid gland enlargement
		Systemic extraglandular manifestations
		Hypergammaglobulinemia/cryoglobulinemia
		Neonatal lupus congenital heart block
Antinuclear antibodies (ANA)	59–85	Parotid gland enlargement
		Systemic extraglandular manifestations
		Hypergammaglobulinemia
Rheumatoid factor	36–74	Younger age at diagnosis
		Positive salivary gland biopsy
		Parotid gland enlargement
		Systemic extraglandular manifestations
		Articular involvement
Cryoglobulins	9–15	Lymphomagenesis
		Younger age at diagnosis
		Parotid gland enlargement
		Systemic extraglandular manifestations
		↓ C3/C4, monoclonal gammopathy
Centromere (ACA)	4–27	Overlap with systemic sclerosis
		Milder disease, with higher risk for lymphoma
Cyclic citrullinated peptides (anti-CCP)	3–10	Articular involvement
Mitochondria (AMA)	1.7–27	Primary biliary cirrhosis
Muscarinic 3 receptor	11	Sicca symptoms
Carbonic anhydrases	12.5–20.8	Renal tubular acidosis
Smooth muscle	30–62	Autoimmune hepatitis

the American-European classification criteria [9]. The Ro/La RNP complex includes four small hY RNAs (human cYtoplasmic RNAs), known as hY1, hY3, hY4, and hY5 RNAs, and the Ro52/TRIM21, Ro60/TROVE2, and La/SSB proteins, with the latter directly interacting with hY RNA.

Ro52 (also known as TRIM21) is a member of the tripartite motif (TRIM) family. Two main functions have been attributed to Ro52/TRIM21 molecule. First, it acts as an Fc-receptor mediating intracellular antiviral immunity and the decoy of antibody-mediated pathogens [10, 11]. Second, it has been identified as an E3 ubiquitin-protein ligase [12]. Ro52/TRIM21 has been implicated in the regulation of cell proliferation and apoptosis and in the regulation of TLR signaling with subsequent IFN production [13]. Besides, Ro60/TROVE2 and La/SSB are RNA-binding proteins involved in the quality control of nascent transcripts. The ring-shaped Ro60/TROVE2 participates in the recognition and degradation of misfolded/defective RNAs [14]. Ro60/TROVE2 has also been shown to promote cell survival after ultraviolet (UV) irradiation, possibly by assisting the decay of the UV-induced damaged RNA [15]. La/SSB has been involved in diverse aspects of RNA metabolism: (a) it chaperones or binds to precursor RNA molecules, in order to protect them from nuclease-mediated decay and to facilitate their correct processing, folding, and maturation by specific ribonucleases [16]; (b) it regulates the expression of micro-RNAs (miRNAs) by protecting and stabilizing the pre-miRNAs from nuclease activity [17];(c) it has been implicated in the enhancement of cap-independent translation of viral or human mRNAs that contain internal ribosome entry sites (IRES);(d) it is involved in efficient RNAi, antiviral defense, and transposon silencing by facilitating the release of cleaved mRNA from the RNA-induced silencing complex (RISC) and thus promoting the multiple-turnover of RISC catalysis; and (e) it regulates cell proliferation and tumor progression by promoting the IRES-dependent translation of the cyclin D1 (CCND1) protein [16–18].

The major antigenic regions of Ro52/TRIM21, Ro60/TROVE2, and La/SSB proteins have been extensively studied (reviewed in [19]). The antigenic peptide 190-245aa, residing in the middle coiled-coil region of Ro52/TRIM21 protein, is recognized in the vast majority of anti-Ro52-positive patients. The main B-cell epitopes for Ro60/TROVE2 reside in the central part of the protein (181–320aa, 139–326aa, and 155–295aa), as well as in the areas defined by the spanning amino acids 216–245, 169–190, and 211–232 [19]. The 169–190aa epitope has been primarily associated with systemic lupus erythematosus (SLE), while the 211–232aa epitope with SS. B-cell responses to La/SSB autoantigen are mainly directed against the peptides 147–154aa, 291–302aa, 301–318aa, and 349–364aa [19].

Historically, the term "anti-Ro/SSA antibodies" has been used to describe autoantibodies reacting with the nonhomologous Ro52/TRIM21 and/or Ro60/TROVE2 proteins, respectively, without distinguishing between the two specificities [20]. Depending on detection method, anti-Ro/SSA antibodies have been described in 33–74 % of SS patients, whereas anti-La/SSB in 23–52 % [21–25]. Autoantibodies against both Ro52/TRIM21 and Ro60/TROVE2 proteins can coexist in a significant proportion of patients, but they can also be found alone [26]. Anti-Ro52/TRIM21 seems to be the most common specificity in patients with SS (66.7 %) compared to anti-Ro60/TROVE2 (52.1 %) [13, 27]. In the vast majority of SS patients, anti-Ro/SSA and anti-La/SSB positivity is detectable at diagnosis and remains unaltered during the follow-up [24, 28, 29].

Detection of anti-Ro/SSA and anti-La/SSB autoantibodies in patients' sera has been correlated with early disease onset, severe exocrine gland hypofunction, positive salivary gland biopsy, recurrent or permanent parotid gland enlargement, and severe ocular involvement [21, 23–25, 30–32]. Furthermore, they are associated with extensive lymphocytic infiltration and development of ectopic germinal centers in the lesions of minor salivary glands. A higher prevalence of extraglandular systemic manifestations, including cutaneous vasculitis, renal involvement, peripheral neuropathy, leukopenia and thrombocytopenia, and Raynaud's phenomenon, was observed in SS patients with anti-Ro/SSA and/or anti-La/SSB when compared to seronegative patients [3, 21, 23, 31, 33]. Anti-La/SSB antibody positivity has also been associated with pulmonary involvement [25]. Moreover, anti-Ro/La antibodies in SS patients have been correlated to other laboratory markers, such as antinuclear antibodies (ANA), rheumatoid factor (RF), hypergammaglobulinemia, and cryoglobulins [22, 23].

One of the major implications of anti-Ro/SSA and anti-La/SSB autoantibodies is the development of neonatal lupus syndrome (NLS), where they are considered to have direct pathogenic role. In this syndrome, maternal anti-Ro/SSA and/or anti-La/SSB autoantibodies transplacentally pass to the fetal circulation causing injuries to several organs, mainly the skin and heart. NLS may present with a photosensitive annular transient skin rash, reversible alteration of hematological and hepatic function, as well as irreversible cardiac disease, the major finding of which is heart block with or without cardiomyopathy [34]. Complete heart block occurs in nearly 2 % of children born to mothers with anti-Ro/SSA antibodies. Interestingly, the development of the NLS seems to be regulated by the development of an idiotypic/anti-idiotypic network of antibodies. According to idiotypic-anti-idiotypic network theory, the antibodies recognizing a specific epitope on an antigen are also capable to induce an immune response against them, which in turn leads to the production of anti-idiotypic antibodies that neutralize the former antibodies [35]. Indeed, using complementary peptides to the major epitope of La/SSB, spanning the 349–364aa of the protein, our groups have shown that the sera of patients with SS contain an active idiotypic/anti-idiotypic network of the La/SSB autoantigen and a substantial number of anti-La/SSB responses are blocked and hidden in the conventional immunoassays, by the anti-idiotypic antibodies [36]. Furthermore, anti-La/SSB-positive mothers who gave birth to a healthy child had higher titers of anti-idiotypic antibodies in their sera, compared with mothers who gave birth to a child with NLS, suggesting that anti-idiotypic antibodies may be protective, most probably by binding to pathogenic anti-La/SSB antibodies, thereby blocking their entrance in the fetal circulation [36].

Although it is considered that the development of humoral responses against the Ro52/TRIM21, Ro60/TROVE2, and La/SSB autoantigens is governed by typical antigen-driven immune responses, the exact mechanisms mediating their generation and the sites of production are not delineated. Anti-Ro/SSA and/or anti-La/SSB responses have been associated with certain HLA alleles, including HLA-A1, HLA-B8, HLA-DR2, HLA-DR3, HLA-DQ1, and HLA-DQ2 [31, 37–39]. In a multicenter European study, anti-Ro/SSA and anti-La/SSB autoantibodies were associated with HLA-DRB1*03 and HLA-DQB1*02, as well as HLA-DQA1*0501 in patients with autoantibodies to the p301-318, p291-302, and p147-154 La/SSB B-cell epitopes [31]. Recently, high-resolution HLA analysis revealed that anti-Ro/SSA positivity was associated with HLA-B*51:01 and HLA-DRB1*03:01 alleles, whereas anti-La/SSB with HLA-A*01:01 allele was associated with positivity [40].

Although the sites of autoantibody formation are not known, the affected salivary glands most likely serve as such, as indicated by the following: (a) lymphocytic infiltrates in approximately 20 % of SS patients form germinal center-like aggregates in the salivary glands and contain autoreactive B cells; (b) the saliva of SS patients contains high levels of IgG, as well as anti-Ro/SSA and anti-La/SSB autoantibodies; (c) many of the infiltrating plasma cells contain intracytoplasmic immunoglobulins with anti-Ro/SSA activity; and (d) the autoantigens are overexpressed in the salivary gland epithelia of SS patients, whereas they translocate to the cytoplasm and the cellular membrane during ductal cell apoptosis [33, 41–46].

The epithelial expression of autoantigens is considered to have a key role in the development of anti-Ro/SSA and anti-La/SSB responses. Epithelial cells are thought to participate in the exposure of Ro52/TRIM21, Ro60/TROVE2, and La/SSB autoantigens in SS through the release of autoantigen-loaded apoptotic blebs [41, 47] or exosomes [8]. The epithelial capacity to regulate B-cell survival and differentiation [1] and the epithelial expression of the autoantigens acquire particular significance in the pathogenesis of SS. Recently, our group has shown that TLR3 signaling regulates the expression and distribution of Ro52/TRIM21 in salivary gland epithelial cells, partially through the production of IFNβ [48]. Furthermore, the disregulated expression of miR16, miR200b-3p, miR223, and miR483-5p that are thought to target Ro52/TRIM21, Ro60/TROVE2, and La/SSB mRNAs in SS suggests that miRNAs may also be implicated in the regulation of autoantigen expression in SS [49]. The pivotal role of epithelial cells in autoantibody production has been recently confirmed in an experimental mouse model lacking the transcriptional regulator IκB-ζ [50]. The IκB-ζ-deficient mice, which are prompted to epithelial apoptosis, were found to spontaneously develop an SS-like inflammation, manifested as dacryoadenitis associated with the development of lymphocytic infiltrates in the affected tissue and production of high titers of the SS-associated autoantibodies Ro/SSA and La/SSB. This phenotype was found to specifically correlate with increased apoptosis of epithelial, but not immune, cells, demonstrating the significance of epithelial cells in autoimmune humoral responses.

21.2.2 Antinuclear Antibodies (ANA)

Up to 85 % of SS patients has antinuclear antibodies (ANA), which similarly to anti-Ro/SSA and anti-La/SSB autoantibodies, are detectable at diagnosis and do not change thereafter [21–25, 28]. Positivity for ANA has been associated with parotid gland enlargement; systemic extraglandular manifestations; such as Raynaud's phenomenon, cutaneous vasculitis, articular and renal involvement, fever, adenopathies, and cytopenias; as well as various laboratory markers, including hypergammaglobulinemia, positive RF, and anti-Ro/SSA, anti-La/SSB, and antiphospholipid antibodies [21, 23, 25, 51].

21.2.3 Rheumatoid Factor

Rheumatoid factors (RF) are antibodies directed against the Fc portion of IgG immunoglobulin. RF is detected in the sera of 36–74 % of patients with primary SS [21–25, 52, 53]. In the majority of SS patients, RF is detected at diagnosis, but its prevalence tends to increase during the follow-up [24, 28, 53]. RF positivity is associated with younger age and positive salivary gland biopsy, as well as other serologic features, such as anti-Ro/SSA and anti-La/SSB autoantibodies, ANA, cryoglobulins, hypocomplementemia, and hypergammaglobulinemia [22–25, 51]. Both the presence and the titers of RF have been positively correlated with extraglandular manifestations of SS, such as articular manifestations, cutaneous vasculitis, salivary gland enlargement, cytopenias, Raynaud's phenomenon, renal involvement, and central nervous system involvement [22, 23, 25].

21.2.4 Cryoglobulins

Cryoglobulins are immunoglobulins that become reversibly insoluble in temperatures below normal body temperature and undergo precipitation, whereas they redissolve at 37 °C. They are classified in three types: type I which is composed by a single monoclonal immunoglobulin (usually IgM); type II by a polyclonal component, usually IgG, and a monoclonal component, usually IgM or IgA; and type III by polyclonal IgM and IgG molecules. Often, type II and type III cryoglobulins have RF activity. Cryoglobulins are associated with various lymphoproliferative diseases, viral infections, and autoimmune diseases, including SS. They are found in 9–15 % of SS patients, and although they are often present at diagnosis, their prevalence increases during the follow-up [21, 24, 25, 28]. The detection of cryoglobulins outlines a high risk for poor disease outcome and lymphomagenesis [28, 54, 55]. Cryoglobulins have also been correlated with younger age at diagnosis; parotid gland enlargement; cytopenias and extraglandular features, such as Raynaud's phenomenon, vasculitis, renal involvement, peripheral neuropathy, and lymphoma; as well as other serologic markers including RF, anti-Ro/SSA antibodies, hypocomplementemia, and monoclonal gammopathy [23–25].

21.2.5 Anti-centromere Antibodies (ACA)

The anti-centromere antibodies (ACA) are often observed in patients with the limited form of systemic sclerosis (SSc). They usually recognize the CENP-A (17 kDa), CENP-B (80 kDa), and CENP-C (140 kDa) centromere proteins, even though activity against the 50 kDa CENP-D, the 312 kDa CENP-E, the 400 kDa CENP-F, the 95 kDa CENP-G, and the 28 kDa CENP-H has also been described. The prevalence of ACA in SS patients is 4–27 % [56–61]. The pattern of CENP recognition differs significantly between pSS and SSc, with the majority of pSS sera recognizing CENP-C alone (70 % of SS vs. 6 % of SSc) and the majority of SSc sera recognizing both CENP-B and CENP-C (83 % of SSc vs. 0 % of SS) [62]. ACA-positive patients with SS seem to comprise a distinct clinical subgroup, characterized by overlapping clinical manifestations with systemic sclerosis and milder disease compared to ACA-negative SS patients or patients with systemic sclerosis. Compared to ACA-negative SS patients, the ACA-positive patients had a higher mean age at disease onset and a greater prevalence of Raynaud's phenomenon; keratoconjunctivitis sicca; peripheral neuropathy; concomitant autoimmune disorders, such as primary biliary cirrhosis; as well as risk for lymphoma. ACA-positive patients with SS presented lower rates of anti-Ro/SSA and anti-La/SSB antibodies, rheumatoid factor positivity, leukocytopenia, and hypergammaglobulinemia [58, 60, 61, 63–65].

21.2.6 Anti-cyclic Citrullinated Peptides Antibodies (Anti-CCP)

The antibodies against cyclic citrullinated peptides (anti-CCP) are autoantibodies that are directed against peptides and proteins that are citrullinated. Although they are considered specific markers for the diagnosis of rheumatoid arthritis, their prevalence in SS patients has been estimated to range between 3 and 10 % [66–69]. Anti-CCP reactivity is correlated with nonerosive arthritis in SS patients, whereas there is a controversy about its association with joint synovitis [67–70]. A cohort study including 405 patients with primary SS revealed that 52.6 % of the patients with positive anti-CCP antibodies developed RA during a 60-month follow-up, compared to none of the anti-CCP-negative SS group [71], suggesting that anti-CCP-positive SS patients may develop RA. Interestingly, it has been reported that patients with anti-CCP antibodies, with SS and nonerosive arthritis, might fulfill the ACR classification criteria for RA [67, 68].

21.2.7 Antimitochondrial Antibodies (AMA)

Antimitochondrial antibodies (AMA) mainly recognize the ketoacid dehydrogenase multiprotein complex consisting by three major antigens, namely, pyruvate dehydrogenase (PDH), branched-chain ketoacid dehydrogenase (BCKD), and ketoglutarate dehydrogenase (OGD). This complex is responsible for catalyzing the oxidative decarboxylation of ketoacids [72]. AMA characterize primary biliary cirrhosis (PBC), with the 74 kDa E2-subunit of the pyruvate dehydrogenase complex to be the predominant autoantigen in 95 % of all North American and European PBC sera [72]. Sicca symptoms have a high prevalence (up to 81 %) among PBC patients, and liver involvement associated with AMA positivity might be observed in patients with SS [28, 73–75]. AMA are present in 2–27 % of SS patients, depending on the diagnostic method employed [76]. AMA positivity in SS patients has been associated with liver involvement, Raynaud's phenomenon, peripheral neuropathy, and hypergammaglobulinemia [76]. The histopathologic profile of liver and salivary gland lesions is comparable. In both disorders, the tissue lesion is characterized by periductal lymphocytic infiltrates, which primarily consist of $CD4^{+}$ T cells. Moreover, in both conditions, the histopathologic lesions present slow or no progression during disease course [73, 77], whereas the epithelial cells seem to be the "inflamed tissue," supporting the notion of "autoimmune epithelitis" [1].

21.2.8 Antibodies to Muscarinic Receptors

Muscarinic receptors (MRs) are acetylcholine receptors that form G protein-coupled receptor complexes in the plasma membranes of certain neurons or other cells. Numerous functions have been described, the most noteworthy being their function as the main receptors stimulated by acetylcholine released from post-ganglionic fibers in the parasympathetic nervous system [78, 79]. Muscarinic receptors received their name from their higher affinity to muscarine than to nicotine and have been further categorized in five subgroups (M1R-M5R) depending on their reactions with several selective agonists and antagonists. From these muscarinic receptors, M3R has a fundamental role in the parasympathetic regulation of saliva secretion [80]. Anti-M3R autoantibodies in SS sera mainly target the second extracellular loop of M3R. Their presence has been correlated to decreased saliva production, possibly associated with direct blockade of neurotransmission or inhibition of aquaporin 5 trafficking [81–86]. However, the poor detection capacity of conventional immunologic techniques impeded the evaluation of their diagnostic utility and possible associations with clinical features in SS [87, 88].

21.2.9 Antibodies to Carbonic Anhydrases

Carbonic anhydrases comprise a family of enzymes that catalyze the conversion of carbon dioxide and water to bicarbonate and protons and vice versa. They are classified as metalloproteases, since their active site contains a zinc ion and they are mainly involved in the regulation of acid-base balance in the blood and other tissues and in aiding carbon dioxide transport out of tissues. Thirteen isoenzymes of carbonic anhydrase have been described in mammals [89]. Autoantibodies targeting carbonic anhydrase II (anti-CAII) have been described in the serum of patients with various conditions, such as renal disease, cancer, and several autoimmune diseases. In SS, they have been detected in up to 20 % of patients [89–91]. Although their role is not clear, the expression of anti-CAII antibodies has been associated with distal renal tubular acidosis in SS patients [92], whereas intradermal immunization of PL/J mice with human carbonic anhydrase II provoked the development of autoimmune sialadenitis, suggesting that anti-CAII antibodies may have a role in SS pathogenesis [93]. Furthermore, higher levels of autoantibodies to carbonic anhydrases I, II, VI, and VII were found in the sera of SS patients compared to controls [89]. Autoantibodies to other carbonic anhydrases rather than CAII were not correlated with renal tubular acidosis or proteinuria. However, levels of anti-CA II, VI, and XIII antibodies correlated significantly with urinary pH, and inversely with serum sodium concentrations, suggesting a possible implication in renal acidification capacity [89].

21.2.10 Anti-smooth Muscle Antibodies (ASMA)

Anti-smooth muscle antibodies (ASMA) recognize various elements of the cytoskeleton, including actin, microfilaments, microtubules, or intermediate filaments [94]. They are usually detected in patients with type 1 autoimmune hepatitis in association with ANA positivity [95]. The prevalence of autoimmune hepatitis in patients with pSS is rather low (1.7–4 %) [96, 97], whereas ASMA have been described in the sera of 30–62 % of patients with SS [21, 98, 99]. ASMA have been associated with the development of autoimmune hepatitis, and they possibly have a prognostic value for liver disease in SS [30, 96, 98]. Furthermore, higher levels of ASMA have been found in SS patients with bronchiectasis compared to those without [100].

21.2.11 Other Autoantibodies

Several other autoantibodies have been implicated in SS, without clear associations and contradictory results from diagnostic and clinical perspectives. Autoantibodies directed against alpha-fodrin, an intracellular, actin-binding, organ-specific protein of the cytoskeleton, were involved in the pathogenesis of murine models of Sjögren's syndrome and were initially described as a highly specific and sensitive marker for the diagnosis of SS [101]. However, subsequent studies failed to confirm the association in humans [102]. Recently, antibodies to salivary gland protein 1 (SP1) have been described in an animal model and patients with SS; however, their diagnostic or clinical value remains to be validated [103, 104].

21.3 Laboratory Markers and Clinical Associations

Beside cryoglobulins, several laboratory, clinical, and histologic parameters have been shown to serve as predictors of adverse outcome and future lymphoma development in SS. Other clinical parameters that have been reported to predict lymphomagenesis include lymphadenopathy, parotid gland enlargement, palpable purpura, and splenomegaly [28, 55, 105, 106]. Furthermore, the formation of germinal center-like structures in the salivary gland lesions, as well as the infiltration by certain cell types, such as macrophages, has been recognized as predictors of lymphomagenesis [2, 105, 107].

Lymphopenia and neutropenia, as well as low serum C4 and C3 levels, have been described to predict the development of lymphoma [28, 55, 105, 106]. C4 hypocomplementemia is the most consistent adverse prognostic factor for lymphoma in SS. C4 hypocomplementemia also correlates with peripheral neuropathy, cutaneous vasculitis, RF, cryoglobulins, as well as increased mortality [108]. Finally, anemia, lymphocytopenia, thrombocytopenia, hypergammaglobulinemia, the presence of monoclonal serum proteins, and cryoglobulinemia have been associated with the presence of extraglandular symptoms, such as palpable purpura, lymphadenopathy, and splenomegaly [55].

21.4 Summary

Sjögren's syndrome is characterized by intense humoral autoimmune responses against a variety of intracellular autoantigens. The mainly involved autoantigens are protein components of the Ro/La ribonucleoprotein complex. Anti-Ro/La antibodies have a crucial diagnostic utility in SS. They have been associated with early disease onset, severe dysfunction/destruction of the glands, and extraglandular manifestations. Other autoantibodies might be detected in patients with SS. The presence of cryoglobulins identifies patients with adverse prognosis and at a higher risk of future lymphoma development. Anti-CCP autoantibodies are associated with articular involvement; ACA characterize a subset of patients with overlapping features between pSS and SSc, whereas AMA and ASMA are associated with liver involvement (PBC and autoimmune hepatitis, respectively).

Finally, several other clinical, histologic, and laboratory parameters have been suggested to have a predictive value for disease severity and future lymphoma development, to include lymphadenopathy, complementemia, parotid gland enlargement, palpable purpura, and splenomegaly.

References

1. Tzioufas AG, Kapsogeorgou EK, Moutsopoulos HM (2012) Pathogenesis of Sjogren's syndrome: what we know and what we should learn. J Autoimmun 39:4–8
2. Christodoulou MI, Kapsogeorgou EK, Moutsopoulos HM (2010) Characteristics of the minor salivary gland infiltrates in Sjogren's syndrome. J Autoimmun 34:400–407
3. Gerli R, Muscat C, Giansanti M, Danieli MG, Sciuto M, Gabrielli A et al (1997) Quantitative assessment of salivary gland inflammatory infiltration in primary Sjogren's syndrome: its relationship to different demographic, clinical and serological features of the disorder. Br J Rheumatol 36:969–975
4. Routsias JG, Vlachoyiannopoulos PG, Tzioufas AG (2006) Autoantibodies to intracellular autoantigens and their B-cell epitopes: molecular probes to study the autoimmune response. Crit Rev Clin Lab Sci 43:203–248
5. Routsias JG, Kyriakidis N, Latreille M, Tzioufas AG (2010) RNA recognition motif (RRM) of La/SSB: the bridge for interparticle spreading of autoimmune response to U1-RNP. Mol Med 16:19–26
6. Yiannaki E, Vlachoyiannopoulos PG, Manoussakis MN, Sakarellos C, Sakarellos-Daitsiotis M, Moutsopoulos HM et al (2000) Study of antibody and T cell responses in rabbits immunized with synthetic human B cell epitope analogues of La (SSB) autoantigen. Clin Exp Immunol 121:551–556
7. Cohen JJ, Duke RC, Fadok VA, Sellins KS (1992) Apoptosis and programmed cell death in immunity. Annu Rev Immunol 10:267–293
8. Kapsogeorgou EK, Abu-Helu RF, Moutsopoulos HM, Manoussakis MN (2005) Salivary gland epithelial cell exosomes: a source of autoantigenic ribonucleoproteins. Arthritis Rheum 52:1517–1521
9. Vitali C, Bombardieri S, Jonsson R, Moutsopoulos HM, Alexander EL, Carsons SE et al (2002) Classification criteria for Sjogren's syndrome: a revised version of the European criteria proposed by the American-European Consensus Group. Ann Rheum Dis 61:554–558
10. Mallery DL, McEwan WA, Bidgood SR, Towers GJ, Johnson CM, James LC (2010) Antibodies mediate intracellular immunity through tripartite motif-containing 21 (TRIM21). Proc Natl Acad Sci U S A 107:19985–19990

11. McEwan WA, James LC (2015) TRIM21-dependent intracellular antibody neutralization of virus infection. Prog Mol Biol Transl Sci 129:167–187
12. Higgs R, Ni Gabhann J, Ben Larbi N, Breen EP, Fitzgerald KA, Jefferies CA (2008) The E3 ubiquitin ligase Ro52 negatively regulates IFN-beta production post-pathogen recognition by polyubiquitin-mediated degradation of IRF3. J Immunol 181:1780–1786
13. Oke V, Wahren-Herlenius M (2012) The immunobiology of Ro52 (TRIM21) in autoimmunity: a critical review. J Autoimmun 39:77–82
14. Chen X, Wolin SL (2004) The Ro 60 kDa autoantigen: insights into cellular function and role in autoimmunity. J Mol Med (Berlin) 82:232–239
15. Chen X, Smith JD, Shi H, Yang DD, Flavell RA, Wolin SL (2003) The Ro autoantigen binds misfolded U2 small nuclear RNAs and assists mammalian cell survival after UV irradiation. Curr Biol 13:2206–2211
16. Wolin SL, Cedervall T (2002) The La protein. Annu Rev Biochem 71:375–403
17. Liu Y, Tan H, Tian H, Liang C, Chen S, Liu Q (2011) Autoantigen La promotes efficient RNAi, antiviral response, and transposon silencing by facilitating multiple-turnover RISC catalysis. Mol Cell 44:502–508
18. Sommer G, Dittmann J, Kuehnert J, Reumann K, Schwartz PE, Will H et al (2011) The RNA-binding protein La contributes to cell proliferation and CCND1 expression. Oncogene 30:434–444
19. Routsias JG, Tzioufas AG (2010) B-cell epitopes of the intracellular autoantigens Ro/SSA and La/SSB: tools to study the regulation of the autoimmune response. J Autoimmun 35:256–264
20. Itoh K, Itoh Y, Frank MB (1991) Protein heterogeneity in the human Ro/SSA ribonucleoproteins. The 52- and 60-kD Ro/SSA autoantigens are encoded by separate genes. J Clin Invest 87:177–186
21. Nardi N, Brito-Zeron P, Ramos-Casals M, Aguilo S, Cervera R, Ingelmo M et al (2006) Circulating auto-antibodies against nuclear and non-nuclear antigens in primary Sjogren's syndrome: prevalence and clinical significance in 335 patients. Clin Rheumatol 25:341–346
22. ter Borg EJ, Risselada AP, Kelder JC (2011) Relation of systemic autoantibodies to the number of extraglandular manifestations in primary Sjogren's Syndrome: a retrospective analysis of 65 patients in the Netherlands. Semin Arthritis Rheum 40:547–551
23. Ramos-Casals M, Solans R, Rosas J, Camps MT, Gil A, Del Pino-Montes J et al (2008) Primary Sjogren syndrome in Spain: clinical and immunologic expression in 1010 patients. Medicine (Baltimore) 87:210–219
24. Fauchais AL, Martel C, Gondran G, Lambert M, Launay D, Jauberteau MO et al (2010) Immunological profile in primary Sjogren syndrome: clinical significance, prognosis and long-term evolution to other auto-immune disease. Autoimmun Rev 9:595–599
25. Martel C, Gondran G, Launay D, Lalloue F, Palat S, Lambert M et al (2011) Active immunological profile is associated with systemic Sjogren's syndrome. J Clin Immunol 31:840–847
26. Schulte-Pelkum J, Fritzler M, Mahler M (2009) Latest update on the Ro/SS-A autoantibody system. Autoimmun Rev 8:632–637
27. Routsias JG, Tzioufas AG (2007) Sjogren's syndrome – study of autoantigens and autoantibodies. Clin Rev Allergy Immunol 32:238–251
28. Skopouli FN, Dafni U, Ioannidis JP, Moutsopoulos HM (2000) Clinical evolution, and morbidity and mortality of primary Sjogren's syndrome. Semin Arthritis Rheum 29:296–304
29. Davidson BK, Kelly CA, Griffiths ID (1999) Primary Sjogren's syndrome in the North East of England: a long-term follow-up study. Rheumatology (Oxford) 38:245–253
30. Ramos-Casals M, Sanchez-Tapias JM, Pares A, Forns X, Brito-Zeron P, Nardi N et al (2006) Characterization and differentiation of autoimmune versus viral liver involvement in patients with Sjogren's syndrome. J Rheumatol 33:1593–1599
31. Tzioufas AG, Wassmuth R, Dafni UG, Guialis A, Haga HJ, Isenberg DA et al (2002) Clinical, immunological, and immunogenetic aspects of autoantibody production against Ro/SSA, La/SSB and their linear epitopes in primary Sjogren's syndrome (pSS): a European multicentre study. Ann Rheum Dis 61:398–404

32. Toker E, Yavuz S, Direskeneli H (2004) Anti-Ro/SSA and anti-La/SSB autoantibodies in the tear fluid of patients with Sjogren's syndrome. Br J Ophthalmol 88:384–387
33. Jonsson MV, Skarstein K, Jonsson R, Brun JG (2007) Serological implications of germinal center-like structures in primary Sjogren's syndrome. J Rheumatol 34:2044–2049
34. Izmirly PM, Buyon JP, Saxena A (2012) Neonatal lupus: advances in understanding pathogenesis and identifying treatments of cardiac disease. Curr Opin Rheumatol 24:466–472
35. Jerne NK (1974) Towards a network theory of the immune system. Ann Immunol (Paris) 125C:373–389
36. Stea EA, Routsias JG, Clancy RM, Buyon JP, Moutsopoulos HM, Tzioufas AG (2006) Anti-La/SSB antiidiotypic antibodies in maternal serum: a marker of low risk for neonatal lupus in an offspring. Arthritis Rheum 54:2228–2234
37. Harley JB, Reichlin M, Arnett FC, Alexander EL, Bias WB, Provost TT (1986) Gene interaction at HLA-DQ enhances autoantibody production in primary Sjogren's syndrome. Science 232:1145–1147
38. Whittingham S, Mackay IR, Tait BD (1983) Autoantibodies to small nuclear ribonucleoproteins. A strong association between anti-SS-B(La), HLA-B8, and Sjogren's syndrome. Aust N Z J Med 13:565–570
39. Wilson RW, Provost TT, Bias WB, Alexander EL, Edlow DW, Hochberg MC et al (1984) Sjogren's syndrome. Influence of multiple HLA-D region alloantigens on clinical and serologic expression. Arthritis Rheum 27:1245–1253
40. Hernandez-Molina G, Vargas-Alarcon G, Rodriguez-Perez JM, Martinez-Rodriguez N, Lima G, Sanchez-Guerrero J (2015) High-resolution HLA analysis of primary and secondary Sjogren's syndrome: a common immunogenetic background in Mexican patients. Rheumatol Int 35:643–649
41. Ohlsson M, Jonsson R, Brokstad KA (2002) Subcellular redistribution and surface exposure of the Ro52, Ro60 and La48 autoantigens during apoptosis in human ductal epithelial cells: a possible mechanism in the pathogenesis of Sjogren's syndrome. Scand J Immunol 56:456–469
42. Salomonsson S, Jonsson MV, Skarstein K, Brokstad KA, Hjelmstrom P, Wahren-Herlenius M et al (2003) Cellular basis of ectopic germinal center formation and autoantibody production in the target organ of patients with Sjogren's syndrome. Arthritis Rheum 48:3187–3201
43. Tengner P, Halse AK, Haga HJ, Jonsson R, Wahren-Herlenius M (1998) Detection of anti-Ro/SSA and anti-La/SSB autoantibody-producing cells in salivary glands from patients with Sjogren's syndrome. Arthritis Rheum 41:2238–2248
44. Yannopoulos DI, Roncin S, Lamour A, Pennec YL, Moutsopoulos HM, Youinou P (1992) Conjunctival epithelial cells from patients with Sjogren's syndrome inappropriately express major histocompatibility complex molecules, La(SSB) antigen, and heat-shock proteins. J Clin Immunol 12:259–265
45. Tzioufas AG, Hantoumi I, Polihronis M, Xanthou G, Moutsopoulos HM (1999) Autoantibodies to La/SSB in patients with primary Sjogren's syndrome (pSS) are associated with upregulation of La/SSB mRNA in minor salivary gland biopsies (MSGs). J Autoimmun 13:429–434
46. Maier-Moore JS, Koelsch KA, Smith K, Lessard CJ, Radfar L, Lewis D et al (2014) Antibody-secreting cell specificity in labial salivary glands reflects the clinical presentation and serology in patients with Sjogren's syndrome. Arthritis Rheumatol 66:3445–3456
47. Manoussakis MN, Kapsogeorgou EK (2010) The role of intrinsic epithelial activation in the pathogenesis of Sjogren's syndrome. J Autoimmun 35:219–224
48. Kyriakidis NC, Kapsogeorgou EK, Gourzi VC, Konsta OD, Baltatzis GE, Tzioufas AG (2014) Toll-like receptor 3 stimulation promotes Ro52/TRIM21 synthesis and nuclear redistribution in salivary gland epithelial cells, partially via type I interferon pathway. Clin Exp Immunol 178:548–560
49. Kapsogeorgou EK, Gourzi VC, Manoussakis MN, Moutsopoulos HM, Tzioufas AG (2011) Cellular microRNAs (miRNAs) and Sjogren's syndrome: candidate regulators of autoimmune response and autoantigen expression. J Autoimmun 37:129–135

50. Okuma A, Hoshino K, Ohba T, Fukushi S, Aiba S, Akira S et al (2013) Enhanced apoptosis by disruption of the STAT3-IkappaB-zeta signaling pathway in epithelial cells induces Sjogren's syndrome-like autoimmune disease. Immunity 38:450–460
51. Huo AP, Lin KC, Chou CT (2010) Predictive and prognostic value of antinuclear antibodies and rheumatoid factor in primary Sjogren's syndrome. Int J Rheum Dis 13:39–47
52. Higgs R, Lazzari E, Wynne C, Ni Gabhann J, Espinosa A, Wahren-Herlenius M et al (2010) Self protection from anti-viral responses – Ro52 promotes degradation of the transcription factor IRF7 downstream of the viral Toll-Like receptors. PLoS One 5:e11776
53. Pertovaara M, Pukkala E, Laippala P, Miettinen A, Pasternack A (2001) A longitudinal cohort study of Finnish patients with primary Sjogren's syndrome: clinical, immunological, and epidemiological aspects. Ann Rheum Dis 60:467–472
54. Bournia VK, Vlachoyiannopoulos PG (2012) Subgroups of Sjogren syndrome patients according to serological profiles. J Autoimmun 39:15–26
55. Baimpa E, Dahabreh IJ, Voulgarelis M, Moutsopoulos HM (2009) Hematologic manifestations and predictors of lymphoma development in primary Sjogren syndrome: clinical and pathophysiologic aspects. Medicine (Baltimore) 88:284–293
56. Hsu TC, Chang CH, Lin MC, Liu ST, Yen TJ, Tsay GJ (2006) Anti-CENP-H antibodies in patients with Sjogren's syndrome. Rheumatol Int 26:298–303
57. Gonzalez-Buitrago JM, Gonzalez C, Hernando M, Carrasco R, Sanchez A, Navajo JA et al (2003) Antibodies to centromere antigens measured by an automated enzyme immunoassay. Clin Chim Acta 328:135–138
58. Bournia VK, Diamanti KD, Vlachoyiannopoulos PG, Moutsopoulos HM (2010) Anticentromere antibody positive Sjogren's Syndrome: a retrospective descriptive analysis. Arthritis Res Ther 12:R47
59. Salliot C, Gottenberg JE, Bengoufa D, Desmoulins F, Miceli-Richard C, Mariette X (2007) Anticentromere antibodies identify patients with Sjogren's syndrome and autoimmune overlap syndrome. J Rheumatol 34:2253–2258
60. Caramaschi P, Biasi D, Carletto A, Manzo T, Randon M, Zeminian S et al (1997) Sjogren's syndrome with anticentromere antibodies. Rev Rhum Engl Ed 64:785–788
61. Katano K, Kawano M, Koni I, Sugai S, Muro Y (2001) Clinical and laboratory features of anticentromere antibody positive primary Sjogren's syndrome. J Rheumatol 28:2238–2244
62. Gelber AC, Pillemer SR, Baum BJ, Wigley FM, Hummers LK, Morris S et al (2006) Distinct recognition of antibodies to centromere proteins in primary Sjogren's syndrome compared with limited scleroderma. Ann Rheum Dis 65:1028–1032
63. Kitagawa T, Shibasaki K, Toya S (2012) Clinical significance and diagnostic usefulness of anti-centromere antibody in Sjogren's syndrome. Clin Rheumatol 31:105–112
64. Nakamura H, Kawakami A, Hayashi T, Iwamoto N, Okada A, Tamai M et al (2010) Anti-centromere antibody-seropositive Sjogren's syndrome differs from conventional subgroup in clinical and pathological study. BMC Musculoskelet Disord 11:140
65. Baldini C, Mosca M, Della Rossa A, Pepe P, Notarstefano C, Ferro F et al (2013) Overlap of ACA-positive systemic sclerosis and Sjogren's syndrome: a distinct clinical entity with mild organ involvement but at high risk of lymphoma. Clin Exp Rheumatol 31:272–280
66. Barcelos F, Abreu I, Patto JV, Trindade H, Teixeira A (2009) Anti-cyclic citrullinated peptide antibodies and rheumatoid factor in Sjogren's syndrome. Acta Reumatol Port 34:608–612
67. Gottenberg JE, Mignot S, Nicaise-Rolland P, Cohen-Solal J, Aucouturier F, Goetz J et al (2005) Prevalence of anti-cyclic citrullinated peptide and anti-keratin antibodies in patients with primary Sjogren's syndrome. Ann Rheum Dis 64:114–117
68. Iwamoto N, Kawakami A, Tamai M, Fujikawa K, Arima K, Aramaki T et al (2009) Determination of the subset of Sjogren's syndrome with articular manifestations by anticyclic citrullinated peptide antibodies. J Rheumatol 36:113–115
69. Tobon GJ, Correa PA, Anaya JM (2005) Anti-cyclic citrullinated peptide antibodies in patients with primary Sjogren's syndrome. Ann Rheum Dis 64:791–792

70. Atzeni F, Sarzi-Puttini P, Lama N, Bonacci E, Bobbio-Pallavicini F, Montecucco C et al (2008) Anti-cyclic citrullinated peptide antibodies in primary Sjogren syndrome may be associated with non-erosive synovitis. Arthritis Res Ther 10:R51
71. Ryu YS, Park SH, Lee J, Kwok SK, Ju JH, Kim HY et al (2013) Follow-up of primary Sjogren's syndrome patients presenting positive anti-cyclic citrullinated peptides antibody. Rheumatol Int 33:1443–1446
72. Bogdanos DP, Komorowski L (2011) Disease-specific autoantibodies in primary biliary cirrhosis. Clin Chim Acta 412:502–512
73. Hatzis GS, Fragoulis GE, Karatzaferis A, Delladetsima I, Barbatis C, Moutsopoulos HM (2008) Prevalence and longterm course of primary biliary cirrhosis in primary Sjogren's syndrome. J Rheumatol 35:2012–2016
74. Tsianos EV, Hoofnagle JH, Fox PC, Alspaugh M, Jones EA, Schafer DF et al (1990) Sjogren's syndrome in patients with primary biliary cirrhosis. Hepatology 11:730–734
75. Hansen BU, Lindgren S, Eriksson S, Henricsson V, Larsson A, Manthorpe R et al (1988) Clinical and immunological features of Sjogren's syndrome in patients with primary biliary cirrhosis with emphasis on focal sialadenitis. Acta Med Scand 224:611–619
76. Selmi C, Meroni PL, Gershwin ME (2012) Primary biliary cirrhosis and Sjogren's syndrome: autoimmune epithelitis. J Autoimmun 39:34–42
77. Kapsogeorgou EK, Christodoulou MI, Panagiotakos DB, Paikos S, Tassidou A, Tzioufas AG et al (2013) Minor salivary gland inflammatory lesions in Sjogren syndrome: do they evolve? J Rheumatol 40:1566–1571
78. Eglen RM (2006) Muscarinic receptor subtypes in neuronal and non-neuronal cholinergic function. Auton Autacoid Pharmacol 26:219–233
79. Ishii M, Kurachi Y (2006) Muscarinic acetylcholine receptors. Curr Pharm Des 12:3573–3581
80. Nakamura T, Matsui M, Uchida K, Futatsugi A, Kusakawa S, Matsumoto N et al (2004) M(3) muscarinic acetylcholine receptor plays a critical role in parasympathetic control of salivation in mice. J Physiol 558:561–575
81. Bacman S, Sterin-Borda L, Camusso JJ, Arana R, Hubscher O, Borda E (1996) Circulating antibodies against rat parotid gland M3 muscarinic receptors in primary Sjogren's syndrome. Clin Exp Immunol 104:454–459
82. He J, Guo JP, Ding Y, Li YN, Pan SS, Liu Y et al (2011) Diagnostic significance of measuring antibodies to cyclic type 3 muscarinic acetylcholine receptor peptides in primary Sjogren's syndrome. Rheumatology (Oxford) 50:879–884
83. Koo NY, Li J, Hwang SM, Choi SY, Lee SJ, Oh SB et al (2008) Functional epitope of muscarinic type 3 receptor which interacts with autoantibodies from Sjogren's syndrome patients. Rheumatology (Oxford) 47:828–833
84. Kovacs L, Marczinovits I, Gyorgy A, Toth GK, Dorgai L, Pal J et al (2005) Clinical associations of autoantibodies to human muscarinic acetylcholine receptor 3(213-228) in primary Sjogren's syndrome. Rheumatology (Oxford) 44:1021–1025
85. Li J, Ha YM, Ku NY, Choi SY, Lee SJ, Oh SB et al (2004) Inhibitory effects of autoantibodies on the muscarinic receptors in Sjogren's syndrome. Lab Invest 84:1430–1438
86. Lee BH, Gauna AE, Perez G, Park YJ, Pauley KM, Kawai T et al (2013) Autoantibodies against muscarinic type 3 receptor in Sjogren's syndrome inhibit aquaporin 5 trafficking. PLoS One 8:e53113
87. Roescher N, Kingman A, Shirota Y, Chiorini JA, Illei GG (2011) Peptide-based ELISAs are not sensitive and specific enough to detect muscarinic receptor type 3 autoantibodies in serum from patients with Sjogren's syndrome. Ann Rheum Dis 70:235–236
88. Dawson LJ, Allison HE, Stanbury J, Fitzgerald D, Smith PM (2004) Putative anti-muscarinic antibodies cannot be detected in patients with primary Sjogren's syndrome using conventional immunological approaches. Rheumatology (Oxford) 43:1488–1495
89. Pertovaara M, Bootorabi F, Kuuslahti M, Pasternack A, Parkkila S (2011) Novel carbonic anhydrase autoantibodies and renal manifestations in patients with primary Sjogren's syndrome. Rheumatology (Oxford) 50:1453–1457

90. Itoh Y, Reichlin M (1992) Antibodies to carbonic anhydrase in systemic lupus erythematosus and other rheumatic diseases. Arthritis Rheum 35:73–82
91. Ono M, Ono M, Watanabe K, Miyashita Y, Inagaki Y, Ueki H (1999) A study of anti-carbonic anhydrase II antibodies in rheumatic autoimmune diseases. J Dermatol Sci 21:183–186
92. Takemoto F, Hoshino J, Sawa N, Tamura Y, Tagami T, Yokota M et al (2005) Autoantibodies against carbonic anhydrase II are increased in renal tubular acidosis associated with Sjogren syndrome. Am J Med 118:181–184
93. Nishimori I, Bratanova T, Toshkov I, Caffrey T, Mogaki M, Shibata Y et al (1995) Induction of experimental autoimmune sialaadenitis by immunization of PL/J mice with carbonic anhydrase II. J Immunol 154:4865–4873
94. Toh BH (1979) Smooth muscle autoantibodies and autoantigens. Clin Exp Immunol 38:621–628
95. Bogdanos DP, Invernizzi P, Mackay IR, Vergani D (2008) Autoimmune liver serology: current diagnostic and clinical challenges. World J Gastroenterol 14:3374–3387
96. Lindgren S, Manthorpe R, Eriksson S (1994) Autoimmune liver disease in patients with primary Sjogren's syndrome. J Hepatol 20:354–358
97. Karp JK, Akpek EK, Anders RA (2010) Autoimmune hepatitis in patients with primary Sjogren's syndrome: a series of two-hundred and two patients. Int J Clin Exp Pathol 3:582–586
98. Manthorpe R, Permin H, Tage-Jensen U (1979) Auto-antibodies in Sjogren's syndrome. With special reference to liver-cell membrane antibody (LMA). Scand J Rheumatol 8:168–172
99. Csepregi A, Szodoray P, Zeher M (2002) Do autoantibodies predict autoimmune liver disease in primary Sjogren's syndrome? Data of 180 patients upon a 5 year follow-up. Scand J Immunol 56:623–629
100. Soto-Cardenas MJ, Perez-De-Lis M, Bove A, Navarro C, Brito-Zeron P, Diaz-Lagares C et al (2010) Bronchiectasis in primary Sjogren's syndrome: prevalence and clinical significance. Clin Exp Rheumatol 28:647–653
101. Haneji N, Nakamura T, Takio K, Yanagi K, Higashiyama H, Saito I et al (1997) Identification of alpha-fodrin as a candidate autoantigen in primary Sjogren's syndrome. Science 276:604–607
102. Witte T (2005) Antifodrin antibodies in Sjogren's syndrome: a review. Ann N Y Acad Sci 1051:235–239
103. Shen L, Kapsogeorgou EK, Yu M, Suresh L, Malyavantham K, Tzioufas AG et al (2014) Evaluation of salivary gland protein 1 antibodies in patients with primary and secondary Sjogren's syndrome. Clin Immunol 155:42–46
104. Shen L, Suresh L, Lindemann M, Xuan J, Kowal P, Malyavantham K et al (2012) Novel autoantibodies in Sjogren's syndrome. Clin Immunol 145:251–255
105. Nishishinya MB, Pereda CA, Munoz-Fernandez S, Pego-Reigosa JM, Rua-Figueroa I, Andreu JL et al (2015) Identification of lymphoma predictors in patients with primary Sjogren's syndrome: a systematic literature review and meta-analysis. Rheumatol Int 35:17–26
106. Baldini C, Pepe P, Luciano N, Ferro F, Talarico R, Grossi S et al (2012) A clinical prediction rule for lymphoma development in primary Sjogren's syndrome. J Rheumatol 39:804–808
107. Theander E, Vasaitis L, Baecklund E, Nordmark G, Warfvinge G, Liedholm R et al (2011) Lymphoid organisation in labial salivary gland biopsies is a possible predictor for the development of malignant lymphoma in primary Sjogren's syndrome. Ann Rheum Dis 70:1363–1368
108. Ramos-Casals M, Brito-Zeron P, Yague J, Akasbi M, Bautista R, Ruano M et al (2005) Hypocomplementaemia as an immunological marker of morbidity and mortality in patients with primary Sjogren's syndrome. Rheumatology (Oxford) 44:89–94

Parotid and Submandibular Involvement in Sjögren's Syndrome

22

Savino Sciascia, Andrea De Marchi, and Dario Roccatello

22.1 Introduction

Sjögren's syndrome (SS) is a chronic autoimmune condition characterized by diminished lacrimal and salivary gland function with associated lymphocytic infiltrates of the affected glands. SS may occur in a primary form when it is not associated with other autoimmune disorders or in a secondary form when it complicates another underlying rheumatic disease. Among others, rheumatoid arthritis and systemic lupus erythematosus are the most common diseases associated with SS.

Reduced exocrine gland function is the main pathogenic mechanism underlying the principal clinical manifestations of SS, such as a combination of dry eyes (keratoconjunctivitis sicca [KCS]) and dry mouth (xerostomia) [1, 2].

S. Sciascia
Center of Research of Immunopathology and Rare Diseases, Coordinating Center of the Network of Rare Diseases of Piedmont and Aosta Valley, Department of Rare, Immunologic, Hematologic and Immunohematologic Diseases, Giovanni Bosco Hospital and University of Turin, Piazza del donatore di Sangue 3, Turin 10154, Italy
e-mail: savino.sciascia@unito.it

A. De Marchi
Pathology Department, Giovanni Bosco Hospital, Piazza del donatore di Sangue 3, Turin 10154, Italy

D. Roccatello (✉)
Center of Research of Immunopathology and Rare Diseases, Coordinating Center of the Network of Rare Diseases of Piedmont and Aosta Valley, Department of Rare, Immunologic, Hematologic and Immunohematologic Diseases, Giovanni Bosco Hospital and University of Turin, Piazza del donatore di Sangue 3, Turin 10154, Italy

SCDU Nephrology and Dialysis, Giovanni Bosco Hospital and University of Turin, Piazza del donatore di Sangue 3, Turin 10154, Italy
e-mail: dario.roccatello@unito.it

D. Roccatello, L. Emmi (eds.), *Connective Tissue Disease: A Comprehensive Guide-Volume 1*, Rare Diseases of the Immune System 5,
DOI 10.1007/978-3-319-24535-5_22

For classification purposes, the clinical manifestations of SS are usually divided into the exocrine gland features and the extraglandular disease features [3]. Indeed, a wide variety of extraglandular manifestations can occur in SS and they are described elsewhere in this book.

A retrospective analysis including 80 patients with primary SS with a long follow-up period (median follow-up more than 7 years) showed that KCS and xerostomia occurred in all patients and were the only disease manifestations in 31 % of the patients. Other manifestations included extraglandular involvement in 25 %, while non-Hodgkin lymphoma developed in 2.5 % [3].

Various classification criteria have been proposed to define and characterize SS [4–6]. The 2002 American–European Consensus Group (AECG) classification criteria was the most commonly used classification tool following publication. However, in 2012, another set of criteria was proposed by the American College of Rheumatology (ACR) that differed from the AECG criteria in several points, including the exclusion of subjective ocular or oral dryness from the ACR criteria set and the lack of a distinction between primary and secondary SS [6]. Thus, differences in estimates of the frequency and severity of various clinical manifestations may be observed and are related to the criteria that were used to identify the patients in the analysis [6, 7] (Figs. 22.1 and 22.2).

The main signs of exocrine gland involvement are dry eyes (keratoconjunctivitis sicca) and dry mouth (xerostomia), but other manifestations may also be seen. The ocular symptoms of dry eyes mainly include irritation, grittiness, and a foreign body sensation, and they are described separately in this book.

22.2 Oral Symptoms and Signs

22.2.1 Xerostomia

The effects of SS on the oral cavity result from chronic salivary hypofunction. Dry mouth or xerostomia is a common symptom, particularly in older adults [8], but objective evidence of reduced salivary flow is less frequent [9]. It is described as dryness of the mouth that makes swallowing of food and even talking difficult owing to the dryness of the buccal mucosa. However, a dry mouth is not necessarily painful. A sudden development of pain in the mouth suggests a differential diagnosis with angular chellitis or erythematous petechial-type lesions on the palate (commonly under dentures); such findings suggest oral candidosis. However, one should keep in mind that the onset of these conditions may be triggered by dryness of the mouth itself [10]. Similarly, xerostomia increases the rate of dental caries and periodontal complications and may often be associated with a decrease in the sense of taste and a change in oral flora [11–13].

The pathogenic mechanisms causing xerostomia in SS are described in Chap. 20. For the purpose of this chapter, it is worth noting that the histological features of parotid and submandibular involvement include extensive lymphocytic infiltration, accompanied by glandular and ductal atrophy. This lymphocytic infiltration is

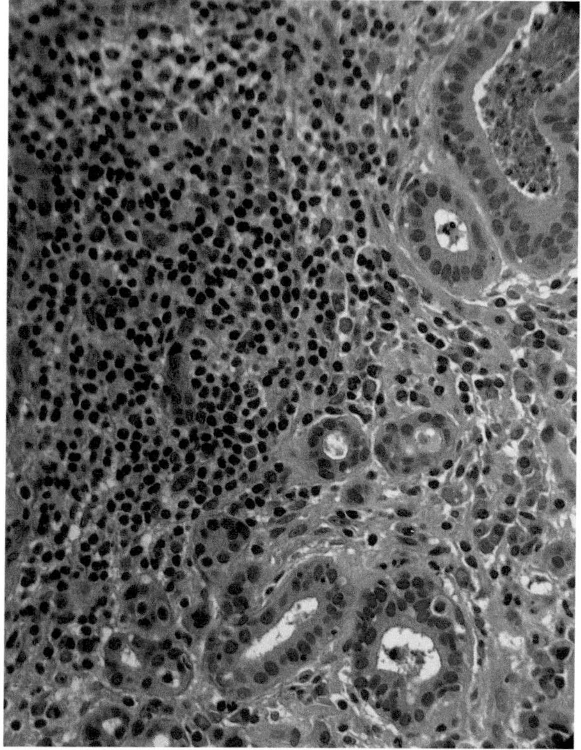

Fig. 22.1 Glandular parenchyma with lymphoplasmacellular infiltrates, showing a reduction of acinar structures and intraepithelial lymphocytes (hematoxylin and eosin stain, 400×)

organized in germinal center-like structures [14]. However, most biopsy samples from patients with SS show that dryness of the mouth cannot simply be attributed to the total destruction of the gland. The residual glandular elements in the salivary gland appear dysfunctional even though they maintain their neural innervation and upregulation of their muscarinic receptors.

22.2.2 Salivary Gland Enlargement

Salivary gland enlargement is common and occurs in 30–50 % of patients with SS at some point during the course of the disease. The parotid, submandibular, and other salivary glands may all undergo hypertrophy in SS. Upon physical examination, the glands are non-tender, and enlargement is firm and diffuse. These changes are most obvious in the parotid glands, but the submandibular glands may be affected to the same degree. Salivary gland enlargement may be either chronic or episodic, with swelling followed by a reduction over a few weeks. A particularly hard or nodular gland may suggest a neoplasm, mainly a lymphoproliferative disease.

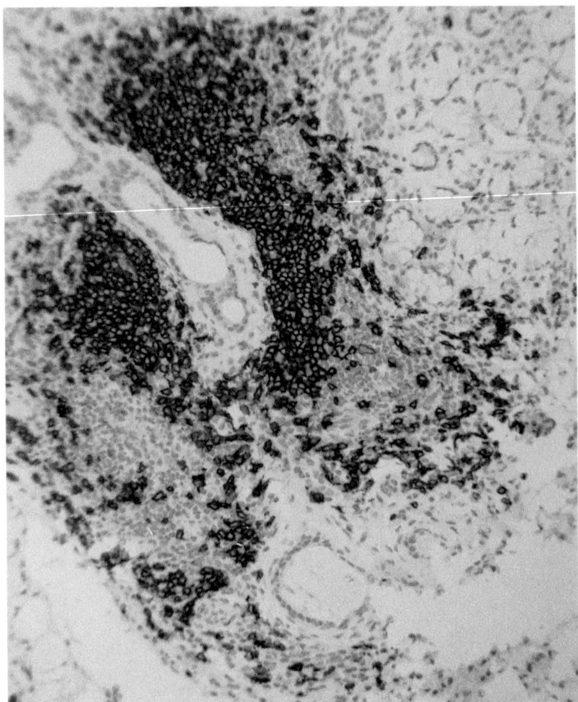

Fig. 22.2 Immunostaining for CD20, showing B-cell lymphocytes with periductal disposition (200×)

22.3 Diagnosis

Confirmation that the symptoms of dryness are caused SS often requires a salivary gland biopsy. This procedure is performed routinely on an outpatient basis. However, salivary gland biopsy is not necessary in all patients. Primary SS is often associated with autoantibodies directed against either the Ro/SSA or La/SSB antigens (see Chap. 21). The combination of clinical features consistent with SS and the finding of anti-Ro/SSA or anti-La/SSB antibodies may generally preclude the need for salivary gland biopsy.

Imaging investigation may enrich the diagnostic pathway for SS. It consists of several tools, including oral examination with sialography or a combination of sialometry (chewing gum test or Saxon test) and salivary scintigraphy. The oldest imaging procedure has maintained its position as sialography is still the method of choice for exploring the ductal system of the salivary glands because of its high diagnostic reliability [15].

Since the 1990s, CT, MRI, MR sialography, and ultrasonography have also been used to diagnose SS. In the assessment of salivary gland involvement in SS, ultrasonography of the major salivary glands warrants special attention as a noninvasive, inexpensive, widely available, easily accessible, and non-irradiating imaging modality [16]. Ultrasonography enables visualization of deep structures of the body by recording the reflections or echoes of ultrasonic pulses directed into the tissues. Frequencies ranging from 1.6 to 22 MHz are used for diagnostic imaging. B-mode is the most widely used ultrasonography mode and the use of color Doppler sonography may contribute to increase the specificity for glandular involvement [16, 17].

However, it has also been reported that the sensitivity of the diagnosis of SS by ultrasonography ranges from 40 to 100 % and that it is not necessarily superior to other methods of examination with regard to diagnostic reliability [17]. A recent meta-analysis evaluating the diagnostic usefulness of ultrasonography for SS concluded that available studies have a high risk of bias in "conduct and interpretation of ultrasound" and that studies evaluating parenchymal homogeneity alone have the best level degree of reproducibility.

22.3.1 Salivary Gland Biopsy

Salivary gland biopsy is usually performed under three circumstances: presence of sicca syndrome, suspicion of SS, and suspicion of another systemic disease. Moreover, parotid biopsy is employed in the diagnosis of lymphoma arising in a patient with SS.

The accuracy of salivary gland biopsy is well established and focal sialoadenitis in minor salivary gland biopsy is one of the main criteria of the revised classification criteria proposed by the American–European Consensus Group. Although the submandibular gland shows the most diagnostic alterations regarding salivary flow rates in SS, there are no studies reporting submandibular biopsy, likely due to the invasiveness of the procedure and to the need for general anesthesia.

Sublingual salivary gland biopsy is reported by a few authors [18–20]. Adam et al. [19] proposed biopsy of the sublingual gland because of the abundance of obtainable tissue [20]. Complications reported with sublingual salivary gland biopsy are scant and involve only swelling of the floor of the mouth.

Parotid biopsy is reported in several studies [21–23]; complications of this procedure include a temporary change in sensation in the pre-auricular area, recovering within 6 months. In experienced hands, sialocele and facial nerve damage are seldom reported.

22.3.2 Differential Diagnosis

The differential diagnosis of xerostomia and enlarged parotid glands are shown in Boxes 22.1 and 22.2, respectively.

Box 22.1: Dry Mouth

Systemic diseases
- Amyloidosis
- Sarcoidosis
- Viral infection (e.g., HIV and HCV)

Drugs
- Antidepressants
- Antihistamines
- Anticholinergics
- Diuretics
- Neuroleptics

Psychogenic
- Anxiety

Radiation therapy

Dehydration

Box 22.2: Salivary Gland Enlargement

Usually unilateral

Acute
- Bacterial infection
- Actinomycosis
- Obstruction

Chronic
- Chronic sialadenitis
- Primary neoplasm (adenoma, adenocarcinoma, lymphoma, mixed salivary gland tumors)

Usually bilateral

Acute
- Acute viral infections (EBV, mumps, CMV, Coxsackie A virus)

Chronic
- Chronic viral infections (HIV, HCV)
- IgG4-related sialadenitis
- Amyloidosis
- Granulomatous diseases (sarcoidosis, tuberculosis)
- HIV infection
- Hyperlipidemia
- Diabetes mellitus
- Alcoholism
- Malnutrition
- Acromegaly
- Anorexia and bulimia

Dryness in patients with neurological conditions such as Alzheimer's disease or multiple sclerosis has been associated with a dysfunction of the subcortical white matter that signals the lacrimatory and salivatory nuclei [24]. The so-called dry burning mouth sensation has often been described in association with depression and anxiety [24], as a result of possible cortical factors to the functional circuit that regulates glandular function and the cortical sensation of dryness.

A sudden onset of swelling of a single gland suggests infection, and the presence of swollen glands or lymphadenopathy raises the possibility of lymphoma, a process that is much more frequent in patients with SS than in the general population. Indeed, lymphoproliferative disease is a particular concern in SS because the risk of lymphoma is 40 times greater than in the general population.

22.4 Complications

Patients may complain directly of oral dryness or of complications such as dysphagia, adherence of food to buccal surfaces, problems with dentures, changes in taste, or an inability to eat dry food or to speak continuously for long periods.

Chronic xerostomia resulting from parotid and submandibular involvement may result in a number of complications, including: dental caries (affecting up to 65 % of SS patients [25]), gingival recession [26], oral candidiasis (affecting up to 40 % of patients with SS [27–29]), and other types of oral infections such as bacterial infections of Stensen's duct.

Moreover, laryngotracheal reflux due to decreased salivary flow may occur, which may lead to frequent throat clearing, cough, substernal pain, and nocturnal awakening that simulate panic attacks [30, 31]. The absence of the normal gastric acid buffer related to decreased salivary flow and of reflux of gastric acid into the esophagus and trachea result in laryngotracheal reflux and chronic esophagitis. Finally, weight loss, due to difficulty with chewing and swallowing, may be present.

Conclusion

Parotid and submandibular involvement is present in virtually all patients with SS, and salivary gland enlargement may be either chronic or episodic. It most often affects the parotid glands, but the submandibular glands may be similarly involved. They are usually firm, diffuse, and not painful on physical examination. The presence of features such as a hard or nodular gland requires ruling out any underlying lymphoproliferative disease.

References

1. Ramos-Casals M, Tzioufas AG, Font J (2005) Primary Sjogren's syndrome: new clinical and therapeutic concepts. Ann Rheum Dis 64(3):347–354
2. Pertovaara M, Korpela M, Uusitalo H, Pukander J, Miettinen A, Helin H et al (1999) Clinical follow up study of 87 patients with sicca symptoms (dryness of eyes or mouth, or both). Ann Rheum Dis 58(7):423–427

3. Asmussen K, Andersen V, Bendixen G, Schiodt M, Oxholm P (1996) A new model for classification of disease manifestations in primary Sjogren's syndrome: evaluation in a retrospective long-term study. J Intern Med 239(6):475–482
4. Vitali C, Bombardieri S, Jonsson R, Moutsopoulos HM, Alexander EL, Carsons SE et al (2002) Classification criteria for Sjogren's syndrome: a revised version of the European criteria proposed by the American-European Consensus Group. Ann Rheum Dis 61(6):554–558
5. Vitali C (2003) Classification criteria for Sjogren's syndrome. Ann Rheum Dis 62(1):94–95; author reply 5
6. Shiboski SC, Shiboski CH, Criswell L, Baer A, Challacombe S, Lanfranchi H et al (2012) American College of Rheumatology classification criteria for Sjogren's syndrome: a data-driven, expert consensus approach in the Sjogren's International Collaborative Clinical Alliance cohort. Arthritis Care Res 64(4):475–487
7. Malladi AS, Sack KE, Shiboski SC, Shiboski CH, Baer AN, Banushree R et al (2012) Primary Sjogren's syndrome as a systemic disease: a study of participants enrolled in an international Sjogren's syndrome registry. Arthritis Care Res 64(6):911–918
8. Schein OD, Hochberg MC, Munoz B, Tielsch JM, Bandeen-Roche K, Provost T et al (1999) Dry eye and dry mouth in the elderly: a population-based assessment. Arch Intern Med 159(12):1359–1363
9. Hochberg MC, Tielsch J, Munoz B, Bandeen-Roche K, West SK, Schein OD (1998) Prevalence of symptoms of dry mouth and their relationship to saliva production in community dwelling elderly: the SEE project. Salisbury Eye Evaluation. J Rheumatol 25(3):486–491
10. Daniels TE (2000) Evaluation, differential diagnosis, and treatment of xerostomia. J Rheumatol Suppl 61:6–10
11. Schiodt M, Christensen LB, Petersen PE, Thorn JJ (2001) Periodontal disease in primary Sjogren's syndrome. Oral Dis 7(2):106–108
12. Wu AJ (2003) The oral component of Sjogren's syndrome: pass the scalpel and check the water. Curr Rheumatol Rep 5(4):304–310
13. Soto-Rojas AE, Villa AR, Sifuentes-Osornio J, Alarcon-Segovia D, Kraus A (1998) Oral candidiasis and Sjogren's syndrome. J Rheumatol 25(5):911–915
14. Jonsson MV, Skarstein K, Jonsson R, Brun JG (2007) Serological implications of germinal center-like structures in primary Sjogren's syndrome. J Rheumatol 34(10):2044–2049
15. Kalk WW, Vissink A, Spijkervet FK, Bootsma H, Kallenberg CG, Roodenburg JL (2002) Parotid sialography for diagnosing Sjogren syndrome. Oral Surg Oral Med Oral Pathol Oral Radiol Endod 94(1):131–137
16. Hocevar A, Ambrozic A, Rozman B, Kveder T, Tomsic M (2005) Ultrasonographic changes of major salivary glands in primary Sjogren's syndrome. Diagnostic value of a novel scoring system. Rheumatology 44(6):768–772
17. Carotti M, Salaffi F, Manganelli P, Argalia G (2001) Ultrasonography and colour doppler sonography of salivary glands in primary Sjogren's syndrome. Clin Rheumatol 20(3): 213–219
18. Pennec YL, Leroy JP, Jouquan J, Lelong A, Katsikis P, Youinou P (1990) Comparison of labial and sublingual salivary gland biopsies in the diagnosis of Sjogren's syndrome. Ann Rheum Dis 49(1):37–39
19. Adam P, Haroun A, Billet J, Mercier J (1992) Biopsy of the salivary glands. The importance and technic of biopsy of the sublingual gland on its anterio-lateral side. Rev Stomatol Chir Maxillofac 93(5):337–340
20. Berquin K, Mahy P, Weynand B, Reychler H (2006) Accessory or sublingual salivary gland biopsy to assess systemic disease: a comparative retrospective study. Eur Arch Oto-Rhino-Laryngol: Off J Eur Fed Oto-Rhino-Laryngol Soc 263(3):233–236
21. Baurmash H (2005) Parotid biopsy technique. J Oral Maxillofac Surg: Off J Am Assoc Oral Maxillofac Surg 63(10):1556–1557
22. McGuirt WF Jr, Whang C, Moreland W (2002) The role of parotid biopsy in the diagnosis of pediatric Sjogren syndrome. Arch Otolaryngol Head Neck Surg 128(11):1279–1281

23. Marx RE, Hartman KS, Rethman KV (1988) A prospective study comparing incisional labial to incisional parotid biopsies in the detection and confirmation of sarcoidosis, Sjogren's disease, sialosis and lymphoma. J Rheumatol 15(4):621–629
24. Fox RI (2005) Sjogren's syndrome. Lancet 366(9482):321–331
25. Daniels TE, Silverman S Jr, Michalski JP, Greenspan JS, Sylvester RA, Talal N (1975) The oral component of Sjogren's syndrome. Oral Surg Oral Med Oral Pathol 39(6):875–885
26. Rhodus NL, Michalowicz BS (2005) Periodontal status and sulcular Candida albicans colonization in patients with primary Sjogren's Syndrome. Quintessence Int 36(3):228–233
27. van der Reijden WA, Vissink A, Veerman EC, Amerongen AV (1999) Treatment of oral dryness related complaints (xerostomia) in Sjogren's syndrome. Ann Rheum Dis 58(8):465–474
28. Rhodus NL, Bloomquist C, Liljemark W, Bereuter J (1997) Prevalence, density, and manifestations of oral Candida albicans in patients with Sjogren's syndrome. J Otolaryngol 26(5):300–305
29. Tapper-Jones L, Aldred M, Walker DM (1980) Prevalence and intraoral distribution of Candida albicans in Sjogren's syndrome. J Clin Pathol 33(3):282–287
30. Belafsky PC, Postma GN (2003) The laryngeal and esophageal manifestations of Sjogren's syndrome. Curr Rheumatol Rep 5(4):297–303
31. Postma GN, Belafsky PC, Aviv JE, Koufman JA (2002) Laryngopharyngeal reflux testing. Ear Nose Throat J 81(9 Suppl 2):14–18

Extraglandular Involvement in Sjögren's Syndrome

23

Roberta Priori, Antonina Minniti, Giovanna Picarelli, and Guido Valesini

23.1 Introduction

Although primary Sjögren's syndrome (pSS) mainly affects the exocrine glands, resulting in a wide range of disturbing sicca symptoms (such as dry mouth, dry eyes, xerotrachea, dry vagina), extraglandular disease manifestations also occur in a non-negligible percentage of patients.

As a matter of fact, more than two-thirds of patients present systemic features [1–3] which are severe in about 10–20 % [4–8]. A comparison of the prevalence of extraglandular manifestations in several pSS cohorts reveals substantial variability which can be linked to disparities in the specific study populations, recruitment sources, classification criteria used for pSS, and methods for assessing and defining such complications (Table 23.1).

The spectrum of pSS may therefore range from a benign, slowly progressive, autoimmune exocrinopathy to a heterogeneous and potentially fatal systemic disorder characterized by an increased risk of non-Hodgkin's lymphoma (NHL). In some patients the disease starts with nonspecific manifestations such as arthralgias, Raynaud's phenomenon, purpura, or other uncommon systemic manifestations [9]. Longer disease duration and younger age at diagnosis are associated with severe extraglandular pSS complications. It seems that the presence of multiple serological markers, such as low C3/C4, hypergammaglobulinemia, cryoglobulins, and rheumatoid factor positivity can help in the early identification of patients prone to present non-exocrine manifestations [7, 10, 11]. Similarly, a high focus score for ectopic and germinal center formation in minor salivary glands, which occurs in

R. Priori • A. Minniti • G. Picarelli • G. Valesini (✉)
UOC Reumatologia, Sapienza Università di Roma, Via Policlinico 155, Rome 00161, Italy
e-mail: guido.valesini@uniroma1.it

D. Roccatello, L. Emmi (eds.), *Connective Tissue Disease: A Comprehensive Guide-Volume 1*, Rare Diseases of the Immune System 5,
DOI 10.1007/978-3-319-24535-5_23

Table 23.1 Patients' demographic and extraglandular features

	Baldini et al. [7]	Pertovaara et al. [4]	Garcìa-Carrasco et al. [2]	Alamanos et al. [5]	Ramos-Casals et al. [1]	Martel et al. [6]
Patients *N*	1115	110	400	422	1010	445
Sex (female)	1067 (95.7 %)	107 (97 %)	373 (93 %)	402 (95 %)	937 (93 %)	400 (90 %)
Age at diagnosis (mean ± SD)	51.6 ± 13.8	62 ± 13	52.7 ± 0.85	55.4 (12.5)	53 ± 0.48	53.6 ± 1.4
Age at inclusion (mean ± SD)	57.5 ± 13.7	–	58.7 ± 0.72	–	58.7 ± 0.46	–
Follow up mean (mean ± SD, years)	5.8 ± 6.5	–	–	–	6 ± 0.3	
Arthralgias	683 (61.3)	82 (75 %)	147 (37 %)	165 (39 %)	490 (48 %)	222 (50 %)
Arthritis	123 (11 %)	24 (22 %)	–	–	150 (15 %)	–
Raynaud's phenomenon	239 (21.4)	55 (50 %)	62 (16 %)	146 (34.6 %)	187 (18 %)	189 (42 %)
Lung involvement	60 (5.4)	–	37 (9 %)	–	112 (11 %)	55 (12 %)
PNS involvement	59 (5.3)	23 (21 %)	29 (7 %)	–	110 (11 %)	70 (16 %)
Skin involvement	106 (9.5)	22 (20 %)	47 (12 %)	20 (4.7 %)	91 (9 %)	70 (16 %)
Lymphoma	50 (4.5)	–	–	–	–	18 (4 %)

PNS peripheral nervous system

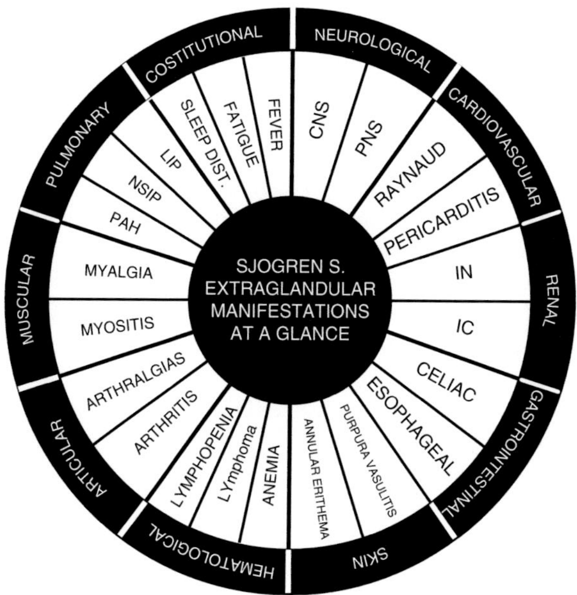

Fig. 23.1 Extraglandular manifestations in pSS

about one-quarter of patients with pSS, is associated with more severe disease and the risk of developing lymphoma [12–16]. All these features can be useful aids for screening possible candidates to more aggressive treatment.

Several attempts have been made to draft a sound classification system for the disease features that would be useful for patient monitoring and scientific communication as well as for distinguishing clinically relevant disease subsets. Clinical manifestations can be classified as glandular and extraglandular [17], or more accurately, taking the concept of autoimmune epithelitis into account [18], into exocrine and non-exocrine, and thereafter assembled into subgroups (Fig. 23.1) [19, 20].

More simply, systemic manifestations can be divided into four groups: non specific, those caused by the extension of lymphocytic infiltration into parenchimal organs, those immune complexes mediated and lymphoproliferative complications [9].

23.2 Constitutional Signs and Symptoms

Constitutional symptoms such as chronic fatigue, sleep disturbance, low-grade fever, myalgias, and widespread pain are frequent and can have a negative impact on the patients' daily life. As a matter of fact, pSS patients experience significant functional disability compared to age-matched healthy controls [21]. Fatigue, tiredness, and widespread pain are, without a doubt, among the most common symptoms in pSS and are reported by 68–85 % of patients [22–25]. Their underlying mechanisms are still unknown. An association between fibromyalgia (FM) and SS has been reported, though with conflicting evidence [25–28], while others have described mild histopathological signs of myositis in patients affected by SS [29]. Psychosocial variables are determinants of fatigue, but only partially account for it, and the relationship between fatigue and depression in pSS is not clear [30]. Lastly, some authors have hypothesized that fatigue, widespread pain, anxiety, and depression, so frequently affecting SS patients, may be explained by autonomic nervous system disturbances [31]. Patients describe their fatigue as an ever-present, fluctuating, and non-relievable lack of vitality [32].

Sleep disturbances and excessive daytime sleepiness have been reported in patients with pSS [33–36] related to a wide spectrum of causes: fibromyalgia, mood disorders, muscle and joint pain, night sleep restriction linked to the need to awake up and drink water because of the xerostomia, restless leg symptoms, and a concomitant obstructive sleep apnea syndrome (OSAS), which has been reported with a higher prevalence in pSS patients [37–40]. Fever has been reported in 6–41 % of pSS cases, more often at onset in those with neurological involvement or other extraglandular features [41, 42].

23.3 Neurological Manifestations

Nervous system complications are part of the clinical spectrum of pSS and can be peripheral or, to a lesser extent, central. The prevalence of neurological involvement is controversial mainly because of differences in the methodological approach used to assess it and in the criteria adopted to classify patients; however, it ranges between 11 and 70 %. Neurological manifestations can precede pSS diagnosis, thus representing a diagnostic challenge in the absence of other clear symptoms [43, 44].

While peripheral nervous system (PNS) dysfunction is a well-known aspect of pSS that usually appears in older patients, central nervous system (CNS) involvement is more frequently overlooked and misdiagnosed even if it has recently gained more attention than in the past. Diffuse, non-focal neurological manifestations are the most frequent manifestations and include a variety of features, such as cognitive deficits, psychiatric abnormalities, and migraine; however, focal defects associated with meningoencephalitis, transverse myelitis, and subarachnoid hemorrhage may also occur. In patients with a relapsing–remitting course of disease, CNS involvement may be indistinguishable from multiple sclerosis [45, 46]. Both migraine and tension-type headaches are very common in pSS patients [47]. Anti-Ro/SSA antibodies have been related to more severe and progressive cases and to the presence of MRI, CT, and angiographic abnormalities, while other autoantibodies, such as antiphospholipid and anti-P ribosomal protein, appear to play a secondary role in SS.

The clinical spectrum of PNS complications is broad and includes (1) pure sensory neuropathy, which presents with distal symmetric sensory loss due to axonal degeneration of sensory fibers, sensory ataxia due to loss of proprioceptive large fibers associated with dorsal root ganglionitis, or small fiber sensory neuropathy due to degeneration of cutaneous axons, which presents with painful dysesthesias (a skin biopsy to evaluate the loss or reduction of nerve fiber density is required to diagnose the latter, which appears to be the most common neuropathy in pSS); (2) sensorimotor polyneuropathy affecting sensory and motor axons, generally associated with palpable purpura and cryoglobulinemia and a higher risk of developing lymphoma; and (3) more infrequent forms, including autoimmune demyelinating neuropathy, mononeuropathy, mononeuropathy multiplex, and autonomic neuropathy.

The clinical heterogeneity of PNS involvement and the lack of a standardized approach for diagnosis make it difficult to accurately calculate prevalence and to determine clinical associations and risk factors [48, 49].

23.4 Cardiovascular Manifestations

More than 10 % of patients with pSS present Raynaud's phenomenon (RP), which is probably its most common vascular feature. RP may represent the first clinical sign at onset suggesting a diagnosis of pSS, but it may also identify a specific subset of patients with anti-centromere (ACA) antibodies, suggestive of overlapping systemic sclerosis (SSc) [50, 51].

The links between pSS and cardiovascular (CV) disease have only recently been evaluated, though with conflicting results. SS patients seem to be more likely to experience known CV risk factors, such as hypertension, diabetes mellitus, and dyslipidemia, than age- and sex-matched healthy controls. Such features do not completely explain subclinical accelerated atherosclerosis, a recently recognized feature of the disease, which might predispose to CV death [52–54]. However, it is not clear whether an increase in CV death occurs in pSS, even if a recent study demonstrated a higher risk of cerebrovascular events and myocardial infarction [55].

Clinically overt heart disease is infrequent. However, recent echocardiographic studies showed that asymptomatic cardiac involvement, mainly pericarditis and diastolic dysfunction, is not rare in pSS [56–60].

23.5 Renal Manifestations

Renal involvement in pSS is relatively rare and may precede the onset of sicca symptoms. Renal involvement in pSS consists primarily of interstitial nephritis and, less commonly, immune complex glomerulonephritis. Interstitial nephritis (IN) is characterized by the presence of lymphocytes, plasma cells, and monocytes in the interstitium combined with tubular atrophy and fibrosis. The majority of the infiltrating cells have a CD4+ cell phenotype, resembling the lesions in the salivary glands [61]. The clinical presentation may include hyposthenuria, overt or latent distal renal tubular acidosis (RTA) (type I), and, less commonly, Fanconi syndrome (RTA) (type II). RTA may be present in 22–30 % of pSS patients [62]. Unlike interstitial nephritis, glomerulonephritis (GN) is a late sequela in the course of the disease and is strongly correlated to more generalized small-vessel involvement. GN presents as palpable purpura, peripheral neuropathy, or B-cell lymphoma [63].

In addition, chronic interstitial cystitis (IC) may occur in pSS. IC, also known as painful bladder syndrome, is a chronic inflammatory disease of the bladder of unknown etiology, occurring mainly in women and primarily during middle age. Patients usually present with irritative symptoms, such as urinary frequency, urgency, nocturia, and suprapubic, urethral, and perineal pain, but no infectious organisms are detected in the urine. Histopathological study of the bladder shows mucosal edema and mononuclear cell infiltration of the interstitium [64].

23.6 Gastrointestinal Manifestations

Any part of the gastrointestinal (GI) system, from the mouth, esophagus, and bowel to the liver and pancreas, can be involved in pSS as it is an epithelitis, which primarily affects exocrine glands. Dysphagia, occurring in 30–80 % of cases, is partly due to xerostomia, but also to esophageal dysfunction. Dyspepsia is less common; mild atrophic changes in the antrum may be observed more frequently in patients with pSS than in controls, but severe mucosal atrophy is rare [65]. Whether the incidence of *Helicobacter pylori* is higher in pSS is still controversial, but this organism has been associated with MALT lymphomas in pSS [66]. Documented intestinal involvement is rare to absent in large series [65]. Hepatomegaly and abnormal liver function tests (LFT) have been found in up to 25 % of pSS patients [67]. The most frequent causes of liver disease in pSS are primary biliary cirrhosis (PBC), autoimmune hepatitis (AH), nonalcoholic fatty liver disease, and, above all, chronic hepatitis C virus (HCV) infection [68]. Hepatomegaly occurs in 11–21 % of patients, while abnormal LFTs are found in 10–49 % of patients, although usually mild and without clinical significance. PBC and pSS share several features (skewed sex prevalence, common effector mechanisms acting on the same target, i.e., the epithelium), and they occasionally overlap [69]; in such cases, PBC tends to be pathologically mild, with a propensity for slow progression, as assessed clinically, biochemically, and histologically [70]. AH has been reported in 0–7 % of patients with pSS [65]. HCV infection may be associated with sicca complaints and the presence of serum cryoglobulins. As a matter of fact, besides hepatocytes and lymphocytes, HCV seems to show a special tropism for lacrimal and salivary epithelial cells, while chronic focal sialoadenitis, resembling what is seen in pSS, may be observed in approximately 50 % of HCV-infected patients eliminare [71]. However, sicca symptoms seem to be less frequent and milder in HCV-infected patients. Histological examination of salivary glands in HCV-infected patients shows different aspects compared to what is observed in pSS patients: lymphocytic infiltrates are often located in the pericapillary area rather than around the glandular ducts and the lymphocytic subpopulations that are present in the glandular infiltrates appear to be different and sometimes show a predominance of CD8+ T lymphocytes. Lastly, specific autoantibodies for pSS are not detectable in the sera of HCV-infected patients. As compared to the healthy population, a higher percentage of patients with either chronic HCV infection associated with mixed cryoglobulinemia and hypocomplementemia or patients with pSS may develop B-cell lymphomas [72, 73]. The possible relationship between frank SS and HCV infections is still under debate, thus leading the American–European Consensus Group for the Classification of SS to list HCV infections among the exclusion criteria for SS [74]. However, a true overlap between HCV infection and pSS is possible, and various studies reported an HCV prevalence of 3–14 % among patients with previously identified pSS, which is significantly higher than in the general population (1.2 %) [75]. These findings suggest that HCV might be involved in SS pathogenesis [76, 77].

On the contrary, HBV infection does not seem to be higher in SS patients.

Since the pancreas is, in part, an exocrine gland, it can be affected in pSS patients. Alterations of pancreatic enzymes and pancreatic exocrine dysfunction have been reported in less than 40 % of patients; however, the latter is usually both mild and subclinical [78]. Celiac disease (CD) has also been reported to occur in 4.5–14.7 % of pSS patients [79, 80], and identifying patients who present mild or atypical symptoms is necessary [81].

23.7 Skin Manifestations

Cutaneous manifestations, which are generally classified as vasculitic and non-vasculitic, are part of the spectrum of the extraglandular features of pSS, even if they are responsible for increased disease activity in only 8.6 % of patients at diagnosis and in 13.4 % at any time during the disease course [82]. Skin dryness has been shown to be a very common symptom in pSS, with frequency varying from 23 to 68 % and usually presenting with 2 non-specific pruritus and a sensation of dryness. The mechanism that is responsible for skin xerosis has not been fully elucidated, but since decreased sweating has been reported in pSS patients, impairment of the sweat glands has been hypothesized [83].

The most common vasculitic lesion is palpable purpura. This usually appears in the lower limbs as recurrent crops of round, pink, separated, or confluent lesions turning purple and brown within a few days and finally resolving or leaving a pale brown stain. Cryoglobulinemic palpable purpura has been associated with lymphoma development and mortality. Hypergammaglobulinemic purpura is relatively common in patients with pSS and may be associated with sensory peripheral neuropathy. The skin lesions are non-palpable and are often associated with a higher prevalence of anemia, elevated eritrosedimentation rate (ESR), hypergammaglobulinemia, rheumatoid factor, antinucleaar antibodies (ANA), and anti-Ro/SSA antibodies [84]. The second most common form of inflammatory vascular disease is urticarial vasculitis, which is characterized by smaller stinging or burning lesions that usually persist for 24 h and often resolve in hyperpigmentation, indicating red blood cell extravasation [85, 86]. Patients with pSS may also present a wide range of non-vasculitic lesions. One of the most characteristic is annular erythema, which is primarily reported in Asian patients with pSS [87, 88]. These cutaneous lesions are annular, polycyclic, and photosensitive and are clinically identical to those seen in patients with subacute cutaneous lupus erythematosus with anti-Ro/SSA antibodies. Some patients diagnosed with isolated, subacute cutaneous lupus erythematosus may actually have underlying pSS. On the other hand, pSS patients with annular erythema should be followed up to detect the possible evolution to systemic lupus erythematosus [89]. Other manifestations include vitiligo, alopecia, angular cheilitis, eyelid dermatitis, anetoderma, and cutaneous lymphoma [90].

23.8 Hematological Manifestations

Hematological abnormalities are rather common in pSS. Normocytic normochromic anemia is frequently observed, and various abnormalities can be observed in the leukocyte counts, above all leukopenia, which is observed in 15–30 % of patients with pSS [90]. Lymphopenia is quite often found, and granulocytopenia can be observed as well. When the various lymphocyte subpopulations are considered, it has been shown that 5–6 % of patients with pSS have CD4+ T lymphocytopenia [91, 92]. Lympoma development is the subject of other chapters.

23.9 Articular and Muscular Involvement

Musculoskeletal manifestations are very common in pSS patients; indeed, it is estimated that up to 90 % of patients experience arthralgias, myalgias, fatigue, or morning stiffness. Authors report arthralgias in 48–73.5 % of patients, whereas arthritis is observed in up to 17 % of them. Joint symptoms may also appear prior to the classical sicca manifestations in 30 % of cases. The pattern of joint involvement is usually that of intermittent, symmetrical, polyarticular arthropathy affecting both small and large joints [93]. The small joints of the hand, such as the metacarpophalangeal and interphalangeal joints, are frequently affected, resembling rheumatoid arthritis (RA) when accompanied by synovitis. Unlike RA, arthritis in pSS is often non-erosive, even in the presence of antibodies against cyclic citrullinated peptides (anti-CCP). Indeed, while anti-CCP antibodies are an independent and predictive factor in the development of erosions in RA, in pSS patients, this positivity along with other signs of an active immunological profile (rheumatoid factor, SSA or SSB isolation, cryoglobulinemia) seems to be correlated to the presence of musculoskeletal involvement alone [94]. In contrast, other authors demonstrated the presence of severe polyarthritis with features of RA, including erosions, especially in patients with anti-CCP and selected alleles of major histocompatibility complex (MHC) class II molecules [95]. Therefore, the erosive nature of arthritis in the course of pSS remains controversial. Using ultrasonography, which is a more sensitive method than classical radiology, the most frequently observed sign is moderate–mild degree synovitis mainly involving the small joints of the hand, wrists, and knees, although the ankles, hips, and shoulders may be involved as well. Subclinical synovitis may also be observed in patients without any symptoms of articular involvement [96], thus suggesting a higher prevalence of joint involvement in the course of pSS. Myalgia and muscular weakness are other recurrent symptoms in pSS patients, but to date, only a few studies have examined the prevalence of muscular involvement. Although myositis occurs only in about 1.2–3 % of patients, higher percentages of subclinical myositis diagnosed by muscular biopsy may be observed (5–73 %), and the histopathology is often characterized by perivascular inflammation or interstitial myositis without the involvement of muscle fibers [29]. These features, however, are common in several connective tissue diseases, and the clinical significance is uncertain. There is some evidence that inflammatory myopathy in the course of pSS could be interpreted as an overlapping syndrome [97–99] with a generally good outcome and that only a low percentage of patients are resistant to therapy.

23.10 Pulmonary Involvement

The frequency of pulmonary involvement reportedly varies from 9 to 75 %, depending on the detection method that is employed, on ethnic or environmental factors, or on underdiagnosis due to few symptoms. The main findings include small airway abnormalities and interstitial lung disease (ILD), which is often subclinical or is accompanied by dry cough or dyspnea if symptomatic. An early study [100] showed that lung involvement was common and mostly subclinical, with lesions of the small bronchioles leading to significantly lower expiratory flow values. Most patients complained of dry cough without specific clinical findings. Histological examination in 10 patients out of 61 in this cohort revealed the presence of peribronchial lymphocytic infiltrates, similar to those described in the exocrine glands. In the course of pSS, many ILD patterns may occur; it seems that the most common features are: a diffuse, cellular interstitial pneumonia that can be classified as non-specific interstitial pneumonia (NSIP) or lymphocytic interstitial pneumonia (LIP) on the basis of the intensity of the inflammatory infiltrate (which is greater in LIP) [101]. LIP is a lymphoproliferative disease with benign behavior, characterized by polyclonal proliferation of lymphocytes and plasma cells in the interstitium. LIP typically appears as ground-glass opacities with thin-walled cysts on radiographic images. It was considered the most common pulmonary pSS manifestation, but now its prevalence is lower, perhaps because of the revisions in the histopathological criteria for ILD, so that many cases that would previously have been diagnosed as LIP are now diagnosed as NSIP [102]. Other patterns of ILD include organizing pneumonia (OP), usual interstitial pneumonia (UIP), and diffuse interstitial amyloidosis; moreover, the lung can also be the site of a primary pulmonary lymphoma in pSS. Although lung involvement is relatively frequent in pSS, there are limited data on prognosis. Some studies have suggested that pulmonary manifestations of pSS do not worsen the prognosis. Indeed, a 10-year follow-up of 30 British patients [103] showed that most of them had stable pulmonary function with low mortality (15.4 %), while two Asian studies reported that the mortality rate seems to be higher (27.3–30.3 %) [104, 105]. Therefore, more studies are needed to explore the relationship between pulmonary involvement and mortality rate among pSS patients. Pulmonary arterial hypertension (PAH), a type of lung involvement that is rarely observed in pSS, is a disease characterized by vascular proliferation and remodelling of the small pulmonary arteries which results in a progressive increase in pulmonary vascular resistance, thus leading to right ventricular failure and death.

References

1. Ramos-Casals M, Solans R, Rosas J et al (2008) Primary Sjogren syndrome in Spain: clinical and immunologic expression in 1010 patients. Medicine 87:210–219
2. Garcia-Carrasco M, Ramos-Casals M, Rosas J et al (2002) Primary Sjogren syndrome: clinical and immunologic disease patterns in a cohort of 400 patients. Medicine 81:270–280
3. Lin DF, Yan SM, Zhao W et al (2010) Clinical and prognostic characteristics of 573 cases of primary Sjögren's syndrome. China Med J 123:3252–3257
4. Pertovaara M, Pukkala E, Laippala P et al (2001) A longitudinal cohort study of Finnish patients with primary Sjogren's syndrome: clinical, immunological, and epidemiological aspects. Ann Rheum Dis 60:467–472
5. Alamanos Y, Tsifetaki N, Voulgari PV et al (2006) Epidemiology of primary Sjogren's syndrome in north-west Greece, 1982–2003. Rheumatology 45:187–191
6. Martel C, Gondran G, Launay D et al (2011) Active immunological profile is associated with systemic Sjogren's syndrome. J Clin Immunol 31:840–847
7. Baldini C, Pepe P, Quartuccio L et al (2014) Primary Sjogren's syndrome as a multi-organ disease: impact of the serological profile on the clinical presentation of the disease in a large cohort of Italian patients. Rheumatology 53:839–844
8. Li X, Xu B, Ma Y et al (2015) Clinical and laboratory profiles of primary Sjogren's syndrome in a Chinese population: a retrospective analysis of 315 patients. Int J Rheum Dis 18:439–446
9. Moutsopoulos HM (2014) Sjögren's syndrome: a forty-year scientific journey. J Autoimmun 51:1–9
10. Baldini C, Pepe P, Luciano N et al (2012) A clinical prediction rule for lymphoma development in primary Sjogren's syndrome. J Rheumatol 39:804–808
11. Voulgarelis M, Ziakas PD, Papageorgiou A et al (2012) Prognosis and outcome of non-Hodgkin lymphoma in primary Sjogren syndrome. Medicine 91:1–9
12. Daniels TE, Cox D, Shiboski CH et al (2011) Associations between salivary gland histopathologic diagnoses and phenotypic features of Sjögren's syndrome among 1,726 registry participants. Arthritis Rheum 63:2021–2030
13. Theander E, Vasaitis L, Baecklund E et al (2011) Lymphoid organization in labial salivary gland biopsies is a possible predictor for the development of malignant lymphoma in primary Sjögren's syndrome. Ann Rheum Dis 70:1363–1368
14. Risselada AP, Looije MF, Kruize AA et al (2013) The role of ectopic germinal centers in the immunopathology of primary Sjögren's syndrome: a systematic review. Semin Arthritis Rheum 42:368–376
15. Risselada AP, Kruize AA, Goldschmeding R et al (2014) The prognostic value of routinely performed minor salivary gland assessments in primary Sjogren's syndrome. Ann Rheum Dis 73:1537–1540
16. Carubbi F, Alunno A, Cipriani P et al (2015) A retrospective, multicenter study evaluating the prognostic value of minor salivary gland histology in a large cohort of patients with primary Sjögren's syndrome. Lupus 24:315–320
17. Fox RI, Howell FV, Bone RC, Michelson P (1984) Primary Sjogren's syndrome: clinical and immunopathological features. Semin Arthritis Rheum 14:7–103
18. Mitsias DI, Kapsogeorgou EK, Moutsopoulos HM (2006) Sjogren's syndrome: why autoimmune epithelitis? Oral Dis 12:523–532
19. Oxholm P, Asmunssen K (1996) Primary Sjogren's syndrome: the challenge for classification of disease manifestations. J Intern Med 239:467–474
20. Asmunssen K, Andersen V, Bendixen G et al (1996) A new model for classification of disease manifestations in primary Sjogren's syndrome: evaluation in a retrospective long-term study. J Intern Med 239:475–482
21. Hackett KL, Newton JL, Frith J et al (2012) Impaired functional status in primary Sjogren's syndrome. Arthritis Care 64:1764–1767
22. Ng W, Bowman SJ (2010) Primary Sjogren's syndrome: too dry and too tired. Rheumatology 49:844–853

23. Barendregt PJ, Visser M, Smets E et al (1998) Fatigue in primary Sjögren's syndrome. Ann Rheum Dis 57:291–295
24. Tensing EK, Solovieva SA, Tervahartiala T et al (2001) Fatigue and health profile in sicca syndrome of Sjögren's and non-Sjogren's syndrome origin. Clin Exp Rheumatol 19:313–316
25. Priori R, Iannuccelli C, Alessandri C et al (2010) Fatigue in Sjögren's syndrome: relationship with fibromyalgia, clinical and biological features. Clin Exp Rheumatol 28(Suppl 63):S82–S86
26. Ostuni P, Botsios C, Sfriso P et al (2002) Fibromyalgia in Italian patients with primary Sjögren's syndrome. Joint Bone Spine 69:51–57
27. Giles I, Isemberg D (2000) Fatigue in primary Sjögren's syndrome: is there a link with the fibromyalgia syndrome? Ann Rheum Dis 59:875–878
28. Tishler M, Barak Y, Paran D, Yaron M (1997) Sleep disturbances, fibromyalgia and primary Sjögren's syndrome. Clin Exp Rheumatol 15:71–74
29. Lindvall B, Bengtsson A, Ernerudh J et al (2002) Subclinical myositis is common in primary Sjögren's syndrome and is not related to muscle pain. J Rheumatol 29:717–725
30. Segal B, Thomas W, Rogers T et al (2008) Prevalence, severity and predictors of fatigue in primary Sjögren's syndrome. Arthritis Rheum 59:1780–1787
31. Mandl T, Hammar O, Theander E et al (2010) Autonomic nervous dysfunction development in patients with primary Sjögren's syndrome: a follow up study. Rheumatology 49:1101–1106
32. Mengshoel AM, Norheim KB, Omdal R (2014) Primary Sjögren's syndrome: fatigue is an ever-present, fluctuating, and uncontrollable lack of energy. Arthritis Care Res (Hoboken) 66:1227–1232
33. Gudbjörnsson B, Broman JE, Hetta J, Hällgren R (1993) Sleep disturbances in patients with primary Sjögren's syndrome. Br J Rheumatol 32:1072–1076
34. Godaert GL, Hartkamp A, Geenen R et al (2002) Fatigue in daily life in patients with primary Sjögren's syndrome and systemic lupus erythematosus. Ann N Y Acad Sci 966:320–326
35. Walker J, Gordon T, Lester S et al (2003) Increased severity of lower urinary tract symptoms and daytime somnolence in primary Sjögren's syndrome. J Rheumatol 30:2406–2412
36. Iannuccelli C, Spinelli FR, Guzzo MP et al (2012) Fatigue and widespread pain in systemic lupus erythematosus and Sjögren's syndrome: symptoms of the inflammatory disease or associated fibromyalgia? Clin Exp Rheumatol 30(6 Suppl 74):117–121
37. Westhoff G, Dörner T, Zink A (2012) Fatigue and depression predict physician visits and work disability in women with primary Sjögren's syndrome: results from a cohort study. Rheumatology 51:262–269
38. Segal BM, Pogatchnik B, Holker E et al (2012) Primary Sjogren's syndrome: cognitive symptoms, mood, and cognitive performance. Acta Neurol Scand 125:272–278
39. Goodchild CE, Treharne GJ, Booth DA, Bowman SJ (2010) Daytime patterning of fatigue and its associations with the previous nights discomfort and poor sleep among women with primary Sjögren's syndrome or rheumatoid arthritis. Musculoskeletal Care 8:107–117
40. Usmani ZA, Hlavac M, Rischmueller M et al (2012) Sleep disordered breathing in patients with primary Sjögren's syndrome: a group controlled study. Sleep Med 13:1066–1070
41. Wang HC, Chang K, Lin CY et al (2012) Periodic fever as the manifestation of primary Sjogren's syndrome: a case report and literature review. Clin Rheumatol 31:1517–1519
42. Fernandez-Molina G, Michel-Peregrina M, Bermúdez-Bermejo P et al (2012) Early and late extraglandular manifestations in primary Sjögren's syndrome. Clin Exp Rheumatol 30:455
43. Massara A, Bonazza S, Castellino G et al (2010) Central nervous system involvement in Sjogren' syndrome: unusual, but non unremarkable-clinical, serological characteristics and outcomes in a large cohort of Italian patients. Rheumatology 49:1540–1549
44. Delalande S, de Seze J, Fauchais AL et al (2004) Neurologic manifestations in primary Sjögren syndrome: a study of 82 patients. Medicine (Baltimore) 83:280–291
45. Moreira I, Teixeira F, Martins Silva A et al (2015) Frequent involvement of central nervous system in primary Sjögren syndrome. Rheumatol Int 35:289–294
46. Morgen K, McFarland HF, Pillemer SR (2004) Central nervous system disease in primary Sjogren's syndrome: the role of magnetic resonance imaging. Semin Arthritis Rheum 34:623–630

47. Gokcay F, Oder G, Celebisoy N et al (2008) Headache in primary Sjogren's syndrome: a prevalence study. Acta Neurol Scand 118:189–192
48. Mori K, Iijima M, Koike H et al (2005) The wide spectrum of clinical manifestations in Sjögren's syndrome-associated neuropathy. Brain 128:2518–2534
49. Pavlakis PP, Alexopoulos H, Kosmidis ML et al (2012) Peripheral neuropathies in Sjögren's syndrome: a critical update on clinical features and pathogenetic mechanisms. J Autoimmun 39:27–33
50. Garcia-Carrasco M, Siso A, Ramos-Casals M et al (2002) Raynaud's phenomenon in primary Sjogren's syndrome. Prevalence and clinical characteristics in a series of 320 patients. J Rheumatol 29:726–730
51. Bournia VK, Vlachoyiannopoulos PG (2012) Subgroups of Sjögren syndrome patients according to serological profiles. J Autoimmun 39:15–26
52. Vaudo G, Bocci EB, Shoenfeld Y et al (2005) Precocious intima-media thickening in patients with primary Sjogren's syndrome. Arthritis Rheum 52:3890–3897
53. Juarez M, Toms TE, De Pablo M et al (2014) Cardiovascular risk factors in women with primary Sjögren's syndrome: United Kingdom primary Sjögren's syndrome registry results. Arthritis Care Res 66:757–764
54. Perez-De-Lis M, Akasbi M, Siso A et al (2010) Cardiovascular risk factors in primary Sjogren's syndrome: a case–control study in 624 patient. Lupus 19:941–948
55. Bartoloni E, Baldini C, Schillaci G et al (2015) Cardiovascular disease risk burden in primary Sjogren's syndrome: results of a population-based multicentre cohort study. J Intern Med 278(2):185–192
56. Rantapää-Dahlqvist S, Backman C, Sandgren H, Östberg Y (1993) Echocardiographic findings in patients with primary Sjögren's syndrome. Clin Rheumatol 12:214–218
57. Mita S, Akizuki S, Koido N et al (1994) Cardiac involvement in Sjögren's syndrome detected by two dimensional ultrasonic cardiography. In: Homma M, Sugai S, Tojo T, Miyasaka N, Akizuki M (eds) Sjögren's syndrome – state of the art. Kugler, Amsterdam, pp 427–430
58. Gyöngyösi M, Pokorny G, Jambrik Z et al (1996) Cardiac manifestations in primary Sjögren's syndrome. Ann Rheum Dis 55:450–454
59. Manganelli P, Bernardi P, Taliani U et al (1997) Echocardiographic findings in primary Sjögren's syndrome. Ann Rheum Dis 56:568
60. Vassiliou VA, Moyssakis I, Boki KA, Moutsopoulos HM et al (2008) Is the heart affected in primary Sjögren's syndrome? An echocardiographic study. Clin Exp Rheumatol 26:109–112
61. Goules AV, Tatouli IP, Moutsopoulos HM et al (2013) Clinically significant renal involvement in primary Sjögren's syndrome: clinical presentation and outcome. Arthritis Rheum 65:2945–2953
62. Skopouli FN, Dafni U, Ioannidis JPA et al (2000) Clinical evolution and morbidity and mortality of primary Sjogren's syndrome. Semin Arthritis Rheum 29:296–304
63. Goules A, Masouridi S, Tzioufas AG et al (2000) Clinically significant and biopsy documented renal involvement in primary Sjogren's syndrome. Medicine 79:241–249
64. Emmungil H, Kalfa M, Zihni FY et al (2012) Interstitial cystitis: a rare manifestation of primary Sjögren's syndrome, successfully treated with low dose cyclosporine. Rheumatol Int 32:1215–1218
65. Ebert EC (2012) Gastrointestinal and hepatic manifestations of Sjogren syndrome. J Clin Gastroenterol 46:25–30
66. Raderer M, Osterreicher C, Machold K et al (2001) Impaired response of gastric MALT-lymphoma to Helicobacter pylori eradication in patients with autoimmune disease. Ann Oncol 12:937–939
67. Abraham S, Begum S, Isenberg D (2004) Hepatic manifestations of autoimmune rheumatic diseases. Ann Rheum Dis 63:123–129
68. Ramos-Casals M, Sánchez-Tapias JM, Parés A et al (2006) Characterization and differentiation of autoimmune versus viral liver involvement in patients with Sjögren's syndrome. J Rheumatol 33:1593–1599

69. Selmi C, Meroni PL, Gershwin ME (2012) Primary biliary cirrhosis and Sjogren's syndrome: autoimmune epithelitis. J Autoimmun 39:34–42
70. Hatzis GS, Fragoulis GE, Karatzaferis A et al (2008) Prevalence and long term course of primary biliary cirrhosis in primary Sjögren's syndrome. J Rheumatol 35:2012–2016
71. Loustaud-Ratti V, Riche A, Liozon E et al (2001) Prevalence and characteristics of Sjögren's syndrome or Sicca syndrome in chronic hepatitis C virus infection: a prospective study. J Rheumatol 28:2245–2251
72. Ramos-Casals M, De Vita S, Tzioufas AG (2005) Hepatitis C virus, Sjögren's syndrome and B-cell lymphoma: linking infection, autoimmunity and cancer. Autoimmun Rev 4:8–15
73. Haddad J, Deny P, Munz-Gotheil C et al (1992) Lymphocytic sialadenitis of Sjögren's syndrome associated with chronic hepatitis C virus liver disease. Lancet 8(339):321–323
74. Vitali C, Bombardieri S, Jonsson R, European Study Group on Classification Criteria for Sjögren's Syndrome et al (2002) Classification criteria for Sjögren's syndrome: a revised version of the European criteria proposed by the American-European Consensus Group. Ann Rheum Dis 6:554–558
75. Garcia-Carrasco M, Ramos M, Cervera R et al (1997) Hepatitis C virus infection in 'primary' Sjogren's syndrome: prevalence and clinical significance in a series of 90 patients. Ann Rheum Dis 56:173–175
76. Ceribelli A, Cavazzana I, Cattaneo R et al (2008) Hepatitis C virus infection and primary Sjögren's syndrome: a clinical and serologic description of 9 patients. Autoimmun Rev 8:92–94
77. Jadali Z, Alavian SM (2010) Autoimmune diseases co-existing with hepatitis C virus infection. Iran J Allergy Asthma Immunol 9:191–206
78. Hernández-Molina G, Michel-Peregrina ML (2011) Sjögren's syndrome and pancreatic affection. Reumatol Clin 7:130–134
79. Iltanen S, Collin P, Korpela M, Holm K et al (1999) Celiac disease and markers of celiac disease latency in patients with primary Sjogren's syndrome. Am J Gastroenterol 94:1042–1046
80. Szodoray P, Barta Z, Lakos G et al (2004) Coeliac disease in Sjögren's syndrome – a study of 111 Hungarian patients. Rheumatol Int 24:278–282
81. Roblin X, Helluwaert F, Bonaz B (2004) Celiac disease must be evaluated in patients with Sjögren syndrome. Arch Intern Med 164:2387
82. Ramos-Casals M, Brito-Zerón P, Solans R, SS Study Group, Autoimmune Diseases Study Group (GEAS) of the Spanish Society of Internal Medicine (SEMI) et al (2014) Systemic involvement in primary Sjogren's syndrome evaluated by the EULAR-SS disease activity index: analysis of 921 Spanish patients (GEAS-SS Registry). Rheumatology 53:321–331
83. Roguedas AM (2004) Cutaneous manifestations of primary Sjogren's syndrome are underestimated. Clin Exp Rheumatol 22:632–636
84. Quartuccio L, Isola M, Baldini C et al (2015) Clinical and biological differences between cryoglobulinaemic and hypergammaglobulinaemic purpura in primary Sjögren's syndrome: results of a large multicentre study. Scand J Rheumatol 44(1):36–41
85. Abdallah M, Darghouth S, Hamzaoui S et al (2010) McDuffie hypocomplementemic urticarial vasculitis associated with Sjögren's syndrome. Rev Med Interne 31(7):e8–e10
86. Ramos-Casals M, Anaya JM, García-Carrasco M, Rosas J, Bové A, Claver G, Diaz LA, Herrero C, Font J (2004) Cutaneous vasculitis in primary Sjögren syndrome: classification and clinical significance of 52 patients. Medicine (Baltimore) 83(2):96–106
87. Brito-Zerón P, Retamozo S, Akasbi M et al (2014) Annular erythema in primary Sjogren's syndrome: description of 43 non-Asian cases. Lupus 23(2):166–175
88. De Winter S, van Buchem MA, Vermeer MH (2006) Annular erythema of Sjögren's syndrome. Lancet 367(9522):1604
89. Albrecht J, Atzeni F, Baldini C et al (2006) Skin involvement and outcome measures in systemic autoimmune diseases. Clin Exp Rheumatol 24:S52–S59
90. Ramakrishna R, Chandhuri K, Sturgess A et al (1992) Haematological manifestations of primary SS: a clinico-pathological study. Q J Med New Ser 84:547–554

91. Ferraccioli GF, Tonutti E, Casatta L (1996) CD4 cytopenia and occasional expansion of CD4+CD8+ lymphocytes in Sjögren's syndrome. Clin Exp Rheumatol 14:125–130
92. Mandl T, Bredberg A, Jacobsson LT et al (2004) CD4+ T-lymphocytopenia a frequent finding in anti-SSA antibody seropositive patients with primary Sjögren's syndrome. J Rheumatol 31:726–728
93. Fauchais AL, Ouattara B, Gondran G et al (2010) Articular manifestations in primary Sjögren's syndrome: clinical significance and prognosis of 188 patients. Rheumatology 49:1164–1172
94. Atzeni F, Sarzi-Puttini P, Lama N et al (2008) Anti-cyclic citrullinated peptide antibodies in primary Sjögren syndrome may be associated with non-erosive synovitis. Arthritis Res Ther 10(3):R51
95. Mohammed K, Pope J, Le Riche N et al (2009) Association of severe inflammatory polyarthritis in primary Sjogren's syndrome: clinical, serologic, and HLA analysis. J Rheumatol 36(9):1937–1942
96. Iagnocco A, Modesti M, Priori R et al (2010) Subclinical synovitis in primary Sjögren's syndrome: an ultrasonographic study. Rheumatology (Oxford) 49(6):1153–1157
97. Colafrancesco S, Priori R, Gattamelata A et al (2015) Myositis in primary Sjögren's syndrome: data from a multicentre cohort. Clin Exp Rheumatol 33(4):457–64
98. Giroux M, Dequatre N, Zéphir H, Lacour A, Vermersch P (2010) Polymyositis revealing a Sjogren's syndrome. Rev Neurol (Paris) 166(1):96–99
99. Monteiro P, Coutinho M, Salvador MJ et al (2009) Primary Sjögren syndrome and inclusion body myositis. Acta Reumatol Port 34(2A):261–265
100. Spyros A, Papiris MM, Stavros H et al (1999) Lung involvement in primary Sjögren's syndrome is mainly related to the small airway disease. Ann Rheum Dis 58:61–64
101. Parambil JG, Myers JL, Lindell RM et al (2006) Interstitial lung disease in primary Sjögren syndrome. Chest 130(5):1489–1495
102. Schneider F, Gruden J, Tazelaar HD, Leslie KO (2012) Pleuropulmonary pathology in patients with rheumatic disease. Arch Pathol Lab Med 136(10):1242–1252
103. Davidson BK, Kelly CA, Griffiths ID (2000) Ten year follow up of pulmonary function in patients with primary Sjogren's syndrome. Ann Rheum Dis 59:709e12
104. Ito I, Nagai S, Kitaichi M et al (2005) Pulmonary manifestations of primary Sjogren's syndrome: a clinical, radiologic, and pathologic study. Am J Respir Crit Care Med 171(6):632–638
105. Chen MH, Chou HP, Lai CC et al (2014) Lung involvement in primary Sjögren's syndrome: correlation between high-resolution computed tomography score and mortality. J Chin Med Assoc 77:75–82

Dry Eye in Sjögren Syndrome: Diagnostic Tools and Therapy

24

Rita Mencucci, E. Favuzza, and L. Terracciano

Dry eye is a multifactorial disease of the tears and ocular surface that results in symptoms of discomfort, visual disturbance and tear film instability with potential damage to the ocular surface. It is accompanied by increased osmolarity of the tear film and inflammation of the ocular surface.
DEWS 2007

24.1 Epidemiology and Risk Factors

Dry eye disease (DED) is one of the most common ophthalmological conditions seen in clinical practice. A healthy tear film is needed for normal function of the eyes, and dry eye occurs when an unstable tear film cannot ensure the ocular surface homeostasis, causing inflammation and symptoms of ocular discomfort. The exact prevalence of dry eye is difficult to establish, mainly because of differences in the diagnostic criteria used and the lack of established protocols for the diagnosis. Many of the clinical tests lack repeatability, and there is often poor correlation between patients' symptoms and clinical findings.

It has been estimated that about 3.2 million women and 1.7 million men ≥50 years old in the USA have dry eye. However, occasional subjective symptoms of dry eye can occur in up to 33 % of ≥45 years [1]. When objective measurements are applied, the prevalence decreases to 17–25 %, and when combining subjective symptoms with an objectively reduced Schirmer test, it further decreases to 2 %.

Older age, perimenopausal stages in women, hormonal diseases, and several drug therapies are risk factors that can lead to DED.

Men ≥75 years were more likely to have DED: recent data show that prevalence rises from 3.9 % among men aged 50–54 years to 7.7 % among men ≥80. However,

R. Mencucci (✉) • E. Favuzza • L. Terracciano
Ophthalmology Center AOU Careggi, Largo Brambilla, 3, Florence 50134, Italy
e-mail: rita.mencuccini@unifi.it

D. Roccatello, L. Emmi (eds.), *Connective Tissue Disease: A Comprehensive Guide-Volume 1*, Rare Diseases of the Immune System 5,
DOI 10.1007/978-3-319-24535-5_24

Table 24.1 Medications that could lead to dry eye syndrome

Antidepressants	Muscular spasm
Amitriptyline	Cyclobenzaprine
Imipramine	Methocarbamol
Doxepin	
Blood pressure control	Parkinson's disease
Clonidine	Trihexyphenidyl
Prazosin	Benztropine
Propranolol	Biperiden
Reserpine	Procyclidine
Cardiac antiarrhythmics	Decongestants
Disopyramide	Ephedrine
Mexiletine	Pseudoephedrine

Modified from Taylor et al. [3]

after controlling for age and other variables, there were no substantial differences in the prevalence of DED among men by either race or geographic origin. Similarly, there was also no significant association between dry eye and diabetes mellitus. In contrast, men with treated or untreated hypertension and men with benign prostatic hyperplasia were significantly more susceptible to have dry eye [2].

Older age is associated with the development of meibomian gland dysfunction (MGD), which leads to tear film instability and evaporative dry eye. It seems that androgen deficiency can be the basis of some of the anatomical and physiological modifications of the meibomian gland. Both the observations of a higher prevalence of dry eye among women and an increasing prevalence of DED with aging in both sexes strengthen the hypothesis that androgen fall contributes to an increased risk of dry eye [2].

It is important to consider that many drugs can induce, through different mechanisms (e.g., anticholinergic effects), a dry eye syndrome (examples are shown in Table 24.1).

24.2 Tear Film and Control of Tear Secretion

The ocular surface and tear-secreting glands are a complex integrated functional system that is interconnected by sensory and autonomic nerves. This functional unit maintains the health of the ocular surface balancing tear production and its evaporation, absorption, and drainage.

Tear fluid is disposed to form a film of about 4–11 μm over the ocular surface, consisting of three qualitatively different interlacing layers that are in interaction with each other: an interior mucin mucous matrix, a middle aqueous layer, and an anterior lipid layer.

Mucous matrix consists of mucins, which are water-retaining, high-molecular-weight glycoproteins essential for the homeostasis of the ocular surface. On the ocular surface and in tear fluid, there are two groups of mucins: transmembrane, mainly MUC1, MUC4 and MUC16, and secreted gel forming, such as MUCA5C. Epithelial cells of both cornea and conjunctiva produce MUC1 and

MUC16, but only conjunctival epithelial cells and limbal corneal epithelial cells produce MUC4; gel-forming mucins are produced by the conjunctival goblet cells [4]. It seems that mucous matrix could increase the hydrophilic nature of the epithelium, thereby enhancing the wetting properties of the ocular surface.

The aqueous layer contains electrolytes, proteins, and metabolites. This composition is guaranteed by the secreting action of the lacrimal glands and of the ocular surface epithelial cells. Tear fluid is rich in protein: the typical concentration is 7–10 mg/mL, with as many as 500 different types of proteins identified in tear fluid. Many of these are involved in wound healing and inflammatory processes and play a vital role in protecting the cornea from pathogens. Tear film also contains group II phospholipase A2, an hydrolytic antibacterial enzyme that degrades the cell walls of gram-positive bacteria and therefore is involved in the host defense mechanism of the ocular surface. It also contains enzymes able to interact with lipids, such as acidic and neutral sphingomyelinases, acidic and neutral ceramidases, and PC-specific phospholipase C secreted by the epithelial cells. It appears, therefore, that protein-lipid interactions have a function in maintaining the lipid homeostasis of the tear film, interacting with the lipid layer, and thus, it seems to have a biophysical function in its stabilization and organization [4].

The lipids forming the external layer are secreted by the meibomian glands in the lids margins. The bulk of the lipid layer adjacent to the aqueous-mucin gel is composed of hydrophilic polar lipids, including phospholipids, sphingomyelin, ceramides, and cerebrosides, whereas the bulk of the tear lipid layer consists of overlying nonpolar hydrophobic lipids, including wax esters, cholesterol esters, triglycerides, free fatty acids, and hydrocarbons [3]. Hydrophobic lipids at the air-water interface possess a tendency to aggregate (thus minimizing the contact area with the polar water molecules) and therefore do not form a homogenous lipid layer; amphipathic phospholipids, thanks to their physicochemical properties, are able to form a homogeneous monolayer, thereby ensuring hydrophobic interface and providing a suitable interface for nonpolar lipid spreading. It is thought that lipid layer stabilizes the tear film by lowering the aqueous tear surface tension and retards the evaporation of water from the ocular surface.

The majority of tear secretion by the lacrimal glands is reflexive, ensuring hydrophobic interface impulses from these tissues reach the superior salivary nucleus in the pons via the ophthalmic branch of the trigeminal nerve, and efferent fibers pass to the pterygopalatine ganglion synapsing with the postganglionic fibers that innervate the lacrimal gland, nasopharynx, and vessels of the orbit.

Another neural pathway controls the blink reflex via trigeminal afferents and the somatic efferent fibers of the facial nerve, and there is also a rich activity of higher centers that feed into the brainstem nuclei (providing "emotional" input) [3].

24.3 Causative Mechanisms of Dry Eye and Classification

There are two core mechanisms which can be considered capable of initiate, amplify, and change the character of dry eye over time: tear hyperosmolarity and tear film instability.

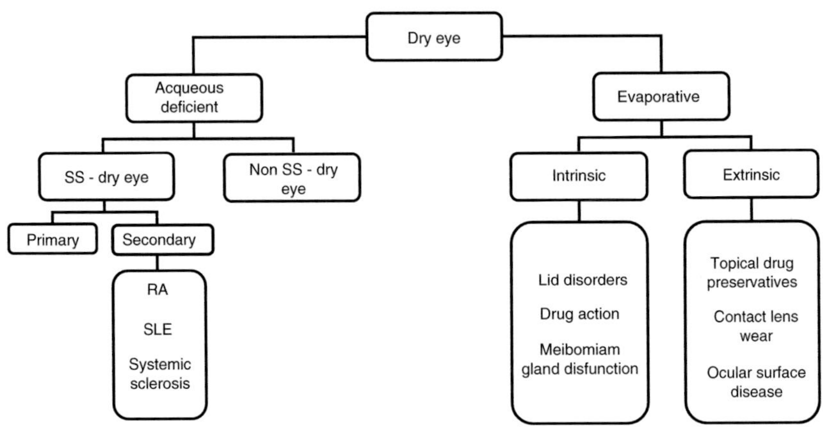

Fig. 24.1 Schematic classification of dry eye (Modified from 2007 Report of the International Dry Eye Workshop)

Tear hyperosmolarity is considered the central mechanism determining ocular surface inflammation, damage and symptoms, and the initiation of compensatory mechanisms in dry eye. It can result from water evaporation from the exposed ocular surface in situations of low aqueous tear flow, or from excessive evaporation, or as a combination of these events.

It has been demonstrated that hyperosmolarity can stimulate an inflammatory cascade involving MAP kinases and NFκB signaling pathways, leading to the production of pro-inflammatory cytokines such as IL-1α, IL-1β, TNF-α, and MMP-9. There are several evidences that these mediators cause the apoptotic death of surface epithelial cells, including goblet cells, and also of the importance of activity of corneal and conjunctival epithelial cells in the pathogenesis of dry eye [5].

Some forms of dry eye can be due to tear film instability as initiating event; when the tear film breaks up during the blink interval, it cause local drying and hyperosmolarity of the exposed surface, resulting in inflammation and epithelial surface damage.

Dysfunction in dry eye can be classified by mechanism (see Fig. 24.1): aqueous-deficient dry eye, evaporative dry eye, or mixed mechanism. In aqueous-deficient dry eye, an insufficient volume of tears is produced, due to either dysfunction or anatomical destruction of the lacrimal glands; the latter group is mostly associated with autoimmune diseases such as Sjögren's disease. In evaporative dry eye, poor tear quality and tear film hyperosmolarity derive from lack of meibomian gland activity, lagophthalmos, or decreased blink rate or function [6].

Aqueous-deficient dry eye can be divided into two major subclasses, Sjögren syndrome (SS) dry eye, and non-SS dry eye. In SS, the lacrimal and salivary glands are infiltrated by activated T cells, resulting in acinar and ductular cell death and hyposecretion of tears or saliva. If the glands are affected by an inflammatory process, it can results in an upregulation of the expression of MHC class II molecules and of autoantigens at the surface of epithelial cells, as fodrin, Ro, and La, as well as the retention of tissue-specific CD4+ and CD8+ T cells [3].

In primary SS, aqueous-deficient dry eye syndrome occurs in combination with symptoms and signs of dry mouth in the presence of specific autoantibodies. In secondary SS, the signs of primary SS occur together with the features of a systemic autoimmune connective tissue disease.

Non-SS dry eye is a form of aqueous deficiency due to lacrimal dysfunction where the systemic autoimmune features have been excluded.

24.4 Mechanisms of Pathogenesis in Autoimmune-Mediated Dry Eye

Pathogenesis of DED is likely multifactorial with genetic and environmental components capable of eliciting an autoimmune response in predisposed patients.

Certain human leukocyte antigen (HLA) genes, such as HLA-DRβ1, encode specific MHC class II molecules and are upregulated in patients with Sjögren's disease. The upregulation of such HLA alleles is thought to genetically predispose individuals to Sjögren's disease and thus is useful for clinical diagnosis [6].

Autoantibodies have long been used as diagnostic tools for Sjögren's disease. Anti-Ro/SSA, anti-La/SSB, and anti-nuclear antibodies (ANA) are often detected at high levels in patients with Sjögren's disease. Several studies comparing SS-related DED with dry eye patients without Sjögren's disease have shown that anti-Ro and anti-La antibodies are only detected in Sjögren's-associated DED. It should be stressed, however, that autoantibodies alone cannot be used as exclusive diagnostic tools or as predictor of the development of autoimmune disease, since autoantibodies can be detected in healthy patients due to tolerance mechanisms to self-antigens [7].

Several viruses can also set off an autoimmune response in a process called molecular mimicry, where antigen epitopes on microbial proteins cross-react with mammalian self-antigens. It is hypothesized that molecular mimicry mediates post-viral dry eye syndrome. The herpes simplex virus has been shown to react with La/SSB antigen in Sjögren's patients, and Coxsackie virus 2B can cross-react with the Rh60 autoantigen. Interestingly, these two viruses have also been shown to cross-react with autoantigens in systemic lupus erythematosus (SLE) patients [6].

An accelerated rate of apoptosis has been observed in Sjögren's disease. Increased corneal epithelial cell apoptosis has been observed in both Sjögren syndrome- and non-Sjögren syndrome-associated DED.

DNA and/or RNA fragments from apoptotic cells also have the ability to activate toll-like receptors (TLRs). TLRs are found on macrophages and dendritic cells, where they respond to pathogen-associated molecular patterns to break out an immune response. Specific toll-like receptors such as TLR3, TLR7/8m, and TLR9 are activated in systemic autoimmune diseases like Sjögren's disease. On the corneal surface of SS-dry eye patients, increased apoptosis is observed with chromatic and small ribonuclear particles (snRNPs) likely activating TLRs [8]. Another apoptotic pathway likely involved in Sjögren's disease and dry eye syndrome is death receptor Fas/Fas ligand (FasL) binding. In apoptosis, the Fas/FasL interaction activates caspases and proteinases that result in DNA fragmentation and cell death. Higher levels of Fas-positive cells and soluble FasL were detected in the serum of Sjögren syndrome-associated DED than in non-Sjögren syndrome-associated DED patients. However, a direct correlation has not been established between increased serum Fas/FasL and increased rate of apoptosis [6].

In dry eye syndrome, all these afore mentioned antigens are presented to immature antigen-presenting cells (APCs), which are then activated by major histocompatibility complex (MHC) class II cell surface receptors. Mature APCs then present antigen to T cells to generate an inflammatory and immune response.

Because of injury to the ocular surface in dry eye syndrome, MHC class II and co-stimulatory molecules are overexpressed, further perpetuating the cycle of antigen recognition, immune response, and inflammation. Several molecular pathways involving MHC class II have been established. These pathways involve TGF-β, the actomyosin cytoskeleton, and the regulation by GTPases. The role of TGF-β in MHC II presentation is particularly important because of its activity in Sjögren syndrome-associated DED; in a mouse model of dry eye, disruption of TGF-β was found to suppress APC maturation in the cornea, leading to an improvement in dry eye clinical expression and in conjunctival inflammation [6].

Cell-mediated immunity is important in the pathogenesis of autoimmune diseases such as Sjögren's disease: desiccating stress in mice has been shown to elicit T cell-mediated inflammation, specifically in the cornea, conjunctiva, and lacrimal gland.

In Sjögren's disease, such as in several autoimmune syndromes (SLE, rheumatoid arthritis, type I diabetes, and multiple sclerosis), B cell dysfunction and the resultant disruption of host immune tolerance have been observed. B cells are necessary for the development of Sjögren's disease. B cell hyper-reactivity followed by hypergammaglobulinemia has been observed in Sjögren's disease [9]. Notably, upregulation of B cell activating factors, BAFF and APRIL, has been detected in the lacrimal glands of Sjögren's patients. BAFF (BLyS or B lymphocyte stimulator) is a B cell activating factor of the tumor necrosis factor family: it has been established that this protein is significantly overexpressed in salivary glands of Sjögren's disease patients, and it seems to be able to prevent the apoptosis of autoreactive B cells [6].

Helper or effector T cells are activated after APC stimulation and facilitate cytokine secretion; TH17 induces the secretion of IL-17 in response to TGF-β or IL-6, which then stimulates the production of pro-inflammatory cytokines and matrix metallo-proteinases (MMP). Matrix metallo-proteinases are upregulated in the lacrimal and salivary glands in Sjögren's disease, leading to significant tissue injury and destruction. The TH17-centric cytokine IL-17 has been analyzed in the tear film, revealing highest levels in Sjögren syndrome-associated DED as well as increased levels in non-Sjögren syndrome-associated DED versus control subjects. TH17 has been implicated in other autoimmune diseases such as Crohn's disease and collagen-induced arthritis. Thus, the regulation of pro-inflammatory cytokines and matrix metallo-proteinases could play a main role in dry eye syndrome, resulting in dysfunction of exocrine glands [6].

Dysfunction of regulatory T cells (Treg) is observed in autoimmune diseases such as Sjögren's disease. Treg deficiency could predispose to Sjögren's disease and DED. Interestingly, TH17 cells (aforementioned – implicated in the pathogenesis of dry eye syndrome) seem to be resistant to Treg-mediated suppression; a demonstrated imbalance between Treg cells and IL-17, with an increase in IL-17 activity, could lead to tissue injury in Sjögren's disease [6].

24.5 Clinical Findings

Patients who have dry eye often suffer from eye irritation, a gritty or foreign body sensation, burning, tearing, photophobia, stinging, or intermittent sharp pain. Blurry vision that improves with blinking or instillation of nonviscous artificial tears is also referred. Depending on severity and sensitivity of each one, dry eye patients may have all, some, or none of these symptoms.

For the majority of DED patients, there is some relation between symptoms and clinical signs. However, it is also well established that perceived symptom severity may not correlate to clinical signs of disease, and there exists a significant proportion of patients who can have seemingly conflicting signs and symptoms. In fact, in early or mild DED, the presence of hyperalgesia can cause significant ocular discomfort without any signs of tissue damage; in more severe or chronic disease, decreased corneal sensation due to compensatory reflex mechanisms can actually reduce discomfort [10].

As mentioned before, dry eye can be part of more complex rheumatologic syndromes, among which the most common is the Sjögren syndrome.

Primary SS is a systemic autoimmune disease of unknown cause that is characterized by progressive lymphocytic and plasma cell infiltration of the exocrine glands, mainly salivary and lacrimal glands (see classification criteria in Table 24.2); it shows a sexual dimorphism, with women 10–20 times more frequently affected than men.

It is important to consider that about 4–10 % of patients with SS develop non-Hodgkin's B cell lymphomas, some of which become high-grade malignancies.

Secondary SS is marked by the targeting of either the lacrimal and/or salivary glands together with a systemic autoimmune disease as follows. Up to 20 % of patients with rheumatoid arthritis may develop DED. The dry eye manifestations usually follow joint involvement and frequently occur in patients with quiescent and well-controlled joint manifestations. Dryness prevalence increases approximately 10 % every 10 years and was associated with systemic disease therapy [3]. Dry eye symptoms are also frequent in patients with systemic lupus erythematosus, showing two peaks of incidence, the first one in patients aged 20–30 and the second one in those aged over 50 [12]. In a recent study, it has been shown that these patients have a recognized genetic predisposition (HLA-DR3) and autoantibody production (ANA, SS-A, SS-B) [3].

SS may also occur in patients with graft versus host disease, typically 6 months after hematopoietic stem cell transplantation. Immune system responds against a

Table 24.2 Revised international classification criteria for ocular manifestations of Sjögren syndrome

Ocular symptoms: a positive response to at least one of the following questions:
Have you had daily, persistent, troublesome dry eyes for more than 3 months?
Do you have a recurrent sensation of sand or gravel in the eyes?
Do you use tear substitutes more than 3 times a day?
Oral symptoms: a positive response to at least one of the following questions:
Have you had a daily feeling of dry mouth for more than 3 months?
Have you had recurrently or persistently swollen salivary glands as an adult?
Do you frequently drink liquids to aid in swallowing dry food?
Ocular signs: that is, objective evidence of ocular involvement defined as a positive result for at least one of the following two tests:
Schirmer test performed without anesthesia (≤5 mm in 5 min)
Rose bengal score or other ocular dye score (≥4 according to van Bijsterveld's scoring system)
Histopathology: In minor salivary glands (obtained through normal-appearing mucosa), focal lymphocytic sialoadenitis, evaluated by an expert histopathologist, with a focus score >1, defined as a number of lymphocytic foci (which are adjacent to normal-appearing mucous acini and contain more than 50 lymphocytes) per 4 mm^2 of glandular tissue
Salivary gland involvement: objective evidence of salivary gland involvement defined by a positive result for at least one of the following diagnostic tests:
Unstimulated whole salivary flow (≤1.5 ml in 15 min)
Parotid sialography showing the presence of diffuse sialectasis (punctate, cavitary, or destructive pattern), without evidence of obstruction in the major ducts
Salivary scintigraphy showing delayed uptake, reduced concentration, and/or delayed excretion of tracer
Autoantibodies; presence in the serum of the following autoantibodies:
Antibodies to Ro(SSA) or La(SSB) antigens or both

Modified from Vitali et al. [11]

wide range of host antigens, including histocompatibility antigens, leading to lacrimal gland fibrosis due to co-localization of periductal CD4+ and CD8+ T cells with antigen-presenting fibroblasts [3]. Other associated disorders include polyarteritis nodosa, Wegener's granulomatosis, systemic sclerosis, primary biliary cirrhosis, and mixed connective tissues disease [13].

24.6 Diagnosis of Ocular Involvement

Slit-lamp examination should be performed before any other tests, which may alter or mask some of the relevant findings on examination and lead to a possible misdiagnosis. Dry eye signs identified on slit-lamp examination include superficial corneal erosions, inadequate tear lake volume, reduced tear film breakup time, conjunctival hyperemia, conjunctival surface irregularities, and meibomian gland dysfunction.

The main diagnostic tests currently used include:

Schirmer test. First described in 1903 by Schirmer, this test is still one of the most commonly used to measure tear production. The Schirmer I test measures total tear secretion (reflex and basal tears). Avoiding anesthetic drops, a Schirmer paper strip (a Whatman no. 41 filter paper 5 mm wide by 35 mm long) should be inserted over the lower lid margin at the junction of its middle and outer thirds. The eye is kept closed and the amount of wetting is measured after 5 min. Normal values range from 8 to 33 mm, but an accepted normal value is greater than 10 mm. A variant of the test just described involves the use of anesthetic drop and is useful for evaluating the only basal tear secretion (Jones' Test). The Schirmer II test is similar but uses an irritant stimulus, such as a cotton bud wetted with NaCl 5 % inserted into the nose, capable to stimulate reflex tear secretion. Topical anesthesia is not used and an abnormal test result on this test is considered to be <15 mm of wetting in 5 min. Notably, inferior gaze of the eye could produce a falsely higher result. Although the Schirmer test is one of the most widely used tools in diagnosing dry eye, the lengthy nature of the test, the fact that most patients find the test irritating and invasive, and its unreliable and largely irreproducible nature may explain a high risk of underdiagnosis [14].

Tear film breakup time (tBUT). This test measures the time required for the tear film to break from being a confluent film using 5 μL fluorescein drops instilled alone without the anesthetic. tBUT is the time interval after a patient blinks to the first appearance of dryness in the tear film, and the patient can be classified as dry eye-affected if this dry area appears before 10 s [14].

Fluorescein staining. 2–5 μL of fluorescein sodium can be used to identify corneal epithelial defects. The corneal surface will stain if there is a disruption of cell-to-cell junctions. The staining can show corneal superficial punctate epithelial erosions in patterns that are suggestive of certain causes of dry eye [14].

Rose bengal (RB) staining, widely used in the past, has lost much of its value as a diagnostic tool because of the significant and well-documented corneal toxicity of this substance.

Lissamine green (LG) is another dye similar to RB (in which staining occurs in areas on the cornea or conjunctiva that lack membrane-associated mucins). Both types of dyes have similar staining patterns and can be interchangeable. But unlike RB, LG is not toxic to the corneal epithelium and is better tolerated. Ten microliters of 1 % LG was found to give the best reliability, especially when using a red filter [14].

Questionnaires can help establish cases of dry eye that are subclinical and represent a valuable tool for measuring the impact of dry eye on the quality of daily life of patients. The Standard Patient Evaluation of Eye Dryness questionnaire is a repeatable and effective measure that can help identify a patient's symptoms. This tool uses a scale ranging from 0 to 4 focusing on frequency and severity of symptoms. Another questionnaire is the Ocular Surface Disease Index according to which score values range from 0 to 100, with higher scores signifying associated to higher disability. Other questionnaires such as the Dry Eye Questionnaire and its variations (DEQ, DEQ-8, Contact Lens Dry Eye Questionnaire), the National Eye Institute Visual Functioning Questionnaire, and the Impact of Dry Eye on Everyday

Table 24.3 Simple diagnostic algorithm for dry eye

Clinical history
Symptom questionnaire
Slit-lamp examination
Fluorescein tBUT
Ocular surface staining grading with fluorescein
Schirmer I test without anesthetic, or I with anesthetic, and/or Schirmer II with nasal stimulation
Other tests may be added according to availability

Table 24.4 Step-by-step treatment options for DED

Step-by-step treatment options in DED
Education and environmental/dietary modifications
Elimination of environmental DED-related factors
Artificial tear substitutes
Eyelid therapy
If treatments are inadequate, add
Anti-inflammatories
Tetracyclines (for meibomianitis, rosacea)
Absorbable punctal plugs
Secretagogues
If treatments are inadequate, add
Autologous serum
Contact lenses
Permanent punctal occlusion
If treatments are still inadequate, add:
Systemic anti-inflammatory agents
Surgery

Life Questionnaire can help distinguish between symptomatic and asymptomatic patients. A recent study showed that only the Ocular Surface Disease Index and Impact of Dry Eye on Everyday Life Questionnaire are validated, unlike the others that have not been tested for reliability [15].

A practical approach to DED is represented in Tables 24.3 and 24.4.

24.7 Therapy of Ocular Involvement

24.7.1 Tear Supplementation: Artificial Tears

The main objectives in caring for patients with dry eye disease are to improve the patient's ocular comfort and quality of life and to reestablish homeostasis of the ocular surface and tear film.

Although certain artificial tears have demonstrated more success than others in reducing symptoms of irritation or decreasing ocular surface dye staining, there have been no large-scale comparative clinical trials to evaluate the wide variety of ocular lubricants.

Ocular lubricants are characterized by hypotonic or isotonic buffered solutions containing electrolytes, surfactants, and several types of viscosity agents. Ideal artificial lubricant should be preservative-free; contain potassium, bicarbonate, and other electrolytes; and have a polymeric system to increase its retention time. Physical properties should include a neutral or few alkaline pH. Osmolarities of artificial tears have been measured to range from about 181 to 354 mOsm/L.

The single most critical advance in the treatment of dry eye has been the elimination of preservatives, such as benzalkonium chloride (BAK), from lubricants. Because of the risk of contamination of multidose products, most lubricants contain a preservative or employ some mechanism for minimizing contamination. Benzalkonium chloride is the most frequently used preservative in topical ophthalmic preparations: its epithelial toxic effects have been well established and it is related to its concentration, the frequency of dosing, the level or amount of tear secretion, and the severity of the ocular surface disease. In patients with mild dry eye, BAK-preserved drops are usually well tolerated when used four to six times a day or less. In patients with moderate-to-severe dry eye, side effect risk for BAK toxicity is high, because of decreased tear secretion cell turnover [16]. Preservative-free formulations are absolutely necessary for patients with severe dry eye with ocular surface disease and dysfunction of lacrimal gland secretion or for patients that use multiple preserved topical medications for any chronic eye disease. Another additive used in artificial tears formulations is disodium (EDTA). It amplifies the preservative efficacy of BAK but it is not a sufficient preservative when used alone. Used in some non-preserved solutions, it may help limit microbial growth in opened unit-dose vials. Although use of EDTA may allow a lower concentration of preservative, EDTA shows an important toxicity, by itself, to the ocular surface epithelium. Less toxic preservatives, such as polyquad (polyquaternium-1), sodium chlorite, and sodium perborate, have been developed to allow the use of multidose bottled lubricants and to avoid the known toxicity of BAK-/EDTA-containing solutions [16].

As aforementioned, tears of patients with dry eye have a higher tear film osmolarity (crystalloid osmolarity) than normal tears. Protection against the adverse effects of increased osmolarity has led to development of lubricant drops incorporating compatible solutes (such as glycerin, erythritol, and levocarnitine) in which these substances are distributed between the tears and into intracellular fluids to protect against potential cellular damage from hyperosmolarity.

However, ocular lubricants, which have been shown to provide some protection of the ocular surface epithelium and some improvement in patient symptoms and objective findings, have not been demonstrated in controlled clinical trials to be sufficient to resolve the ocular surface disorder and inflammation seen in most dry eye sufferers [16].

24.7.2 Tear Retention

24.7.2.1 Punctal Occlusion

Punctal plugs are divided into two main types: absorbable and nonabsorbable. The former are made of collagen or polymers and last for variable periods of time (3 days to 6 months). It has been established that the use of these devices has been associated with objective and subjective improvement in patients with both Sjögren and non-Sjögren aqueous tear-deficient dry eye. Beneficial outcome in dry eye symptoms has been reported in 74–86 % of patients treated with punctal plugs. Objective indices of improvement include improved corneal staining, prolonged tBUT, decrease in tear osmolarity, and increase in goblet cell density. Punctal plugs are indicated in symptomatic dry eye patients with Schirmer test result (with anesthesia) less than 5 mm at 5 min and show evidence of ocular surface dye staining [17]. Contraindications to the use of punctal plugs include allergy to the materials used in the plugs, punctal ectropion, pre-existing nasolacrimal duct obstruction, and acute or chronic infection of the lacrimal canaliculus or lacrimal sac; treatment of the ocular surface inflammation prior to plug insertion has been recommended [16].

24.7.2.2 Contact Lenses

Contact lenses may help to protect and hydrate the corneal surface in severe dry eye conditions. Improved visual acuity and comfort such as decreased corneal epitheliopathy and healing of corneal epithelial defects have been reported [18]. There is a risk of corneal vascularization and possible corneal infection associated with the use of these devices for a long time.

24.7.2.3 Tear Stimulation

There are some secretogogue agents currently under investigation by pharmaceutical companies, such as diquafosol (one of the P2Y2 receptor agonists), rebamipide, gefarnate, sodium (mucous secretion stimulants), and 15(S)-HETE (MUC1 stimulant). Among them, 2 % diquafosol eye drop is the only one to have been thoroughly evaluated positively in clinical trials, proving to be effective in the treatment of dry eye in a randomized, double-blind trial in humans to reduce ocular surface staining [19].

Two orally administered cholinergic agonists, pilocarpine and cevimeline, have been evaluated in clinical trials for treatment of Sjögren syndrome-associated DED. Patients who were treated with pilocarpine at a dose of 5 mg showed a significantly greater overall improvement than placebo-treated patients. The most commonly reported side effects from this medication were excessive sweating, which occurred in over 40 % of patients [20], diarrhea, and flushing.

Cevimeline is another oral cholinergic agonist that seems able to significantly improve symptoms of dryness and aqueous tear production and ocular surface disease compared to placebo when taken in doses of 15 or 30 mg. This agent may have fewer adverse systemic side effects than oral pilocarpine [16].

24.7.3 Biological Tear Substitutes

24.7.3.1 Autologous Serum (AS)

Autologous serum eye drops have been recommended for the treatment of several ocular surface disturbances, such as Sjögren's syndrome-related tear deficiency, graft-versus-host disease-associated tear deficiency, neurotrophic keratitis, persistent epithelial defects, superior limbic keratoconjunctivitis, and postoperative dry eye induced by LASIK. Subjective improvement in dry eye symptoms in patients treated with 20–50 % AS, four to eight times a day, has been reported; objective improvement based on fluorescein staining and breakup time tests also was observed. AS is usually well tolerated, and patients usually report improvement of ocular discomfort. Side effects occasionally occur, in terms of increased discomfort, slight epitheliopathy, bacterial conjunctivitis, or eyelid eczema [21].

24.7.3.2 Salivary Gland Autotransplantation

This procedure, indicated only in end-stage dry eye disease with an absolute aqueous tear deficiency (Schirmer test wetting of 1 mm or less), a conjunctivalized surface epithelium, and persistent severe pain despite punctal occlusion and at least hourly application of unpreserved tear substitutes, requires collaboration between an ophthalmologist and a maxillofacial surgeon. With appropriate microvascular anastomosis, 80 % of grafts survive [16].

24.7.4 Anti-inflammatory Therapy

24.7.4.1 Cyclosporine (CsA)

CsA is able to significantly decrease conjunctival rose bengal staining, superficial punctate keratitis, and ocular irritation symptoms. There was no clear dose response; CsA 0.1 % produces the most consistent improvement in objective endpoints, whereas CsA 0.05 % shows the most consistent improvement in patient-subjective symptoms; CsA 0.05 % treatment proved able to significantly greater improvements ($P<0.05$) in three subjective measures of dry eye disease (blurred vision symptoms, need for concomitant artificial tears, and the global response to treatment). No dose-response effect was noted. No CsA was detected in patients' blood treated with this topical immunosuppressant medication for 12 months. Treated eyes had an approximately 200 % increase in conjunctival goblet cell density, with decreased expression of immune activation and apoptosis markers and of inflammatory cytokine IL-6 by the conjunctival epithelial cells. The numbers of CD3-, CD4-, and CD8-positive T lymphocytes in the conjunctiva decreased in cyclosporine-treated patients [22].

24.7.4.2 Topical Corticosteroids

Corticosteroids are the standard anti-inflammatory agent for numerous basic research studies of inflammation. Corticosteroids are an effective anti-inflammatory therapy also in dry eye disease: several corticosteroid formulations have obtained

Level I evidence. In a 4-week, double-blind, randomized study in 64 patients with DED and delayed tear clearance, loteprednol etabonate 0.5 % ophthalmic suspension was found to be more effective than placebo in improving some signs and symptoms [23], and it has been established that clinical improvement of dry eye syndrome can be observed after therapy with corticosteroids [16].

24.7.4.3 Tetracyclines

Tetracyclines and their analogues are effective in the treatment of ocular rosacea, for which a single daily dose of doxycycline may be safe and effective. In addition to the anti-inflammatory effects of tetracyclines, their ability to inhibit angiogenesis may contribute to their efficacy in rosacea-related disorders. Despite tetracyclines have been used for a long time for management of this disease, no randomized, placebo-controlled clinical trials have been performed to establish their efficacy [16].

Meibomian gland dysfunction (MGD) has been associated with apparent aqueous-deficient dry eye. Use of tetracycline in patients with MGD has been shown to decrease lipase production by tetracycline-sensitive as well as resistant strains of staphylococci, leading to clinical improvement. Tetracycline derivatives have been recommended as treatment options for chronic blepharitis because of their high concentration in tissues, low renal clearance, long half-life, high level of binding to serum proteins, and decreased risk of photosensitization [16].

The optimal dosing schedule has not been established; however, a variety of dose regimens have been proposed including 50 or 100 mg doxycycline once a day or an initial dose of 50 mg a day for the first 2 weeks followed by 100 mg a day for a period of 2.5 months, in an intermittent therapeutic-protocol; a recent study suggested that a 3-month course of 100 mg of minocycline might be effective in controlling of significant meibomianitis, as continued control was maintained for at least 3 months after therapy cessation [24].

However, factors that may decrease tear production or increase tear evaporation, such as the use of systemic anticholinergic medications and desiccating environmental stresses (e.g., low humidity and air conditioning drafts), should be minimized or eliminated. Video display terminals should be lowered and patients should be encouraged to take periodic breaks with eye closure when reading or working on a computer. A humidified environment could reduce tear evaporation and lead to an improvement in ocular discomfort symptoms [16] (see Table 24.3).

References

1. The epidemiology of dry eye disease: report of the Epidemiology Subcommittee of the International Dry Eye Workshop (2007) Ocul Surf 5(2):93–107
2. Schaumberg DA, Dana R, Buring JE, Sullivan DA (2009) Prevalence of dry eye disease among US men: estimates from the Physicians' Health Studies. Arch Ophthalmol 127(6):763–768
3. Taylor S, Pacheco P, Lightman S (2011) Dry eyes in rheumatic disease. Curr Rheumatol Rev 7:3–14
4. Rantamäki AH (2014) Tear film lipid layer – from composition to function implications of the anti-evaporative effect. Helsinki Eye Lab, Department of Ophthalmology, University of Helsinki

5. The definition and classification of dry eye disease: report of the definition and classification Subcommittee of the International Dry Eye Workshop (2007) Ocul Surf 5(2):75–92
6. Liu KC, Huynh K, Grubbs J Jr, Davis RM (2014) Autoimmunity in the pathogenesis and treatment of Keratoconjunctivitis Sicca. Curr Allergy Asthma Rep 14(1):403
7. Mimori T (1999) Autoantibodies in connective tissue diseases: clinical significance and analysis of target autoantigens. Intern Med 38(7):523–532
8. Yeh S, Song XJ, Farley W, Li DQ, Stern ME, Pflugfelder SC (2003) Apoptosis of ocular surface cells in experimentally induced dry eye. Invest Ophthalmol Vis Sci 44(1):124–129
9. Voulgarelis M, Moutsopoulos HM (2003) Lymphoproliferation in autoimmunity and Sjogren's syndrome. Curr Rheumatol Rep 5(4):317–323
10. Badouin C, Aragona P, Van Setten G et al (2014) Diagnosing the severity of dry eye: a clear and practical algorithm. Br J Ophthalmol 98:1168–1176
11. Vitali C, Bombordieri S, Jonnson R et al (2002) Classification criteria for Sjogren's syndrome: a revised version of the European criteria proposed by the American-European Consensus Group. Ann Rheum Dis 1:554–558
12. Hochberg MC, Boyd RE, Ahearn JM et al (1985) Systemic lupus erythematosus: a review of clinico-laboratory features and immunogenetic markers in 150 patients with emphasis on demographic subsets. Medicine (Baltimore) 64(5):285–295
13. Wiik A, Cervera R, Haass M et al (2006) European attempts to set guidelines for improving diagnostics of autoimmune rheumatic disorders. Lupus 15(7):391–396
14. Ben-Zeev SM, Miller DD et al (2014) Diagnosis of dry eye disease and emerging technologies. Clin Ophthalmol 8:581–590
15. Grubbs JR Jr, Tolleson-Rinehart S, Huynh K, Davis RM (2014) A review of quality of life measures in dry eye questionnaires. Cornea 33(2):215–218
16. 2007 Report of the Dry Eye Workshop (DEWS) (2007) Ocul Surf 5(2)
17. Baxter SA, Laibson PR (2004) Punctal plugs in the management of dry eyes. Ocul Surf 2:255–265
18. Pullum KW, Whiting MA, Buckley RJ (2005) Scleral contact lenses: the expanding role. Cornea 24:269–277
19. Tauber J, Davitt WF, Bokosky JE et al (2004) Double-masked, placebo-controlled safety and efficacy trial of diquafosol tetrasodium (INS365) ophthalmic solution for the treatment of dry eye. Cornea 23:784–792
20. Vivino FB, Al-Hashimi I, Khan K et al (1999) Pilocarpine tablets for the treatment of dry mouth and dry eye symptoms in patients with Sjogren's syndrome. Arch Intern Med 159:174–181
21. Pan Q, Angelina A, Zambrano A et al (2013) Autologous serum eye drops for dry eye. Cochrane Database Syst Rev (8):CD009327
22. Turner K, Pflugfelder SC, Ji Z et al (2000) Interleukin-6 levels in the conjunctival epithelium of patients with dry eye disease treated with cyclosporine ophthalmic emulsion. Cornea 19:492–496
23. Flugfelder SC, Maskin SL, Anderson B et al (2004) A randomized, doublemasked, placebo-controlled, multicenter comparison of loteprednol etabonate ophthalmic suspension, 0.5%, and placebo for treatment of keratoconjunctivitis sicca in patients with delayed tear clearance. Am J Ophthalmol 138:444–457
24. Aronowicz JD, Shine WE, Oral D et al (2006) Short term oral minocycline treatment of meibomianitis. Br J Ophthalmol 90:856–860

Neurological Involvement in Sjögren's Syndrome

25

Roberto Cavallo, Maria Roberta Bongioanni, and Paola Richiardi

Sjögren's syndrome (SS) is a systemic autoimmune disease characterized by xerophthalmia and xerostomia. Besides sicca syndrome, neurological manifestations involving both the central nervous system (CNS) and the peripheral nervous system (PNS) may be present in SS.

25.1 Epidemiology of Neurological Involvement in SS

The prevalence of neurological manifestations ranges from 10 to 70 % [1].

The wide spectrum of prevalence data is related to several factors: the different diagnostic criteria that were used before and after 2002, definition of the disease, differences in study populations, and definition and method of detection of neurological involvement [2, 3]. Central nervous system involvement is far less common and varies from 2 to 25 % [2]. The male/female ratio of patients with neurological manifestations of SS ranges from 3.8 to 31 [2]. Neurological involvement may precede the development of sicca syndrome in 25–65 % of cases [4]. Disability is more frequent in cases of CNS involvement than in cases of PNS involvement [1].

25.2 Pathophysiology of Neurological Involvement in SS

The pathogenetic mechanisms responsible for neurological manifestations of SS are still unknown.

R. Cavallo (✉) • M.R. Bongioanni • P. Richiardi
Neurology Department and Center of Research of Immunopathology and Rare Diseases, Department of Rare, Immunologic, Hematologic and Immunohematologic Diseases, Giovanni Bosco Hospital, University of Turin, Piazza donatore di Sangue 3, Turin 10154, Italy
e-mail: roberto.cavallo@unito.it

D. Roccatello, L. Emmi (eds.), *Connective Tissue Disease: A Comprehensive Guide-Volume 1*, Rare Diseases of the Immune System 5,
DOI 10.1007/978-3-319-24535-5_25

Many hypotheses have been put forth to explain the wide range of neurological disorders. As far as PNS involvement is concerned, ganglionitis has been hypothesized in sensory ataxic, autonomic, painful, and trigeminal neuropathy, whereas vasculitis is the cause of multiple mononeuropathies and multiple cranial neuropathies [2]. Cryoglobulins may play a pathogenetic role in sensory-motor neuropathy [1].

Several studies have suggested that there is an ischemic mechanism in CNS involvement [3]. However, multiple sclerosis-like manifestations are not consistent with this explanation. Mononuclear cell infiltration of the CNS is another hypothesis. Other mechanisms, such as immunologically mediated vascular damage, the action of antineural antibodies, or a direct role of anti-SSA antibodies, have also been suggested [1].

25.3 Diagnosis

The typical autoantibodies associated with SS (anti-SSA and anti-SSB) are observed in only 40 % of patients with neurological involvement, whereas positivity may be as high as 60 % in patients without neurological involvement [3].

Some autoantibodies (anti-GW182, anti-alpha-fodrin, anti-3 muscarinic receptor) have been described as potential serological markers, but their usefulness is uncertain [3].

Schirmer's test is positive in 56–89 % of patients with SS-associated neuropathy, and Rose Bengal testing is also positive in 69–92 % of patients with SS-associated neuropathy [4].

Biopsy of the minor salivary glands of the lip may be diagnostic in 37–75 % of patients with PNS involvement in SS [4].

Non-serological ancillary testing is more sensitive than autoantibodies in neurological involvement in SS [4].

25.4 Peripheral Nervous System Involvement

Various neuropathy subtypes have been reported in SS patients. Sensory neuropathies are the most common manifestations (e.g., small fiber involvement and sensory ataxic neuropathy), but other subtypes like multiple mononeuropathy, polyradiculopathy, sensory-motor neuropathy, cranial neuropathy, and autonomic neuropathy have been described [2, 3].

The course of the disease can be subacute or chronic; in some cases it may be indolent for many years [2].

The onset of neuropathy can precede the diagnosis of SS by several years. This chronological pattern is more characteristic of ganglionitis-related neuropathies, suggesting that, as well as salivary and lacrimal glands, neural tissues, especially sensory dorsal root ganglion cells and autonomic ganglion cells, are the primary targets in SS.

25.4.1 Sensory Neuropathies

25.4.1.1 Sensory Ataxic Neuronopathy/Sensory Ganglionopathy

Sensory ataxic neuronopathy is due to posterior spinal root involvement with lymphocytic infiltration without vasculitis of the dorsal root ganglia [2, 3, 5].

This neuropathy is characterized by sensory ataxia without substantial motor symptoms. Distal, asymmetrical paresthesias are the heralding symptom. Onset of the symptoms ranges from subacute to chronic. Impaired proprioception can go from gait instability to severe incapacitation and wheelchair confinement. Pseudoathetosis may be present. Autonomic symptoms have been reported [5].

Conduction studies indicate axonal damage with reduced amplitude or absent sensory nerve action potentials with preservation of compound motor action potentials [5]. In some patients a posterior column high-intensity signal on T2-weighted MRI is observed due to retrograde degeneration of the large afferent fibers in the posterior columns [5].

Sural nerve biopsy predominantly demonstrates large fiber loss [5].

Several treatments have been reported, but randomized controlled trials are lacking. There are reports of the use of intravenous immunoglobulins, plasmapheresis, D-penicillamine, infliximab, interferon alpha, and rituximab [5].

25.4.2 Painful Small Fiber Neuropathy

It is a painful, sensory neuropathy affecting the nociceptive A-alpha and unmyelinated C-fibers that relay nociceptive and temperature stimuli [5]. A burning sensation in the feet is the typical symptom, but some patients present patchy burning paresthesias in the thighs and legs. This fact suggests a small fiber sensory neuronopathy, rather than a dying-back sensory axonopathy [5].

Impairment of the superficial sensation of pain, temperature, and light touch is associated with pain or painful dysesthesia. Deep sensation is well preserved, as is motor function. Nerve conduction studies are normal. Sural nerve biopsy shows small fiber loss, but skin biopsy is the standard tool for recognizing painful, small fiber neuropathy by demonstrating the decrease of intraepidermal nerve fiber density [2, 4, 5].

Treatment is generally symptomatic using antiepileptic agents or tricyclic antidepressants and avoiding agents with more anticholinergic side effects. A small, uncontrolled trial showed an improvement in neuropathic pain with the use of intravenous immunoglobulins [5].

25.4.3 Sensory Axonal Polyneuropathy

This neuropathy presents with distal, symmetric sensory deficits of chronic or subacute onset in a glove and stocking distribution [5]. It is the most characteristic peripheral involvement in SS and mainly affects the lower limbs [3], though the upper limbs may be affected in 20 % of cases [5]. Electrophysiological studies show axonal impairment of the sensory nerves. Sural nerve biopsy reveals a varying degree of reduction of fiber density, mainly a dying-back axonal degeneration of thinly myelinated fibers without vasculitis [3]. Treatment is symptomatic with anti-epileptic agents or tricyclic antidepressants [5].

25.4.4 Sensory-Motor Neuropathies

25.4.4.1 Sensory-Motor Polyneuropathy/Polyradiculoneuropathy

There is a wide range in the reported prevalence of sensory-motor polyneuropathy in SS patients (6–68 %) depending on whether subclinical motor abnormalities are taken into consideration or not. Large-diameter fibers are involved [2].

Some patients show a chronic inflammatory demyelinating polyneuropathy pattern in electrophysiological studies. Muscle weakness and sensory symptoms are present.

Sensory-motor polyneuropathy may be accompanied by palpable purpura, low C4 complement factor and cryoglobulinemia, and an increased risk of developing lymphoma [5].

Polyradiculoneuropathy has an average prevalence of 4–15 % in patients with SS neuropathy [2]. F-wave prolongation with abnormal motor distal latencies is a common finding in nerve conduction studies. Selective abnormal gadolinium enhancement of the dorsal spinal roots and cauda equina are found in the MRI of the lumbar spine [2].

Cerebrospinal fluid protein concentration is raised. Sural nerve biopsy shows demyelinating changes [2]. Symptomatic treatment is administered for positive sensory symptoms. Remission of neuropathic manifestations has been reported in patients with lymphoma who were treated with CHOP (cyclophosphamide, doxorubicin, vincristine, prednisone) and/or rituximab [5].

25.4.5 Multiple Mononeuropathy

Although relatively uncommon, the prevalence of multiple mononeuropathy in SS patients is reportedly between 6 and 12 % [2].

Typically, onset is acute or subacute with asymmetric multifocal paresthesias or dysesthesias and weakness in the distal limbs [2].

Trigeminal and autonomic fibers may be involved as well. Electrophysiological studies demonstrate a marked reduction of compound motor action potentials and sensory nerve action potentials. Sural nerve biopsy shows a depletion of both large and small myelinated fibers along with axonal degeneration and typical vasculitic lesions with perivascular cellular invasion [6].

Rapid immunosuppressive treatment is needed to prevent permanent axonal damage due to ischemic nerve insult in vasculitis [5].

Along with corticosteroids, cyclophosphamide is the mainstay of treatment. Rituximab has been reported as being an effective alternative treatment [5].

25.4.6 Cranial Neuropathies

Trigeminal neuropathy is present in 17 % of patients with SS, and typically, the sensory branch is involved. The progression of symptoms is indolent [2].

Besides trigeminal neuropathy, recurrence of other cranial nerve neuropathies, mainly facial and cochlear nerve neuropathy, may occur [2].

25.4.7 Autonomic Neuropathy

Autonomic symptoms can occur in up to 50 % of patients with SS-associated neuropathy [2, 5, 6]. However, isolated autonomic involvement is rare (about 3 %). Symptoms range from pupillary constriction abnormalities (Adie's pupils likely caused by neuronitis in the ciliary ganglion cells) to severe postural hypotension and may include anhidrosis and urinary dysfunction [2].

Antibodies against type 3 muscarinic acetylcholine receptors have been described in SS as a partial explanation for the autonomic dysfunction seen in some patients [5].

25.4.8 Myopathy

Muscle pain is common in SS, but symptomatic myopathy is uncommon with prevalence ranging from 2.4 to 14 % of SS patients. It is often subclinical with normal muscle strength and normal serum creatine kinase levels [2].

Muscle biopsy reveals perivascular inflammation with perimysial or endomysial infiltrates [2].

Treatment with steroids and immunosuppressive drugs is similar to inflammatory myopathies not associated with SS.

25.5 Central Nervous System Involvement

CNS involvement in SS is controversial, and its prevalence ranges from 0 to 68 %, depending on the heterogeneity of inclusion criteria of each study [3]. PNS manifestations are present in 30–63 % of patients presenting with CNS involvement [2, 3].

Clinical manifestations can be focal or diffuse [8].

25.5.1 Focal Manifestations

25.5.1.1 Multiple Sclerosis-Like Manifestations

Patients with a syndrome resembling multiple sclerosis have been reported. MRI usually shows white matter lesions in the brain and spinal cord [2, 3]. Oligoclonal bands are present in cerebrospinal fluid analysis [2]. Many patients are seronegative for anti-SSA and anti-SSB and do not complain of sicca syndrome [8]. The course of the disease may be relapsing-remitting or progressive.

25.5.1.2 Neuromyelitis Optica

There is an emerging relationship between neuromyelitis optica (NMO) and SS. In about 2 % of NMO patients, a diagnosis of SS is also present [4].

NMO is a demyelinating disease with relapsing, longitudinally extended transverse myelitis and recurrent optic neuritis. Characteristically, autoantibodies to aquaporin-4 are present. Brain lesions are distributed in the hypothalamus, brain stem, and periventricular regions, and spinal cord lesions span multiple segments unlike what is observed in multiple sclerosis [4].

Patients affected by NMO and patients affected by NMO and SS have similar features which differ only with regard to age at onset (patients with SS are older than those with NMO alone).

25.5.2 Transverse Myelitis

Transverse myelitis is an inflammatory disorder of the spinal cord that presents acutely or subacutely [4, 8]. The incidence of myelitis in SS is unknown but at least 60 cases have been reported in the literature. Transverse myelitis accompanying SS usually spans more than three levels of the spinal cord [4].

Intravenous corticosteroids are the first-line treatment, and monthly cyclophosphamide can be administered to patients who do not improve with corticosteroids [4, 8].

25.5.3 Focal Encephalic Manifestations

In SS, focal manifestations mainly occur with stroke-like features such as hemiplegia, aphasia, cerebellar ataxia, or internuclear ophthalmoplegia. An ischemic mechanism has been hypothesized [1, 3].

Moreover, dystonia, chorea, parkinsonism, seizures, and spastic tetraparesis have been reported.

25.5.4 Meningoencephalitis

Meningoencephalitis has been reported as a neurological complication of SS. Brain MRI can be normal or may show inflammatory changes both in white and gray matter or vasculitis. CSF analysis reveals aseptic lymphocytic meningitis [3, 8].

25.6 Diffuse Manifestations

Diffuse CNS involvement is considered to be more frequent than focal involvement [7].

Headache, cognitive dysfunction, mood disorders, and fatigue are the symptoms.

Brain MRI is normal in 80 % of cases, but SPECT can show cortical hypoperfusion in the frontal and temporal lobes [7].

References

1. Delalande S, de Seze J, Fauchais AL et al (2004) Neurologic manifestations in primary Sjoegren syndrome – a study of 82 patients. Medicine 83:280–291
2. Chai J, Logigian EL (2010) Neurological manifestations of primary Sjoegren's syndrome. Curr Opin Neurol 23:509–513
3. Tobon GJ, Pers JO, Devauchelle-Pensec V, Youinou P (2012) Neurological disorders in primary Sjogren's syndrome. Autoimmun Dis 2012:645967
4. Berkowitz AL, Samuels MA (2014) The neurology of Sjoegren's syndrome and the rheumatology of peripheral neuropathy and myelitis. Pract Neurol 14:14–22
5. Pavlakis PP, Alexopoulos H, Kosmidis ML et al (2012) Peripheral neuropathies in Sjogren's syndrome: a critical update on clinical features and pathogenetic mechanisms. J Autoimmun 39:27–33
6. Mori K, Iijima M, Koike H et al (2005) The wide spectrum of clinical manifestations in Sjoegren's syndrome-associated neuropathy. Brain 128:2518–2534
7. Morreale M, Marchione P, Giacomini P et al (2014) Neurological involvement in primary Sjogren syndrome: a focus on central nervous system. PLoS One 9:1–8
8. Fauchais AL, May L, Vidal E (2012) Central and peripheral neurological complications of primary Sjogren's syndrome. PresseMed 41:e485–e493

Lymphoproliferative Disorders Associated with Sjögren Syndrome

26

Corrado Tarella, Safaa Ramadan, Angela Gueli, Simona Sammassimo, and Stefano Pileri

Sjögren syndrome (SS) is one of the most common chronic, slowly progressing systemic autoimmune diseases. It occurs in 0.1–3.0 % of the general population with a prevalence of 0.2–1.4 %. Therefore, it is the second most prevalent autoimmune disease after rheumatoid arthritis. The disease predominantly affects women with female-to-male ratio of 9:1. It develops mainly between the fourth and sixth decades of life [1–5]. Exocrinopathy with keratoconjunctivitis sicca and xerostomia are the hallmarks of the disease. However, the diversity of the clinical spectrum and disease complications is broad, and approximately half of the patients develop systemic disorders during their disease course [1–4, 6]. SS is referred to as "primary SS" if it is not associated with other autoimmune diseases; otherwise it is indicated as a secondary disease. Most of the work reviewed in this chapter refers to the primary form unless otherwise specified.

26.1 Lymphoproliferative Disorders and Sjögren Syndrome

A broad spectrum of lymphoproliferative activity has been recognized in patients with Sjögren syndrome (SS patients) over the past decades. This spectrum ranges from benign to malignant lymphoproliferation [6–14]. A series of case reports and studies demonstrated increased levels of circulating monoclonal immunoglobulins and free light chains, circulating CD5-positive B cells, and mixed monoclonal cryoglobulinemia and more importantly a high incidence of malignant non-Hodgkin lymphoma (NHL) [6, 8, 15–18]. There is considerable evidence that Sjögren syndrome carries a greater risk of developing NHL compared with other autoimmune

C. Tarella (✉) • S. Ramadan • A. Gueli • S. Sammassimo • S. Pileri
Haemato-Oncology Division, Istituto Europeo di Oncologia, European Institute of Oncology, Via Ripamonti, 435, Milan 20141, Italy
e-mail: corrado.tarella@ieo.it

D. Roccatello, L. Emmi (eds.), *Connective Tissue Disease: A Comprehensive Guide-Volume 1*, Rare Diseases of the Immune System 5,
DOI 10.1007/978-3-319-24535-5_26

diseases [6, 10–14, 19–21]. Moreover, NHL has a detrimental effect on the survival of SS patients [6, 10–14, 19, 20].

26.2 Lymphoma and Sjögren Syndrome

The association between lymphoma and autoimmunity has been known for several decades [19–22]. The first report of lymphoma in patients with Sjögren syndrome was in 1963 [15]. Thereafter, a number of case reports and studies raised concerns about the risk of lymphoma as a major complication in Sjögren syndrome [6, 18–21].

Smedby et al. conducted a population-based, case-control study in Denmark and Sweden which included 3,055 NHL patients and 3,187 matched controls who were interviewed about their history of autoimmune and chronic inflammatory disorders, markers of severity, and treatment. The overall risk (OR) for NHL was high in Sjögren syndrome, rheumatoid arthritis (RA), systemic lupus erythematosus (SLE), and celiac disease. SS patients had a sixfold increased risk of NHL, which is the highest among the four autoimmune diseases (OR was 6.1, 1.5, 4.6, and 2.1, respectively) [23].

Subsequently, a meta-analysis of five studies conducted between 1987 and 2000 showed that SS patients had an 18.8 times increased risk of developing NHL compared to the general population. Similarly, NHL risk in SS patients was higher than in RA and SLE patients with a standardized incidence ratio (SIR) of 3.9 and 7.4, respectively [23].

26.3 The Incidence of Non-Hodgkin Lymphoma in Patients with Sjögren Syndrome

The exact incidence of NHL in SS patients is not well defined and has been variably reported over the years. This is largely due to disparity in the included number of patients and in the duration of follow-up in each series. The main studies are summarized in the following sections (Table 26.1).

Five main studies reported a very high risk of NHL in SS patients with an SIR ranging between 33 and 44. In an early work by the National Institutes of Health (NIH), 7 out of 136 female SS patients developed NHL 6 months to 13 years after being seen at the NIH. Compared to women in the same age range in the general population at that time, women with SS had a 43.8 times higher incidence than expected [24]. Similarly, in an Italian series of 331 SS patients, 9 were diagnosed with NHL with a relative risk (RR) of 33.3. The incidence rate of NHL was also relatively variable, 5.4/1,000 per year in the north and 4.8/1,000 per year in the center-south of the country [8].

In the third study, Davidson et al. identified 3 NHL cases among 100 SS patients within 10 years of follow-up. Considering the whole cohort, the relative risk of NHL was 14.4. SS patients express autoantibodies targeting the Ro and La

Table 26.1 Studies on the risk of non-Hodgkin lymphoma (NHL) in patients with Sjögren syndrome

Reference	No. of SS patients	No. of observed lymphomas	SIR (95 % CI)
Kassan et al. [24]	142	7	44.4 (16.7–118.4)
Kauppi et al. [30]	676	11	8.7 (4.3–15.5)
Valesini et al. [8]	295	9	33.3 (17.3–64.0)
Davidson et al. [25]	100	3	14.4 (4.7–44.7)
Pertovaara et al. [28]	110	13	13 (2.7–3.8.0)
Lazarus et al. [26]	112	11	37.5 (20.7–67.6)
Theander et al. [29]	286	11 + 1	15.57 (777–2785)
Zhang et al. [27]	1,320	8	48.1 (20.7–94.8)
Weng et al. [3]	6,911	23	7.1 (425–103)
Johnsen et al. [31]	443	7	9.0 (71–253)
Fallah et al. [32]	14,570	143	4.9 (42–58)

components of a ribonucleoprotein. These antibodies are involved in the systemic inflammation of the disease [25]. In this study, NHL occurred only in the Ro/La-seropositive patients. Therefore, by restricting the analysis to this subgroup of patients, the RR was 49.7, comparable to the level of risk indicated by Kassan et al. [24, 25]. Likewise, a significant increase in lymphoma incidence (SIR 37.5) was estimated among 112 patients with SS treated at the University College Hospital, London [26]. The fifth study retrospectively assessed malignancy risk in 1,320 SS Chinese patients. With an average follow-up of 4.4 years, patients were found to be at higher risk of malignancy compared to the general population. The SIRs for all malignancies and for lymphomas were 3.25 and 48.1, respectively [27].

In two other SS series, higher incidences of NHL in SS patients compared to the corresponding matched general population were observed (SIR = 13 and 15.57, respectively) [28, 29]. In the Finish series, 3 NHL (2 B-cell and 1 T-cell lymphoma) cases occurred compared to 0.23 expected among 110 SS patients within 2, 4, and 10 years from SS diagnosis [28], while the follow-up period was of about 7 years in the Swedish series during which 11 NHL cases were observed compared to 0.71 expected [29].

On the other hand, and compared to the previously mentioned risk rates, four studies indicated a lower NHL risk rate in SS (SIR range: 4–9), which was still significant compared to the general population. For example, the SIR for NHL was 8.7 and 4.5 in a cohort of 676 primary SS patients and 709 secondary SS patients collected from the Finnish hospitals' national discharge registry, respectively [30]. In accordance, 7 of 443 Norwegian SS patients were found to have NHL with an estimated SIR of 9.0. NHL occurred at a median time of 9.3 years (range: 6.8–18.2 years) after the diagnosis of SS [31].

In the third study, Weng et al. analyzed the SIR of NHL among 6,911 Taiwanese women affected by SS. Twenty-three patients were documented with NHL resulting in an SIR of 7.1 [3]. More recently, Fallah et al. observed 143 NHL cases after an average 9 years of follow-up of 4,570 SS patients with an SIR of 4.9 [32].

The results of the main studies addressing the relative risk of NHL occurrence in SS are summarized in Table 26.1.

26.4 Predictive Factors for the Development of Non-Hodgkin Lymphoma

Several clinical and laboratory factors are thought to be correlated with an increased risk of NHL in SS patients.

Clinical factors are mainly related to the duration and severity of the disease. This may reflect chronic antigenic stimulation, a mechanism thought to be involved in the pathogenesis of lymphoma development. These factors include prolonged parotid gland enlargement, lymphadenopathy [33, 34], vasculitis such as purpura [29, 33, 34], and inflammatory neuropathy [28]. The onset of SS at a young age has also been linked to greater NHL risk [35, 36]. In a series of 387 Italian SS patients, Baldini et al. found that salivary gland enlargement and disease duration are independent risk factors [21, 37]. This is supported by the results of a recent study by Solans-Laqué et al. who showed that the cumulative risk of developing lymphoma increased from 3.4 % in the first 5 years to 9.8 % at 15 years [38].

In another retrospective study involving 536 SS patients, the presence of neutropenia, cryoglobulinemia, splenomegaly, lymphadenopathy, and low C4 levels at diagnosis predicted a fivefold increased risk of marginal zone (MZ) lymphomas compared to patients with no risk factors, whereas lymphocytopenia was a risk factor for diffuse large B-cell (DLBC) lymphoma [39].

Theander et al. also showed that low CD4+ (hazard ratio, HR = 8.14) and a low CD4+/CD8+ ratio (HR = 10.92) are strong predictors of being diagnosed with lymphoma [29].

Other laboratory biomarkers that are considered to be risk factors for NHL include mixed monoclonal (type II) cryoglobulinemia, low serum complement (C4) levels, and the presence of monoclonal gammopathy in the serum or free light chains in the urine [22, 28, 34, 40–43]. Solans-Laqué et al. found that only hypocomplementemia and lymphocytopenia are independent risk factors. Moreover, hypocomplementemia was correlated to higher mortality [38].

Other more recently identified biologic markers are the presence of germinal center-like (GC-like) structures [44] and the focus score of lymphocytic infiltration of the minor salivary glands of SS patients. The latter is determined by the number of lymphocyte foci per 4 mm^2 of glandular tissue [45].

Theander et al. examined 175 minor salivary gland biopsies performed at baseline in SS patients. GC-like structures were significantly more frequent in patients who later developed NHL versus those without subsequent NHL (86 % versus 22 %, respectively). It is worth noting that the GC-like structures are detectable more than 7 years before lymphoma occurs [44]. However, they are not part of the routine assessment of SS patients. Therefore, measuring the focus score (high $\geq$3) could be an alternative biomarker for identifying patients at NHL risk [45].

26.5 Subtypes of Sjögren Syndrome-Associated Non-Hodgkin Lymphomas

A remarkable association between mucosa-associated lymphoid tissue (MALT) lymphomas and Sjögren syndrome is well recognized [31, 32, 40, 46, 47]. Conversely, in more recent studies, DLBC lymphoma was either as frequent as MALT or actually the most frequent subtype [29, 32, 48, 49].

Voulgarelis et al. described 33 cases of NHL in 765 SS patients. SS and NHL were diagnosed at the same time in 2 patients and in 31 others at intervals ranging from 1 to 36 years after diagnosis. Twenty-three patients (69.7 %) had low-grade lymphomas, of which 12 were MALT, 8 were small lymphocytic/plasmacytoid, 1 was small lymphocytic, 1 was monocytoid B cell, and 1 was follicular mixed large and small cell. Ten patients had intermediate- or high-grade lymphomas. Among them, three had MALT, five had large-cell immunoblastic, one had DLBC, and one had follicular lymphoma subtypes. Median survival of patients in the high/intermediate and low histological grades was 1.83 years and 6.33 years, respectively [40].

In a population-based study by Smedby et al., 12 cases of NHL occurred over a range of 2–30 years after SS diagnosis. There was a significant increase in the risk of MZ (RR=28) and DLBC lymphomas (RR=11) [47].

Six of the seven SS-associated lymphomas in the Norwegian series were of the MALT type. Johnsen et al. reported that among them, four were located in the parotid gland and the others in the labial salivary glands, the thymus gland, and the lingual tonsil. The seventh presented with concomitant B-cell chronic lymphocytic leukemia (B-CLL) and extranodal marginal zone (ENMZ) lymphomas [29]. Similarly, Lazarus et al. found that 8 of the 11 patients with SS-associated NHL were MALT type, 1 was high-grade NHL, and 2 were of unknown subtype [26].

More recently, Papageorgiou et al. evaluated the medical records of all consecutive patients with an initial diagnosis of primary SS at the University of Athens between 1993 and September 2013. Of the 77 patients diagnosed with NHL, MALT lymphoma constituted the majority (51/77, 66.2 %) of NHL subtypes, followed DLBC (12/77, 15.6 %) and nodal marginal zone (NMZ) lymphomas (8/77, 10.4 %). Compared to patients with DLBC, MALT lymphoma patients were significantly younger (median age was 55 versus 69 years, respectively) and developed lymphoma much earlier (median time from SS diagnosis to MALT development was 65.80 versus 97.54 months, respectively) [50].

In contrast to the above data, six other studies suggested that the incidence of SS-associated diffuse large B-cell NHL is higher than previously estimated [27, 29, 32, 48, 49, 51]. Tonami et al. reviewed 27 reported lymphoma cases in 463 patients with Sjögren syndrome. The calculated prevalence of lymphoma in patients with Sjögren syndrome was 5.8 %. Twenty-six were NHL and one was Hodgkin disease. Of the 26, only 6 were MALT, while the others were diffuse medium ($n=10$) and diffuse large [49].

In the second study, Vasaitis et al. examined 70 SS-associated lymphomas occurring at a mean follow-up time of 13 years (3–35 years) in 236 SS patients whose data were retrieved from the national Swedish patient registry. The percentage of

MALT ($n=24$) and DLBC ($n=22$) lymphomas was quite similar (34.3 % versus 31.4 %, respectively). Involvement of the parotid gland was common among the MALT ($n=18/24$; 75 %), but not among the DLBC lymphomas ($n=2/22$; 9 %). There were only a few cases of other lymphoma subtypes: follicular mixed type and angioimmunoblastic T cell (two cases each) and follicular medium and T cell-rich B-cell type (one case each) [48].

Theander et al. also revised 12 SS-associated lymphomas, and diffuse large B cell was the most frequent subtype (7/12; 58 %), while the other 5 were small lymphocytic lymphomas ($n=3$) and follicular and anaplastic large T-cell NHL (1 case each) [29].

Fallah et al. confirmed this observation in his recent Swedish series of 143 SS-associated lymphomas. Diffuse large B-cell lymphoma was the main histological subtype ($n=41$ cases), followed by follicular cell ($n=28$), mantle cell ($n=4$), and T-cell and small lymphocytic lymphomas (one each). In addition, this cohort included 15 other unspecified NHL subtypes [32].

Voulgarelis and colleagues evaluated 584 SS patients who were diagnosed between 1980 and 2010, of whom 53 subsequently presented NHL, the majority of which were MALT (59 %) lymphomas. Nodal marginal zone lymphoma and DLBC lymphoma made up 15 % each. The remaining 11 % ($n=6$) were lymphoplasmacytic NHL ($n=2$) and small lymphocytic NHL, follicular NHL, peripheral T-cell NHL unspecified, and classic Hodgkin disease (one case each) [51].

In the Chinese cohort, seven of the eight SS-associated NHL patients had B-cell NHL and only one had T-cell NHL. Four B-cell NHLs were confirmed by parotid biopsy.

A similar number of pathologic subtypes of B-cell type, including diffuse large B-cell lymphoma and lymphomas of mucosa-associated lymphoid tissue (two cases each), one intravascular large B-cell lymphoma, and two B-cell lymphomas, unclassifiable, were seen [27].

26.6 Pathologic Features and Underlying Mechanisms

Any type of malignant lymphoma can affect the salivary glands, either primarily or secondarily [52, 53]. A further distinction should be made between tumors involving the gland parenchyma and those affecting the lymph nodes comprised within it, the latter being at times erroneously considered primary events. Herein, only "de novo" lymphoid tumors of the salivary glands will be discussed. These are indeed rare (about 7 % of all lymphomas of the head and neck) and more frequently affect the parotid gland (78 %) [54, 55]. The histotype can vary from follicular lymphoma [56] to Hodgkin lymphoma [57], although ENMZ/MALT lymphoma represents the most common variety [58, 59], thus warranting a detailed description also in the light of its shared association with SS and hepatitis C virus (HCV) infection [7, 58, 59].

From a morphologic point of view [58], ENMZ lymphoma consists of small- to medium-sized cells that display variable profiles. They may resemble centrocytes with cleaved nuclei, monocytoid B cells with a wide rim of clear cytoplasm and distinct borders, or more rarely, small mature lymphocytes. The number of mitotic figures is usually low. Features of plasma cell differentiation are commonly seen, at times becoming prominent. Some blasts are always scattered throughout: they do not affect the clinical behavior unless they form either clusters consisting of at least 20 elements or sheetlike proliferations which are regarded as indicative of transformation into a DLBC lymphoma. Such population most often develops around reactive secondary follicles in a marginal zone distribution. Importantly, the follicles can be colonized by neoplastic cells. In the most common situation, tumoral elements overrun the lymphoid follicles, leaving behind scattered germinal center cell fragments and dispersed mantle zone cells resulting in a vague nodular pattern. At times, they may selectively infiltrate, replace, and expand germinal centers, resulting in an appearance that mimics follicular lymphoma.

An important diagnostic feature of MALT lymphomas is usually the presence of lymphoepithelial lesions, defined by the infiltration and distortion of epithelial structures by aggregates of (usually three or more) neoplastic cells [58]. This is not the case in the setting of the salivary glands. In fact, the tumor generally develops on a background of a myoepithelial sialadenitis/benign lymphoepithelial lesion [58]. When fully developed, the latter comprises atrophic acinar tissue infiltrated by small lymphocytes and plasma cells, often with reactive lymphoid follicles and characteristically with numerous epimyoepithelial islands. The first morphologic manifestation of ENMZ lymphoma is the presence of halos or collars of neoplastic cells around the epimyoepithelial islands. Such infiltrates usually show immunoglobulin light chain restriction and clonal IgVH rearrangement by polymerase chain reaction (PCR) (see below). More advanced lymphomas reveal expansile, often destructive proliferations of neoplastic MZ cells “cavitating” preexisting benign lymphoepithelial lesions.

Immunohistochemistry shows that neoplastic cells bear the following profile: CD20+, IgM (>IgA > IgG) +, W>IgD-, CD5-, CD10-, BCL6-, and cyclin D1 (1, 7). Such phenotype allows to exclude mantle cell lymphoma and follicular lymphoma but is not per se pathognomonic. The IRTA1 monoclonal antibody is the only currently existing specific marker that reacts with more than 90 % EMZLs [60]. In particular, the “balls” of neoplastic cells growing within the lymphoepithelial lesions display very strong staining. Unfortunately, although extensively applied in some centers, the IRTA1 monoclonal antibody is not yet commercially available. Aberrant CD43 expression occurs in about half of the cases. In properly fixed material, monotypic restriction of Ig light chains is easily detected in both the perinuclear spaces of neoplastic cells and the associated plasma cell component, which also expresses IRF4/MUM1. The stains for CD21 and CD23 highlight remnants of follicular dendritic cells. Lastly, in case of follicular colonization, lymphomatous elements progressively lose IRTA1 and acquire BCL6 in the absence of CD10 staining [60]. The latter finding is indeed useful for distinguishing colonized follicles from residual follicles (CD10+ BCL6+).

PCR studies based on the BIOMED-2 approach detect a monoclonal Ig rearrangement in most, if not all, cases [58]. Ig sequencing shows a high load of somatic mutations, which can become ongoing in case of follicular colonization. Conversely to what is seen in lymphoplasmacytic lymphoma, MYD88 mutations rarely occur [61].

Three chromosomal translocations [t(11;18)(q21;q21)/API2-MALT1, t(14;18)(q32;q21)/IgH-MALT1, t(1;14)(p22;q32)/(IgH-BCL10)] can be detected in the ENMZLs of the salivary glands, while to the best of the authors' knowledge, the t(3;14)(p14;q32)/IgH-FOXP1 has not never been detected [58]. The three translocations seem to promote lymphoma development by a shared mechanism. In particular, they trigger NF-kB activation, a transcription factor that controls lymphocyte proliferation and apoptosis via the deregulation of BCL10 or MALT1 expression. The t(14;18)(q32;q21)/IgH-MALT1 represents the most commonly reported translocation in the setting of salivary gland MALT lymphoma, the remaining two being much rarer or even exceptional [58].

26.7 The Outcome of Patients with Sjögren Syndrome-Associated Lymphomas

The prognosis of lymphoma is widely variable depending on the histological subtype and grade as well as other factors such as disease stage. In general, low-grade lymphomas such as MALT lymphomas have a very good prognosis, and 5-year survival is approximately 90 %. On the other hand, aggressive forms like diffuse large B-cell lymphoma have a 5-year survival of 60 %.

Three relatively large studies examined the outcome of patients with SS-associated lymphomas [39, 40, 62].

In 1999, Voulgarelis et al. investigated the survival of 33 SS-related lymphoma patients categorized by histological subtype and showed that the median survival of patients with the high/intermediate histological grades was 1.83 years, while of low grades it was 6.33 years. The presence of B symptoms and largest tumor diameter >7 cm, along with histological classification, were associated with worse survival [40].

Pollard et al. explored the clinical course of patients with localized MALT lymphoma of the parotid gland that is linked to Sjögren syndrome. Lymphoma occurred in 35 cases out of 329 SS patients at a median follow-up of 76 months (range 16–153 months). Treatment was "watchful waiting" ($n=10$), surgery ($n=3$), radiotherapy ($n=1$), surgery combined with radiotherapy ($n=2$), rituximab alone ($n=13$), or rituximab combined with chemotherapy ($n=6$). Fourteen patients achieved complete CR, while stable disease was achieved by 20 patients and partial response by 1 patient. High SS disease activity was a poor prognostic factor for the progression of lymphoma and/or SS. The authors suggested that such patients should receive treatment despite having localized indolent lymphoma [62].

Papageorgiou and colleagues analyzed overall and event-free survival (OS and EFS) in the largest and most recent cohort of 77 SS-associated NHL patients. Events were lymphoma relapse, treatment failure, disease progression, histological transformation, or death. Ten patients died, five suffered a relapse, two experienced progression/transformation, and five patients developed other hematological malignancies that included T-cell NHL (two cases) and multiple myeloma, Hodgkin disease, and thymoma (one case each). Seven of the deaths were due to neutropenic sepsis, two were due to relapse, and one death was attributed to reasons other than lymphoma or treatment-related causes. The 5-year OS and EFS for the entire NHL cohort was 90.91 % and 77.92 %, respectively. Depending on NHL subtypes, the 5-year OS was 94.12 % for MALT versus 87.5 % for NMZ, 75.0 % for DLBC, and 100 % for other lymphoma subtypes. The 5-year EFS was 86.27 % for patients with MALT, 62.5 % for patients with NMZ lymphoma, 50.0 % in DLBC lymphoma patients, and 83.3 % for other lymphoma subtypes. Survival differences between MALT and DLBC lymphomas were statistically significant [50]. The studies also revealed that the severity of SS disease (using the disease activity score) negatively impacts on the prognosis of NHL patients. Compared to patients with low SS disease activity, those with high disease activity had a greater risk of death (OR = 5.241) or of an event (OR = 4.317). Consequently, they had significantly worse EFS and OS. The authors also recognized additional predictors of lymphoma prognosis, such as an elevated the lymphoma international prognostic index (IPI) score and bone marrow involvement. After adjustment for identified risk factors, IPI score retained a significant effect on survival outcomes followed by a strong trend for SS disease activity score [50].

A diagnosis of lymphoma worsens expected survival in SS patients [32, 38, 51, 63]. Horvath and colleagues showed that having a lymphoproliferative disease during the course of SS disease increased the risk of mortality. Likewise, Voulgarelis and coworkers found that lymphoma was the main cause of death in patients with SS with a standardized mortality ratio of 3.25 in patients with lymphoma and 1.08 in patients without lymphoma [51].

A number of studies examined the outcome of SS-related lymphomas with specific types of therapy [39, 40, 64]. Ambrosetti and colleagues observed no significant differences in outcomes between SS patients with salivary MALT lymphomas who had undergone a variety of treatment modalities and those who were only observed [39]. This is consistent with a previous study which demonstrated that both SS and SS-associated salivary MALT lymphoma patients have a similar clinical course with a median overall survival of 6.4 years [40].

Voulgarelis and coauthors reported a 75 % CR rate with the purine analog 2-chloro-2-deoxyadenosine (2-CdA) in four SS-associated B-cell lymphoma patients during a 4-year follow-up. Interestingly, SS manifestations improved as well. Authors suggested that pronounced 2-CdA-induced T-cell depletion exerts an additional therapeutic effect in SS patients. Due to the small cohort and short follow-up, investigators could not come to any definitive conclusions on the therapeutic role of 2-CdA in SS-associated lymphoma [65].

Rituximab is a therapeutic agent used in the treatment of SS, with or without associated MALT lymphoma. Fifteen patients with primary SS were included in a phase II trial exploring the safety and efficacy of rituximab in SS patients ($n = 8$) and SS-related MALT lymphomas ($n = 7$). Of the seven patients with MALT lymphomas, CR was achieved in three, stable disease in three, while one patient progressed [64].

On the other hand, R-CHOP is the treatment of choice in SS-related aggressive NHL [66, 67]. Six SS patients with DLBC lymphoma were assigned to receive eight cycles of R-CHOP in a phase II trial. Patients were compared to a historic control of nine DLBC lymphoma patients treated with CHOP alone. A significant difference was observed in OS between the two groups, with a 2-year OS of 100 % in the R-CHOP-treated group versus 37 % in the control group. SS-related symptoms were also better in the study group, thus reflecting the immunogenic effect of rituximab on SS [67].

Conclusions

In summary, the risk of developing lymphoma in SS patients is considerably higher than in the general population. The majority of SS patients develop low-grade, usually ENMZ/MALT lymphoma subtype. High-grade DLBC lymphoma is seen in 10–15 % of SS-related lymphoma patients. The incidence of DLBC lymphoma seems to be underestimated in SS patients, and some studies showed that DLBC subtypes occur at rates similar to or even higher than that of low-grade lymphomas. Several clinical features and laboratory biomarkers are correlated to the risk of lymphoma in SS patients. However, there is currently not enough evidence to support their use in routine clinical practice. SS patients who are diagnosed with lymphoma have worse survival compared to SS patients who have no lymphoma. Studies on the mechanisms underlying lymphomagenesis in SS patients are ongoing.

References

1. Kassan SS, Moutsopoulos HM (2004) Clinical manifestations and early diagnosis of Sjogren syndrome. Arch Intern Med 164:1275–1284
2. Goules AV, Tzioufas AG, Moutsopoulos HM (2014) Classification criteria of Sjogren's syndrome. J Autoimmun 48–49:42–45
3. Weng MY, Huang YT, Liu MF, Lu TH (2011) Incidence and mortality of treated primary Sjogren's syndrome in Taiwan: a population-based study. J Rheumatol 38:706–708
4. Qin B, Wang J, Yang Z et al (2015) Epidemiology of primary Sjogren's syndrome: a systematic review and meta-analysis. Ann Rheum Dis 74:1983–1989
5. Reksten TR, Jonsson MV (2014) Sjogren's syndrome: an update on epidemiology and current insights on pathophysiology. Oral Maxillofac Surg Clin N Am 26:1–12
6. Nocturne G, Mariette X (2015) Sjogren syndrome-associated lymphomas: an update on pathogenesis and management. Br J Haematol 168:317–327
7. Quartuccio L, Isola M, Baldini C et al (2014) Biomarkers of lymphoma in Sjogren's syndrome and evaluation of the lymphoma risk in prelymphomatous conditions: results of a multicenter study. J Autoimmun 51:75–80
8. Valesini G, Priori R, Bavoillot D et al (1997) Differential risk of non-Hodgkin's lymphoma in Italian patients with primary Sjogren's syndrome. J Rheumatol 24:2376–2380
9. Youinou P, Mackenzie L, le Masson G et al (1988) CD5-expressing B lymphocytes in the blood and salivary glands of patients with primary Sjogren's syndrome. J Autoimmun 1:185–194
10. Hansen A, Daridon C, Dorner T (2010) What do we know about memory B cells in primary Sjogren's syndrome? Autoimmun Rev 9:600–603
11. Jonsson R, Nginamau E, Szyszko E, Brokstad KA (2007) Role of B cells in Sjogren's syndrome–from benign lymphoproliferation to overt malignancy. Front Biosci 12:2159–2170

12. Skarstein K, Nerland AH, Eidsheim M et al (1997) Lymphoid cell accumulation in salivary glands of autoimmune MRL mice can be due to impaired apoptosis. Scand J Immunol 46:373–378
13. Talal N, Sokoloff L, Barth WF (1967) Extrasalivary lymphoid abnormalities in Sjogren's syndrome (reticulum cell sarcoma, "pseudolymphoma," macroglobulinemia). Am J Med 43:50–65
14. Yamasaki S, Matsushita H, Tanimura S et al (1998) B-cell lymphoma of mucosa-associated lymphoid tissue of the thymus: a report of two cases with a background of Sjogren's syndrome and monoclonal gammopathy. Hum Pathol 29:1021–1024
15. Talal N, Bunim JJ (1964) The development of malignant lymphoma in the course of Sjoegren's syndrome. Am J Med 36:529–540
16. Talal N, Aufdemorte TB, Kincaid WL et al (1988) Two patients illustrating lymphoma transition and response to therapy in Sjogren's syndrome. J Autoimmun 1:171–184
17. Voulgarelis M, Skopouli FN (2007) Clinical, immunologic, and molecular factors predicting lymphoma development in Sjogren's syndrome patients. Clin Rev Allergy Immunol 32:265–274
18. Routsias JG, Goules JD, Charalampakis G et al (2013) Malignant lymphoma in primary Sjogren's syndrome: an update on the pathogenesis and treatment. Semin Arthritis Rheum 43:178–186
19. Smedby KE, Askling J, Mariette X, Baecklund E (2008) Autoimmune and inflammatory disorders and risk of malignant lymphomas – an update. J Intern Med 264:514–527
20. Zintzaras E, Voulgarelis M, Moutsopoulos HM (2005) The risk of lymphoma development in autoimmune diseases: a meta-analysis. Arch Intern Med 165:2337–2344
21. Tarella C, Gueli A, Ruella M, Cignetti A (2013) Lymphocyte transformation and autoimmune disorders. Autoimmun Rev 12:802–813
22. Martin DN, Mikhail IS, Landgren O (2009) Autoimmunity and hematologic malignancies: associations and mechanisms. Leuk Lymphoma 50:541–550
23. Smedby KE, Baecklund E, Askling J (2006) Malignant lymphomas in autoimmunity and inflammation: a review of risks, risk factors, and lymphoma characteristics. Cancer Epidemiol Biomarkers Prev 15:2069–2077
24. Kassan SS, Thomas TL, Moutsopoulos HM et al (1978) Increased risk of lymphoma in sicca syndrome. Ann Intern Med 89:888–892
25. Davidson BK, Kelly CA, Griffiths ID (1999) Primary Sjogren's syndrome in the North East of England: a long-term follow-up study. Rheumatology (Oxford) 38:245–253
26. Lazarus MN, Robinson D, Mak V et al (2006) Incidence of cancer in a cohort of patients with primary Sjogren's syndrome. Rheumatology (Oxford) 45:1012–1015
27. Zhang W, Feng S, Yan S et al (2010) Incidence of malignancy in primary Sjogren's syndrome in a Chinese cohort. Rheumatology (Oxford) 49:571–577
28. Pertovaara M, Pukkala E, Laippala P et al (2001) A longitudinal cohort study of Finnish patients with primary Sjogren's syndrome: clinical, immunological, and epidemiological aspects. Ann Rheum Dis 60:467–472
29. Theander E, Henriksson G, Ljungberg O et al (2006) Lymphoma and other malignancies in primary Sjogren's syndrome: a cohort study on cancer incidence and lymphoma predictors. Ann Rheum Dis 65:796–803
30. Kauppi M, Pukkala E, Isomaki H (1997) Elevated incidence of hematologic malignancies in patients with Sjogren's syndrome compared with patients with rheumatoid arthritis (Finland). Cancer Causes Control 8:201–204
31. Johnsen SJ, Brun JG, Goransson LG et al (2013) Risk of non-Hodgkin's lymphoma in primary Sjogren's syndrome: a population-based study. Arthritis Care Res (Hoboken) 65:816–821
32. Fallah M, Liu X, Ji J et al (2014) Autoimmune diseases associated with non-Hodgkin lymphoma: a nationwide cohort study. Ann Oncol 25:2025–2030
33. Anaya JM, McGuff HS, Banks PM, Talal N (1996) Clinicopathological factors relating malignant lymphoma with Sjogren's syndrome. Semin Arthritis Rheum 25:337–346
34. Nishishinya MB, Pereda CA, Munoz-Fernandez S et al (2015) Identification of lymphoma predictors in patients with primary Sjogren's syndrome: a systematic literature review and meta-analysis. Rheumatol Int 35:17–26

35. Ramos-Casals M, Solans R, Rosas J et al (2008) Primary Sjogren syndrome in Spain: clinical and immunologic expression in 1010 patients. Medicine (Baltimore) 87:210–219
36. Ramos-Casals M, Brito-Zeron P, Siso-Almirall A, Bosch X (2012) Primary Sjogren syndrome. BMJ 344:e3821
37. Baldini C, Pepe P, Quartuccio L et al (2014) Primary Sjogren's syndrome as a multi-organ disease: impact of the serological profile on the clinical presentation of the disease in a large cohort of Italian patients. Rheumatology (Oxford) 53:839–844
38. Solans-Laque R, Lopez-Hernandez A, Bosch-Gil JA et al (2011) Risk, predictors, and clinical characteristics of lymphoma development in primary Sjogren's syndrome. Semin Arthritis Rheum 41:415–423
39. Ambrosetti A, Zanotti R, Pattaro C et al (2004) Most cases of primary salivary mucosa-associated lymphoid tissue lymphoma are associated either with Sjoegren syndrome or hepatitis C virus infection. Br J Haematol 126:43–49
40. Voulgarelis M, Dafni UG, Isenberg DA, Moutsopoulos HM (1999) Malignant lymphoma in primary Sjogren's syndrome: a multicenter, retrospective, clinical study by the European concerted action on Sjogren's syndrome. Arthritis Rheum 42:1765–1772
41. Muller K, Oxholm P, Mier-Madsen M, Wiik A (1989) Circulating IgA- and IgM-rheumatoid factors in patients with primary Sjogren syndrome. Correlation to extraglandular manifestations. Scand J Rheumatol 18:29–31
42. Brito-Zeron P, Ramos-Casals M, Nardi N et al (2005) Circulating monoclonal immunoglobulins in Sjogren syndrome: prevalence and clinical significance in 237 patients. Medicine (Baltimore) 84:90–97
43. Brito-Zeron P, Kostov B, Solans R et al (2014) On behalf of the SS Study Group, Autoimmune Diseases Study Group (GEAS), Spanish Society of Internal Medicine (SEMI). Systemic activity and mortality in primary Sjogren syndrome: predicting survival using the EULAR-SS Disease Activity Index (ESSDAI) in 1045 patients. Ann Rheum Dis doi:10.1136/annrheumdis-2014-206418
44. Theander E, Vasaitis L, Baecklund E et al (2011) Lymphoid organisation in labial salivary gland biopsies is a possible predictor for the development of malignant lymphoma in primary Sjogren's syndrome. Ann Rheum Dis 70:1363–1368
45. Risselada AP, Kruize AA, Goldschmeding R et al (2014) The prognostic value of routinely performed minor salivary gland assessments in primary Sjogren's syndrome. Ann Rheum Dis 73:1537–1540
46. Baimpa E, Dahabreh IJ, Voulgarelis M, Moutsopoulos HM (2009) Hematologic manifestations and predictors of lymphoma development in primary Sjogren syndrome: clinical and pathophysiologic aspects. Medicine (Baltimore) 88:284–293
47. Smedby KE, Hjalgrim H, Askling J et al (2006) Autoimmune and chronic inflammatory disorders and risk of non-Hodgkin lymphoma by subtype. J Natl Cancer Inst 98:51–60
48. Vasaitis L Nordmark G, Askling J, Ekström-Smedby K, Backlin C, Rönnblom L (2012) Diffuse large B-cell lymphoma. An underestimated subtype and cause of death in primary Sjögren's syndrome. Abstract EULAR
49. Tonami H, Matoba M, Kuginuki Y et al (2003) Clinical and imaging findings of lymphoma in patients with Sjogren syndrome. J Comput Assist Tomogr 27:517–524
50. Papageorgiou A, Ziogas DC, Mavragani CP et al (2015) Predicting the outcome of Sjogren's syndrome-associated non-hodgkin's lymphoma patients. PLoS ONE 10:e0116189
51. Voulgarelis M, Ziakas PD, Papageorgiou A et al (2012) Prognosis and outcome of non-Hodgkin lymphoma in primary Sjogren syndrome. Medicine (Baltimore) 91:1–9
52. Jaffe ES (2009) The 2008 WHO classification of lymphomas: implications for clinical practice and translational research. Hematol Am Soc Hematol Educ Prog 2009:523–531
53. Revanappa MM, Sattur AP, Naikmasur VG, Thakur AR (2013) Disseminated non-Hodgkin's lymphoma presenting as bilateral salivary gland enlargement: a case report. Imaging Sci Dent 43:59–62

54. Mian M, Capello D, Ventre MB et al (2014) Early-stage diffuse large B cell lymphoma of the head and neck: clinico-biological characterization and 18 year follow-up of 488 patients (IELSG 23 study). Ann Hematol 93:221–231
55. Anacak Y, Miller RC, Constantinou N et al (2012) Primary mucosa-associated lymphoid tissue lymphoma of the salivary glands: a multicenter rare cancer network study. Int J Radiat Oncol Biol Phys 82:315–320
56. Shashidara R, Prasad PR, Jaishankar JT (2014) Follicular lymphoma of the submandibular salivary gland. J Oral Maxillofac Pathol 18:S163–S166
57. Agaimy A, Wild V, Markl B et al (2015) Intraparotid classical and nodular lymphocyte-predominant hodgkin lymphoma: pattern analysis with emphasis on associated lymphadenoma-like proliferations. Am J Surg Pathol 39:1206–1212
58. Bacon CM, Du MQ, Dogan A (2007) Mucosa-associated lymphoid tissue (MALT) lymphoma: a practical guide for pathologists. J Clin Pathol 60:361–372
59. Zinzani PL (2012) The many faces of marginal zone lymphoma. Hematol Am Soc Hematol Educ Prog 2012:426–432
60. Falini B, Agostinelli C, Bigerna B et al (2012) IRTA1 is selectively expressed in nodal and extranodal marginal zone lymphomas. Histopathology 61:930–941
61. Voulgarelis M, Mavragani CP, Xu L et al (2014) Absence of somatic MYD88 L265P mutations in patients with primary Sjogren's syndrome. Genes Immun 15:54–56
62. Pollard RP, Pijpe J, Bootsma H et al (2011) Treatment of mucosa-associated lymphoid tissue lymphoma in Sjogren's syndrome: a retrospective clinical study. J Rheumatol 38:2198–2208
63. Horvath IF, Szanto A, Papp G, Zeher M (2014) Clinical course, prognosis, and cause of death in primary Sjogren's syndrome. J Immunol Res 2014:647507
64. Pijpe J, van Imhoff GW, Spijkervet FK et al (2005) Rituximab treatment in patients with primary Sjogren's syndrome: an open-label phase II study. Arthritis Rheum 52:2740–2750
65. Voulgarelis M, Petroutsos G, Moutsopoulos HM, Skopouli FN (2002) 2-chloro-2′-deoxyadenosine in the treatment of Sjogren's syndrome-associated B cell lymphoproliferation. Arthritis Rheum 46:2248–2249
66. Voulgarelis M, Giannouli S, Tzioufas AG, Moutsopoulos HM (2006) Long term remission of Sjogren's syndrome associated aggressive B cell non-Hodgkin's lymphomas following combined B cell depletion therapy and CHOP (cyclophosphamide, doxorubicin, vincristine, prednisone). Ann Rheum Dis 65:1033–1037
67. Voulgarelis M, Giannouli S, Anagnostou D, Tzioufas AG (2004) Combined therapy with rituximab plus cyclophosphamide/doxorubicin/vincristine/prednisone (CHOP) for Sjogren's syndrome-associated B-cell aggressive non-Hodgkin's lymphomas. Rheumatology (Oxford) 43:1050–1053

Pathogenetic Aspects of Sjögren's Syndrome: Relationships with Cryoglobulinemia and Lymphoproliferation of MALT

27

Salvatore De Vita and Luca Quartuccio

27.1 Introduction

Sjögren's syndrome (SS) is defined both as an autoimmune and a lymphoproliferative disease [1, 2]: in fact, B cells are overexpanded since the onset of the disease. SS is a disorder of mucosa-associated lymphoid tissue (MALT). Autoimmune epithelitis is also a crucial event [3].

The risk of B-cell lymphoma evolution is markedly increased in SS [4] (about 5 % of patients), and B-cell overexpansion represents a predisposing factor for non-Hodgkin's lymphoma (NHL), usually involving MALT tissue. Of note, patients may progress from a fully benign lymphoproliferation to an overt B-cell NHL through intermediate stages [5].

This wide spectrum of manifestations offers the opportunity to analyze in detail the etiopathogenetic events involved in the process of B-cell lymphomagenesis, by using SS as a model.

Cryoglobulinemia, with or without a concomitant cryoglobulinemic vasculitis (CV), and the persistent swelling of the major salivary glands (usually the parotids) represent the two main risk factors for B-cell NHL evolution in SS.

Understanding the mechanisms involved in the transition from B-cell overexpansion to lymphoproliferation might lead to the development of more effective and targeted treatments still currently lacking in SS.

S. De Vita (✉) • L. Quartuccio
Department of Medical and Biological Science, Clinic of Rheumatology,
University Hospital of "Santa Maria della Misericordia",
Piazza S. Maria della Misericordia 15, 33010 Udine, Italy
e-mail: devita.salvatore@aoud.sanita.fvg.it

D. Roccatello, L. Emmi (eds.), *Connective Tissue Disease: A Comprehensive Guide-Volume 1*, Rare Diseases of the Immune System 5,
DOI 10.1007/978-3-319-24535-5_27

27.2 The Classification of SS-Related Lymphoproliferation of MALT

The diagnosis of B-cell malignancy is based on tissue biopsy, and the B-cell malignancy in SS is classified according to the current standards [6]. The integration of clinical, pathologic, and molecular results is crucial in difficult cases. The proposed classification, discussed at international levels [7], distinguishes between fully benign lymphoproliferation (a feature of SS) and nonmalignant lymphoproliferative disorder (a more advanced stage toward B-cell malignancy). These processes may involve different MALT sites, the lymph nodes, and more rarely the bone marrow, and may be associated with hypergammaglobulinemia, positive M-component, and/or cryoglobulinemia (polyclonal, oligoclonal, or monoclonal).

Fully benign lymphoproliferation is usually represented either by infiltrates without histological sign of malignancy in MALT sites or reactive lymphadenopathy in the absence of serum M-component [7].

In lymphoepithelial or myoepithelial sialadenitis (MESA) with benign lymphoid infiltrates, the lobular architecture of the gland is preserved. Lymphoepithelial lesions are characterized by monocytoid and marginal zone B cells (centrocyte-like). Reactive follicles without expansion of the mantle or marginal zones are also present, and small lymphocytes and plasma cells (usually not in broad sheets) are prominent in the interfollicular regions.

Several MALT sites may be involved, including gastric MALT lesions up to a grade 2 [8, 9].

The nonmalignant lymphoproliferative disorder includes the cases of "lymphoproliferative lesion" in MALT sites, nodal atypical lymphoproliferative disorder [10], and monoclonal cryoglobulinemia or M-component in biologic fluids [7].

In MESA with "lymphoproliferative lesions," the process is diffuse or multifocal within the gland. Islands of acini are often preserved, while aggregates of centrocyte-like cells may be present within a diffuse lymphoid infiltrate. Nonconfluent centrocyte-like cell "halos" surrounding the lymphoepithelial lesions are often observed. Lymphoepithelial aggressiveness may be pronounced. Areas of immunoglobulin light-chain restriction may be also present.

Conversely, in **low-grade MALT-type marginal zone B-cell lymphomas**, a dense lymphoid infiltrate diffusely involving the gland is usually observed. It can occur as a localized mass, with obliteration of acini. Lymphoid cells and plasma cells present monotypic immunoglobulin expression. Plasmacytic differentiation may occur. A large cell component may be detected. Reactive lymphoid follicles and lymphoepithelial lesions are usually prominent as observed in MESA. However, in contrast with MESA, centrocyte-like cells form broad interconnecting strands between lymphoepithelial lesions (key feature) and broad "halos" around the epithelial cell nests.

Gastric MALT lesions of grades 3 and 4 according to Wotherspoon and Isaacson [8] and lymphoproliferative lesions not presenting definite malignant features are considered SS-related nonmalignant lymphoproliferative disorders [9].

An accurate pathologic evaluation is critical in distinguishing between nonmalignant and low-grade malignant lymphoproliferation of MALT. B-cell monoclonality alone is not a criterion to establish B-cell malignancy [7]. Different patterns of tissue B-cell expansion can be identified by molecular analyses in SS-related MALT lesions by studying synchronous and metachronous tissue lesions, implying a different risk of lymphoma progression: polyclonal, oligoclonal or monoclonal expansion without clonal persistence, monoclonal expansion with clonal persistence, and monoclonal expansion with dissemination. Then, molecular analyses of B-cell clonal expansion proved to be of major value for prognosis, rather than for diagnosis [7].

27.3 The Pathogenesis of SS-Related Lymphomas of MALT: Lessons from Infection-Related Lymphomas

Gastric B-cell NHL of MALT, associated with *H. pylori* infection, is the most important model of infection-related acquisition of lymphoid tissue and B lymphomagenesis [8]. Other infection-related B-cell NHLs include those related to hepatitis C virus (HCV), *Chlamydia psittaci* (ocular adnexa), *Borrelia burgdorferi* (skin), and *Campylobacter jejuni* (small intestine) [11]. These associations support the role of an infectious trigger in boosting the expansion of a B-cell clone. However, subsequent stochastic oncogenetic events are necessary to make the clone proliferation in part or fully independent from the initial infectious trigger. Thus, the observation that infection-related NHLs may often respond to the eradication of the infectious trigger, though the expanded B-cell clone persists in tissues (as detected by molecular studies), is not surprising. In addition, the malignant B-cell clone is not directed toward the infectious agent, supporting the concept that autoreactivity is implicated in infection-related B-cell lymphomagenesis [11].

Overall, one can speculate that mechanisms occurring in MALT lesions of SS share some similar pathogenic events in infection-related lymphomagenesis.

27.4 Rheumatoid Factor Specificity of SS-Related Lymphomas

SS-related lymphomas and also a fraction of B-cell lymphomas related to infection (see above) appear to derive from B cells involving immunoglobulin genes associated with autoantibody production [12, 13].

The expansion of anti-SSA/SSB and rheumatoid factor (RF)-positive clones in SS salivary glands is frequently observed also in the absence of a frank lymphoproliferation. In MESA and in B-cell lymphomas in SS, the expanded clones often show a biased VH and Vk gene usage (e.g., VH1-69, VH3-7, VH4-59, Kv325, and Kv328), particularly VDJ combinations (e.g., VH1-69/DP10-D-JH4, VH3/DP54-DH21/9-JH3, VH4/DP71-D2-JH2), and similarity with RF database sequences [13–19].

Interestingly, these sequences are similar to those detected in HCV-related lymphomas [20]. Martin and coworkers documented the B-cell NHLs in SS produced RFs [17]. Overall, malignant B-cell lymphoproliferation in SS does not appear to involve the B-cell clones producing anti-SSA/SSB antibodies, but, rather, the RF autoantibodies.

27.5 B-Cell Expansion in MALT Sites in SS

The development of ectopic lymphoid structures (ELSs) in labial salivary gland biopsies of patients with SS has been well described [21–24]. The definition of ELS is based on the presence of periductal lymphomonocytic cell clusters characterized by T and B lymphocytes and the differentiation of CD21+ follicular dendritic cell (FDC) networks. The hypothesis that the lymphoneogenetic process is controlled by reactivation of pathways physiologically involved in secondary lymphoid organ development is supported by the observation of increased levels of lymphoid chemokines CXCL13 and CCL21 in salivary glands (SGs) of patients with SS with lymphoid features.

The identification of lymphoid chemokines in the SG of SS suggests that alternative cell types may express lymphoid chemokines during chronic inflammation. Importantly, both resident, nonlymphoid cells and infiltrating immune cells have been shown to produce lymphoid chemokines in the target organ. Ductal epithelial cells, together with infiltrating mononuclear cells, were the main source of lymphoid chemokines, supporting the notion that the periductal organization of the lymphoid aggregates in SS might be dependent on chemokine gradients displayed by epithelial cells [25–27]. Thus, growing levels of evidence support that subsets of stromal cells and infiltrating immune cells are critical in the development of ELS in the SG of SS.

Lymphomas are the main cause of increased mortality in SS. Evidences that MALT-NHL development is the result of an antigen-driven immune response comes from the observation that in gastric MALT-NHL malignant marginal zone B-cell proliferation is dependent on *H. pylori*-specific T cells [28, 29], and eradication of *H. pylori* may result in tumor regression [30]. Similarly, in SS, the evidence that a common clonal lineage exists between the polyclonal and later monoclonal B-cell population with progression from lymphoepithelial lesions toward SG and extraglandular MALT-NHLs [14, 15, 31] strongly suggests that SS-MALT-NHL is a multistep antigen-driven process. SS-related MESA and MALT-NHLs of the parotids often display IgVH-CDR3 with RF homology [13, 17, 32], suggesting a cross talk between autoimmunity and lymphomagenesis, potentially supported by a chronic antigenic stimulation.

A study analyzing labial SG biopsies obtained at the time of diagnosis of SS patients who later developed parotid MALT-NHL showed that ELSs were present in over 75 % of these patients several years before malignant transformation [33]. These data were confirmed in a large cohort of SS patients, where the presence of ELS in labial SG at diagnosis conferred a 15-fold increased risk of B-cell lymphoma compared to SS patients with a positive biopsy but without features of ELS [34].

Thus, severe lymphoproliferation of salivary MALT is associated with a higher risk of NHL in SS. This might be detectable in labial salivary gland biopsies at the time of diagnosis by routine light microscopy of H&E sections. The assessment of lymphoid features of labial salivary glands should be routinely performed in SS.

The early identification of lymphoproliferation features would also allow the recognition of a subset of SS patients with a more severe disease phenotype, which would potentially benefit from a more intensive follow-up and treatment [35, 36].

27.6 Cryoglobulinemia Developing: Lessons from HCV-Related Cryoglobulinemia

In HCV-related cryoglobulinemic vasculitis, HCV infection triggers the expansion of RF-positive clones. Why this preferentially occurs in the course of HCV infection, when compared to other chronic infections, is still controversial. A study demonstrated that RFs in HCV-related cryoglobulins also recognize the HCV epitope NS3 and reported that NS3 HCV peptide can induce the production of an anti-HCV antibody with RF capacity [37]. These observations support a possible mechanism for infections in triggering autoimmunity, i.e., a double antibody reactivity or a mechanism of molecular mimicry.

Cryoglobulinemia detection is a red flag for lymphoma. Indeed, nearly a half of SS patients with lymphoma present with circulating cryoglobulins, also in the absence of HCV infection. The identification of other triggers in SS deserves additional study.

27.7 The Clinical Picture of Cryoglobulinemic Vasculitis in SS

New classification criteria for cryoglobulinemic vasculitis (CV) have been recently published [38] and validated [39] (Table 27.1). The presence of serum mixed cryoglobulinemia, i.e., serum positivity of cryoglobulins, occurs in about 10–15 % patients with SS [38], while a frank clinical CV is less frequent, though it greatly affects the SS-related morbidity [40].

The biologic and, to some extent, the clinical characteristics of HCV-unrelated CV may be different from HCV-related CV. A sub-analysis of the sensitivity and the specificity of the CV classification criteria was performed in 55 SS patients carrying serum cryoglobulins with or without the clinical picture of CV (CwV) [41]. This sub-analysis demonstrated that sensitivity and specificity of the classification criteria for the CV in SS patients were high: 88.9 % and 91.3 %, respectively [41]. No statistical differences between SS-CV and SS-CwV patients were observed as regard to clinical features of lymphoproliferation, including lymphadenopathy, splenomegaly, salivary gland swelling, lacrimal gland swelling, and B symptoms, while the prevalence of a lymphoproliferative disorder per se was more frequent in CV than in CwV (nonmalignant lymphoproliferative disorder in 13/29 in CV vs.

Table 27.1 Classification criteria for cryoglobulinemic vasculitis

(i) *Questionnaire item*: at least 2 out of the following:	
Do you remember one or more episodes of small red spots on your skin, particularly involving the lower limbs?	
Have you ever had red spots on your lower extremities, which leave a brownish color after their disappearance?	
Has a doctor ever told you that you have viral hepatitis?	
(ii) *Clinical item*: at least 3 out of the following 4 (present or past):	
Constitutional symptoms	Fatigue
	Low-grade fever (37–37.9 °C, >10 days, no other cause)
	Fever (>38 °C, no other cause)
	Fibromyalgia
Articular involvement	Arthralgias
	Arthritis
Vascular involvement	Purpura
	Skin ulcers
	Necrotizing vasculitis
	Hyperviscosity syndrome
	Raynaud's phenomenon
Neurologic involvement	Peripheral neuropathy
	Cranial nerve involvement
	Vasculitic CNS involvement
(iii) *Laboratory item*: at least 2 out of the following 3 (present)[a]:	
Low serum C4	
Presence of serum rheumatoid factor	
Presence of serum monoclonal component	

Satisfied if at least two out of three items (questionnaire, clinical, laboratory) are positive. The patient must be positive for serum cryoglobulins in at least two determinations at ≥12-week interval

CNS central nervous system

[a]The fulfillment of the laboratory item in a patient satisfying the criteria highlights the possible presence of cryoglobulinemic vasculitis even in the absence of serum cryoglobulins by initial testing

4/26 in CwV, malignant lymphoma in 10/29 CV vs. 3/26 CwV). Furthermore, as compared to SS-CwV, SS-CV was more frequently characterized by the presence of type II cryoglobulinemia and NHL [42].

Skin vasculitis in the course of SS was deeply investigated by a recent Italian collaborative network of rheumatologic centers [43]. A total of 652 SS patients were examined, and cryoglobulinemic purpura was well differentiated from hypergammaglobulinemic purpura. Peripheral neuropathy, low C4, leukopenia, serum monoclonal component, and the presence of anti-SSB/La antibodies characterized CV, whereas RF, leukopenia, serum monoclonal component, and anti-SSA/Ro antibodies were significantly associated with hypergammaglobulinemic purpura. A lymphoma was associated only with CV. While hypergammaglobulinemic purpura in SS seems to be related to a benign B-cell proliferation, CV seems to be a systemic immune complex-mediated vasculitis with complement activation and a high risk of lymphoma. CV, but not hypergammaglobulinemic purpura, can be envisaged in SS as a prelymphomatous condition [43].

27.8 Relationship between SS-Associated Cryoglobulinemia and MALT Lymphoproliferation

B-cell NHL is a well-described complication in a subset of patients with CV secondary to HCV infection [44]. However, CV may also occur in HCV-negative patients, including subjects with SS. Of note, HCV-related CV and SS-associated HCV-unrelated CV are both associated with mixed cryoglobulinemia and predispose to B-cell NHL.

While lymphomas complicating the course of HCV-related CV usually involve the bone marrow [44, 45], B-cell NHL complicating the course of SS usually involves the MALT sites [1, 7, 31, 46].

Cryoglobulinemia appears to be linked to MALT lymphoproliferation in SS and shows a different biologic background when compared to HCV-associated cryoglobulinemia.

Recently, our group further elucidated this aspect [47]. First, molecular analyses of bone marrow B-cell clonal expansion were performed in consecutive SS cases with mixed HCV-unrelated cryoglobulinemia and compared with classical HCV-associated CV patients without SS. A polyclonal pattern was more frequently observed in SS patients with type II or type III mixed cryoglobulinemia, while a B-cell oligo-/monoclonal expansion was more frequently detected in HCV-related CV. Furthermore, the bone marrow was rarely involved in SS-related lymphomas supporting the crucial role of chronic inflammation and lymphoproliferation of salivary MALT in predisposing to lymphoma [34, 47]. Lastly, in the patient with SS, CV, and parotid B-cell NHL of MALT, bilateral parotidectomy results in a decrease in serum RF and cryoglobulins, implying a critical role of salivary MALT for the production of cryoglobulins [47].

27.9 Upregulation of B-Lymphocyte Stimulator and Lymphoproliferation

The B-lymphocyte stimulator (BLyS), also called B-cell activating factor (BAFF), was identified in 1999. Transgenic mice overexpressing BLyS developed critical lymphoid proliferation in blood and in the marginal zones of lymph nodes and high titers of immunoglobulins and autoantibodies, such as RF, anti-DNA antibodies, and sometimes cryoglobulins. As these mice aged, they also developed a lupus-like glomerulonephritis or a Sjögren's-like syndrome (with salivary gland inflammatory infiltration) and eventually a B-cell lymphoma [48–50].

Consonant with these observations, high levels of BLyS in the serum and/or in the affected tissue have been detected in SS and in CV [51–53]. Furthermore, a strong BLyS upregulation has been in SS associated with lymphoproliferation, either nonmalignant or malignant [54]. In addition, anti-BLyS therapy with belimumab proved to be effective in a preliminary open study in 30 patients with primary SS, all anti-SSA or anti-SSB positive [55, 56]. These observations strongly support pathogenetic implication of BLyS in SS.

Of note, anti-CD20 therapy with rituximab may not deplete the B-cell infiltrate in the SS salivary tissue [57]. Indeed, the local expression of BLyS in the MALT tissue is crucial for tissue resistance to B-cell depletion as shown in a murine model [58].

Rituximab or belimumab alone is ineffective in inducing a regression of low-grade parotid lymphoma of MALT. However, we recently reported that only a sequential use of rituximab preceded by belimumab resulted in a regression of low-grade parotid lymphoma of MALT [59]. One can speculate that, being effective on MALT, the sequential or combined use of anti-BlyS and anti-CD20 therapy might be effective not only in severe SS but also on sicca manifestations in this disease [59].

Conclusions

In SS, the local MALT microenvironment sustains the local expansion of B cells. A first pathogenic trigger, such as an infection, may lead to local inflammation, which in turn stirs up an autoimmune process.

The chronic stimulation of RF-positive B cells in the MALT microenvironment causes their preferential expansion in SS, leading to an increased risk for B-cell lymphoma. Lymphoma transformation may occur when stochastic oncogenetic events occur. The RF produced by the B-cell clones, either nonneoplastic or neoplastic, may behave as a cryoglobulin and possibly lead to a concomitant vasculitis.

SS can be then considered both an autoimmune and a lymphoproliferative disorder.

Future studies focusing on SS-related B-cell lymphoproliferation may contribute to identify the key pathogenetic events and to develop new therapeutic strategies in SS.

References

1. Anderson LG, Talal N (1971) The spectrum of benign to malignant lymphoproliferation in Sjögren's syndrome. Clin Exp Immunol 9:199–221
2. Talal N (1989–1990) Sjögren's syndrome. Curr Opin Immunol 2(4):622–624
3. Mitsias DI, Kapsogeorgou EK, Moutsopoulos HM (2006) The role of epithelial cells in the initiation and perpetuation of autoimmune lesions: lessons from Sjögren's syndrome (autoimmune epithelitis). Lupus 15(5):255–261
4. Tzioufas AG (1996) B-cell lymphoproliferation in primary Sjögren's syndrome. Clin Exp Rheumatol 14(Suppl 14):S65–S70
5. Tzioufas AG, Katsikis PD, Youinou PY, Moutsopoulos HM (1990) Sjögren's syndrome: an oligo-monoclonal B cell process. Clin Exp Rheumatol 8(Suppl 5):17–21

6. Campo E, Swerdlow SH, Harris NL, Pileri S, Stein H, Jaffe ES (2011) The 2008 WHO classification of lymphoid neoplasms and beyond: evolving concepts and practical applications. Blood 117(19):5019–5032
7. De Vita S, De Marchi G, Sacco S, Gremese E, Fabris M, Ferraccioli G (2001) Preliminary classification of nonmalignant B cell proliferation in Sjögren's syndrome: perspectives on pathobiology and treatment based on an integrated clinico-pathologic and molecular study approach. Blood Cells Mol Dis 27(4):757–766
8. Wotherspoon AC, Doglioni C, Isaacson PG (1992) Low-grade gastric B-cell lymphoma of mucosa-associated lymphoid tissue (MALT): a multifocal disease. Histopathology 20(1):29–34
9. Burke JS (1999) Are there site-specific differences among the MALT lymphomas – morphologic, clinical? Am J Clin Pathol 111(1 Suppl 1):S133–S143
10. Krishnan J, Danon AD, Frizzera G (1993) Reactive lymphadenopathies and atypical lymphoproliferative disorders. Am J Clin Pathol 99(4):385–396
11. Zucca E, Bertoni F, Vannata B, Cavalli F (2014) Emerging role of infectious etiologies in the pathogenesis of marginal zone B-cell lymphomas. Clin Cancer Res 20(20):5207–5216
12. De Vita S, Pivetta B, Ferraccioli GF et al (1997) Immunoglobulin gene usage and somatic mutations in primary Sjögren's syndrome-associated monoclonal B-cell lymphoproliferation, prelymphomatous and frankly malignant. J Rheumatol 24:36 [abstract]
13. De Vita S, Boiocchi M, Sorrentino D et al (1997) Characterization of prelymphomatous stages of B cell lymphoproliferation in Sjögren's syndrome. Arthritis Rheum 40(2):318–331
14. Bahler DW, Swerdlow SH (1998) Clonal salivary gland infiltrates associated with myoepithelial sialadenitis (Sjögren's syndrome) begin as nonmalignant antigen-selected expansions. Blood 91(6):1864–1872
15. Gasparotto D, Pivetta B, De Re V et al (2000) B-cell lymphoproliferation in primary Sjögren's syndrome: an antigen driven expansion employing rheumatoid factor-encoding genes. Clin Exp Rheumatol 18:131
16. Miklos JA, Swerdlow SH, Bahler DW (2000) Salivary gland mucosa-associated lymphoid tissue lymphoma immunoglobulin V (H) genes show frequent use of V1-69 with distinctive CDR3 features. Blood 95(12):3878–3884
17. Martin T, Weber JC, Levallois H et al (2000) Salivary gland lymphomas in patients with Sjögren's syndrome may frequently develop from rheumatoid factor B cells. Arthritis Rheum 43(4):908–916
18. Anderson LG, Cummings NA, Asofsky R et al (1972) Salivary gland immunoglobulin and rheumatoid factor synthesis in Sjögren's syndrome. Natural history and response to treatment. Am J Med 53(4):456–463
19. Kipps TJ, Tomhave E, Chen PP, Fox RI (1989) Molecular characterization of a major autoantibody-associated cross-reactive idiotype in Sjögren's syndrome. J Immunol 142:4261–4268
20. De Re V, De Vita S, Gasparotto D et al (2002) Salivary gland B cell lymphoproliferative disorders in Sjögren's syndrome present a restricted use of antigen receptor gene segments similar to those used by hepatitis C virus-associated non-Hodgkins's lymphomas. Eur J Immunol 32(3):903–910
21. Stott DI, Hiepe F, Hummel M, Steinhauser G, Berek C (1998) Antigen-driven clonal proliferation of B cells within the target tissue of an autoimmune disease. The salivary glands of patients with Sjögren's syndrome. J Clin Invest 102(5):938–946
22. Aziz KE, McCluskey PJ, Wakefield D (1997) Characterisation of follicular dendritic cells in labial salivary glands of patients with primary Sjögren's syndrome: comparison with tonsillar lymphoid follicles. Ann Rheum Dis 56(2):140–143
23. Jonsson MV, Skarstein K, Jonsson R, Brun JG (2007) Serological implications of germinal center-like structures in primary Sjögren's syndrome. J Rheumatol 34(10):2044–2049
24. Barone F, Bombardieri M, Manzo A et al (2005) Association of CXCL13 and CCL21 expression with the progressive organization of lymphoid-like structures in Sjögren's syndrome. Arthritis Rheum 52(6):1773–1784

25. Xanthou G, Polihronis M, Tzioufas AG, Paikos S, Sideras P, Moutsopoulos HM (2001) "Lymphoid" chemokine messenger RNA expression by epithelial cells in the chronic inflammatory lesion of the salivary glands of Sjögren's syndrome patients: possible participation in lymphoid structure formation. Arthritis Rheum 44(2):408–418
26. Amft N, Curnow SJ, Scheel-Toellner D et al (2001) Ectopic expression of the B cell-attracting chemokine BCA-1 (CXCL13) on endothelial cells and within lymphoid follicles contributes to the establishment of germinal center-like structures in Sjögren's syndrome. Arthritis Rheum 44(11):2633–2641
27. Baekkevold ES, Yamanaka T, Palframan RT et al (2001) The CCR7 ligand elc (CCL19) is transcytosed in high endothelial venules and mediates T cell recruitment. J Exp Med 193(9):1105–1112
28. Hussell T, Isaacson PG, Crabtree JE, Spencer J (1996) Helicobacter pylori-specific tumour-infiltrating T cells provide contact dependent help for the growth of malignant B cells in low-grade gastric lymphoma of mucosa-associated lymphoid tissue. J Pathol 178(2):122–127
29. Isaacson PG, Du MQ (2005) Gastrointestinal lymphoma: where morphology meets molecular biology. J Pathol 205(2):255–274
30. Wohrer S, Troch M, Raderer M (2007) Therapy of gastric mucosa-associated lymphoid tissue lymphoma. Expert Opin Pharmacother 8(9):1263–1273
31. Gasparotto D, De Vita S, De Re V et al (2003) Extrasalivary lymphoma development in Sjögren's syndrome: clonal evolution from parotid gland lymphoproliferation and role of local triggering. Arthritis Rheum 48:3181–3186
32. Bende RJ, Aarts WM, Riedl RG, de Jong D, Pals ST, van Noesel CJ (2005) Among B cell non-Hodgkin's lymphomas, MALT lymphomas express a unique antibody repertoire with frequent rheumatoid factor reactivity. J Exp Med 201(8):1229–1241
33. Bombardieri M, Barone F, Humby F et al (2007) Activation-induced cytidine deaminase expression in follicular dendritic cell networks and interfollicular large B cells supports functionality of ectopic lymphoid neogenesis in autoimmune sialoadenitis and MALT lymphoma in Sjögren's syndrome. J Immunol 179(7):4929–4938
34. Theander E, Vasaitis L, Baecklund E et al (2011) Lymphoid organisation in labial salivary gland biopsies is a possible predictor for the development of malignant lymphoma in primary Sjögren's syndrome. Ann Rheum Dis 70(8):1363–1368
35. Carubbi F, Alunno A, Cipriani P et al (2015) A retrospective, multicenter study evaluating the prognostic value of minor salivary gland histology in a large cohort of patients with primary Sjögren's syndrome. Lupus 24(3):315–320
36. Baldini C, Pepe P, Quartuccio L et al (2014) Primary Sjögren's syndrome as a multi-organ disease: impact of the serological profile on the clinical presentation of the disease in a large cohort of Italian patients. Rheumatology (Oxford) 53(5):839–844
37. De Re V, Sansonno D, Simula MP et al (2006) HCV-NS3 and IgG-Fc crossreactive IgM in patients with type II mixed cryoglobulinemia and B-cell clonal proliferations. Leukemia 20(6):1145–1154
38. De Vita S, Soldano F, Isola M et al (2011) Preliminary classification criteria for the cryoglobulinaemic vasculitis. Ann Rheum Dis 70(7):1183–1190
39. Quartuccio L, Isola M, Corazza L et al (2014) Validation of the classification criteria for cryoglobulinaemic vasculitis. Rheumatology (Oxford) 53(12):2209–2213
40. Baimpa E, Dahabreh IJ, Voulgarelis M, Moutsopoulos HM (2009) Hematologic manifestations and predictors of lymphoma development in primary Sjögren syndrome: clinical and pathophysiologic aspects. Medicine (Baltimore) 88:284–293
41. Quartuccio L, Isola M, Corazza L et al (2012) Performance of the preliminary classification criteria for cryoglobulinaemic vasculitis and clinical manifestations in hepatitis C virus-unrelated cryoglobulinaemic vasculitis. Clin Exp Rheumatol 30(1 Suppl 70):S48–S52
42. Quartuccio L, Corazza L, Monti G et al (2011) Lymphoma prevalence in patients with serum cryoglobulins with or without cryoglobulinemic vasculitis: data extrapolated from the cryoglobulinemic vasculitis classification criteria database. Arthritis Rheumatol 63(10):S597

43. Quartuccio L, Isola M, Baldini C et al (2015) Clinical and biological differences between cryoglobulinaemic and hypergammaglobulinaemic purpura in primary Sjögren's syndrome: results of a large multicentre study. Scand J Rheumatol 44(1):36–41
44. Monti G, Pioltelli P, Saccardo F et al (2005) Incidence and characteristics of non-Hodgkin lymphomas in a multicenter case file of patients with hepatitis C virus-related symptomatic mixed cryoglobulinemias. Arch Intern Med 165:101–105
45. Mazzaro C, De Re V, Spina M et al (2009) Pegylated-interferon plus ribavirin for HCV-positive indolent non-Hodgkin lymphomas. Br J Haematol 145:255–257
46. Voulgarelis M, Dafni UG, Isenberg DA, Moutsopoulos HM (1999) Malignant lymphoma in primary Sjogren's syndrome: a multicenter, retrospective, clinical study by the European concerted action on Sjögren's syndrome. Arthritis Rheum 42:1765–1772
47. De Vita S, Quartuccio L, Salvin S, Corazza L, Zabotti A, Fabris M (2012) Cryoglobulinaemia related to Sjogren's syndrome or HCV infection: differences based on the pattern of bone marrow involvement, lymphoma evolution and laboratory tests after parotidectomy. Rheumatology (Oxford) 51(4):627–633
48. Mackay F, Woodcock SA, Lawton P et al (1990) Mice transgenic for BAFF develop lymphocytic disorders along with autoimmune manifestations. J Exp Med 190(11):1697–1710
49. Batten M, Fletcher C, Ng LG et al (2004) TNF deficiency fails to protect BAFF transgenic mice against autoimmunity and reveals a predisposition to B cell lymphoma. J Immunol 172(2):812–822
50. Groom J, Kalled SL, Cutler AH et al (2002) Association of BAFF/BLyS overexpression and altered B cell differentiation with Sjögren's syndrome. J Clin Invest 109(1):59–68
51. Cheema GS, Roschke V, Hilbert DM, Stohl W (2001) Elevated serum B lymphocyte stimulator levels in patients with systemic immune-based rheumatic diseases. Arthritis Rheum 44:1313–1319
52. Mariette X, Roux S, Zhang J et al (2003) The level of BLyS (BAFF) correlates with the titre of autoantibodies in human Sjögren's syndrome. Ann Rheum Dis 62(2):168–171
53. Fabris M, Quartuccio L, Sacco S et al (2007) B-Lymphocyte stimulator (BLyS) up-regulation in mixed cryoglobulinaemia syndrome and hepatitis-C virus infection. Rheumatology (Oxford) 46(1):37–43
54. Quartuccio L, Salvin S, Fabris M et al (2013) BLyS upregulation in Sjögren's syndrome associated with lymphoproliferative disorders, higher ESSDAI score and B-cell clonal expansion in the salivary glands. Rheumatology (Oxford) 52(2):276–281
55. Mariette X, Seror R, Quartuccio L et al (2015) Efficacy and safety of belimumab in primary Sjögren's syndrome: results of the BELISS open-label phase II study. Ann Rheum Dis 74(3):526–531
56. De Vita S, Quartuccio L, Seror R, et al (2015) Efficacy and safety of belimumab given for 12 months in primary Sjögren's syndrome: the BELISS open-label phase II study. Rheumatology (Oxford). pii: kev257. [Epub ahead of print]
57. De Vita S, De Marchi G, Sacco S, Zaja F, Scott CA, Ferraccioli G (2002) Treatment of B-cell disorders of MALT in Sjögren's syndrome with anti-CD20 monoclonal antibody. In: Proceedings of the 8th International Symposium on Sjögren's Syndrome; Kanazawa, Japan. pp 51. P8-2
58. Gong Q, Ou Q, Ye S et al (2005) Importance of cellular microenvironment and circulatory dynamics in B cell immunotherapy. J Immunol 174(2):817–826
59. De Vita S, Quartuccio L, Salvin S et al (2014) Sequential therapy with belimumab followed by rituximab in Sjögren's syndrome associated with B-cell lymphoproliferation and overexpression of BAFF: evidence for long-term efficacy. Clin Exp Rheumatol 32(4):490–494

Systemic Therapy of Sjögren Syndrome 28

Soledad Retamozo, Pilar Brito-Zerón, Hoda Gheitasi, Verónica Saurit, and Manuel Ramos-Casals

28.1 Introduction

Sjögren syndrome (SS) is a systemic autoimmune disease with a wide clinical spectrum that extends from sicca symptoms of the mucosal surfaces to extraglandular manifestations. The histological hallmark of the disease is focal lymphocytic infiltration of the exocrine glands, as shown in minor labial salivary gland biopsy [1]. The main clinical features (dry mouth and dry eyes) are determined by specific oral (salivary flow measurement, parotid scintigraphy) and ocular (fluorescein staining, Schirmer test) tests, respectively [2]. SS patients may develop a large number of

S. Retamozo
Department of Rheumatology, Hospital Privado Centro Médico de Córdoba, Postgraduate Career of Rheumatology Catholic University of Córdoba, Institute University of Biomedical Sciences University of Córdoba (IUCBC), Córdoba, Argentina

Sjögren Syndrome Research Group (AGAUR), Laboratory of Autoimmune Diseases Josep Font, CELLEX-IDIBAPS, Department of Autoimmune Diseases, ICMiD, Hospital Clínic Barcelona, Barcelona, Spain
e-mail: soleretamozo@hotmail.com

P. Brito-Zerón • H. Gheitasi • M. Ramos-Casals (✉)
Sjögren Syndrome Research Group (AGAUR), Laboratory of Autoimmune Diseases Josep Font, CELLEX-IDIBAPS, Department of Autoimmune Diseases, ICMiD, Hospital Clínic Barcelona, Barcelona, Spain
e-mail: mramos@clinic.ub.es

V. Saurit
Department of Rheumatology, Hospital Privado Centro Médico de Córdoba, Postgraduate Career of Rheumatology Catholic University of Córdoba, Institute University of Biomedical Sciences University of Córdoba (IUCBC), Córdoba, Argentina
e-mail: vsaurit@gmail.com

D. Roccatello, L. Emmi (eds.), *Connective Tissue Disease: A Comprehensive Guide-Volume 1*, Rare Diseases of the Immune System 5, DOI 10.1007/978-3-319-24535-5_28

systemic manifestations [3], either as the presenting manifestation or during the evolution. While sicca features primarily affect the quality of life and cause local complications in the mucosa involved, systemic or extraglandular involvement marks the disease prognosis [4]. In addition, patients present a broad spectrum of analytical features (mainly cytopenias) and a plethora of autoantibodies, of which antinuclear antibodies are the most frequently detected, anti-Ro/SS-A the most specific, and cryoglobulins and hypocomplementemia the main prognostic markers. The main complication of the disease is the development of B-cell lymphoma, with a risk 10–40 times higher than that found in the general population [5].

Treatment of primary SS is based on symptomatic management of sicca manifestations and broad-spectrum immunosuppression for extraglandular disease [6]. Over the last decade, research has centered on new therapies with the hope of providing better management approaches [7]. The emergence of biological therapies has recently increased the therapeutic armamentarium available to treat SS, but their use is still limited by the lack of licensing [8]. This chapter summarizes the current pharmacotherapy options and future directions on systemic-targeted therapies in patients with primary SS.

28.2 The Importance of Systemic Disease in Primary SS

28.2.1 Systemic Versus Nonsystemic Involvement

A large percentage of primary SS patients have no systemic involvement, with a clinical pattern totally dominated by the triad of severe dryness, fatigue, and pain, which are not life threatening but have a serious impact on the quality of life [9]. The poor correlation between systemic disease and this triad of symptoms is clearly demonstrated by the lack of correlation between the two EULAR indexes (systemic EULAR-SS disease activity index – ESSDAI – and the patient-orientated EULAR Sjögren's Syndrome Patient Reported Index – ESSPRI) [10] and the results of some recent studies [11–13].

Systemic involvement plays a key role in the prognosis of primary SS. Some recent studies, including more than 2500 European patients, have confirmed that primary SS is, undeniably, a systemic disease [10, 14, 15]. Seror et al. [10] found that 70 % of patients had a history of systemic involvement at enrollment, and Baldini et al. [15] found severe systemic disease in 15 % of patients, especially in those with an immunological profile suggestive of B-cell activation.

28.2.2 Systemic Disease and Prognostic Classification

Ioannidis et al. [16] were the first to propose a prognostic classification of primary SS, dividing patients into two groups according to the presence or absence of factors. The main factors reported in prospective studies include parotid involvement, vasculitis, hypocomplementemia, and cryoglobulins [8]. Baldini et al. [15] have recently identified hypergammaglobulinemia, rheumatoid factor (RF), hypocomplementemia, and cryoglobulinemia as prognostic factors. A practical message for clinical practice is that patients with this "high-risk" presentation should receive a closer follow-up and, probably, an earlier and more robust therapeutic management [17].

28.2.3 Characterization of Systemic Disease in Primary SS

The development of the ESSDAI [18] by the EULAR task force on SS represents a step forward in the evaluation of systemic Sjögren [10, 14]. Systemic involvement has been evaluated using the organ-by-organ ESSDAI definitions in nearly 1000 Spanish patients [14], and, in more than 80 %, the score at diagnosis indicated systemic activity (score ≥1), with the joints, lungs, skin, and peripheral nerves being the most-frequent organs involved, while cytopenias, hypocomplementemia, and cryoglobulinemia were the laboratory abnormalities most-often associated with systemic Sjögren [14]. In addition, a recent study [17] has found that patients who present at diagnosis with high systemic activity (ESSDAI ≥14) and/or predictive immunological markers (especially those with more than one) are at higher risk of death. These studies, together with the robust results demonstrated by the validation study [18], confirm the ESSDAI as a solid instrument for the measurement of systemic activity in the daily practice.

28.3 Therapeutic Management of General Symptoms

28.3.1 Nonbiological Agents

More than 80 % of patients with primary SS present muscle and joint pain, fatigue, and weakness, which may have a much greater impact on the quality of life than sicca features. In these patients, the first step should be a differential diagnosis with associated processes such as hypothyroidism, neoplasia, depression, and, especially, fibromyalgia, which is reported in nearly one third of primary SS patients [19, 20]. After discarding these processes, hydroxychloroquine may be a keystone drug, with clinical benefits being reported beyond fatigue and musculoskeletal pain; uncontrolled studies found additional improvements in subjective and objective sicca features, reduction in parotid enlargement and oral infections, and improvement in analytical and immunological parameters. However, a recent clinical trial [21] found that the use of hydroxychloroquine in comparison with placebo did not improve the main symptoms (dryness, fatigue, and pain) during 24 weeks of treatment. Further studies are needed to evaluate longer-term outcomes of hydroxychloroquine for general symptoms.

28.3.2 Biological Agents

The four biological agents tested in primary SS have been associated with some improvements in fatigue (including one small randomized controlled trial [RCT]) using rituximab (RTX). The results of a large multicenter RCT have recently shown limited benefits for general symptoms. Devauchelle-Pensec et al. [22] evaluated 122 consecutive patients who were assigned to receive either RTX infusions (1 g) or placebo at weeks 0 and 2. The primary end point was improvement (≥30 mm) of two of four visual analogue scale (VAS) that evaluate dryness, pain, fatigue, and global health between weeks 0 and 24. For the composite primary end point, 13/60 (22 %) patients treated with RTX had a favorable overall response in comparison with 11/53 (21 %) patients who received placebo. Statistically significant differences were found in some secondary end points including sicca and fatigue VAS and salivary flow rate, but not in objective measurements (Schirmer test, salivary gland biopsy) or ESSDAI score. We consider that the off-label use of biologics to treat only general symptoms (even when severe) is not warranted.

28.4 Therapeutic Management of Extraglandular Involvement

28.4.1 Nonbiological Agents

As a general rule, the management of extraglandular features in primary SS should be organ specific, mainly using corticosteroids and immunosuppressive agents [1, 4, 8]. However, the main studies analyzing the effects of immunosuppressive agents in primary SS (overwhelmingly uncontrolled) are designed to evaluate their effects on sicca rather than systemic features and have shown poor results with an excess of adverse events.

Some retrospective studies have specifically analyzed the use of corticosteroids and immunosuppressive agents in organ-specific involvements. These studies support the use of corticosteroids and cyclophosphamide in myelitis, azathioprine in interstitial lung disease, and methotrexate in joint involvement [23]. Evidence for the therapeutic management of other extraglandular SS features relies on isolated case reports or small case series [1, 4, 8] suggesting the use of cyclophosphamide for glomerulonephritis, vasculitis, multineuritis and central nervous system (CNS) involvement, and intravenous immunoglobulins for axonal and ataxic neuropathies [1, 4, 8].

In contrast, some extraglandular features, such as interstitial nephritis or ataxic neuronopathy, seem to have a poor response to corticosteroids and immunosuppressive agents [23]. Given the low level of evidence, the choice of drugs for organ-by-organ management is usually heavily influenced by therapeutic strategies accepted in clinically similar, but etiopathogenically different, diseases, such as systemic lupus erythematosus (SLE) or systemic vasculitis.

28.4.2 Biological Agents

The amount and quality of evidence on the off-label use of RTX in SS-related extraglandular features is higher than that reported for the use of the standard options (corticosteroids and immunosuppressive agents), although a reasonable assessment of the risk of serious adverse events versus the potential benefits of treatment should be always made on an individual basis.

The majority of uncontrolled studies have retrospectively collected the results of the use of RTX in real-life patients with extraglandular involvement and have found a clinical response in >80 % of patients with systemic involvement, a significant improvement in several immunological parameters, and a reduction in the mean daily corticosteroid dose [22, 24–28]. More than 20 uncontrolled studies have evaluated the use of RTX in patients with primary SS, including open-label prospective studies [25, 27, 29] and retrospective studies evaluating either systemic involvement or B-cell lymphoma [8, 28, 30–38]. The first study was conducted in 2005 by Gottenberg et al. [30] in six patients with primary SS treated with RTX and reported therapeutic efficacy in five with extraglandular features, with lowering of corticosteroid dosage in four out of five patients. In 2007, Seror et al. [28] made a retrospective analysis of 16 patients with primary SS who received RTX for lymphoma ($n=5$) or systemic manifestations ($n=11$); treatment efficacy was observed in 9 of these 11 patients, with corticosteroid doses being lowered in all cases. Vasil'ev et al. [32] reported the use of RTX in four patients with systemic manifestations, of whom three (75 %) responded to RTX (no response was observed in a patient with cryoglobulinemic glomerulonephritis).

Three multicenter national registries that collected patients with SAD treated with RTX have included patients with primary SS. The BIOGEAS Spanish registry [8, 26] included 16 patients with systemic manifestations, including peripheral neuropathies ($n=5$), CNS involvement ($n=3$), autoimmune cytopenias ($n=3$), refractory arthritis ($n=1$), protein-losing enteropathy ($n=1$), and myasthenia gravis ($n=1$); only three patients with systemic features had no therapeutic response (arthritis, glomerulonephritis, and CNS involvement, respectively). In the Germany GRAID registry [33], four patients with primary SS were included (two had a complete response and the other two a partial response). However, the larger uncontrolled study that has evaluated the therapeutic efficacy of RTX on systemic Sjögren [31] has evaluated the results obtained in 74 patients (42 had more than 1 systemic involvement), including mainly articular involvement ($n=27$), peripheral neuropathies ($n=12$), vasculitis ($n=8$), and pulmonary involvement ($n=9$). At 6 months after the first cycle of RTX, therapeutic response assessed by the global opinion of the physician was observed in 60 % of cases. The ESSDAI score decreased from 11 to 7.5, and the mean daily dose of prednisone decreased from 17.6 to 10.8 mg. No significant differences were found according to the presence of anti-Ro/La antibodies or the concomitant use of immunosuppressant agents. Zhou et al. [34] have reported the successful use of low-dose RTX (100 mg in weeks 0 and 1) combined with high-dose oral prednisone (1–2 mg/kg/day) in four patients with primary SS and severe refractory thrombocytopenia.

28.5 Therapeutic Management of Severe Systemic Involvement

Severe, life-threatening involvement has rarely been reported in primary SS. In nine studies including 2241 patients with primary SS in which mortality rates and causes of death were detailed, only 17 patients died due to SS-related systemic involvement, representing only 8 % of the 221 reported deaths [39]. A recent multicenter study [17] have analyzed the main causes of death in 115 patients, including cardiovascular disease in 35 patients, infections in 21, systemic disease in 18, and hematological neoplasia in 10; survival at 5, 10, 20. and 30 years was 96.0 %, 90.5 %, 80.9 %, and 60.4 %, respectively. The main baseline factors associated with mortality caused by systemic disease were active disease at diagnosis, cytopenias, monoclonal gammopathy, cryoglobulins, and hypocomplementemia.

Vasculitis (overwhelmingly cryoglobulinemic) is the main cause of life-threatening presentation of primary SS, involving vital organs such as the kidneys, the lungs, and the gastrointestinal tract. Other severe involvements included CNS features, progressive ataxic neuronopathy, pulmonary arterial hypertension, and severe cytopenia [3]. Two recent studies have focused on the efficacy and safety of RTX in SS-related neurological involvement. The first study found stabilization or improvement of CNS involvement in 7/11 (64 %) patients treated with RTX [35]. The second study found a better response to RTX in 17 patients with vasculitic neuropathy in comparison with those with non-vasculitic neuropathy [36]. RTX was effective in 9/10 (90 %) patients in comparison with only 2 (29 %) of the non-vasculitic 7 patients.

There are no controlled studies evaluating the therapeutic management of SS patients with life-threatening conditions; at present, there are only some retrospective studies (with <10 patients) and isolated case reports. However, this scarce evidence, taken together with expert review, suggests that methylprednisolone and cyclophosphamide pulses should be used in patients with severe systemic vasculitis or CNS involvement, with plasma exchange being added in the most severe situations [3]. RTX is increasingly reported as a promising therapy, not only in patients with life-threatening situations but also in those with associated B-cell lymphoma [3].

28.6 Therapeutic Guidelines for Systemic Sjögren

For the treatment of severe systemic SS, a combination of glucocorticosteroids and immunosuppressive agents is the classical approach, in spite of the very limited level of scientific evidence supporting their use. However, this approach is often associated with adverse events, and there is growing awareness of infections and cardiovascular involvement in these patients. Systemic life-threatening involvement has rarely been reported in primary SS [6] with cryoglobulinemic vasculitis (involving the kidneys, lungs, or gastrointestinal tract) being the main cause of severe SS presentation [5]. Other severe involvements unrelated to cryoglobulinemia include myelitis, ataxic neuronopathy, and pulmonary arterial hypertension [35]. Therapeutic recommendations are often based on the use of methylprednisolone and cyclophosphamide pulses, with plasma exchange being added in the most severe situations [19].

In the last years, biological therapies have emerged as new therapeutic agents that are increasingly used for systemic primary SS (Table 28.1). B-cell targeted therapies are the most promising agents in primary SS, although their use is significantly limited by the current lack of specific licensing. RTX has been used in more

Table 28.1 Studies evaluating rituximab in patients with primary SS: systemic outcomes

					Outcomes (improvement/total patients)				
Author (year)	N (female)	Mean age (years)	Study design (duration)	Therapeutic regimen (dose)	Systemic features	Lymphoma	ESSDAI score	Prednisone	Serological response
Pijpe et al. (2005)	15 (14)	50	Prospective 12 weeks	375 mg/m^2 Weeks: 0, 1, 2, 3	–	MALT-type lymphoma (parotid gland)	–	Not allowed during the study (except in patients with severe extraglandular manifestations)	Peripheral B cells: reduction in 12/14 IgM-RF levels: reduction in 5 with MALT/ primary SS Levels of IgG, IgA, IgM, 2-microglobulin: stable in all patients HACAs: 4/15 (27 %)
Gottenberg et al. (2005)	6 (6)	57	Retrospective (8 m)	Weeks: 0, 1, 2, 3 (5 cases) Weeks: 0, 1 (1 case) (375 mg/m^2)	Vasculitis (2/2) Parotid + arthritis (2/2)	MALT (1/2)	–	Dose reduction in 4/5 patients	RF titer reduction (4/4) Cryo negativiz (2/2)
Devauchelle-Pensec et al. (2007)	16 (14)	55	Prospective 36 weeks	375 mg/m^2 Weeks: 0, 1	Resolution pulmonary involve ($n=1$)	ND	–	–	RF reduction (0.04)

(continued)

Table 28.1 (continued)

					Outcomes (improvement/total patients)				
Author (year)	N (female)	Mean age (years)	Study design (duration)	Therapeutic regimen (dose)	Systemic features	Lymphoma	ESSDAI score	Prednisone	Serological response
Seror et al. (2007)	16 (16)	58	Retrospective 5 m	375 mg/m^2 Weeks: 0, 1, 2, 3 (n=14) Other regimens (n=2)	Systemic features (9/11) (82 %) Cryog vasculitis (4/5) Thrombocytop (0/1) Pulmonary + arthritis (2/2) Arthritis (2/2) Renal (1/1) Parotid enlargement (3/3)	–	–	Reduced median daily dose of corticosteroids (p=0.003)	ESR (p=0.009), CRP (p=0.02), gamma (p=0.003), beta2 (p=0.003), cryo negativiz (4/4), reduced RF (p=0.004)
Dass et al. (2008)	17 (ND)	52	RCT-d 6 m	1 g/15days (n=8) Placebo (n=9) Week 0 and 2	ND	ND	–	n	ESR, CRP, abs, IgG, RF reduction (p=0.05)
Vasil'ev et al. (2009)	13 (ND) 3 associated	ND	Retrospective	MP 500 mg premedic	Systemic (3/4)	Lymphoma (clinical response): CR 7, PR 2	–	ND	ND

Meijer et al. (2010)	30 (29)	43	RCT-d 48 weeks	1 g/15days ($n=20$) Placebo ($n=10$) Weeks 0 and 2	Extraglandular features: decreased number ($p=0.029$), reduced vasculitis ($p=0.03$)	ND	–	ND	Igs, decreased RF (<0.05)
Tony et al. (2011)	4 (ND)	ND	Retrospective	375 mg/m^2 Weeks: 0, 1, 2, 3 ($n=11$)	ND	ND	–	ND	PR ($n=2$), CR ($n=2$)
St Clair et al. (2013)	12 (12)	51	Prospective 52 weeks	1 g/15days Weeks 0, 2	ND	ND	–	ND	Little effect on the serum levels of anti-Ro/SSA and anti-La/SSB antibodies (data not shown) Decrease in the levels of RF

(continued)

Table 28.1 (continued)

					Outcomes (improvement/total patients)				
Author (year)	N (female)	Mean age (years)	Study design (duration)	Therapeutic regimen (dose)	Systemic features	Lymphoma	ESSDAI score	Prednisone	Serological response
Gottenberg et al. (2013)	78 (67)	60	Retrospective	375 mg/m^2 Weeks: 0, 1, 2, 3 ($n=11$) Rituximab 1 g Weeks: 0, 2 ($n=67$)	Systemic features (44/74) Articular (17/27) (63 %) CNS (2/6) (33 %) PN (6/12) (50 %) Lung (7/9) (78 %) Vasculitis (5/8) (63 %) Renal (5/6) (83 %) Myositis (0/3) (0 %) Cytopenia (2/2) (100 %) Pancreatitis (1/1) (100 %) Glandular enlarge (2/3) (67 %) Sclera vasculitis (0/1) (0 %)	ND	ESSDAI score ($p<0.0001$)	Reduced median daily dose of corticosteroids mg/day ($p=0.1$)	ND

Devauchelle-Pensec et al. (2014)	122 (ND)	ND	RCT-d 24 weeks	1 g/15days ($n=53$) Placebo ($n=60$) Weeks 0 and 2	Resolution of parotid gland enlargement (40/54 patients [74.1 %]) Resolution of joint involvement (47/61 patients [77 %])	ND	ESSDAI glandular item (rituximab group) scored 0 at week 24	ND	ESR, mm/h ($p=0.84$) Serum CRP level, mg/L ($p=0.95$) IgG, mg/L ($p=0.37$) IgA, mg/L ($p=0.026$) IgM, mg/L ($p=0.004$) C4 complement level, g/L ($p=0.32$)

abs autoantibodies, *C4* complement level, *CNS* central nervous system, *CR* complete response, *CRP* C-reactive protein, *cryo* cryoglobulins, *d* day, *ESR* erythrocyte sedimentation rate, *ESSDAI* European activity score, *Gamma* serum gammaglobulins, *HACAs* human antibodies against chimeric antibodies, *Igs* serum immunoglobulins, *m* months, *MALT* mucosa-associated lymphoid tissue, *MP* methylprednisolone, *ND* not detailed, *PN* peripheral neuropathy, *PR* partial response, *RCT* randomized controlled trial, *-d* double blind, *RF* rheumatoid factor, *w* weeks

than 400 patients included in either controlled or uncontrolled studies, with a wide range of outcomes evaluated, including sicca features, fatigue, and, especially, systemic features and lymphoma. Although some studies have reported significant improvements in sicca features and fatigue, we consider that the off-label use of these new drugs to treat only these symptoms (even when severe) is not currently warranted [2]. In contrast, RTX is the most widely used biological agent in patients with severe involvements refractory to standard treatment in an off-label context and is increasingly used in patients with associated B-cell lymphoma. Therefore, current scientific evidence suggests that RTX may be considered in patients with involvements refractory to standard treatment (lack of response or intolerance to corticosteroids and immunosuppressive agents) [40].

28.7 Future Directions

The most recent therapeutic advances in patients with systemic autoimmune diseases are searching for new highly selective biological therapies without the adverse effects often associated with the standard, less-selective current therapeutic options (corticosteroids, immunosuppressants). The emergence of biological agents targeting molecules and receptors involved in the etiopathogenesis of primary SS has opened up a new era in the therapeutic management of the disease. The excellent results of tumor necrosis factor (TNF)-targeted therapies in rheumatoid arthritis led to these agents being tested in patients with primary SS [8], although RCTs showed a lack of efficacy.

B cells are central in the pathogenesis of primary SS. The disease is characterized by a marked B-cell polyclonal hyperactivity, which may turn on monoclonal B-cell expansion leading, in some patients, to the development of B-cell lymphoma, which is the worst complication of primary SS. B-cell targeted therapies, including RTX, epratuzumab, and belimumab, seem to be the most promising agents tested so far [40].

The close association between B lymphocyte stimulator (BLyS) levels and the key features of primary SS are paving the ground for further investigations about the therapeutic utilities around this molecule [14, 41]. Unfortunately, controlled data of the use of B-cell activating factor (BAFF)-targeted therapies in patients with primary SS are not yet available, and two clinical trials with belimumab are underway (NCT01160666 and NCT01008982) [42]. The recently revealed preliminary results of the BELISS trial [43], the first open-label study of belimumab in primary SS patients, are promising [43, 44]. These patients had to have at the time of inclusion either systemic complications, early disease ($\leq$5 years), or the presence of altered biomarkers. Patients were treated with 10 mg/kg of belimumab (weeks 0, 2, and 4, and then every 4 weeks until week 24). The primary end point was evaluated at week 28 and consisted of improvement of at least two of the five following items: $\geq$30 % reduction of VAS for dryness, fatigue, musculoskeletal pain, and physician's systemic activity and $\geq$25 % reduction of any of the abovementioned B-cell activation biomarkers. The percentage of responders was 8/11 (73 %) in patients with early disease and 7/15 (47 %) in those with systemic disease. A specific subanalysis of the therapeutic response in patients with parotid involvement at week 28 found that the glandular domain improved in 10/13 (77 %) patients [44], while no improvement was reported in two patients with parotid low-grade lymphoma. The ESSDAI score decreased from 8.8 to 5.59 and the ESSPRI score from 6.44 to 5.56. Only one severe adverse event was reported (pneumococcus meningitis) after six infusions of the drug.

Conclusions

Dryness of the mucosal surfaces is the pivotal, but not the only, clinical involvement characterizing primary SS. This has strongly influenced how the diagnosis of SS is made, since the classification criteria currently used (AECG) or under evaluation (ACR) only evaluate glandular involvement and fail to capture the full spectrum of SS involvement. Although a long list of extraglandular features involving most organs and systems has been reported in the last 30 years, few studies have attempted to characterize systemic involvement. However, there is growing interest in systemic SS after the appearance of the ESSDAI score. Therapeutically, direct and indirect B-cell blocking seems to be the most promising approach, although others, such as abatacept [45, 46] and biosimilars [47], are under investigation. However, the variable results obtained with RTX in the two main clinical components of the disease must be taken into account: the results are often good for systemic involvement, but should be considered, at most, modest for the triad of dryness, pain, and fatigue. The great influence of personal and environmental factors on the intensity of these symptoms, which are measured subjectively using visual analogue scales, may account, in part, for the lack of significant differences detected in the two largest RCTs carried out in patients with primary SS [22, 48]. Better understanding of the influence of factors external to the disease, the etiopathogenic mechanisms of extraglandular damage, active international collaborations promoting multicenter registries to enroll and characterize large cohorts of patients with primary SS, and the development of an international consensus on a homogeneous diagnostic and therapeutic approach may help improve the prognosis of patients with systemic Sjögren disease. The current off license use of biological agents should be accompanied by a reasonable assessment of the risk of serious adverse events versus the potential benefits of treatment.

References

1. Fox RI (2005) Sjogren's syndrome. Lancet 366(9482):321–331
2. Ramos-Casals M, Brito-Zeron P, Siso-Almirall A, Bosch X (2012) Primary Sjogren syndrome. BMJ 344:e3821
3. Ramos-Casals M, Brito-Zeron P, Bové A (2011) Sjögren's syndrome: beyond sicca involvement. In: Khamashta MA, Ramos-Casals M (eds) Autoimmune diseases acute and complex situations. I Springer-Verlag, London, pp 45–66
4. Kassan SS, Moutsopoulos HM (2004) Clinical manifestations and early diagnosis of Sjogren syndrome. Arch Intern Med 164(12):1275–1284

5. Theander E, Baecklund E (2012) Cancer. In: Ramos-Casals M, Stone JH, Moutsopoulos HM (eds) Sjögren syndrome: diagnosis and therapeutics. Springer, London, pp 477–492
6. Ramos-Casals M, Brito-Zeron P, Siso-Almirall A, Bosch X, Tzioufas AG (2012) Topical and systemic medications for the treatment of primary Sjogren's syndrome. Nat Rev Rheumatol 8(7):399–411
7. Coca A, Sanz I (2012) Updates on B-cell immunotherapies for systemic lupus erythematosus and Sjogren's syndrome. Curr Opin Rheumatol 24(5):451–456
8. Ramos-Casals M, Tzioufas AG, Stone JH, Siso A, Bosch X (2010) Treatment of primary Sjogren syndrome: a systematic review. JAMA 304(4):452–460
9. Lendrem D, Mitchell S, McMeekin P, Bowman S, Price E, Pease CT et al (2014) Health-related utility values of patients with primary Sjogren's syndrome and its predictors. Ann Rheum Dis 73(7):1362–1368
10. Seror R, Gottenberg JE, Devauchelle-Pensec V, Dubost JJ, Le Guern V, Hayem G et al (2013) European league against rheumatism Sjogren's syndrome disease activity index and European League Against Rheumatism Sjogren's syndrome patient-reported index: a complete picture of primary Sjogren's syndrome patients. Arthritis Care Res 65(8):1358–1364
11. Gandia M, Morales-Espinoza EM, Martin-Gonzalez RM, Retamozo S, Kostov B, Belenguer-Prieto R et al (2014) Factors influencing dry mouth in patients with primary Sjogren syndrome: usefulness of the ESSPRI index. Oral Health Dent Manag 13(2):402–407
12. Segal BM, Pogatchnik B, Henn L, Rudser K, Sivils KM (2013) Pain severity and neuropathic pain symptoms in primary Sjogren's syndrome: a comparison study of seropositive and seronegative Sjogren's syndrome patients. Arthritis Care Res 65(8):1291–1298
13. ter Borg EJ, Kelder JC (2014) Lower prevalence of extra-glandular manifestations and anti-SSB antibodies in patients with primary Sjogren's syndrome and widespread pain: evidence for a relatively benign subset. Clin Exp Rheumatol 32(3):349–353
14. Ramos-Casals M, Brito-Zeron P, Solans R, Camps MT, Casanovas A, Sopena B et al (2014) Systemic involvement in primary Sjogren's syndrome evaluated by the EULAR-SS disease activity index: analysis of 921 Spanish patients (GEAS-SS Registry). Rheumatology 53(2):321–331
15. Baldini C, Pepe P, Quartuccio L, Priori R, Bartoloni E, Alunno A et al (2014) Primary Sjogren's syndrome as a multi-organ disease: impact of the serological profile on the clinical presentation of the disease in a large cohort of Italian patients. Rheumatology 53(5):839–844
16. Ioannidis JP, Vassiliou VA, Moutsopoulos HM (2002) Long-term risk of mortality and lymphoproliferative disease and predictive classification of primary Sjogren's syndrome. Arthritis Rheum 46(3):741–747
17. Brito-Zeron P, Kostov B, Solans R, Fraile G, Suarez-Cuervo C, Casanovas A et al (2014) Systemic activity and mortality in primary Sjogren syndrome: predicting survival using the EULAR-SS Disease Activity Index (ESSDAI) in 1045 patients. Ann Rheum Dis. pii: annrheumdis-2014-206418
18. Seror R, Theander E, Brun JG, Ramos-Casals M, Valim V, Dorner T et al (2015) Validation of EULAR primary Sjogren's syndrome disease activity (ESSDAI) and patient indexes (ESSPRI). Ann Rheum Dis 74(5):859–866
19. Belenguer R, Ramos-Casals M, Brito-Zeron P, del Pino J, Sentis J, Aguilo S et al (2005) Influence of clinical and immunological parameters on the health-related quality of life of patients with primary Sjogren's syndrome. Clin Exp Rheumatol 23(3):351–356
20. Ostuni P, Botsios C, Sfriso P, Punzi L, Chieco-Bianchi F, Semerano L et al (2002) Fibromyalgia in Italian patients with primary Sjogren's syndrome. Joint Bone Spine Rev Rhum 69(1):51–57
21. Gottenberg JE, Ravaud P, Puechal X, Le Guern V, Sibilia J, Goeb V et al (2014) Effects of hydroxychloroquine on symptomatic improvement in primary Sjogren syndrome: the JOQUER randomized clinical trial. JAMA 312(3):249–258
22. Devauchelle-Pensec V, Mariette X, Jousse-Joulin S, Berthelot JM, Perdriger A, Puechal X et al (2014) Treatment of primary Sjogren syndrome with rituximab: a randomized trial. Ann Intern Med 160(4):233–242

23. Mavragani CP, Kassan S (2012) Classic immunosuppressive and immunomodulatory drugs. In: Ramos-Casals M, Stone J, Moutsopoulos HM (eds) Sjögren's syndrome diagnosis and therapeutics. Springer-Verlag, Berlin, p 565
24. Dass S, Bowman SJ, Vital EM, Ikeda K, Pease CT, Hamburger J et al (2008) Reduction of fatigue in Sjogren syndrome with rituximab: results of a randomised, double-blind, placebo-controlled pilot study. Ann Rheum Dis 67(11):1541–1544
25. Devauchelle-Pensec V, Pennec Y, Morvan J, Pers JO, Daridon C, Jousse-Joulin S et al (2007) Improvement of Sjogren's syndrome after two infusions of rituximab (anti-CD20). Arthritis Rheum 57(2):310–317
26. Meijer JM, Meiners PM, Vissink A, Spijkervet FK, Abdulahad W, Kamminga N et al (2010) Effectiveness of rituximab treatment in primary Sjogren's syndrome: a randomized, double-blind, placebo-controlled trial. Arthritis Rheum 62(4):960–968
27. Pijpe J, van Imhoff GW, Spijkervet FK, Roodenburg JL, Wolbink GJ, Mansour K et al (2005) Rituximab treatment in patients with primary Sjogren's syndrome: an open-label phase II study. Arthritis Rheum 52(9):2740–2750
28. Seror R, Sordet C, Guillevin L, Hachulla E, Masson C, Ittah M et al (2007) Tolerance and efficacy of rituximab and changes in serum B cell biomarkers in patients with systemic complications of primary Sjogren's syndrome. Ann Rheum Dis 66(3):351–357
29. St Clair EW, Levesque MC, Prak ET, Vivino FB, Alappatt CJ, Spychala ME et al (2013) Rituximab therapy for primary Sjogren's syndrome: an open-label clinical trial and mechanistic analysis. Arthritis Rheum 65(4):1097–1106
30. Gottenberg JE, Guillevin L, Lambotte O, Combe B, Allanore Y, Cantagrel A et al (2005) Tolerance and short term efficacy of rituximab in 43 patients with systemic autoimmune diseases. Ann Rheum Dis 64(6):913–920
31. Gottenberg JE, Cinquetti G, Larroche C, Combe B, Hachulla E, Meyer O et al (2013) Efficacy of rituximab in systemic manifestations of primary Sjogren's syndrome: results in 78 patients of the AutoImmune and Rituximab registry. Ann Rheum Dis 72(6):1026–1031
32. Vasil'ev VI, Logvinenko OA, Kokosadze NV, Gaiduk IV, Varlamova E, Kovrigina AM et al (2009) [First experience with the application of rituximab for the treatment of patients with Sjogren's syndrome and disease]. Vestnik Rossiiskoi akademii meditsinskikh nauk/Rossiiskaia akademiia meditsinskikh nauk. (2):3–10
33. Tony HP, Burmester G, Schulze-Koops H, Grunke M, Henes J, Kotter I et al (2011) Safety and clinical outcomes of rituximab therapy in patients with different autoimmune diseases: experience from a national registry (GRAID). Arthritis Res Ther 13(3):R75
34. Zhou L, Xin XF, Wu HX (2012) The efficacy and safety of low-dose rituximab in treatment of primary Sjogren's syndrome with thrombocytopenia. Zhonghua nei ke za zhi 51(1): 37–41
35. Mekinian A, Ravaud P, Hatron PY, Larroche C, Leone J, Gombert B et al (2012) Efficacy of rituximab in primary Sjogren's syndrome with peripheral nervous system involvement: results from the AIR registry. Ann Rheum Dis 71(1):84–87
36. Mekinian A, Ravaud P, Larroche C, Hachulla E, Gombert B, Blanchard-Delaunay C et al (2012) Rituximab in central nervous system manifestations of patients with primary Sjogren's syndrome: results from the AIR registry. Clin Exp Rheumatol 30(2):208–212
37. Pollard RP, Abdulahad WH, Vissink A, Hamza N, Burgerhof JG, Meijer JM et al (2013) Serum levels of BAFF, but not APRIL, are increased after rituximab treatment in patients with primary Sjogren's syndrome: data from a placebo-controlled clinical trial. Ann Rheum Dis 72(1):146–148
38. Voulgarelis M, Ziakas PD, Papageorgiou A, Baimpa E, Tzioufas AG, Moutsopoulos HM (2012) Prognosis and outcome of non-Hodgkin lymphoma in primary Sjogren syndrome. Medicine 91(1):1–9
39. Brito-Zeron P, Ramos-Casals M (2008) Prognosis of patients with primary Sjogren's syndrome. Med Clin 130(3):109–115
40. Engel P, Gomez-Puerta JA, Ramos-Casals M, Lozano F, Bosch X (2011) Therapeutic targeting of B cells for rheumatic autoimmune diseases. Pharmacol Rev 63(1):127–156

41. Quartuccio L, Salvin S, Fabris M, Maset M, Pontarini E, Isola M et al (2013) BLyS upregulation in Sjogren's syndrome associated with lymphoproliferative disorders, higher ESSDAI score and B-cell clonal expansion in the salivary glands. Rheumatology 52(2):276–281
42. Brito-Zeron P, Siso-Almirall A, Bove A, Kostov BA, Ramos-Casals M (2013) Primary Sjogren syndrome: an update on current pharmacotherapy options and future directions. Expert Opin Pharmacother 14(3):279–289
43. Mariette X, Seror R, Quartuccio L, Baron G, Salvin S, Fabris M et al (2015) Efficacy and safety of belimumab in primary Sjogren's syndrome: results of the BELISS open-label phase II study. Ann Rheum Dis 74(3):526–531
44. De Vita S, Seror R, Quartuccio L et al (2012) Efficacy of belimumab on non-malignant parotid swelling and systemic manifestations of Sjögren's syndrome: results of the beliss study. Arthritis Rheum 64(Suppl 2189):S926
45. Meiners PM, Vissink A, Kroese FG, Spijkervet FK, Smitt-Kamminga NS, Abdulahad WH et al (2014) Abatacept treatment reduces disease activity in early primary Sjogren's syndrome (open-label proof of concept ASAP study). Ann Rheum Dis 73(7):1393–1396
46. Adler S, Korner M, Forger F, Huscher D, Caversaccio MD, Villiger PM (2013) Evaluation of histologic, serologic, and clinical changes in response to abatacept treatment of primary Sjogren's syndrome: a pilot study. Arthritis Care Res 65(11):1862–1868
47. Cuadrado MJ, Sciascia S, Bosch X, Khamashta MA, Ramos-Casals M (2013) Is it time for biosimilars in autoimmune diseases? Autoimmun Rev 12(10):954–957
48. Mariette X, Ravaud P, Steinfeld S, Baron G, Goetz J, Hachulla E et al (2004) Inefficacy of infliximab in primary Sjogren's syndrome: results of the randomized, controlled Trial of Remicade in Primary Sjogren's Syndrome (TRIPSS). Arthritis Rheum 50(4):1270–1276

Index

D. Roccatello, L. Emmi (eds.), *Connective Tissue Disease: A Comprehensive Guide-Volume 1*, Rare Diseases of the Immune System 5,
DOI 10.1007/978-3-319-24535-5

T